Hip Preservation Surgery in Children and Adolescents

Hip Preservation Surgery in Children and Adolescents

Young-Jo Kim, MD, PhD, MHCM
Boston Children's Hospital
Harvard Medical School
Boston, Massachusetts

Eduardo N. Novais, MD
Boston Children's Hospital
Harvard Medical School
Boston, Massachusetts

Sarah D. Bixby, MD
Pierre d'Hemecourt, MD, RMSK
Vivek Dutt, MBBS, MS (Ortho)
Travis H. Matheney, MD
Michael P. McClincy, MD
Michael B. Millis, MD
Benjamin J. Shore, MD, MPH, FRCSC
Andrea Stracciolini, MD, FACSM, FAAP
James D. Wylie, MD, MHS
Yi-Meng Yen, MD, PhD

Wolters Kluwer

Philadelphia • Baltimore • New York • London
Buenos Aires • Hong Kong • Sydney • Tokyo

Acquisition Editor: Matt Hauber
Development Editor: Stacey Sebring
Editorial Coordinator: Cody Adams
Marketing Manager: Phyllis Hitner
Project Production Manager: David Saltzberg
Manufacturing Coordinator: Beth Welsh
Design Coordinator: Steve Druding
Production Service: S4Carlisle Publishing Services

9 8 7 6 5 4 3 2 1

Printed in China

Library of Congress Cataloging-in-Publication Data

ISBN-13: 978-1-4963-9749-2

ISBN-10: 1-4963-9749-5

Library of Congress Control Number: 2020937575

---

shop.lww.com

CCS0720

Contributors

Sarah D. Bixby, MD
Associate Professor of Radiology
Harvard Medical School
Director of Magnetic Resonance Imaging
Department of Radiology
Boston Children's Hospital
Boston, Massachusetts

Pierre d'Hemecourt, MD, RMSK
Assistant Professor of Orthopaedic Surgery
Harvard Medical School
Director, Primary Care Sports Medicine
Department of Orthopaedic Surgery
Division of Sports Medicine
Boston Children's Hospital
Boston, Massachusetts

Vivek Dutt, MBBS, MS (Ortho)
Assistant Professor, Orthopaedic Surgery
Albany Medical College
Department of Orthopaedic Surgery
Albany Medical Center
Albany, New York

Young-Jo Kim, MD, PhD, MHCM
Professor of Orthopaedic Surgery
Harvard Medical School
Director, Child and Young Adult Hip Preservation Program
Department of Orthopaedic Surgery
Boston Children's Hospital
Boston, Massachusetts

Travis H. Matheney, MD
Assistant Professor of Orthopaedic Surgery
Harvard Medical School
Department of Orthopaedic Surgery
Boston Children's Hospital
Boston, Massachusetts

Michael P. McClincy, MD
Assistant Professor of Orthopaedic Surgery
University of Pittsburgh School of Medicine
Division of Pediatric Orthopaedic Surgery
UPMC Children's Hospital of Pittsburgh
Pittsburgh, Pennsylvania

Michael B. Millis, MD
Professor of Orthopaedic Surgery
Harvard Medical School
Founding Director, Adolescent and Young Adult Hip Unit
Department of Orthopaedic Surgery
Boston Children's Hospital
Boston, Massachusetts

Eduardo N. Novais, MD
Associate Professor of Orthopaedic Surgery
Harvard Medical School
Department of Orthopaedic Surgery
Boston Children's Hospital
Boston, Massachusetts

Benjamin J. Shore, MD, MPH, FRCSC
Associate Professor of Orthopaedic Surgery
Harvard Medical School
Co-Director, Cerebral Palsy and Spasticity Center
Department of Orthopedic Surgery
Boston Children's Hospital
Boston, Massachusetts

Andrea Stracciolini, MD, FACSM, FAAP
Assistant Professor of Orthopedic Surgery
Assistant Professor of Pediatrics
Harvard Medical School
Director, Performing Arts Medicine
Department of Orthopaedic Surgery
Division of Sports Medicine
Department of Pediatrics
Division of Emergency Medicine
Boston Children's Hospital
Boston, Massachusetts

James D. Wylie, MD, MHS
Adjunct Assistant Professor of Orthopedic Surgery
University of Utah
Associate Medical Director for Hip and Knee Preservation
Musculoskeletal Clinical Program
Intermountain Healthcare
The Orthopedic Specialty Hospital
Murray, Utah

Yi-Meng Yen, MD, PhD
Associate Professor of Orthopaedic Surgery
Harvard Medical School
Department of Orthopaedic Surgery
Boston Children's Hospital
Boston, Massachusetts

Foreword

Hip disease has been a strong interest for the Department of Orthopaedic Surgery at Boston Children's Hospital since the department's inception early in the 20th century. Arthur Legg used the new modality of radiography to describe a condition affecting children that differed from the then-common synovitis of tuberculosis.

The subsequent decades have seen the development of pediatric orthopedics as a distinct specialty and the further evolution of orthopedics into subspecialty by body regions as well.

The clear association of pediatric and adolescent-onset hip problems with adult hip dysfunction gave impetus to understanding developmental hip disease not only as a cause of childhood dysfunction, but also to understanding their impact on hip function throughout adult life.

John Hall in 1971 brought to Boston Children's Hospital a deep appreciation for the positive role that thoughtful, skillfully applied surgery could play in improving the lives of children and adults with deformity or trauma. Though Dr. Hall has left us in body, he lives on in our culture of open interchange and sharing. All our staff have benefited greatly through both intramural and extramural collaborations. We view this book as such a team effort.

This monograph on the diagnosis and treatment of pediatric, adolescent, and young adult hip conditions reflects contemporary surgical practice in our department. As such, it represents this point in time, with the recognition that the most elegant of techniques described here will be improved upon. Sound principles of treatment, however, we hope will be more durable.

We encourage you not to accept passively this Boston Children's Hospital Orthopaedic Hip Team effort as holy scripture. We look forward to active interchange with you, the reader, in advancing our common goal of continually improving care for those with hip-related dysfunction.

—Michael B. Millis, MD

Acknowledgments

We would like to acknowledge the collaboration from Dr. Daniel Maranho and Dr. Mariana Ferrer who took most of the intraoperative photographs used in this book.

Daniel Augusto Maranho, MD, PhD
Pediatric Orthopaedic Surgeon
Postdoctoral Research Fellow—Boston Children's Hospital (2016–2017)

Mariana Gonçalves Ferrer Oliveira, MD
Pediatric Orthopaedic Surgeon
Postdoctoral Research Fellow—Boston Children's Hospital (2017–2018)

Contents

CHAPTER 1

Infant Hip Dysplasia: Diagnosis and Brace Treatment

EPIDEMIOLOGY, ETIOLOGY, AND PATHOLOGIC ANATOMY

Developmental dysplasia of the hip (DDH) is one of the most common congenital disorders affecting the musculoskeletal system. DDH denotes a wide spectrum of abnormalities ranging from mild acetabular dysplasia, to subluxation, to complete irreducible high-riding dislocation of the hip. Defining the incidence of DDH is challenging and controversial because of variations in the terminology, such as clicking, instability, and dislocation, previously described in the literature. The development of ultrasonographic techniques for screening and diagnosis contributed to the confusion about actual incidence in the literature. For instance, one previous study reported an incidence of 55.1/1000 detected by ultrasound screening.[1] However, the authors suggested the true incidence of DDH was 5/1000 patients, which corresponds to those that remained abnormal and required treatment.

The etiology of DDH remains unknown, although it is most likely multifactorial, including genetic and environmental intrauterine factors. The most universally recognized factors include female gender, breech position at delivery, and history of a first-degree relative affected by DDH. Other reported factors include improper swaddling, oligohydramnios, deformities of the foot, congenital torticollis, first-born birth order, and large birth weight.

The pathophysiology of DDH has been well described, including an abnormality of the posterosuperior acetabular cartilaginous rim that allows the femoral head to subluxate or dislocate. In high-riding untreated dislocation, anatomic obstacles to a concentric reduction include the fibrofatty pulvinar, hypertrophy of the ligamentum teres, a thickened transverse acetabular ligament, an inverted labrum, and an interposed iliopsoas tendon. Concentric reduction of a dislocated hip early in life allows for remodeling of the acetabulum and femur. On the other hand, secondary changes, such as flattening of the acetabular roof, thickening of the medial acetabular wall, and formation of a false acetabulum will develop if a dislocated hip is left untreated.

CLINICAL EXAMINATION

Classically, examination of the hip includes the Barlow and Ortolani maneuvers performed on one hip at a time. The Barlow[2] test is a provocative maneuver to test for hip instability. It was originally described by Le Damany but popularized by Barlow to identify a hip that is reduced but dislocatable. The proximal femur is held between the thumb placed in the groin and the middle finger placed in the greater trochanter. The hip is adducted, and a gentle posteriorly directed force is applied. In a positive test, subluxation or complete dislocation of the hip is noted. It has been our preference to avoid the use of the provocative Barlow maneuver. We favor gently ranging the hip in a flexed position from abduction to adduction without applying an axial pressure to provoke instability. We do not see any benefit in dislocating a reduced hip by a provocative test. Barlow found that 88% of unstable hips in his series eventually became stable without treatment. The Ortolani test[3] assesses whether a dislocated hip can be reduced (**Figure 1.1**). It is performed by abducting the flexed hip with an anteriorly directed force applied at the level of the greater trochanter. If the hip reduces, then a physical sensation can be felt, which is considered a *positive Ortolani test*. It is important to note that negative Ortolani tests do not guarantee a normal hip. In fact, an irreducible dislocated hip may feel stable during the test. However, in fixed dislocated hips, the maximum degree of abduction may be limited. In babies older than 3 to 4 months, both the Barlow and Ortolani tests are typically absent, and restricted hip abduction becomes a more reliable indication for further investigation with imaging. In patients with unilateral hip dislocation, the Galeazzi sign is typically present. The affected limb feels shorter when flexing both the hips and the knees to approximately 90° and comparing the relative levels of the knees. The Klisic test[4] is helpful to identify bilateral dislocation

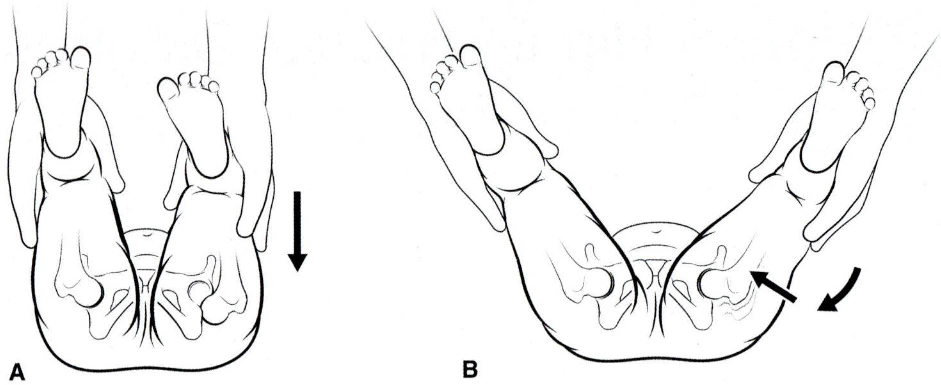

FIGURE 1.1. The Ortolani maneuver assesses whether a dislocated hip can be reduced. In this illustration, the left hip is dislocated, whereas the right hip is normally reduced. A, The first step of the Ortolani test consists in holding the hip in 90° of flexion and neutral abduction and rotation. In this position, the femoral head is dislocated out of the acetabulum. The black arrow represents the effect of gravity and the direction of the dislocation. B, The second step of the Ortolani test is performed by abducting the flexed hip with an anteriorly directed force applied at the level of the greater trochanter. The black arrows represent the direction of the forces applied. A positive Ortolani test consists of a physical sensation of the reduction of the hip.

of the hips. The test is performed by placing the index finger on the anterior superior iliac spine and the middle finger on the greater trochanter. A line between these two points should intersect the umbilicus if the hip is anatomically normal, but it is inferior to the umbilicus if the hip is dislocated.

IMAGING EVALUATION

Ultrasonographic evaluation of the hip is the best imaging modality to assess the hip morphology and dynamic stability during the first 6 months of life. Interpreting hip ultrasonography depends on the quality of the image acquisition, which can be influenced by experience of the examiner that can lead to high variability. Several methods for morphologic and dynamic ultrasonographic examination of the hip have been described.[5-14] Ultrasonography has been used for screening programs resulting in lowering the rate of late diagnosis and surgical interventions. However, application of ultrasonography is limited by patient's age. Once the ossific nucleus of the femoral head ossifies, ultrasonography becomes less reliable and an anteroposterior (AP) pelvic radiograph may be more helpful to evaluate the hip morphology. Our preference is to use ultrasonography up to 6 months of age and radiographs thereafter.

When performing ultrasound for evaluation of hip dysplasia, it is critical that the examination of the hip be performed with experienced sonographers, using a high-frequency linear transducer that penetrates to the level of at least the triradiate cartilage. The unossified femoral head and the unossified portion of the acetabular physis and triradiate cartilage appear as hypoechoic structures (**Figure 1.3**), whereas the ossified pelvic bones and femoral neck are hyperechoic and are useful anatomic landmarks. Various imaging methodologies have been described in the literature and include both static and dynamic maneuvers, which are described in more detail later.

The most widely used method of hip ultrasonography was described by Graf.[5,6] According to Graf, ultrasonography is performed with a linear probe with the baby in lateral decubitus using a pillow for positioning and a lever-arm structure to hold the probe. The hip is in neutral position with about 30° to 55° of flexion. The standard coronal plane should include the lower portion of the osseous ilium, which resembles a straight line and produces strong posterior acoustic shadowing (the iliac line), the entire depth of the acetabular fossa (to the triradiate cartilage), and the acetabular labrum. Graf recommended measurement of the α angle to assess the osseous acetabular roof and the β angle to assess the cartilaginous acetabular roof. The α angle corresponds to the osseous coverage of the femoral head by the acetabular socket, and the smaller the angle, the more severe the degree of dysplasia. The lower limit of normal value for the α angle has been established at 60°.[5] These angles are combined with the morphologic description of the hip for the proposed classification system for ultrasonographic imaging of the hip[5,6] (**Table 1.1**; **Figure 1.2**). Careful imaging acquisition is required to ensure that the standard coronal plane is obtained. The Graf technique has been criticized for its relatively low accuracy and interobserver and intraobserver variability.[15,16] Small changes in probe rotation may change the diagnostic criteria by one or two levels. Notably, the upper limit of agreement of interscan variability has been reported to range from 8° up to 19°.

TABLE 1.1 Graf classification

Type	Description	Morphology characteristics	α angle (degrees)	β angle (degrees)	Age (weeks)	Treatment Recommendation
I	Normal mature hip	Narrow, covers the femoral head, blunt rim	≥60	<55	Any	No
II a	Physiologic immature	Wide roof with round bony rim	50-59	>55	0-12	Depended on α angle[1]
II b	Immature	Wide roof with round bony rim	50-59	>55	>12	Yes
II c	Dysplastic	Wide roof with round or flat bony rim	43-49	<77	Any	Yes
D	Decentered (Subluxated)	The cartilaginous roof is displaced with round or flat bony rim	43-49	>77	Any	Yes
III	Dislocated[2]	Acetabular cartilaginous roof is displaced cranially	<43	-	Any	Yes
IV	Dislocated	Displaced infero-medially (caudally). The labrum may be inverted and interposed	<43	-	Any	Yes

1 – At 6 weeks of age, physiologic immaturity is further classified in II a+ if the α angle is 55°–59° or II a– if the α angle is 50°–54°.
2 – Type III should be divided in III a when the acetabular cartilaginous roof is hypoechoic without major structural alterations and III b when the cartilaginous roof is echogenic.

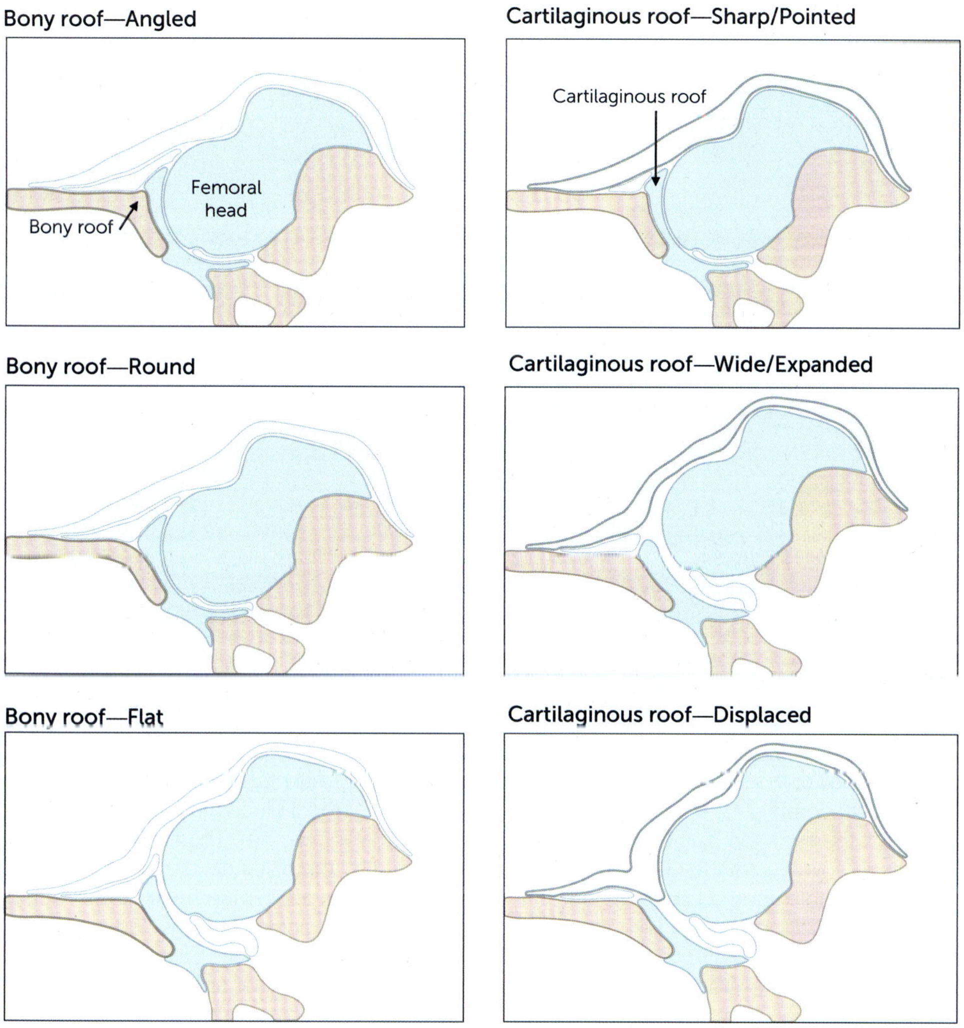

FIGURE 1.2. Illustration showing the Graf criteria to describe the morphology of the acetabulum in hip ultrasonography.

Harcke and colleagues[7,8] developed a technique based on a dynamic multiplanar examination that assesses the hip in positions at rest and under stress. The dynamic assessment of stability includes a coronal view in neutral (15° to 20° of hip flexion) and 90° of hip flexion, and a transverse view in neutral and 90° of hip flexion. The correct coronal view in the mid-acetabular plane should demonstrate the straight iliac line, the transition of bone to cartilage in the depth of the acetabulum, and the tip of the acetabular labrum. This group also proposed measuring the percentage of femoral head that is covered by the bony acetabulum.[17]

Alternative methods described in the literature include the Terjesen method[10,11] as well as other methods using an anterior approach to visualize the hip.[9,12-14] Terjesen[10,11] proposed measurement of the bony rim percentage (BRP) of femoral head coverage by the osseous acetabular roof similar to the description by Harcke's group.[17] Normal coverage has been reported to be at least 50%, that is, the iliac line crosses the femoral head above its center. Treguier et al[18] described the pubofemoral distance (PFD), an important morphologic measurement of the hip for diagnosis and monitoring of treatment. The anatomic landmarks for PFD measurement are the most lateral aspect of the osseous pubis over the acetabular fossa and the most medial aspect of the cartilaginous femoral head. In a normal infant hip, PFD should be less than 6 mm if the ultrasonography is done on the supine position with the hip in flexion and adduction. The upper limit of normal in the lateral decubitus is 4.4 mm, whereas the cutoff value in flexion is 4.9 mm in flexion and 4.6 mm in the neutral position.

Our current ultrasonography protocol is based on the recommendations from the consensus meeting on hip sonography by Harcke, Graf, and Clarke who proposed a dynamic standard minimum examination combining morphologic and stability criteria[19] (**Figure 1.3**).

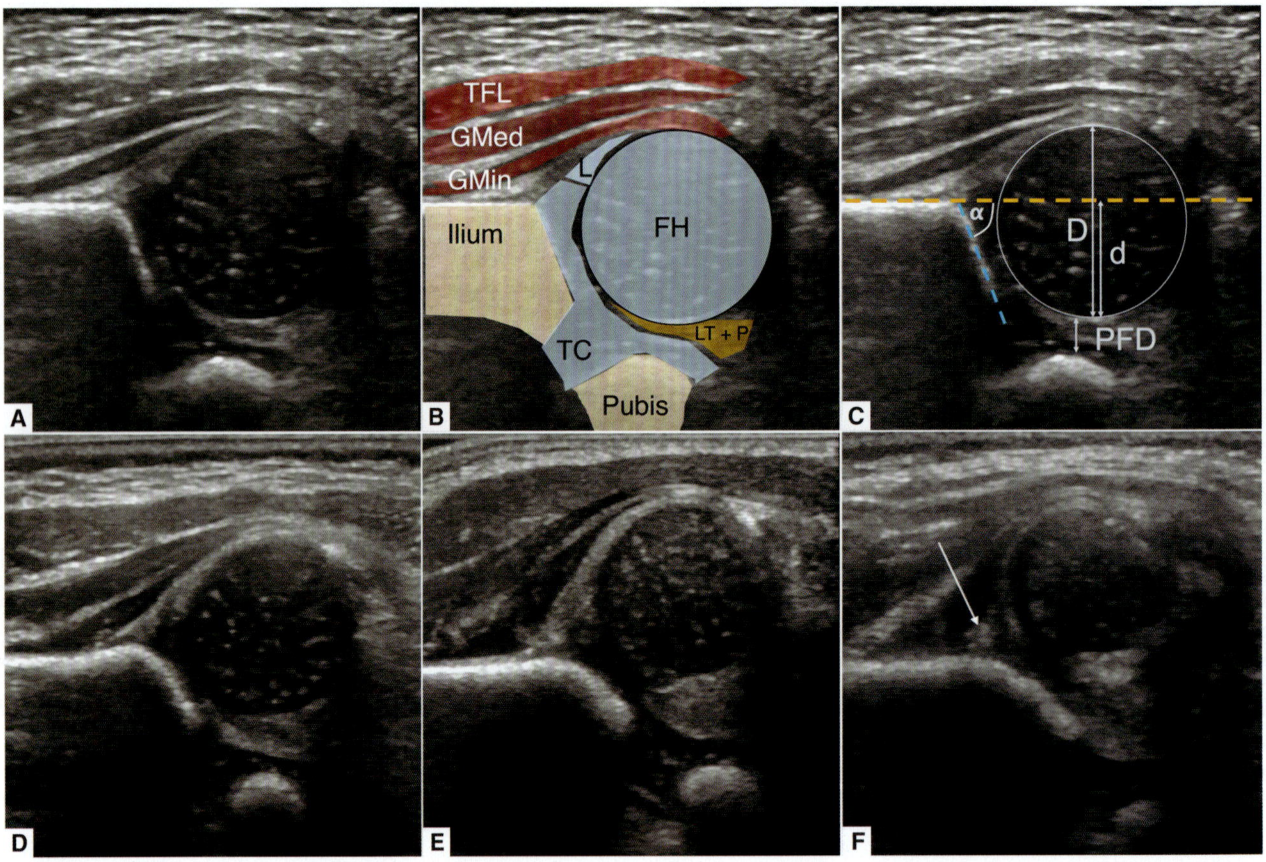

FIGURE 1.3. Ultrasonography of the hip. A, Coronal ultrasound image of a normal hip. B, Illustration showing the normal anatomy of the hip on ultrasonography. C, Measurements obtained from the coronal ultrasound image. The yellow dashed line marks the lateral wall of the ilium; the blue dashed line marks the acetabular bony rim. The angle between these lines is the α angle. The percentage coverage of the femoral head (FH) is calculated by the distance (*d*) divided by the diameter (*D*) of the FH. PFD represents the pubofemoral distance. D, Coronal ultrasonography of a 2.5-month-old female with a stable hip on examination showing an abnormal morphology with abnormal coverage of the FH, increased PFD, and reduced α angle. E, Coronal ultrasonography of a 2-month-old female with unstable hip on examination (positive Ortolani test) showing severe hip abnormality. There is less than 15% coverage of the FH, increased PFD, reduced α angle, and large hypertrophic ligamentum teres and pulvinar (LT+P). F, Coronal ultrasonography of a 4-week-old female with unstable hip on examination (positive Ortolani test) showing severe hip abnormality. The labrum (L) has been pushed cranially by the displaced FH and appears abnormally hyperechoic and blunted (white arrow). TFL, tensor fascia lata; GMed, gluteus medius muscle; GMin, gluteus minimus muscle.

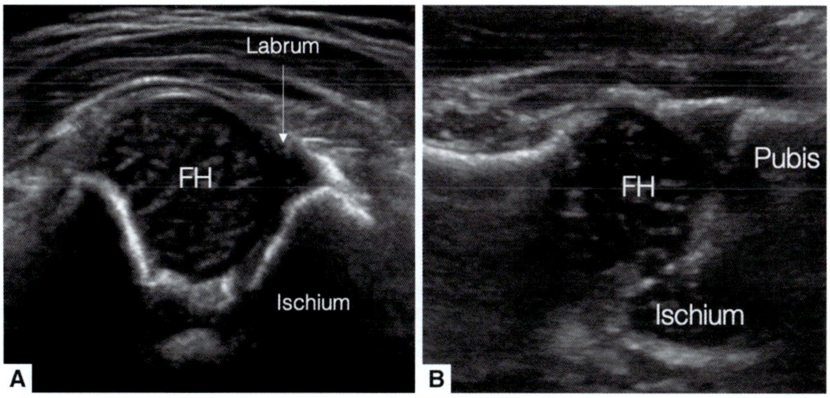

FIGURE 1.4. Alternative views from hip ultrasonography protocol. A, Transverse ultrasound image of a normal hip. The femoral head (FH) is positioned appropriately in the acetabulum with posterior joint stability provided by ischium and posterior labrum. The transverse view allows for dynamic assessment of the hip with and without stress. B, Anterior axial view of the hip. This view is helpful during Pavlik harness treatment to monitor adequate reduction of the FH in the acetabulum.

Notably, this is the most widely used method in North America. We perform standard coronal (frontal) and transverse views of the hip in neutral position in mild flexion. Stress views are then obtained in the transverse plane while simulating a Barlow maneuver. We measure and report the α angle and the percentage of femoral head covered by the bony acetabulum and also note the morphology and echogenicity of the bony and cartilaginous roof along with the PFD. Patients undergoing treatment in the Pavlik harness are scanned carefully without stressing the hip. The anterior axial view is added for patients in Pavlik because it gives a nice view of the hip and is easy to obtain (**Figure 1.4**). The anterior axial view is also helpful to determine concentric reducibility for hips that have been treated in the Pavlik harness but still have slight instability, or hips that failed to reduce. Ultrasound is recommended at the first visit in patients with unstable hips because the morphology of the hip may influence the outcome of treatment[20] (**Figure 1.5**).

TREATMENT OF DEVELOPMENTAL DYSPLASIA OF THE HIP IN INFANTS

The treatment of infants with DDH depends on the severity of the dysplasia assessed by ultrasound and

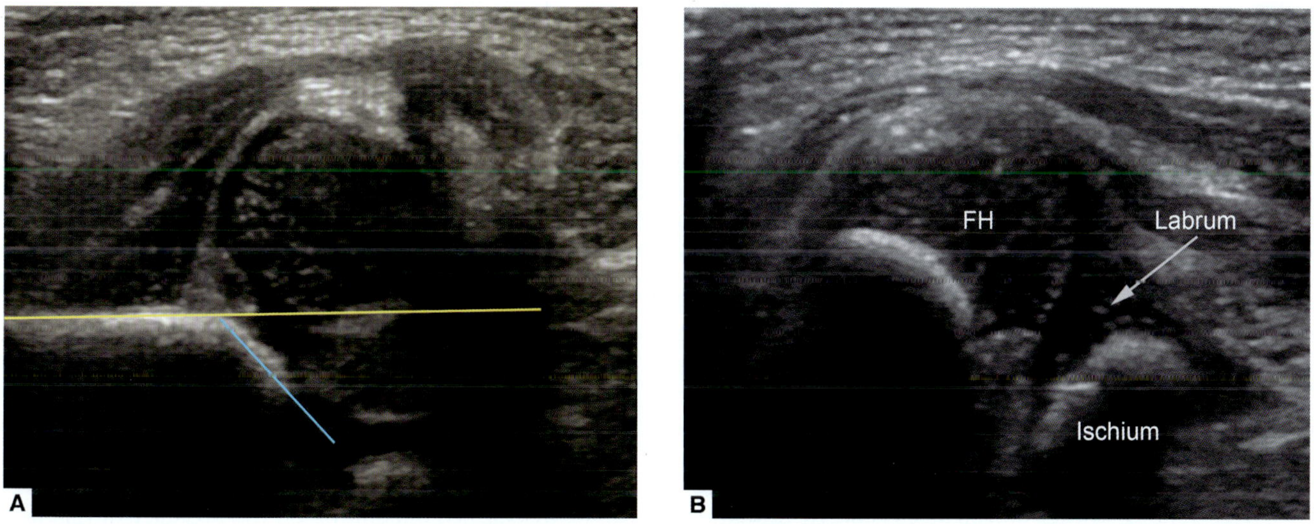

FIGURE 1.5. Ultrasound of the left hip of a 7-day-old male with a dislocated hip at physical examination. A, Coronal image of the hip demonstrates complete superolateral dislocation of the femoral head (FH). The FH is entirely uncovered by the shallow bony acetabulum (blue line) and is positioned lateral to the iliac line (yellow line). B, Transverse image of the left hip demonstrates the FH positioned posterolateral to the ischium even at rest and not seated within the acetabulum, white arrow points to acetabular labrum. Compare with normal position of the hip in Figure 1.4.

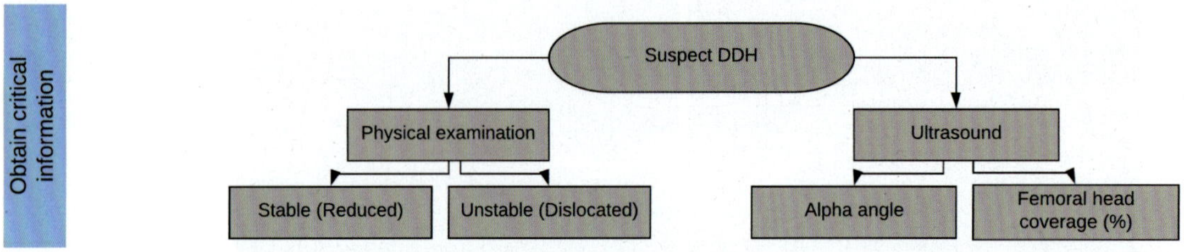

Classification Criteria used at BCH

Hip Classification	Stability	Alpha angle	Femoral head Coverage	Age
Normal	Stable	≥60°	≥50%	Any
Immature, Stable	Stable	50°-60°	≥30%	<3 months
Dysplastic, Stable	Stable	50°-60°	≥30%	>3 months
Dysplastic Subluxated	Stable	43°-50°	10%-30%	Any
Hip Classification	**Stability**	**Ortolani Test**	**-**	**Age**
Dislocated, Reducible	Unstable	Positive	-	Any
Dislocated Irreducible	Unstable	Negative	-	Any

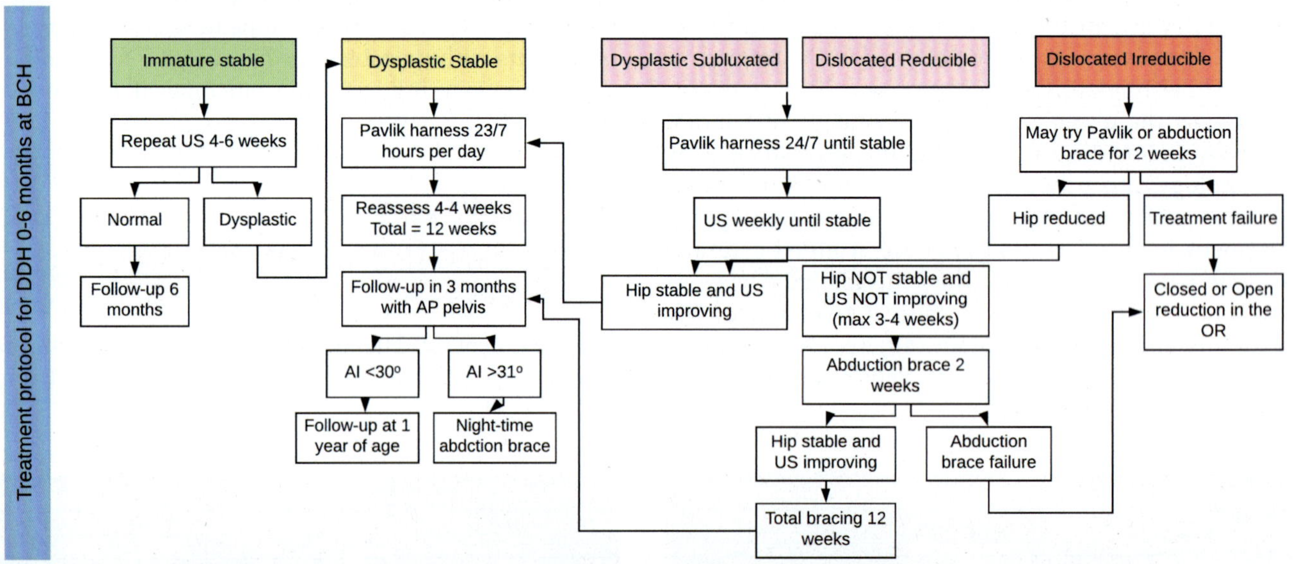

FIGURE 1.6. Algorithm representing the three-step approach for management of patients aged 0 to 6 months with suspected developmental dysplasia of the hip (DDH). The first step is to obtain critical information with a history, physical examination, and ultrasonography (US) of the hip for determination of the femoral head coverage and the morphology of the acetabulum (α angle). Then, the hip is classified according to the findings on examination and US. Finally, each classification follows its treatment protocol, as shown on the bottom part of the figure. AI, acromion index; AP, anteroposterior; OR, operating room.

the ability to reduce the hip with the Ortolani maneuver (**Figure 1.6**). Stable hips with borderline ultrasound findings corresponding to physiologic immaturity (Graf IIA) of the hip in patients less than 12 weeks of age may be carefully monitored. Although some authors may advocate treatment for borderline hip or physiologic immature hips, the potential complications associated with bracing and the burden to the family should be considered and overtreatment avoided. For close monitoring, we recommend a repeat ultrasound in 4 weeks. During this time, we advise avoiding tight swaddling because of its association with dysplasia. We also discuss with the family about carrying the baby with the hips in abduction and avoiding carrying babies with the hip in adducted position. If the ultrasound normalizes in 4 weeks, the patient can be discharged depending on the presence of risk factors for DDH. Female, breech babies and those with positive family history are followed at 6 months of age with an AP pelvis radiograph. Conversely, if the ultrasound is not normalized, a Pavlik harness treatment is instituted.

Pavlik Harness education sheet for families

What is a Pavlik harness?

A soft brace that helps hold your baby's legs in a position that allows their hip joint to be aligned and stable so that it develops correctly. The Pavlik harness is a "dynamic brace," meaning that it is not rigid and allows your baby to move their legs.

The harness is one of the safest, most effective treatment options for developmental dysplasia of the hip (DDH) in infants from birth to six months of age. It is typically worn 24 hours a day, unless otherwise directed by your doctor.

Is treatment painful?

If the harness is properly fitted and cared for, it is a pain-free treatment for infants with DDH. It can take a couple of days for your baby to become accustomed to wearing the harness, so some fussing and crying the first few days is normal.

Within 24 to 72 hours of wearing the harness full-time, your baby will become more comfortable with it, as the treatment itself is gentle.

How long will my child need to wear the harness?

The amount of treatment time varies based upon the severity of your child's DDH. In the majority of cases, the harness is worn 24 hours a day for 8–12 weeks.

Depending on the severity of your baby's dysplasia, for the first few weeks they will usually need to see the doctor every week in order to adjust the harness and receive an ultrasound of their hips. After 3–4 weeks, you will only need to see the doctor fora harness adjustment every 2–4 weeks.

After 6 weeks of treatment, your child will have an ultrasound without wearing the harness. From that assessment, your doctor will determine whether or not your child can stop wearing the harness full-time.

How do i care for the harness?

The Pavlik harness should be kept on your child at all times and should only be removed at the instruction of your doctor.

The harness is worn underneath your baby's clothes. This generally works best with one piece sleep sacks and larger-sized clothing, which help prevent the clothing from restricting your child's ability to move their legs. Clothing that brings the knees in together — such as pants or anything with a waist band — should not be worn.

How do I care for my child while they are wearing the harness?

Bathing

You should not bathe your child in a bath tub while they are wearing the harness full-time. Sponge baths are the best bathing alternative during this time. Once their hip is stable, or your physician permits, you will be able to bathe your child.

Skin care

Do not put lotion on your baby's skin where it comes in contact with the harness, as it could moisten the skin and cause skin breakdown. Also avoid using powders around the harness, as the powder can cause irritation as well.

Pay extra attention to your baby's groin area and behind their knees. Because the harness keeps their legs in a flexed position, these areas often stay moist and can be more easily irritated. A good way to care for this is to wipe behind the knees and in the groin with a dry cloth/paper towel every time you change your child's diaper.

Several times a day, you should check your baby's skin around the edges of the harness to ensure there is no redness or imitation.

Positioning

While your child is wearing the Pavlik harness, it is important that they spend as much time as possible on a flat surface, laying on their back. This helps the knees to fall outward and to the side — allowing the hip socket(s) to properly develop.

If your baby prefers to be swaddled you can swaddle the arms and upper body, but the legs should not be swaddled.

Limit the time your child spends in a bouncy seat or swing to two hours or less per day. The positioning of these activities brings your child's legs inward so that their knees cannot fall outward in the brace.

What are areas of concern that warrant a call to the doctor?

- If your child cries continuously and you are unable to comfort them
- If there are any red and irritated areas of the skin that do not go away with application of moleskin to the harness
- If you notice that your child is not kicking one of his/her legs
- If you have any other questions or concerns

Pavlik Harness
Front view

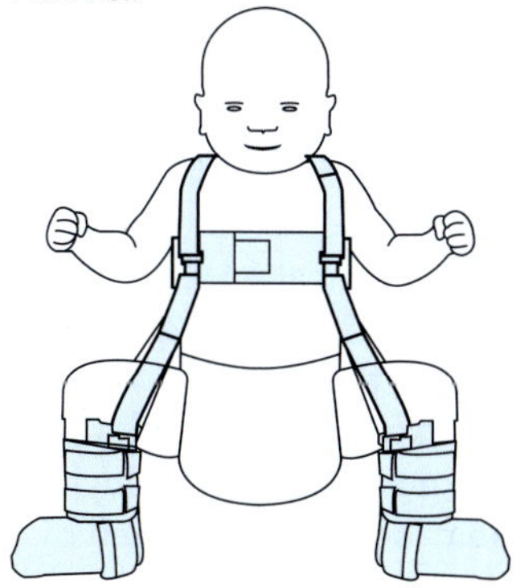

Pavlik Harness
Back and bottom views

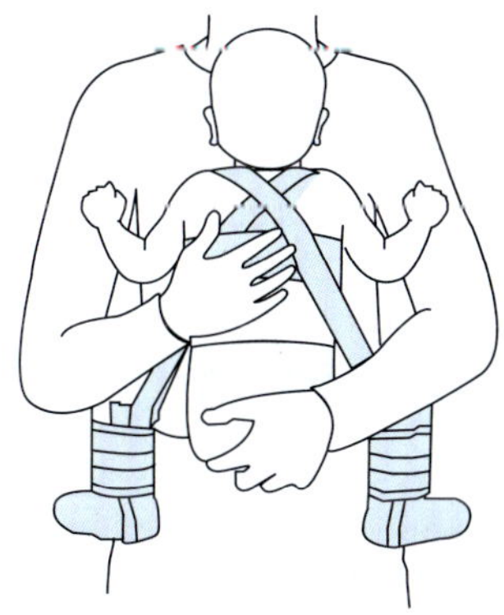

FIGURE 1.7. Education sheet for caregivers with infants treated with a Pavlik harness. The sheet is available at http://www.childrenshospital.org/-/media/Centers-and-Services/Programs/A_E/Child-and-Adult-Hip-Preservation-Program/HipFactSheet_Pavlik.ashx?la=en&hash=03649F108BCE9759929068901F5AB3161E6F14D8.

Treatment with the Pavlik harness in our clinic involves a physician and a dedicated nurse or a nurse practitioner. One of the most crucial aspects of treatment is compliance with the harness to avoid complications. Instruction sheet for families is helpful to maintain safe use and compliance with the brace (**Figure 1.7**).

Stable hips with dysplasia detected on ultrasound are treated with a Pavlik harness typically for 8 to 12 weeks, with regular visits every 4 weeks to check for ultrasound improvement and harness fitting. During treatment for stable hips, parents are allowed to remove the harness for bathing. Treatment of dislocated hips that are reducible by the Ortolani maneuver and stable hips on examination but with ultrasound coverage less than 30% and α angle lower than 50° is initiated immediately with the application of a Pavlik harness. For dislocated reducible hips, we recommend follow-up on a weekly basis until the hip is stabilized and the ultrasound shows morphologic improvement. Once the hip is stable, we then monitor the patient every 4 weeks for a total of 12 weeks in the Pavlik harness. We do not allow the family to remove the harness until the hip is stabilized during the first weeks. Once the hip is stabilized, the caregivers can remove the harness for bathing the patient, and follow-up with ultrasound is done every 4 weeks. Although controversy surrounds the management of the hips that do not become stable with the Pavlik harness, our preference is to monitor patients with unstable hips on a weekly basis until no more than 3 or 4 weeks. If the hip is not stabilized by 3 to 4 weeks, then a dynamic ultrasound is performed to assess whether the hip is reducible. If the hip is still reducible after the Pavlik harness has been used for 3 to 4 weeks, then we recommend an abduction brace. Currently, we use either the rigid abduction brace or the Ilfeld abduction brace because it allows for controlled abduction instead of the fixed wide abduction provided by the plastic brace. After application of the abduction brace, we recommend follow-up in 2 weeks with repeat ultrasound, and if the hip morphology has improved, we will see the patient in clinic every 4 weeks for a minimum of 12 weeks.

Severely dislocated hips with limited abduction, irreducible with the Ortolani maneuver and classified as Graf type IV on ultrasound, are difficult to manage. A type IV hip and male gender have been identified as independent factors for failure of the pelvic harness.[20] However, one recent study reported that about 55% dislocated irreducible hips could be treated with the Pavlik harness, although complications including femoral nerve palsy and osteonecrosis developed in about 10% of those patients. We believe that dislocated irreducible hips treated in the harness have a higher risk of Pavlik harness disease and femoral nerve palsy. Although controversy remains, these hips may be better managed by planned reduction under anesthesia, but further research is necessary.

Clinical outcome following application of the Pavlik harness is in general very good. The success rate of the Pavlik harness to achieve and maintain reduction of a dislocated hip and allow for acetabular remodeling is as high as 90%.[20-22] Both length of treatment and determining whether weaning or immediate discontinuation of the Pavlik harness is preferred after the hip has normalized continue to be topics of controversy. We favor a minimum of 12 weeks of treatment because of the risk of residual dysplasia after harness reported in at least 10% of the patients.[22,23]

Complications of the Pavlik harness method are rare but often prohibit continuation of the treatment. Failure to achieve and maintain stability of the hip with the harness is not recommended because of the risk of so-called "Pavlik harness disease." Pavlik harness disease may develop in hips maintained in the harness despite dislocation of the hip, characterized by a posterolateral deformity of the acetabulum that makes further treatment by closed reduction more difficult. Historically, osteonecrosis of the femoral head following Pavlik has a wide range of incidence reported in the literature of between 1% and 30%.[22] Current literature following a series of patients with close clinical monitoring and serial ultrasound examinations and avoidance of extreme hip positions in the harness demonstrate a lower rate of such complications.[21,24] Femoral nerve palsy is a rare (~2% to 3%) complication that requires immediate discontinuation of the harness. The vast majority of patients who experience this complication will expect full recovery in a few days or 1 to 2 weeks. The sooner the function of the nerve recovers, the better chance the hip has to be treated to cure with the harness or a brace. Although the harness may be reapplied after femoral nerve palsy, we prefer the application of a plastic abduction brace until complete functional recovery of the femoral nerve and confirmatory ultrasound demonstrating satisfactory reduction of the hips. Failure of the Pavlik harness to achieve reduction is a potential complication that is most often observed in patients older than 4 months,[24] male patients,[20] and severely (Graf type IV) dislocated hips.[20,24]

REFERENCES

1. Bialik V, Bialik GM, Blazer S, Sujov P, Wiener F, Berant M. Developmental dysplasia of the hip: a new approach to incidence. *Pediatrics.* 1999;103(1):93-99.
2. Barlow TG. Early diagnosis and treatment of congenital dislocation of the hip. *Proc R Soc Med.* 1963;56:804-806.
3. Mubarak SJ. In search of Ortolani: the man and the method. *J Pediatr Orthop.* 2015;35(2):210-216.
4. Klisic P, Jankovic L. Combined procedure of open reduction and shortening of the femur in treatment of congenital dislocation of the hips in older children. *Clin Orthop Relat Res.* 1976(119):60-69.
5. Graf R. Classification of hip joint dysplasia by means of sonography. *Arch Orthop Trauma Surg.* 1984;102(4):248-255.
6. Graf R. Fundamentals of sonographic diagnosis of infant hip dysplasia. *J Pediatr Orthop.* 1984;4(6):735-740.
7. Harcke HT. The role of ultrasound in diagnosis and management of developmental dysplasia of the hip. *Pediatr Radiol.* 1995;25(3):225-227.
8. Harcke HT, Kumar SJ. The role of ultrasound in the diagnosis and management of congenital dislocation and dysplasia of the hip. *J Bone Joint Surg Am.* 1991;73(4):622-628.
9. Suzuki S. Ultrasound and the Pavlik harness in CDH. *J Bone Joint Surg Br.* 1993;75(3):483-487.
10. Terjesen T, Bredland T, Berg V. Ultrasound for hip assessment in the newborn. *J Bone Joint Surg Br.* 1989;71(5):767-773.
11. Terjesen T, Runden TO, Johnsen HM. Ultrasound in the diagnosis of congenital dysplasia and dislocation of the hip joints in children older than two years. *Clin Orthop Relat Res.* 1991;(262):159-169.
12. van Douveren FQ, Pruijs HE, Sakkers RJ, Nievelstein RA, Beek FJ. Ultrasound in the management of the position of the femoral head during treatment in a spica cast after reduction of hip dislocation in developmental dysplasia of the hip. *J Bone Joint Surg Br.* 2003;85(1):117-120.
13. El Ferzli J, Abuamara S, Eurin D, Le Dosseur P, Dacher JN. Anterior axial ultrasound in monitoring infants with Pavlik harness. *Eur Radiol.* 2004;14(1):73-77.
14. Carlile GS, Woodacre T, Cox PJ. Verification of hip reduction using anterior ultrasound scanning during Pavlik harness treatment of developmental dysplasia of the hip. *J Orthop.* 2014;11(4):174-179.
15. Rosendahl K, Aslaksen A, Lie RT, Markestad T. Reliability of ultrasound in the early diagnosis of developmental dysplasia of the hip. *Pediatr Radiol.* 1995;25(3):219-224.
16. Dias JJ, Thomas IH, Lamont AC, Mody BS, Thompson JR. The reliability of ultrasonographic assessment of neonatal hips. *J Bone Joint Surg Br.* 1993;75(3):479-482.
17. Morin C, Harcke HT, MacEwen GD. The infant hip: real-time US assessment of acetabular development. *Radiology.* 1985;157(3):673-677.
18. Treguier C, Chapuis M, Branger B, et al. Pubo-femoral distance: an easy sonographic screening test to avoid late diagnosis of developmental dysplasia of the hip. *Eur Radiol.* 2013;23(3):836-844.
19. Harcke HT, Graf R, Clarke NM. *Consensus Meeting on Hip Sonography.* Wilmington, DE: Alfred I. duPont Institute; 1993.
20. Novais EN, Kestel LA, Carry PM, Meyers ML. Higher Pavlik harness treatment failure is seen in Graf Type IV Ortolani-positive hips in males. *Clin Orthop Relat Res.* 2016;474(8):1847-1854.
21. Swaroop VT, Mubarak SJ. Difficult-to-treat Ortolani-positive hip: improved success with new treatment protocol. *J Pediatr Orthop.* 2009;29(3):224-230.
22. Omeroglu H. Treatment of developmental dysplasia of the hip with the Pavlik harness in children under six months of age: indications, results and failures. *J Child Orthop.* 2018;12(4):308-316.
23. Novais EN, Sanders J, Kestel LA, Carry PM, Meyers ML. Graf Type-IV hips have a higher risk of residual acetabular dysplasia at 1 year of age following successful Pavlik harness treatment for developmental hip dysplasia. *J Pediatr Orthop.* 2018;38(10):498-502.
24. Omeroglu H, Kose N, Akceylan A. Success of Pavlik harness treatment decreases in patients ≥ 4 months and in ultrasonographically dislocated hips in developmental dysplasia of the hip. *Clin Orthop Relat Res.* 2016;474(5):1146-1152.

CHAPTER 2

Infant Hip Dysplasia: Closed Reduction

FUNDAMENTALS OF DEVELOPMENTAL DYSPLASIA OF THE HIP: TREATMENT BY CLOSED REDUCTION

Treatment of developmental dysplasia of the hip (DDH) between the ages of 0 and 6 months is typically performed using the Pavlik harness method or an abduction brace. One indication for a closed reduction of the hip is failure of these methods to achieve a concentric and stable reduction. Therefore, closed reduction of the hip has been the mainstay for the treatment of DDH in patients who failed bracing or in those presenting during the first year of life. Although closed reduction can be performed in older patients, the likelihood to obtain and maintain hip reduction by closed means decreases with increasing age. After the child starts to walk, the pathologic anatomy of the hip may not allow for a concentric reduction without surgery. The main pathologic factors and structures obstructing the reduction include the adduction contracture with limited hip abduction, an infolded acetabular labrum, hypertrophy of the acetabular roof cartilage (*neolimbus*), the hourglass constriction of the capsule by a tight iliopsoas tendon, excessive fibrofatty pulvinar, hypertrophy of the ligamentum teres, a tight anteromedial joint capsule, and increased thickness of the acetabular transverse ligament that restricts the introitus of the acetabulum. With increasing age, these obstacles to a concentric reduction may not allow the femoral head to seat deep in the acetabulum. Furthermore, acetabular remodeling after closed reduction is directly influenced by age, that is, older patients are more likely to grow with persistent acetabular dysplasia. Hence, closed reduction is preferably performed during the first year of life.

Although closed reduction of a dislocated hip may intuitively seem a simple and straightforward procedure, in reality, it requires attention to detail to avoid immediate complications, such as postoperative subluxation, and long-term complications, including osteonecrosis. The following principles should be considered:

- Closed reduction of a dislocated hip should not be performed as a forceful maneuver.
- The hip should be positioned in ≥90° flexion and gently abducted following the Ortolani maneuver.
- The reduction should be easily felt as the femoral head enters the acetabulum.
- The reduction should be stable. To determine the stability of the reduction, the safe zone or safe arc of motion as described by Ramsey et al[1] should be assessed by comparing the maximum range of abduction to the degree of abduction where the hip redislocates. If the safe zone is wide (≥30°), the reduction is considered stable (**Figure 2.1**).
- Wide abduction must be avoided because of the risk of osteonecrosis to the femoral head. We recommend immobilizing the hip in 10° to 20° less than the maximum abduction, with maximum abduction of 60°.
- The morphology of the reduced hip should be assessed to determine the depth and stability of the reduction. The most common method to assess the morphology of the hip is an arthrogram performed at the time of the reduction (**Figure 2.2**). Alternatively, the hip may be assessed by magnetic resonance imaging (MRI) with or without contrast to evaluate the reduction and, when contrast is used, the perfusion of the femoral head or by ultrasonography. We rarely use computed tomography (CT) scan after closed reduction to assess hip morphology because of the radiation risk and because MRI is better at revealing the anatomy of the structures of interest.
- A hip arthrogram is beneficial to help determine the relationship of the femoral head and the acetabulum

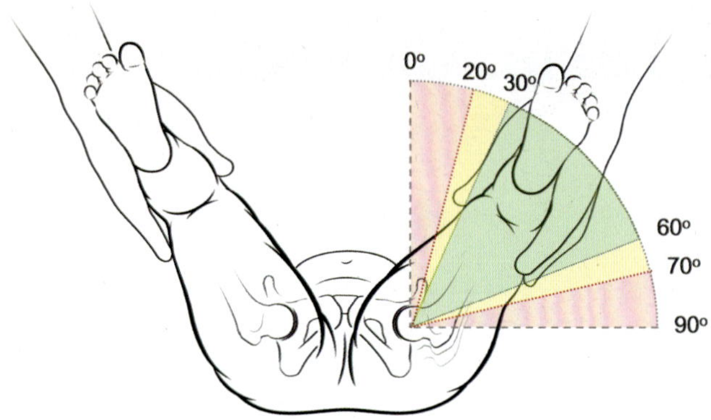

FIGURE 2.1. Illustration showing how to calculate the safe zone of reduction according to Ramsey et al.[1] The safe zone or safe arc is calculated by assessing the maximum unforced abduction of the hip, represented here by 70°. Then, the hip is brought into adduction, and the degree of abduction with the hip dislocated is recorded; here, it is 20°. The safe zone or safe arc of motion is the range of abduction in which the hip maintains stability. It is, therefore, calculated by the maximum and forced abduction minus the degree of abduction at which the hip dislocates; 70° to 20° results in a wide zone of 50°. However, we take about 10° from each end, resulting in a safe zone between 30° and 60°, which is acceptable for closed reduction. Hips with a narrow zone of safety (<30°) are less likely to be stable after closed reduction. A popular method of increasing the safe zone is to perform an abduction tenotomy. The abductor tenotomy theoretically would increase the maximum and forced abduction and increase the safe zone of Ramsey.

before and after closed reduction. Several classification systems have been described to evaluate the hip arthrogram; however, we favor the grading scheme proposed by Tönnis (**Figure 2.3**). The arthrogram should be interpreted after the hip is reduced as follows:

- The percentage or coverage of the femoral head by the acetabulum—at least two-thirds of the femoral head should be covered by the acetabulum.
- The space between the superior labrum and the transverse acetabular ligament (*introitus*) should be larger than 20 mm. The femoral head should be under the superior labrum, which should not be completely infolded and over the transverse acetabular ligament.
- The gap between the femoral head and the acetabular floor should be narrow. Although controversial, we recommend that no more than 4 mm of medial dye pooling should be considered for a closed reduction.

- If gentle closed reduction is stable with a wide safe zone of stability and with adequate coverage of the femoral head on arthrogram, the patient is immobilized in a bilateral spica cast.
- After the spica cast is applied, additional imaging is recommended to confirm a concentric reduction is maintained in the cast.

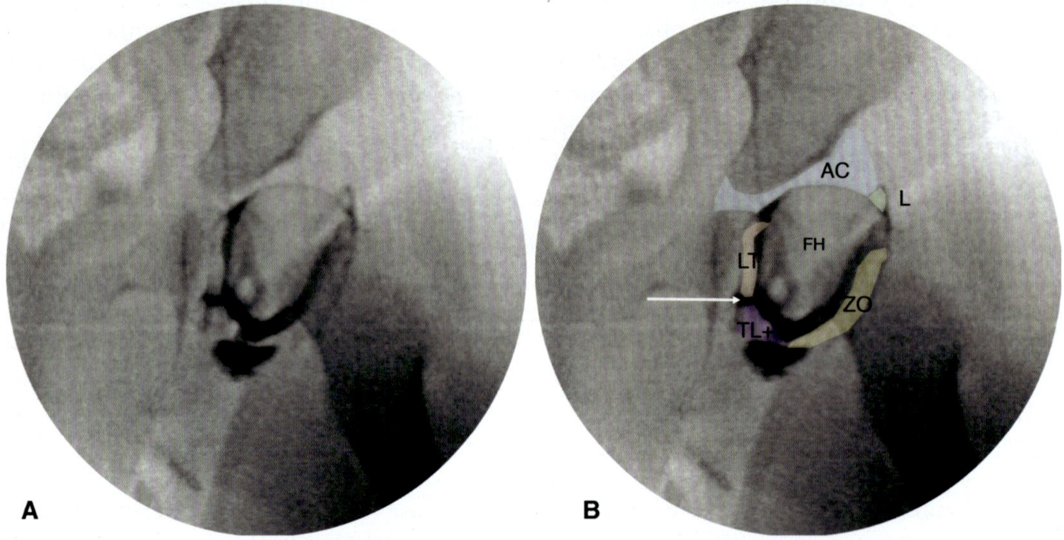

FIGURE 2.2. Hip arthrogram of the pediatric patient for assessment of developmental dysplasia of the hip. A, Intraoperative fluoroscopy image of a previously closed reduced hip in a 7-month-old baby showing normalized parameters of hip arthrogram. In a normal arthrogram, more than two-thirds of the femoral head should be covered by the acetabular cartilage and the labrum. B, Schematic drawing showing the relevant structures outlined in the hip arthrogram: AC, acetabular cartilage; L, the labrum, is a triangular structure that covers the femoral head laterally; ZO, zona orbicularis; LT, ligamentum teres; TL+, transverse ligament + inferior labrum; FH, femoral head.

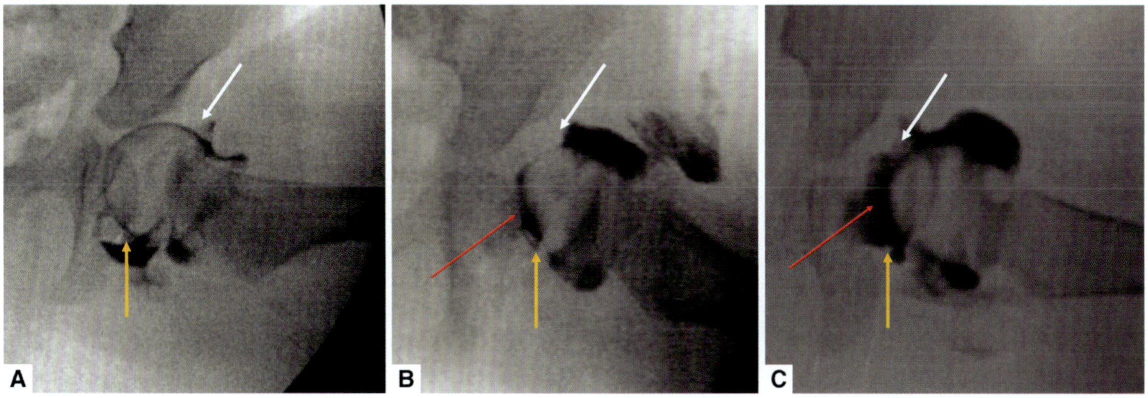

FIGURE 2.3. The Tönnis grading system for assessing the morphology of the hip on an arthrogram after closed reduction. A, Grade I: The femoral head is completely reduced and close to the ischial part of the acetabulum. B, Grade 2: The femoral head is below the labrum but sits more lateral because of the capsular constriction and narrowing of the introitus between the superior labrum and the transverse ligament and inferior labrum. A small amount of medial pooling of the contrast is observed between the femoral head and the acetabular fossa. C, Grade III: The femoral head cannot be positioned under the labrum and sits lateral to the acetabulum introitus. The labrum is typically inverted, and the capsule markedly constricted. White arrows point to the lateral aspect of the acetabular cartilage and labrum. Red arrows point to the medial dye pooling formed between the femoral head and the acetabular fossa. The yellow arrows point to the transverse acetabular ligament.

Clinical Scenario

A 10-month-old female baby presents to clinic after a consultation was requested by the pediatrician who noticed in a recent well-child visit that the legs were asymmetric in length. Family history was negative for hip dysplasia; however, the baby was in breech position during gestation. During physical examination, the patient was found to have a positive Galeazzi sign (left shorter than right). In 90° of hip flexion, the maximum right hip abduction was recorded at 80°, while the left hip had slightly limited abduction recorded at 70°. Anterior pelvic radiographs were obtained in clinic and showed a subluxated left hip with acetabular dysplasia and delayed ossification of the left femoral head (**Figure 2.4**).

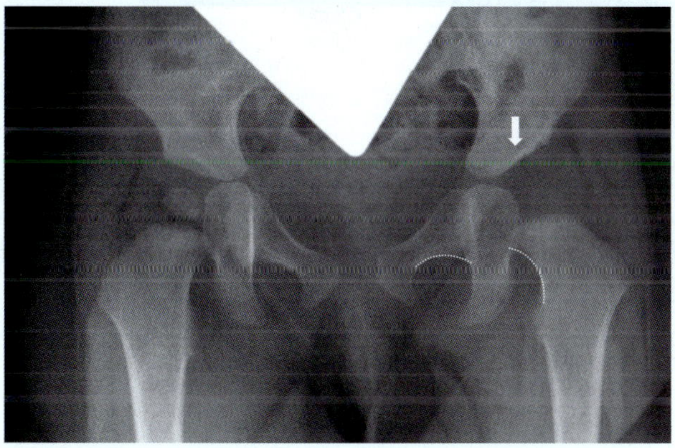

FIGURE 2.4. Anteroposterior pelvic radiograph showing developmental dysplasia and subluxation of the left hip. The Shenton line (white dashed lines) is broken, and the acetabulum is dysplastic.

HIP ARTHROGRAM AND SPICA CAST APPLICATION TECHNIQUE

Closed reduction is performed with the patient under general anesthesia to allow for complete muscle relaxation. The patient is positioned supine in a radiolucent table, and the hips are examined. The affected hip is flexed to 90° and abducted, and a palpable reduction is typically felt. The hip is moved in abduction to adduction to determine the safe zone of Ramsey. This test can also be performed after the arthrogram, but we prefer to fully examine the hip before injecting dye into the hip to avoid any interference from potential joint distention with the injection. In preparation for the hip arthrogram, the patient is positioned with the hips in flexion, abduction, and external rotation. Taping both feet together with the soles facing each other to the operative table helps the hips remain steady for the arthrogram (**Figure 2.5**). The affected hip is prepared and draped in a standard manner. We recommend performing the arthrogram with full preparation of the field in a sterile manner, including applying a sterile cover to the C-arm fluoroscopy machine to avoid any contamination to the field and the risk of a hip infection. For patients younger than 3 years, a 20-gauge spinal needle is routinely used. For older patients, an 18-gauge needle may be used. Several techniques have been described, but we prefer the medial adductor approach. The needle is inserted just distal and inferior to the adductor muscle tendon with an approximately 45° angulation and pointing toward the shoulder (**Figure 2.6**). As the needle advances from the skin through the subcutaneous tissue, it is recommended to obtain a C-arm fluoroscopy image to be certain of the trajectory of the needle. Once the needle reaches the hip capsule, a gentle push through the resistance of the capsule will be felt.

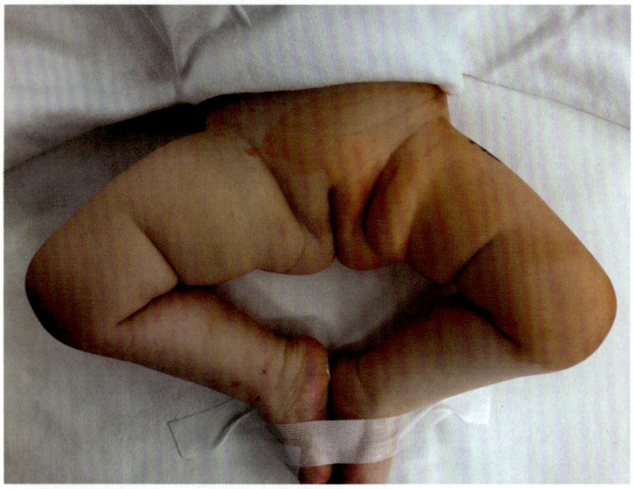

FIGURE 2.5. Intraoperative photograph showing the preparation for left hip arthrogram. Both hips are flexed and abducted, while the soles of both feet are taped together to the table. The entire left groin and left thigh are prepared with ChloraPrep.

At this point, the needle should be in the intra-articular space. Although some surgeons may perform a small air arthrogram, air embolus has been known to occur; therefore, we recommend an injection with saline or ioversol diluted to 50% with sterile saline. The injection should be slow and guided by C-arm fluoroscopy. A very important technical point during an arthrogram is to avoid excessive injection of contrast to avoid distention of the joint. We cannot emphasize enough the importance of only injecting about 1 mL to a maximum of 1.5 mL of the contrast solution to avoid joint distention, which may limit the interpretation of the examination. Another technique pearl involves removing the needle while aspirating the syringe to avoid extravasation of contrast through the path of the needle, which would leave a residual trace of contrast in the adductor musculature. However, even if there is some extravasation, it would be in the adductor muscle, which would not limit the interpretation of the examination. This is an advantage of the medial approach compared to

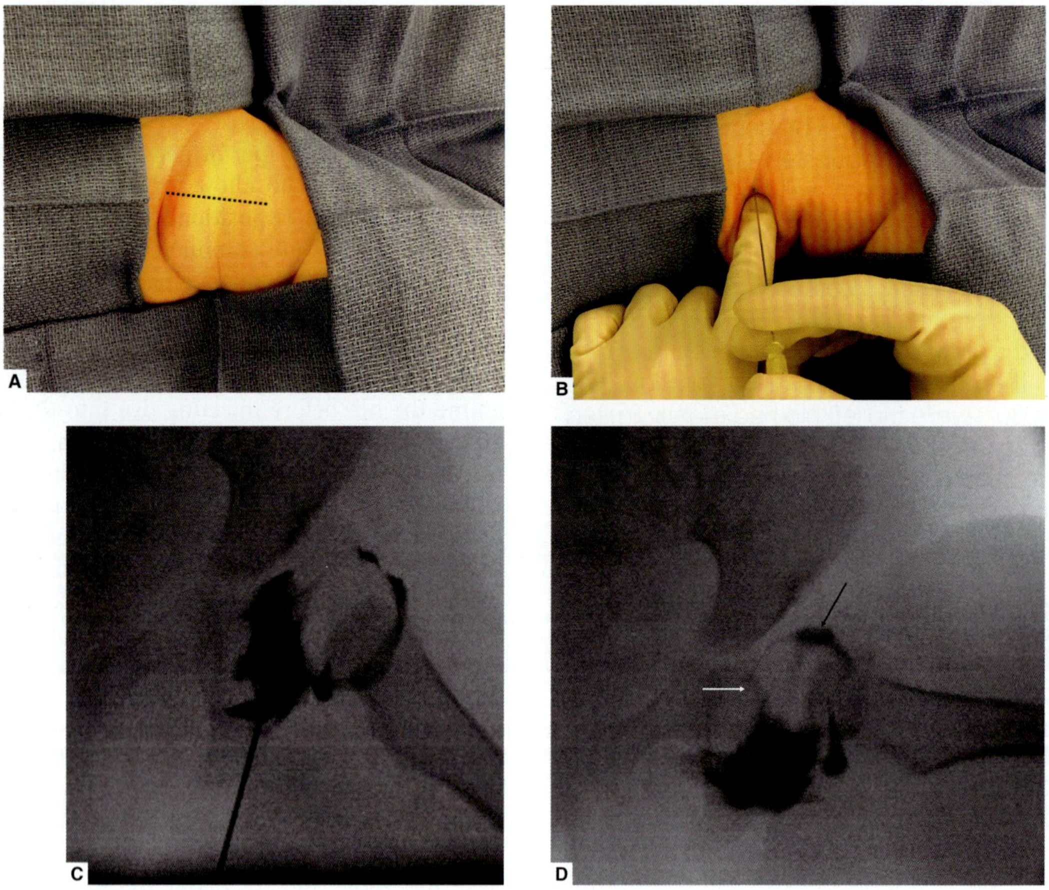

FIGURE 2.6. A, Intraoperative photograph showing the left groin area after the patient is draped. Before introducing the arthrogram needle, we reapply one additional layer of ChloraPrep. The dashed black line marks the level of the adductor longus muscle. B, Intraoperative photograph showing the technique for the arthrogram using a medial approach. The adductor longus tendon is palpated, and the skin is retracted distally. A 20-gauge spinal needle is inserted and advanced cranially and laterally under direct visualization with the C-arm fluoroscopy. C, Intraoperative fluoroscopy view showing the needle being introduced into the left hip and 1.5 mL of the contrast solution injected to the joint. The femoral head is subluxated with a large medial dye pooling with the hip not reduced. D, Intraoperative fluoroscopy view showing the concentric reduction of the femoral head under the acetabulum. Black arrow points to the abnormally shaped labrum that despite the pathologic morphology covers the femoral head entirely. White arrow shows that the femoral head is deeply seated in the acetabulum without pooling of the dye medially.

the anterior approach for arthrogram. Once the needle is removed from the joint, the injection site is protected with sterile dressing and the drapes are removed.

The closed reduction is performed as previously described similar to the Ortolani maneuver, with the affected dislocated femur held with one hand with the thumb in the inner aspect of the thigh while the middle and ring fingers apply pressure in the lateral aspect of the thigh close to the greater trochanter. The hip is then brought into flexion and abduction, and a gentle push is performed from lateral to medial in the lateral aspect of the thigh. Serial fluoroscopy images are obtained with the hip in 90° to 100° of flexion and in different angles of abduction. Once the arthrogram confirms that the femoral head can be concentrically reduced into the acetabulum, the patient is then transferred into the spica cast table and the spica cast is applied (**Figure 2.7**).

Postoperatively, the patient is sent immediately to radiology for MRI of the pelvis, which typically confirms the reduction of the hip (**Figure 2.8**). The patient is then admitted to the orthopedic floor for spica cast care and education by the orthopedic nurse and for safety transportation assessment. Once the patient is comfortable and family is well educated about cast care, the patient is discharged home. We routinely see patients for 2 weeks to assess for the skin condition under the cast and to obtain one anteroposterior (AP) pelvic radiograph in the cast. Six weeks after closed reduction, the patient is brought back to the operating room for a repeat arthrogram and cast change (**Figure 2.9**). Finally, the family is instructed to return in 6 weeks to clinic for cast removal and brace application. An abduction brace is recommended at nighttime for 6 to 12 months following cast removal depending on the remodeling

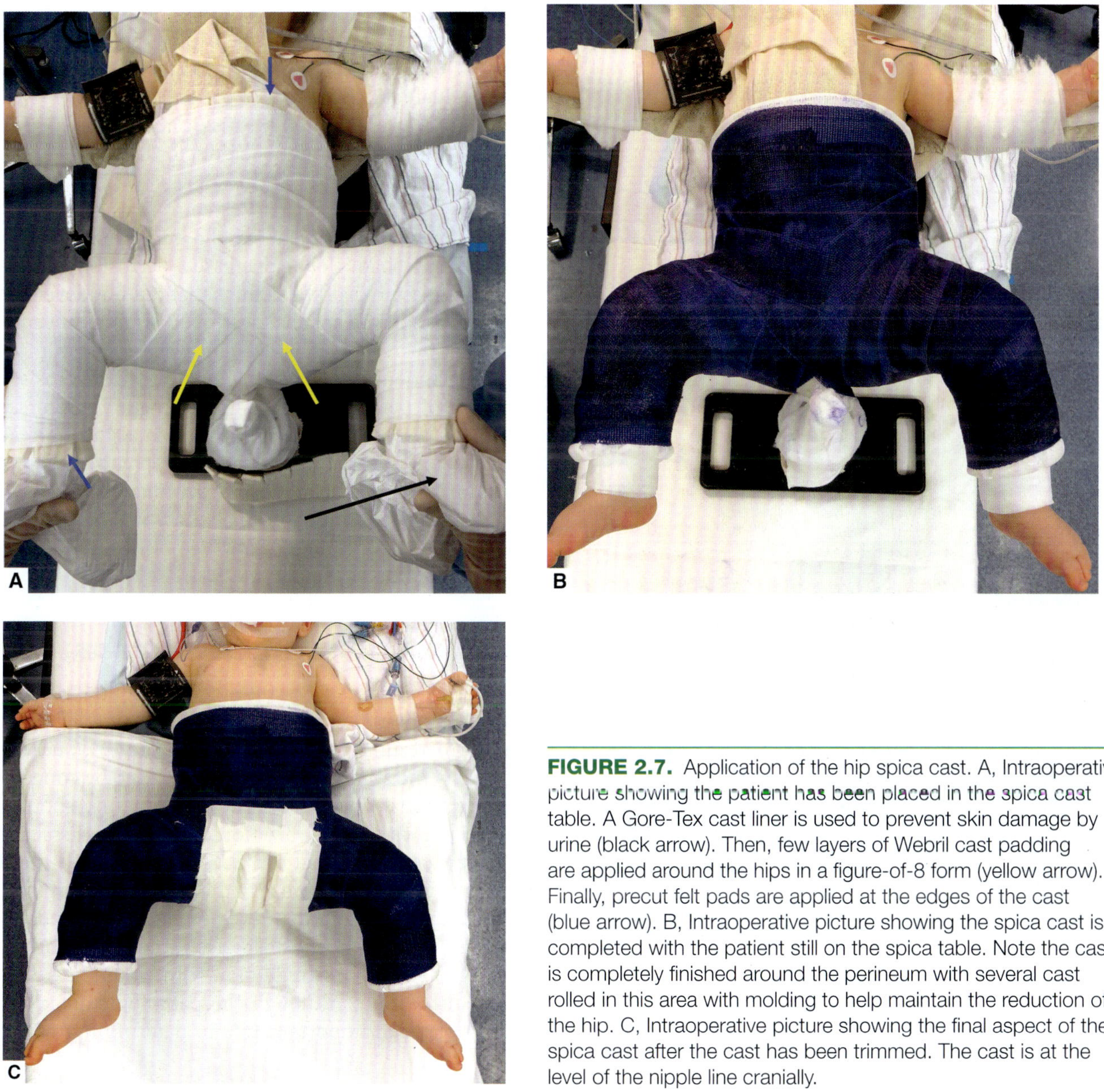

FIGURE 2.7. Application of the hip spica cast. A, Intraoperative picture showing the patient has been placed in the spica cast table. A Gore-Tex cast liner is used to prevent skin damage by urine (black arrow). Then, few layers of Webril cast padding are applied around the hips in a figure-of-8 form (yellow arrow). Finally, precut felt pads are applied at the edges of the cast (blue arrow). B, Intraoperative picture showing the spica cast is completed with the patient still on the spica table. Note the cast is completely finished around the perineum with several cast rolled in this area with molding to help maintain the reduction of the hip. C, Intraoperative picture showing the final aspect of the spica cast after the cast has been trimmed. The cast is at the level of the nipple line cranially.

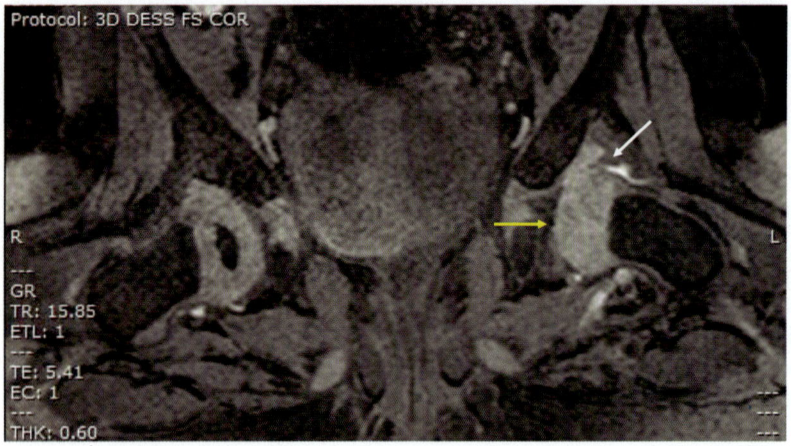

FIGURE 2.8. Postspica magnetic resonance imaging showing the femoral head is concentrically reduced in the acetabulum. The femoral head is completely covered by the labrum (white arrow) and is adjacent to the acetabular floor (yellow arrow).

of the acetabulum (**Figure 2.10**). Patients are routinely followed at 6 and 12 months after reduction and then yearly until age 5 years. At around 5 years of age, or 4 years after closed reduction, there should be enough evidence that the hip has remodeled or if there is persistent acetabular dysplasia.

CLOSED REDUCTION OF THE HIP AUGMENTED BY EVALUATION OF THE BLOOD SUPPLY TO THE FEMORAL HEAD

Osteonecrosis of the hip is the most devastating complication after the treatment of DDH. Assessing the perfusion to the femoral head during and after a closed or open reduction would ideally allow for identification of hips at the risk of developing proximal growth disturbance and deformity associated with osteonecrosis. We have used a protocol for MRI using intravenous gadolinium contrast to evaluate the perfusion of the capital femoral epiphysis after the cast is applied following a closed reduction. We have evaluated 28 hips and 27 patients aged from 1 to 11 months who were treated for dislocated hips by a closed reduction with or without an adductor tenotomy and application of a spica cast.[2] Of the 28 hips, 6 (21%) had evidence of clinically significant osteonecrosis on follow-up radiographs. Fifty percent of the hips that developed osteonecrosis had global decreased perfusion MRI enhancement. Only 2 of the 22 hips that did not develop osteonecrosis showed a global decreased MRI enhancement. Although decreased enhancement was the most important independent factor associated with osteonecrosis, the accuracy of perfusion MRI was not high. Therefore, we have been researching the application of ultrasound technology for assessment of the blood supply to the femoral head during closed reduction. Our initial experience has been positive, but a longitudinal study will be needed to determine the clinical application of ultrasound to guide closed reduction of the hip in DDH.

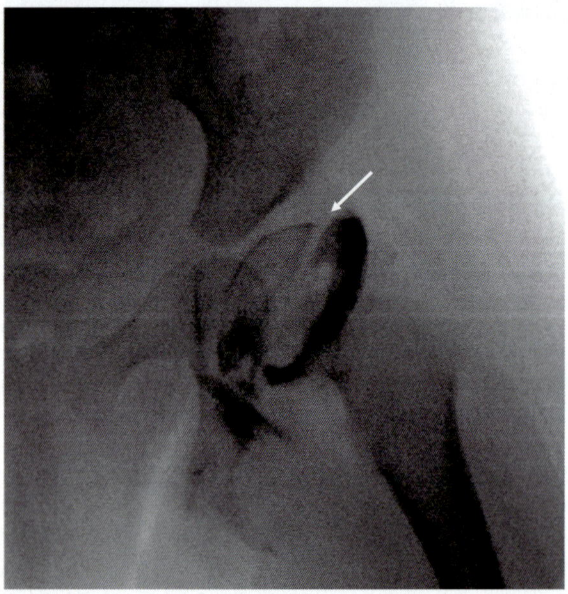

FIGURE 2.9. Intraoperative fluoroscopy obtained 6 weeks after the index closed reduction showing remodeling of the acetabular labrum (white arrow).

Complications and Outcomes

An analysis of the successful outcomes following closed reduction should consider the short-term versus the long-term results. Immediately after surgery, success is defined by the ability of the femoral head to be concentrically reduced into the acetabulum. Reduction should be maintained with immobilization of the hip in a spica cast without excessive abduction. The goal is to gently manipulate the hip and immobilize in the cast without any forceful maneuver to avoid the development of osteonecrosis. In the short term, the most worrisome complication is instability of the hip postreduction with either subluxation or a redislocation. Although the pathologic anatomy of the hip plays an important role in determining whether

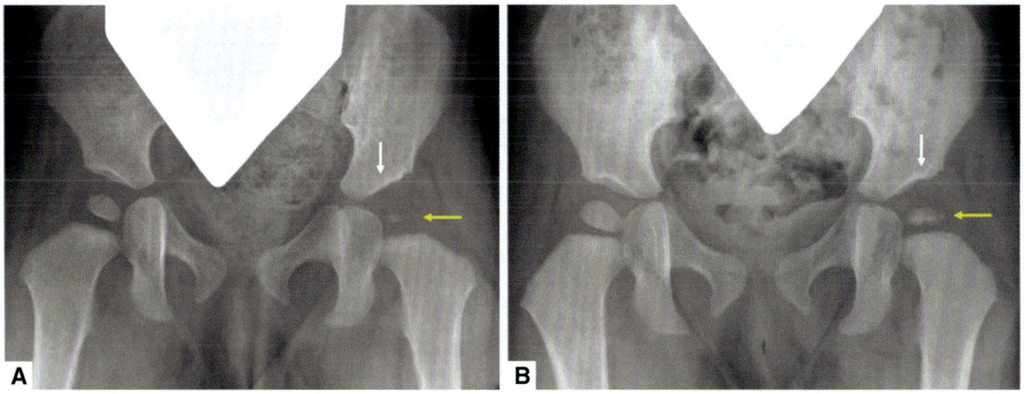

FIGURE 2.10. Postoperative follow-up radiographs showing improvement of the acetabular morphology (white arrow) and ossification of the femoral head (yellow arrow). A, Anteroposterior (AP) pelvic radiograph obtained at 6 months after closed reduction. B, AP pelvic radiograph obtained at 12 months after closed reduction.

or not a hip can be successfully reduced closed, attention to the appropriate surgical technique is crucial to avoid immediate early redislocation.

In the long term, the most worrisome complication is osteonecrosis or the development of pathologic growth disturbance of the proximal femur and residual acetabular dysplasia.

One study from Iowa[3] investigated the outcomes of 119 patients (152 hips) who underwent a closed reduction and who were on average 31 years of age (range 16 to 56 years) at the time of the follow-up. Seventy-five percent of the hips were graded as excellent and 13% as poor by the Iowa hip rating (IHR). The study reported that hips reduced before age 6 months had a better outcome compared to those reduced after 6 months (excellent results, 91% vs. 76%). Residual acetabular dysplasia and deformities of the femur related to osteonecrosis were associated with decreased functional status. Proximal femoral growth deficiency, the terminology used by the authors to describe osteonecrosis changes, was noted in 36% of the hips reduced before 6 months of age compared with 64% of hips treated in patients older than 6 months. However, a higher prevalence of severe deformities was observed in hips reduced under 6 months of age compared to those treated later (type III proximal femoral growth deficiency, 64% vs. 27%). Another long-term study[4] evaluated the results of closed reduction after a period of skin traction in 60 patients (74 hips) with a mean age of 58 years (range 55 to 60 years) and found that good long-term clinical and radiographic outcome occurred in 39 (53%) of 73 hips. One-third of the hips had undergone a total hip replacement, with a mean age of 48 years. A survival analysis considering total hip replacement as an end point showed a reduction in survival for 100% at age 38 years to 62% at age 58 years. Risk factors for poor outcome were age at reduction greater than or equal to 1.5 years and residual acetabular dysplasia (Severin grades 3 and 4) at skeletal maturity.

In summary, closed reduction of the hip is an excellent alternative for the treatment of hips that failed Pavlik harness or abduction bracing or for patients presenting during the first year of life with a dislocated hip. Closed reduction should be performed under general anesthesia combined with assessment of the hip by an arthrogram or intraoperative ultrasound. Closed reduction should not be performed in any circumstance using forceful maneuvers. Rather, closed reduction is a gentle positioning of the hip in flexion and abduction. If a concentric reduction of the hip is achieved, then acetabular remodeling is expected. The long-term results following closed reduction are good and excellent in most patients. However, follow-up until skeletal maturity is recommended because the radiographic morphology of the hip as assessed by the Severin classification is known to be an important factor for the long-term survival of the hip.

REFERENCES

1. Ramsey PL, Lasser S, MacEwen GD. Congenital dislocation of the hip. Use of the Pavlik harness in the child during the first six months of life. *J Bone Joint Surg Am.* 1976;58(7):1000-1004.
2. Tiderius C, Jaramillo D, Connolly S, et al. Post-closed reduction perfusion magnetic resonance imaging as a predictor of avascular necrosis in developmental hip dysplasia: a preliminary report. *J Pediatr Orthop.* 2009;29(1):14-20.
3. Malvitz TA, Weinstein SL. Closed reduction for congenital dysplasia of the hip. Functional and radiographic results after an average of thirty years. *J Bone Joint Surg Am.* 1994;76(12):1777-1792.
4. Terjesen T. Long-term outcome of closed reduction in late-detected hip dislocation: 60 patients aged six to 36 months at diagnosis followed to a mean age of 58 years. *J Child Orthop.* 2018;12(4):369-374.

CHAPTER 3

Open Reduction for the Treatment of Developmental Dysplasia of the Hip

FUNDAMENTALS

Open reduction is the recommended treatment for a dislocated hip when a concentric stable reduction cannot be achieved closed. It should be emphasized that closed reduction should not be forceful, and in order to be accepted as the treatment of choice of a dislocated hip, the following criteria should be present:

- The femoral head should be covered by at least two-thirds of the acetabular labrum in the reduced position without major infolding of the labrum.
- The femoral head should be deeply seated in the acetabulum and proximity to the acetabular fossa, and no more than 5 mm of medial dye pooling should be accepted.
- The hip should have an ample arc of abduction and a wide safe zone (≥30°) of instability.
- The hip should be immobilized in a spica cast without forceful abduction. Abduction in the cast should be less than the maximum degree of abduction (maximum abduction is 60°; ideally at 50°).
- The concentric reduction achieved in the operating room should be confirmed after the application of the spica cast by advanced imaging.

If these criteria are not fulfilled, then the hip should be treated by an open reduction. Moreover, children at walking age with high hip dislocation (grade IV according to the International Hip Dysplasia Institute [IHDI] grading system[1]) may benefit from an open reduction because of the pathologic anatomy of the hip. With time, several intra-articular and periarticular structures may block a concentric closed reduction. These structures, including a tight anterior medial joint capsule, a constricting iliopsoas tendon, a hypertrophic teres ligament, excessive fibrofatty pulvinar, and a tight transverse acetabular ligament, can be released during the open reduction, which would allow the femoral head to articulate deep in the acetabular fossa. Finally, an absolute indication for open reduction is the child with a high hip dislocation when femoral and often pelvic osteotomies are planned.

Open reduction of a dislocated hip may be performed through an anterior approach or various medial approaches. Although the goal for the different approaches is the same, that is, to obtain a concentric reduction of the femoral head into the acetabular cavity, the two approaches have different advantages and disadvantages. Overall, the treating pediatric orthopedic surgeon should consider the severity of the dislocation and pathology, the patient's age, the association with other disorders, and whether previous prolonged brace treatment in a dislocated position was performed. Controversy surrounds the lower and upper age limit for open reduction. In general, medial open reduction is performed from 4 to 12 months of age and the anterior approach is carried out after 6 months of age. We recommend open reduction with femoral and pelvic osteotomies up to 8 years of age, especially in those with unilateral disease.

MEDIAL APPROACH FOR OPEN REDUCTION OF A DISLOCATED HIP

The medial approach for open reduction of the hip was originally described by Ludloff.[2] Since its description, several authors have described slight modifications of the medial approach including a description by Ferguson[3] who used the interval between the adductor longus and the adductor brevis. We use the anteromedial approach through a medial incision with the deep dissection between the neurovascular bundle and the pectineus muscle[4,5] (**Figure 3.1**). Although the medial approach has been used for patients up to age 3 years,

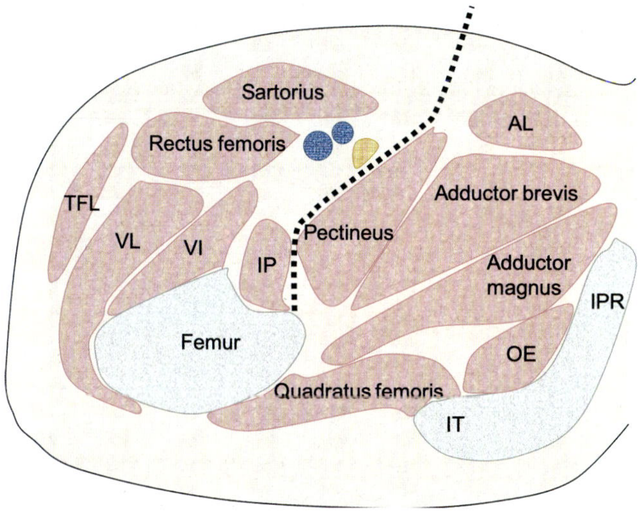

FIGURE 3.1. Illustration of right hemipelvis anatomy in the axial plane showing the plane of dissection of the anteromedial approach to the hip between the pectineus and the neurovascular bundle (black dashed line). Alternatively, the hip may be approached from the medial incision using the plane between the adductor brevis and the adductor magnus or between the adductor brevis and the pectineus. AL, adductor longus; IP, iliopsoas; IPR, inferior pubic ramus; IT, ischial tuberosity; OE, obturator externus; TFL, tensor fascia lata; VI, vastus intermedius; VL, vastus lateralis.

we believe the medial approach should be limited to patients younger than 12 months, especially those with bilateral dislocated hips.[6]

Advantages

- Direct access to the blocks to concentric reduction, including the tight anteromedial joint capsule, the tight transverse acetabular ligament, a hypertrophic ligamentum teres, capsular constriction by a tight iliopsoas tendon, and removal of the fibrofatty pulvinar.
- Cosmetic scar
- Bilateral hip dislocations can be treated with minimal blood loss.
- Easy to perform a *tenodesis* of the ligamentum teres to the anteromedial aspect of the acetabular rim, which may help keep the reduction stable

Disadvantages

- Formal capsulorrhaphy is not possible, although some stiches can be placed in the capsule after reduction.
- The medial femoral circumflex artery (MFCA) crosses the field and is at risk of damage during surgery, raising the concern of high risk of osteonecrosis of the femoral head.
- It is not possible to perform secondary procedures, such as a pelvic osteotomy.

Clinical Scenario

A 12-week-old girl presented to clinic because the pediatrician noted that the hips were asymmetric during her well-child physical examination. She was the first-born child via a C-section owing to breech presentation, and there was no family history of developmental dysplasia of the hip (DDH). Ultrasonography of the hips revealed a severe dislocation of the left hip considered Graf-grade IV, that is, the femoral head was dislocated out of the acetabulum and was pushing against the labrum caudally. The hip was not easily reducible during the Ortolani maneuver, and she was scheduled to undergo closed versus open reduction. Preoperative radiographs obtained at 5 months of age showed dislocation of the left hip (**Figure 3.2**). Arthrogram of the left hip revealed excessive medial dye pooling (>5 mm) and an infolded labrum and a tight transverse acetabular ligament (**Figure 3.3**). The patient underwent treatment by an anteromedial open reduction.

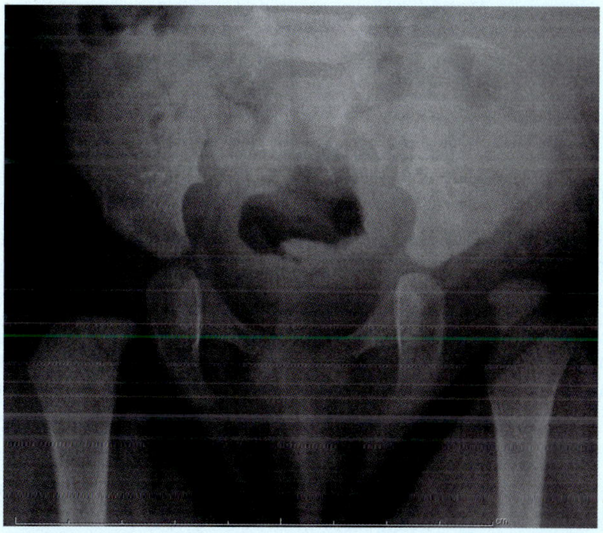

FIGURE 3.2. Preoperative radiograph of a 5-month-old girl born breech who was found to have left irreducible hip during examination showing that the left hip was dislocated

(*continued*)

Clinical Scenario (*continued*)

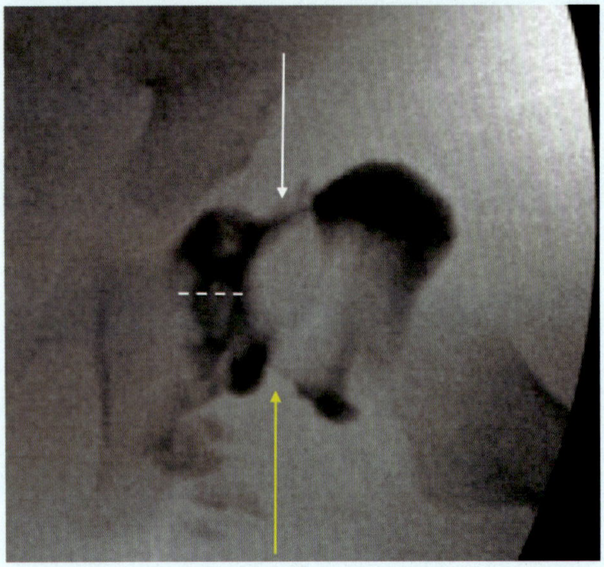

FIGURE 3.3. Left hip arthrogram. Intraoperative fluoroscopy C-arm imaging after left hip arthrogram and attempted closed reduction. The hip was placed in flexion and maximum abduction to about 60° to 70°, but the femoral head was not well covered and the labrum was infolded (white arrow). The femoral head did not pass through the transverse acetabular ligament (yellow arrow), and it was seating laterally, creating a wide (>5 mm) pooling of the dye medially (white dashed lines). The patient was treated with open reduction through the anteromedial approach.

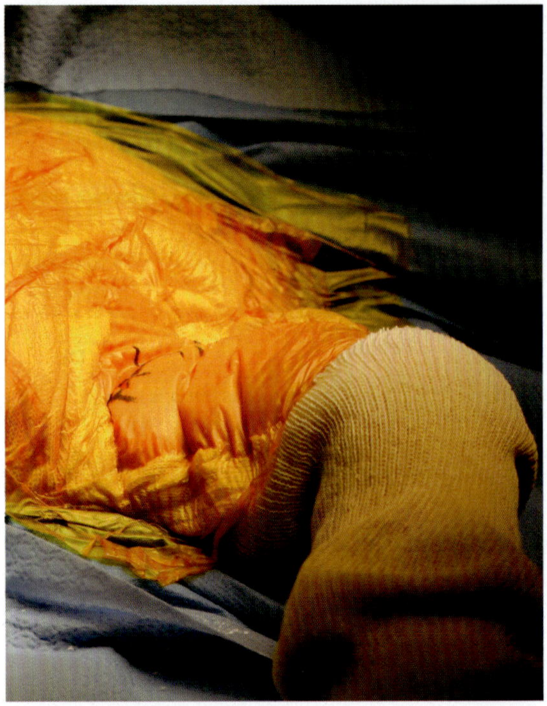

FIGURE 3.4. Patient positioning: intraoperative picture showing the patient is positioned with the left hip in flexion and abduction with external rotation. The entire hemipelvis and lower extremity should be draped free.

Surgical Technique

The medial open reduction is performed with the patient supine on the radiolucent table under general anesthesia and with assisted caudal anesthetic blockage to help with pain management postoperatively. A Foley catheter is inserted and secured in the midline to help in managing the patient and to avoid getting the cast wet during the first 24 hours after surgery. The patient is positioned with the affected hip in flexion, abduction, and external rotation, and the hemipelvis and lower extremity are prepared and draped using standard technique (**Figure 3.4**).

A transverse skin incision is performed from the inferior border of the abductor tendon proximally to the level of the femoral neurovascular bundle parallel to the groin crease. The subcutaneous tissue is dissected exposing the adductor compartment fascia. The fascia on top of the abductor longus tendon is opened longitudinally in line with the tendon. The adductor longus tendon is identified and dissected free (**Figure 3.5**). The adductor longus is released at the muscle–tendon junction and retracted distally (**Figure 3.6**). With retraction of the adductor longus tendon distally, the anterior branch of the obturator nerve is identified crossing on top of the adductor brevis muscle.

The anterior branch of the obturator nerve serves as a reference to identify the pectineus. The nerve is traced proximally where it enters the obturator foramen beneath the pectineus muscle. The neurovascular bundle is identified and dissected free at the proximal or superior border of the wound (**Figure 3.7**). It is our preference to dissect the neurovascular bundle at this time because it is safer to have the femoral artery, vein, and nerve protected and to identify the femoral medial circumflex artery (MFCA) early to avoid damage to the main vascular supply to the femoral head. A vessel loop may be used to protect the neurovascular bundle. The fascia on top of the pectineus is opened in the interval between pectineus, and the neurovascular bundle is dissected, being very careful to avoid damage to the MFCA that courses from superior to inferior. The hip is rotated externally to bring the lesser trochanter toward the operative field. The lesser trochanter is palpated, and the iliopsoas tendon can be identified and dissected with the help of a peanut dissector sponge (**Figure 3.8**). A right-angled clamp is passed underneath the iliopsoas, and the tendon is cut at the insertion on the lesser trochanter (**Figure 3.9**).

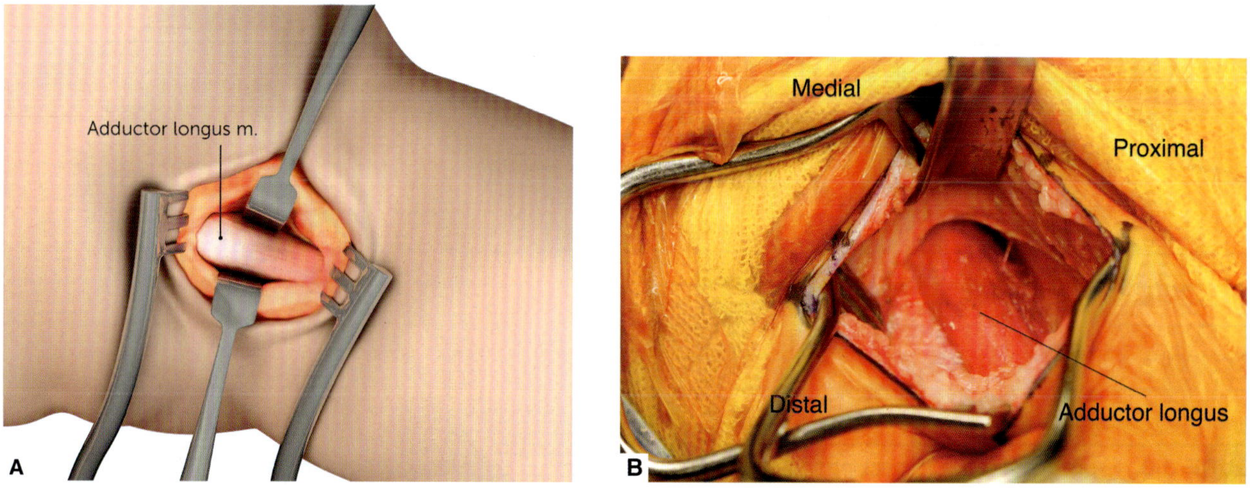

FIGURE 3.5. Superficial dissection: the adductor longus muscle and tendon. (A) Illustration and (B) intraoperative picture showing the adductor longus muscle and tendon should be identified after the fascia is open in line with the muscle.

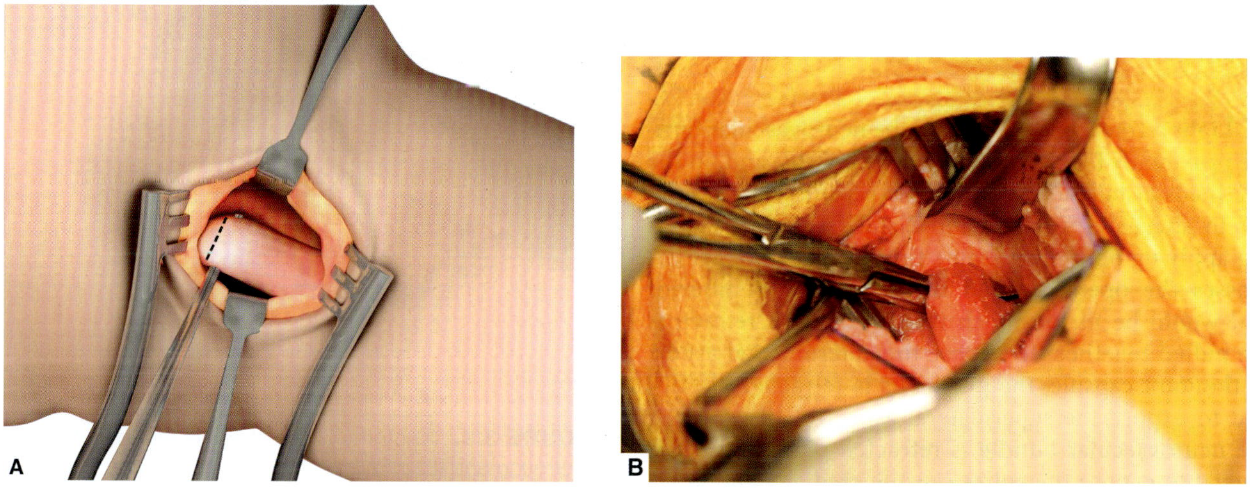

FIGURE 3.6. Tenotomy of the adductor longus. (A) Illustration and (B) intraoperative picture showing that the adductor longus tendon is brought to the surface by a right-angled clamp, and a tenotomy (black dashed line) is performed at the muscle–tendon junction.

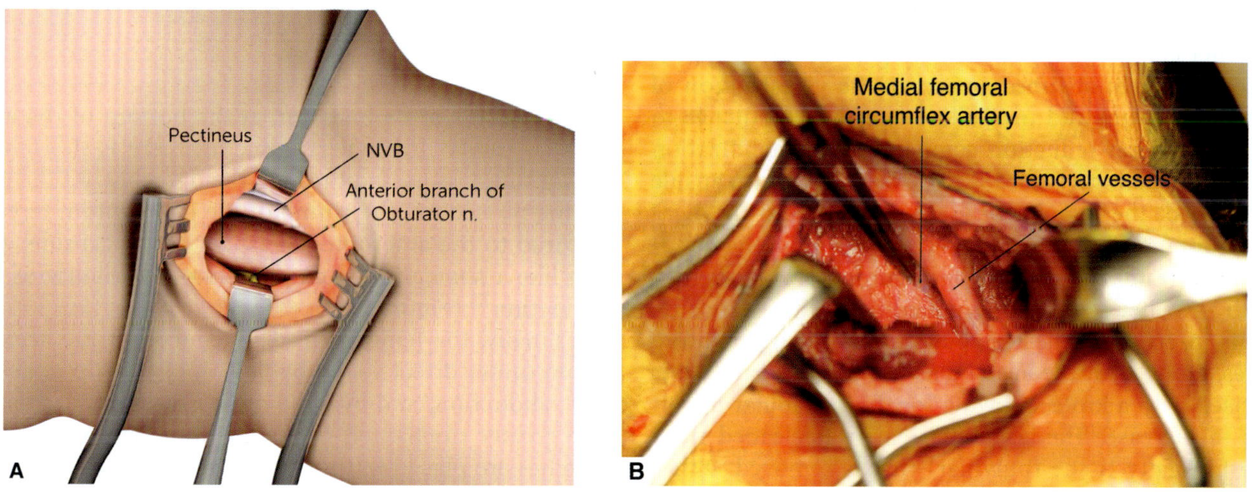

FIGURE 3.7. Identification of the femoral vessels and the medial femoral circumflex artery (MFCA). A, Illustration showing the anterior branch of the obturator nerve crossing under the pectineus. The interval between the pectineus and the neurovascular bundle (NVB) is dissected. B, Intraoperative picture showing the NVB has been fully dissected on the superior or proximal aspect of the operative field, and the MFCA is identified early to protect it during the entire procedure and avoid damage to the main vascular supply to the femoral head.

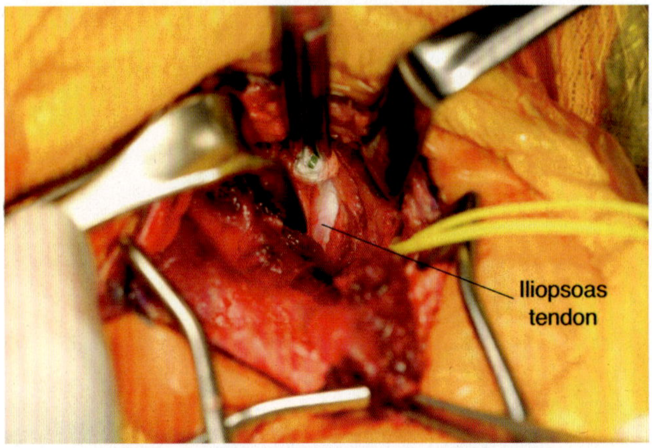

FIGURE 3.8. Exposure of the iliopsoas: intraoperative picture showing a peanut sponge is used to dissect the iliopsoas tendon at the level of the insertion on the lesser trochanter. External rotation of the hip facilitates palpation, and identification of the lesser trochanter before the iliopsoas is dissected free.

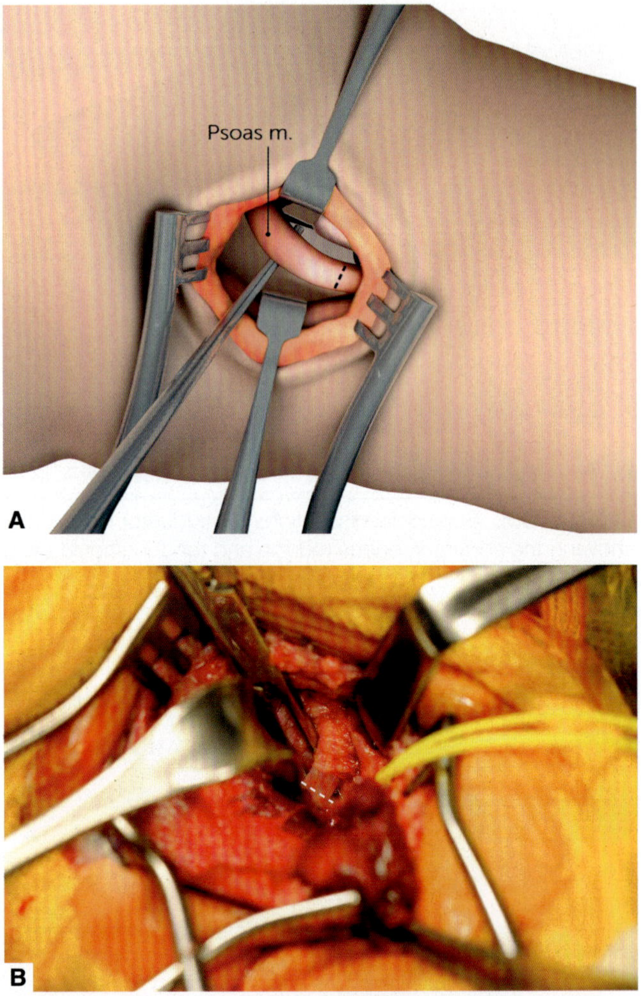

FIGURE 3.9. Tenotomy of the iliopsoas tendon. (A) Illustration and (B) intraoperative picture showing the iliopsoas tendon is isolated with a right-angled clamp, and a tenotomy is performed at the insertion on the lesser trochanter. The white dashed line marks the level of the tenotomy.

Light retraction is applied to the neurovascular bundle proximally (superior portion of the field) and on the pectineus distally to expose the hip capsule. It is important to alternate proximal and distal retraction, avoiding applying both at the same time because the MFCA crosses the operative field from superior to inferior and would be in too much traction if both retractors are pulled together. To expose the anteromedial aspect of the joint capsule, the pectineus is retracted distally, and to expose the superolateral aspect of the capsule, the neurovascular bundle is retracted proximally. It is crucial to expose the entire capsule medially and laterally to the MFCA before the capsulotomy is performed (**Figure 3.10**). Once the capsule is dissected free, an incision is performed in the anteromedial aspect parallel to the acetabular rim. One alternative is to perform another cut to the capsule, creating a "T"-shape capsulotomy, which, at times, improves the visualization of the acetabulum and may allow one to two stitches to be placed after reduction augmenting the stabilization of the reduction (**Figure 3.11**). After the joint capsule is opened, the femoral head is exposed, and the ligamentum teres is cut free from its insertion in the femoral head (**Figure 3.12**). The ligamentum teres is grasped with a Kocher clamp and is pulled to facilitate exposure of its insertion in the acetabular floor. The ligamentum teres, along with the acetabular transverse ligament, is incised with a knife, allowing for the acetabular introitus to increase. The acetabular cavity is cleaned from the fibrofatty tissue (pulvinar) that is removed with a pituitary rongeur (**Figure 3.13**). Alternatively, the ligamentum teres can be left intact in the femoral head, but only resected at its insertion at the bottom of the acetabular cavity. The hypertrophic ligament is shortened, and a suture is passed through the ligament. At the end of the procedure, the stump of the ligamentum teres is sutured to the anteromedial aspect of the capsule, acting like a *tenodesis* and augmenting the stability of the reduction[7,8] (**Figure 3.14**).

Finally, the femoral head is reduced in the acetabulum under direct vision by flexion of the hip to about 90°, abduction, and by applying a gentle push through the greater trochanter. If possible, one or two 0 Vicryl stitches are placed in the capsule to improve the stability postreduction, which can also be improved by the tenodesis of the ligamentum teres. Before the wound

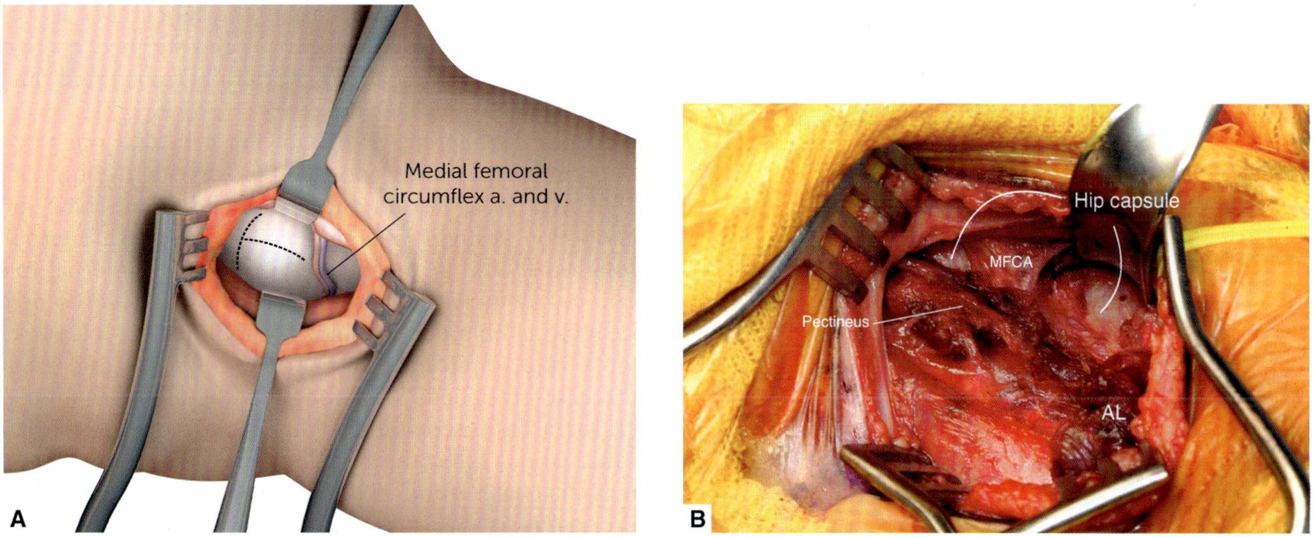

FIGURE 3.10. Complete exposure of the hip capsule medially and laterally to the medial femoral circumflex artery (MFCA). A, Illustration showing the exposure of the hip capsule proximally and distally. The black dashed lines mark the capsulotomy. To expose the proximal aspect of the capsule, a retractor is placed under the neurovascular bundle. To expose the distal aspect, a retractor is placed under the pectineus. Note that the MFCA crosses the field from superior to inferior, and it would be submitted to excessive traction if both retractors are pulled simultaneously. Therefore, exposure of the capsule should be done in a synchronized manner: if one of the retractors is pulling, the other should be relaxed and vice versa. The MFCA should not be placed under excessive tension. (B) Intraoperative picture showing the hip capsule should be visualized both medially and laterally to the MFCA. Lateral exposure is important, especially in higher dislocations. AL, adductor longus.

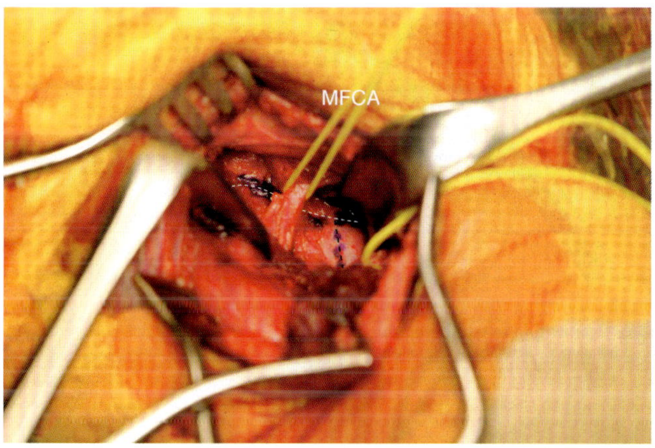

FIGURE 3.11. Capsulotomy. Intraoperative picture showing the capsulotomy is drawn with a marking pen. The medial femoral circumflex artery (MFCA) is protected by a vessel loop. The typical capsulotomy for the medial approach is performed parallel to the acetabular margin (white dashed line). Alternatively, a second cut is added to capsulotomy perpendicular to the first one and in line with the femoral neck axis (black dashed line).

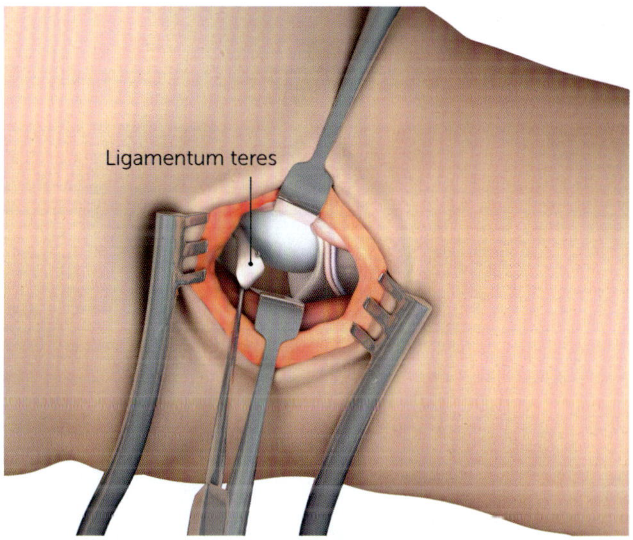

FIGURE 3.12. Ligamentum teres release. Illustration showing that with the hip in external rotation, the femoral head becomes visible in the operative field, and the ligamentum teres is grasped and pulled out. The ligamentum teres is sharply incised from the insertion in the femoral head. A Kocher clamp is used to grasp the ligament toward its insertion (not shown). The ligament is sharply incised at its insertion along with incision of the transverse acetabular ligament.

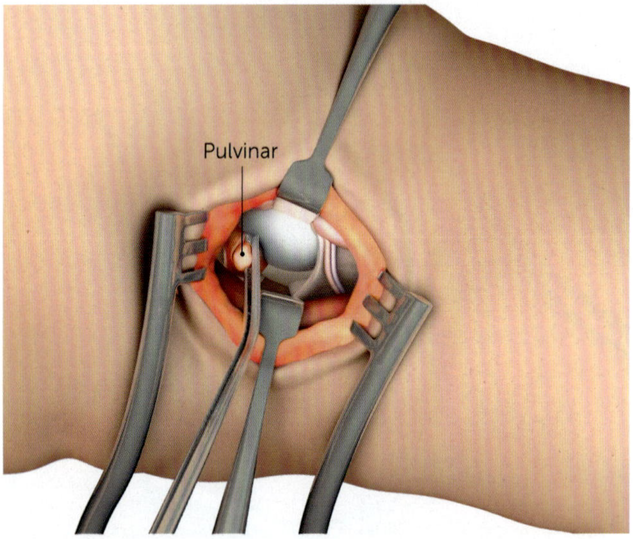

FIGURE 3.13. Preparation of the acetabular cavity: illustration showing a pituitary rongeur is used to clean the fibrofatty pulvinar from the acetabulum. Removal of the pulvinar should be performed with caution to avoid damage to the articular surface.

is closed, we inject about 1 mL of a 50% solution with ioversol and saline to confirm the reduction and to help assess the reduction while applying the spica cast (**Figure 3.15**). The wound is irrigated and closed in layers: the deep adductor fascia, the subcutaneous tissue, and then the skin. Steri-Strips and sterile dressings are applied, and the patient is carefully transferred into a radiolucent spica cast table.

Spica cast application following a medial open reduction: a spica cast will be applied with the hips in 100° to 110° of flexion and 45° of abduction (<60° of abduction is highly recommended). Excessive internal rotation should be avoided; however, slight internal rotation may increase the stability of the hip. Fluoroscopy imaging is obtained through the radiolucent spica cast table after application of the cotton Webril and after the cast is applied. We strongly recommend obtaining a C-arm fluoroscopy during application of the cast because this is often the most critical time when the hip may dislocate. Another important detail while applying the cast is to keep the patient under general anesthesia to avoid any abrupt moving of the hip and knees. After the spica cast is applied, a magnetic resonance imaging (MRI) is obtained to confirm the concentric reduction of the hip. MRI protocol following open reduction does not require the patient to be under full general anesthesia. Often, with the spica cast in place and using rapid MRI sequences, a good detailed examination is possible. The patient is admitted to the orthopedic floor for pain management and spica cast education and is typically discharged the next day following surgery.

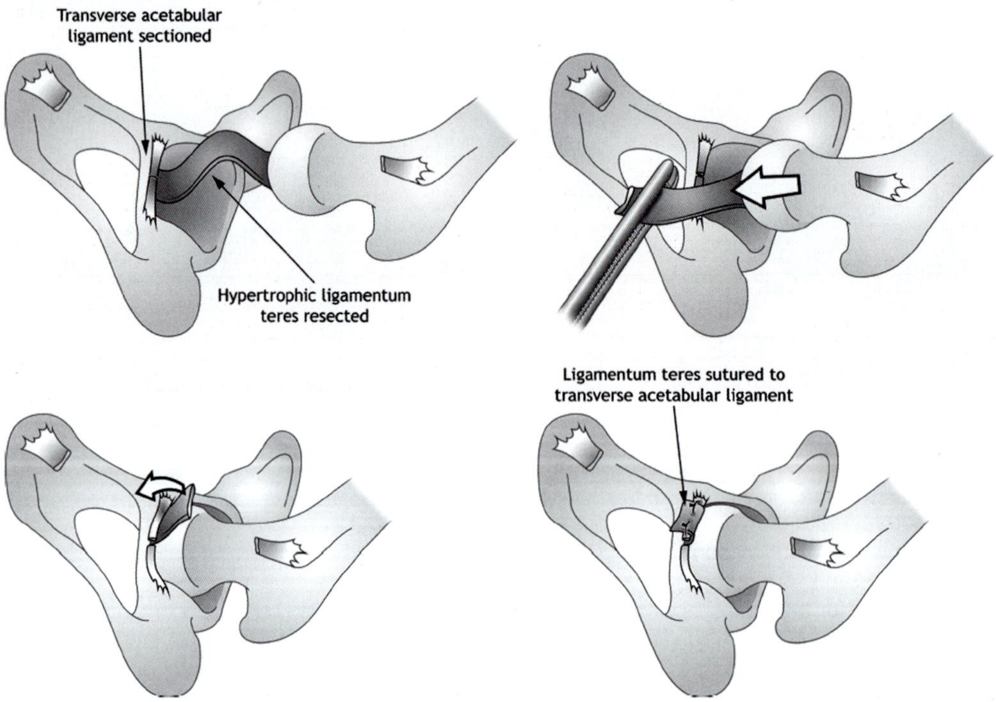

FIGURE 3.14. Illustration showing the steps for the ligamentum teres tenodesis technique. Instead of resecting the ligamentum from the femoral head, the insertion at the transverse acetabular ligament is incised. After the femoral head is reduced in the acetabular cavity, the remaining ligamentum is shortened and sutured back in the acetabular ligament area. Theoretically, this technique augments stability of the hip in the immediate postoperative period. Reproduced with permission from Bache et al.[7]

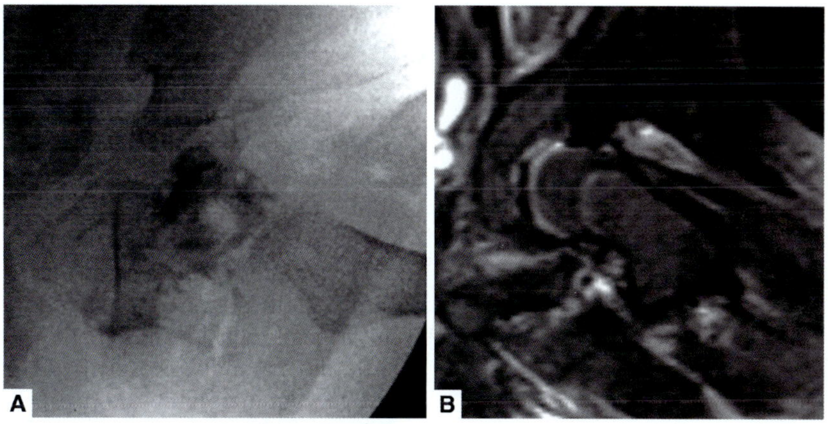

FIGURE 3.15. Postoperative imaging. A, Intraoperative fluoroscopy C-arm imaging obtained just before the spica cast is applied showing the left hip is concentrically reduced and there is minimal dye pooling medially. The arthrogram is performed before the wound is completely closed and helps guiding the application of the cast. B, Postoperative magnetic resonance imaging after anteromedial open reduction and application of spica casting confirming concentric reduction of the hip.

ANTERIOR APPROACH FOR OPEN REDUCTION OF A DISLOCATED HIP

The anterior approach may also leave a cosmetic scar if the modified anterior bikini-type incision is used. Through the anterior approach, a capsulorrhaphy can be performed. Another advantage is that when necessary, a pelvic osteotomy can be performed in the same setting. A potential disadvantage is a relatively higher blood loss compared to the medial approach, which leads to most surgeons avoiding this approach for bilateral open reductions. Bilateral hip dislocations treated through the anterior approach are typically staged 4 to 6 weeks apart. Open reduction of the hip using the anterior approach may be performed in patients older than 6 months. During the first year of life, both medial and anterior open reductions can be used, and the choice should be based on surgeon's experience and comfort with each approach. In general, after 12 months of age, our preference is to use the anterior approach. One relative indication is a hip previously treated by a Pavlik harness with persistent dislocation and deformity of the posterolateral acetabulum—the so-called *Pavlik harness disease.* In such hips, the dissection of the superior and lateral aspects of the capsule and a formal capsulorrhaphy are crucial to keep a concentric and stable reduction.

Clinical Scenario

A 17-month-old girl presented to clinic after she was found to limp and to have asymmetric length of the lower extremities by the pediatrician. Her radiographs showed dislocation of the right hip, and an open reduction of the hip was recommended along with a femoral shortening osteotomy given the high dislocation (IHDI grade IV) (**Figure 3.16**).

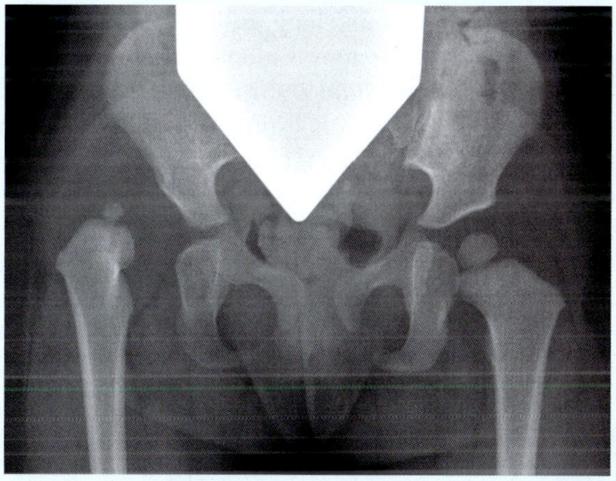

FIGURE 3.16. Preoperative radiograph of a 17-month-old female with right hip dislocation.

SURGICAL TECHNIQUE

Surgery is performed with the patient under general anesthesia with either a single-shot caudal blockade or a lumbar plexus catheter to help with postoperative pain when an osteotomy is planned. The patient is positioned supine with a radiolucent bump under the ipsilateral shoulder and flank. The bump should not be directly under the buttock because this may raise the gluteal musculature, making the approach dissection of the posterior lateral aspect of the capsule more laborious. The entire hemipelvis up to the level of the rib cage is prepared and draped free, including the lower extremity (**Figure 3.17**). Careful preparation of the groin is important because the adductor longus tendon is often released in combination with the open reduction.

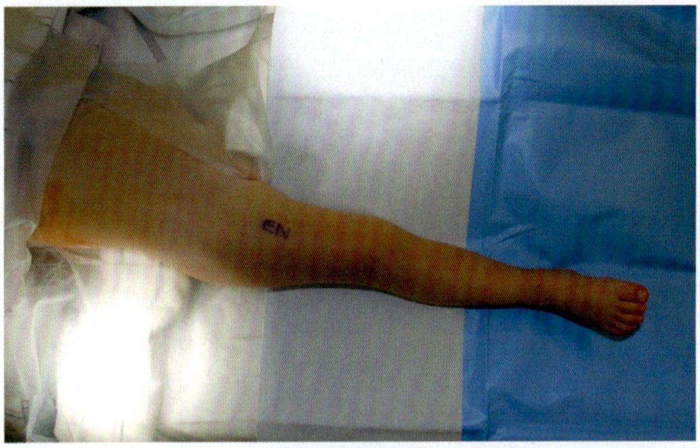

FIGURE 3.17. Patient positioning for anterolateral approach for open reduction. The patient is positioned supine with a radiolucent bump under the ipsilateral scapula to the iliac crest, allowing for 15° to 20° tilt. The bump should not be placed under the gluteus, and the entire hemipelvis, lower extremity, and part of the hemithorax should be prepared and draped free. As a reference, the lower aspect of the rib cage should be in the operative field.

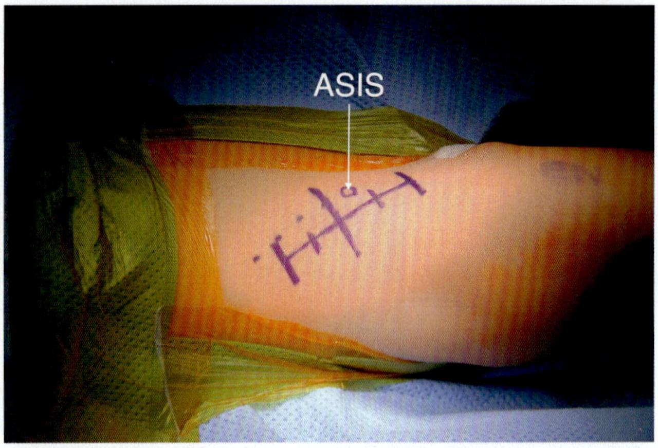

FIGURE 3.19. A modified skin incision following the "biquini" line is more cosmetic than the classic iliofemoral Smith-Petersen incision. Intraoperative picture showing the incision is placed 1 to 2 cm distal and in line with the iliac crest and curved medially about a 3 cm distal and medial to the anterior superior iliac spine (ASIS).

Very often, the first step for an open reduction is release of the adductor longus tendon. Although some surgeons perform a percutaneous tenotomy, our preference is to release the tendon through an open incision (**Figure 3.18**). A small transverse incision is made at the top of the adductor longus tendon. Subcutaneous tissue dissection is performed, and the adductor fascia is exposed. The fascia is opened longitudinally in line with the muscle. The adductor longus is identified, and a right-angled clamp is passed under the muscle tendinous junction. The adductor longus is brought to the surface, and a tenotomy is performed using the cautery. The adductor fascia is sutured after hemostasis, and the subcutaneous tissue and the skin are closed using absorbable sutures.

Next, attention is shifted to the actual open reduction. The incision is placed 1 to 2 cm distal in line with the iliac crest and curved medially about a 3-cm distal and medial to the anterior superior iliac spine (ASIS) (**Figure 3.19**). The subcutaneous tissue is dissected exposing the aponeurosis of the external oblique musculature. We carefully released the insertion of the external oblique muscle of the lateral aspect of the iliac crest to expose the iliac crest apophysis (**Figure 3.20**). Distally in the wound, the interval between the tensor fascia lata and the sartorius muscle is palpated. We recommend against formal dissection of the interval and exposure of the lateral femoral cutaneous nerve. Instead, we open the fascia of the tensor fascia lata muscle (**Figure 3.21**). The tensor fascia lata muscle belly is retracted laterally, preserving the fascia of the sartorius muscle intact and the lateral femoral cutaneous nerve that runs in the sartorius fascia. With further lateral retraction of the tensor fascia lata muscle and medial retraction of the sartorius, the lateral border of the rectus femoris is

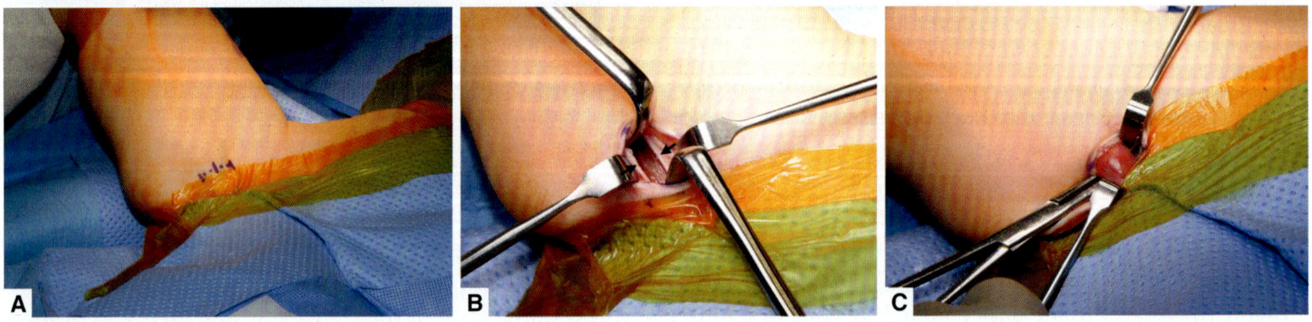

FIGURE 3.18. Adductor longus release. A, Intraoperative picture showing 2- to 3-cm transverse skin is marked on top of the adductor longus about 5 mm from the medial skin crease. B, After the subcutaneous tissue is dissected free, the adductor fascia (black arrows) is exposed and open longitudinally in line with the adductor longus muscle. C, A right-angled clamp is used to bring the muscle out of the wound, and the adductor longus is incised with a cautery at the muscle tendinous junction.

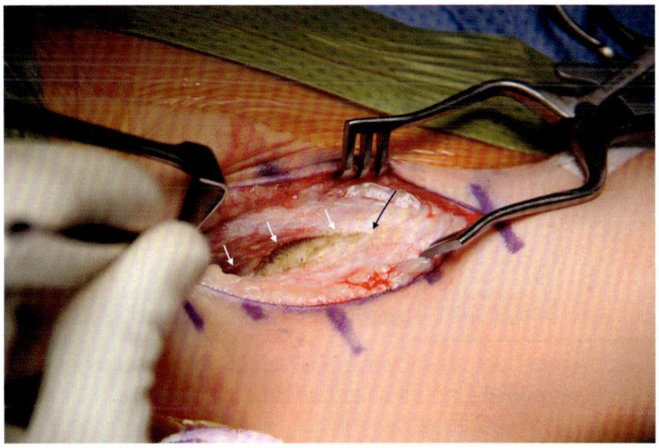

FIGURE 3.20. Release of the external oblique insertion in the iliac crest. The external oblique aponeurosis (white arrows) is incised, and the muscle is released from its insertion in the lateral aspect of the iliac crest to the level of the anterior superior iliac spine (black arrow).

identified (Figure 3.22). The indirect head of the rectus can be identified in the posterior lateral aspect of the hip capsule, whereas the direct head is identified at its insertion into the anterior inferior iliac spine (AIIS).

At this point, the entire iliac crest apophysis, including the ASIS and AIIS, is exposed. The surgeon should pinch the iliac crest between the thumb and the index finger to ensure incising the apophysis in its midline. The iliac crest apophysis is sharply incised from proximal to distal up to the level of the AIIS (Figure 3.23). The apophysis should be carefully popped free by pushing with a sponge before a periosteal elevator is used to expose the inner and outer tables of the ilium. The outer and inner walls of the ilium are dissected subperiosteally with a retractor, and sponges are packed medially and laterally to reduce bleeding. Subperiosteal dissection of the inner wall of the ilium should stop short at the level of the AIIS. The indirect and direct heads of the rectus femoris are identified and released from the capsule and AIIS, respectively (Figure 3.24). Medially to the AIIS, the dissection of the ileum and the pubis should be extraperiosteal to avoid damage to the pubic branch of the triradiate cartilage. A long retractor is placed under the iliopsoas tendon at the pelvic brim. Although release of the iliopsoas tendon can be performed at this time, we prefer to keep the iliopsoas tendon intact until the end of the procedure because it serves as a protection to the femoral neurovascular bundle. A long and thin retractor is placed under the psoas tendon on top of the superior pubic ramus. The iliopsoas is retracted medially, allowing for complete exposure of the anterior medial capsule. It is important to note that the iliocapsularis muscle inserts into the capsule and that it should be completely released to allow full exposure and an adequate capsulotomy.

Once the hip capsule is completely exposed from posterior lateral to the anterior medial, capsulotomy can be performed (Figure 3.25). Capsulotomy is performed sharply about 5 mm distal to the acetabular rim. As soon as the scalpel goes through the capsule, synovial fluid or the contrast previously injected in the case of an arthrogram will extravasate from the joint. We prefer to start a capsulotomy in the anterior medial aspect, which is a crucial part of the capsule to be released. Capsulotomy is then brought proximally and posteriorly parallel to the acetabular rim. Posterolaterally, the capsulotomy is performed up to the level of the insertion of the indirect head of the rectus femoris. Once the capsule is incised, the ligamentum teres becomes visible. However, in high dislocations and in older patients, it is not uncommon to observe

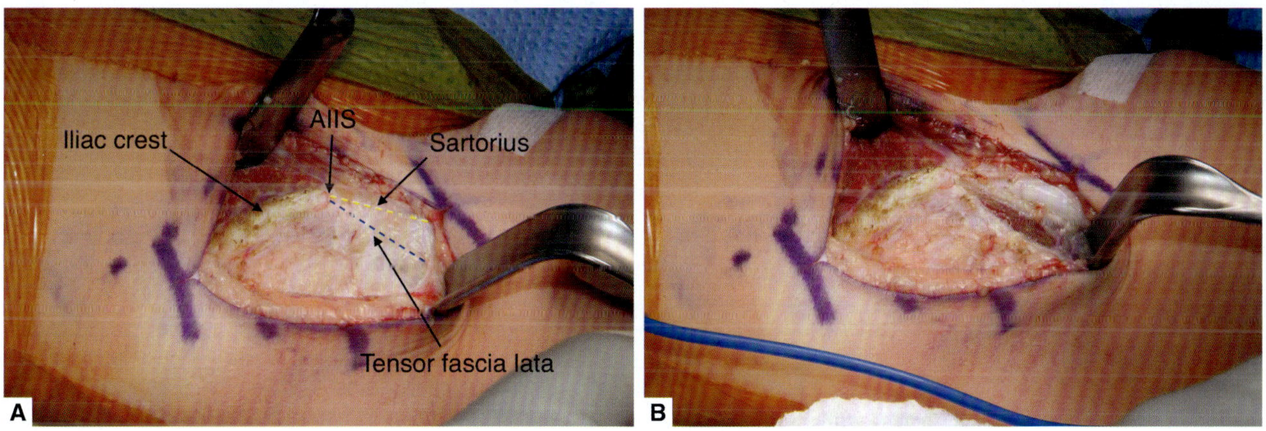

FIGURE 3.21. Distal dissection of the sartorius and tensor fascia lata (TFL) interval. A, Intraoperative picture showing the "classic" plane for exposure of the sartorius–TFL interval (yellow dashed lines). Dissection through this plane exposes the lateral femoral cutaneous nerve that is to be avoided. We prefer to incise the TFL fascia about 30° to 45° distal to the anterior inferior iliac spine (AIIS) (blue dashed line). B, Intraoperative picture showing an incision has been performed over the TFL fascia exposing the muscle belly.

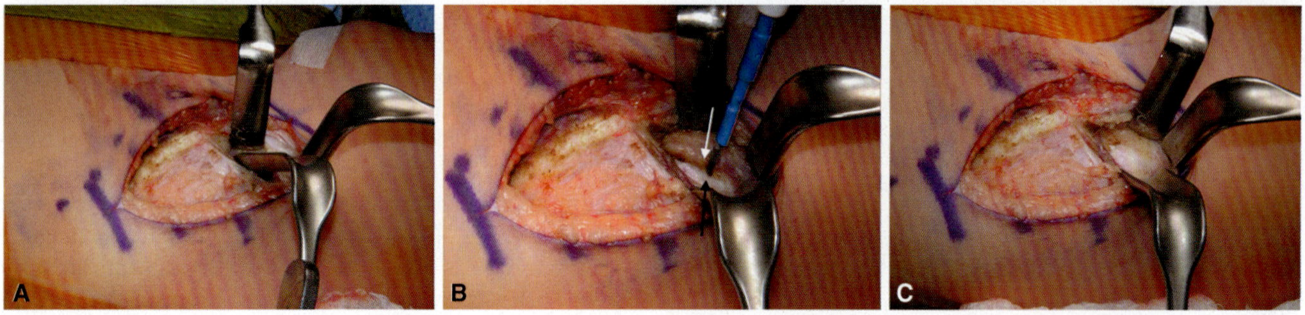

FIGURE 3.22. Distal dissection: exposure of the hip capsule. A, Intraoperative picture showing two retractors placed medially to the tensor fascia lata (TFL): the medial retractor pulls the sartorius muscle medially, and the lateral retractor pulls the TFL laterally. B, Intraoperative picture showing exposure of the rectus femoris muscle (white arrow) medially and the hip capsule (black arrow) laterally to the rectus. C, Further dissection and retraction of the rectus femoris medially and the TFL and gluteus minimus laterally exposes the hip joint capsule.

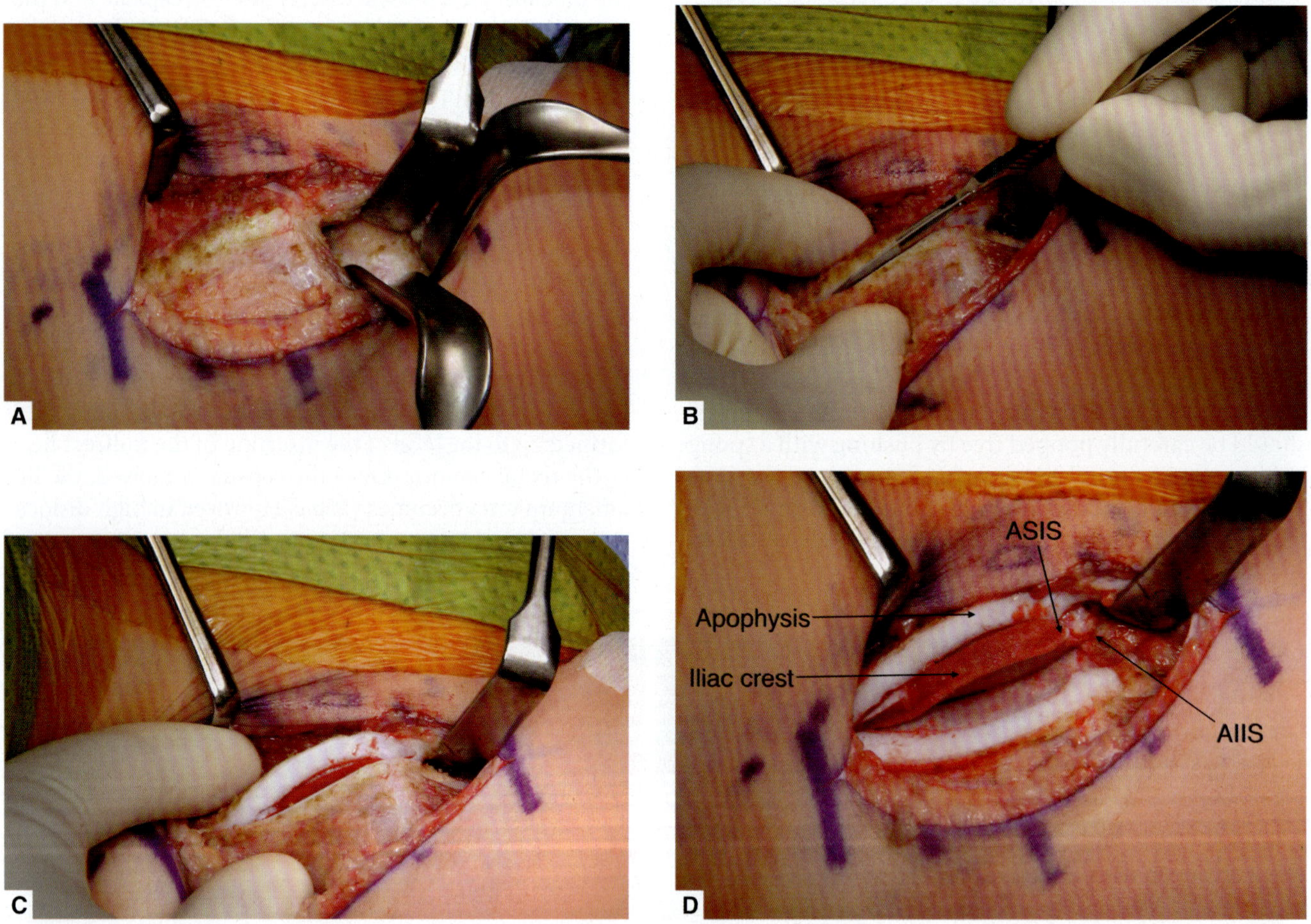

FIGURE 3.23. Proximal dissection: incision of the iliac crest apophysis. A, Intraoperative picture showing complete exposure of the iliac crest including distally the anterior superior iliac spine (ASIS) and the anterior inferior iliac spine (AIIS). B, Intraoperative picture showing the thumb and index finger are used to pinch the iliac crest guiding the scalpel to incise the crest in the midline. C, Intraoperative picture showing the iliac crest apophysis is popped free initially with a gentle push by the thumb with a sponge before using a sharp periosteal elevator. D, Intraoperative picture showing the final aspect after incision of the iliac crest apophysis and dissection of the inner and outer surfaces of the ilium.

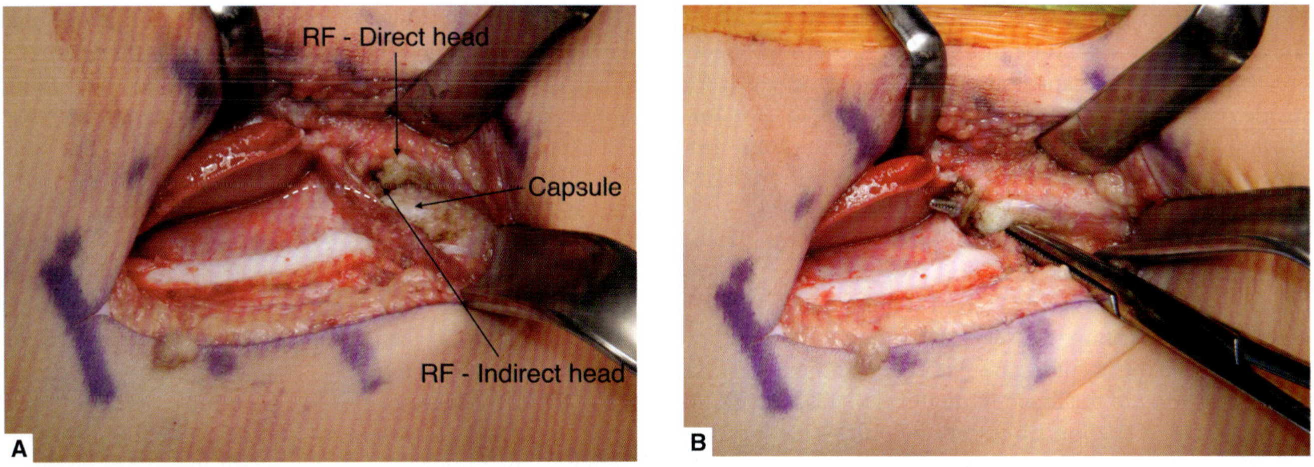

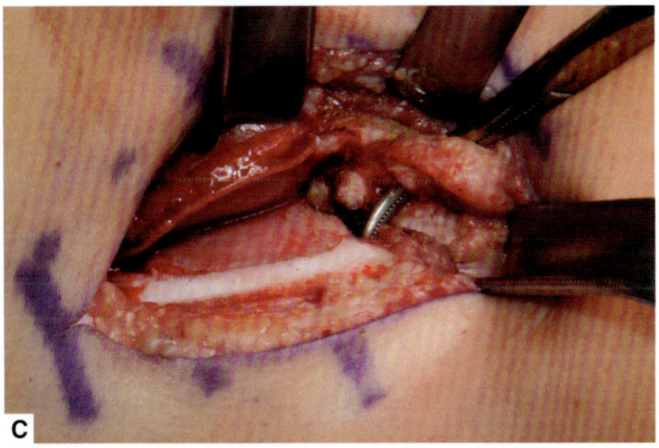

FIGURE 3.24. Connecting the distal and the proximal parts of the dissection. A, Intraoperative picture showing the middle portion of the anterolateral approach. Proximally, the iliac crest apophysis has been split, and the lateral wall of the ilium exposed through subperiosteal dissection. The white dashed line marks the line of incision of the lateral periosteum to allow for complete exposure of the posterolateral aspect of the hip capsule. Distally, the rectus femoris (RF) muscle is retracted medially, and the indirect and direct heads identified and retracted to expose the hip capsule. B, Intraoperative picture showing a right-angled clamp is passed underneath the indirect head of the RF. The indirect head is then sharply incised. C, Intraoperative picture showing a right-angled clamp is passed underneath the direct head of the RF. The direct head is then sharply incised.

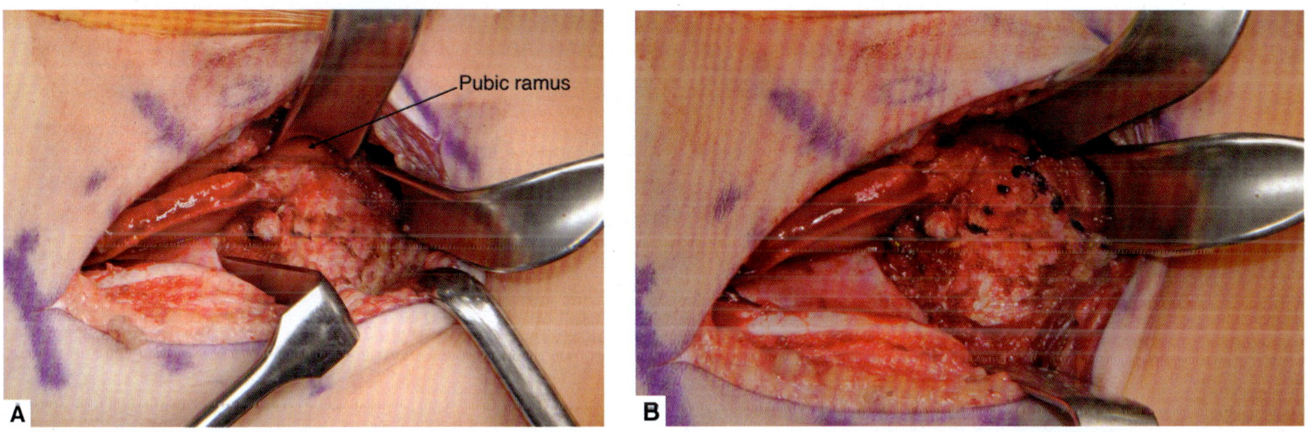

FIGURE 3.25. T-shaped capsulotomy. A, Intraoperative picture showing a retractor is placed under the iliopsoas on top of the superior ramus of the pubis. The periosteum medial to the anterior inferior iliac spine (AIIS) should be preserved to avoid damage to the pubic ramus, contributing to the triradiate cartilage and further growth disturbance of the acetabulum. Another retractor is placed distal, and the iliocapsularis muscle is retracted, allowing complete exposure of the hip capsule. B, Intraoperative picture showing the planned capsulotomy is drawn in the hip joint capsule. The capsulotomy has the shape of the letter "T": the horizontal portion starts as medial as possible at the pubic insertion of the capsule, and it should end posterior and laterally just passed the level of the indirect head of the rectus femoris. This portion of the capsular opening is made in parallel with the acetabular rim and as close as possible to it without damaging the acetabular labrum. The distal extent of the capsulotomy is horizontal in line with the neck.

that the ligamentum teres is absent. The second portion of the capsulotomy should be in line with the femoral neck, creating a T-shaped capsulotomy, and is performed from inside out to avoid damage to the femoral head. It is important to place the second cut of the capsulotomy not excessively lateral because this would make it more laborious to perform an appropriate capsulorrhaphy.

Once the capsulotomy is complete, the femoral head is exposed and the insertion of the ligamentum teres in the femoral head is sharply incised (**Figure 3.26**). The ligamentum teres stump will serve as a guide to the inferior aspect of the true acetabulum. A Kocher clamp is used to grasp the stump of the ligamentum teres that is pulled out. Using a lighted suction tip is very helpful to identify the insertion of the ligamentum teres in the inferior aspect of the acetabulum in very close proximity to the transverse acetabular ligament. The ligamentum teres is sharply excised with a long handle scalpel from its insertion in the inferior aspect of the acetabulum. Incision of the ligamentum teres typically leads to bleeding that can be easily controlled by pressure hemostasis. The acetabular cavity is inspected for the presence of a fibrofatty pulvinar, and the morphology of the acetabular labrum should also be noted. The fibrofatty pulvinar is resected with a pituitary long rongeur. Cleaning of the fibrofatty pulvinar should be performed with caution to avoid damage to the articular cartilage. Often, the acetabular labrum is infolded, and its shape can be improved using a peanut sponge by pulling the labrum underneath it. Cutting the labrum to increase the acetabular opening is not only unnecessary but contraindicated and should not be performed. At this point, the acetabular cavity is cleaned, and the transverse acetabular ligament can be adequately exposed and incised sharply with a long handle scalpel or rongeur. Release of the transverse acetabular ligament is crucial to improve the opening of the acetabulum, which is typically smaller than the femoral head.

After the release of the ligamentum teres and transverse acetabular ligament and cleaning of the fibrofatty pulvinar, the femoral head is reduced in the acetabulum. Reduction is easily performed by flexion, abduction, and by levering the greater trochanter. Assessment of the required force and stability of the reduction is an essential step of the open reduction. Although the hip is typically stable in flexion, abduction, and internal rotation, the position of the hip where stability is lost may serve as a guide for additional procedures. For instance, if instability is noticed by simply extending the hip, we consider that anterior coverage of the femoral head is insufficient, which can be corrected by a pelvic osteotomy. If the stability of

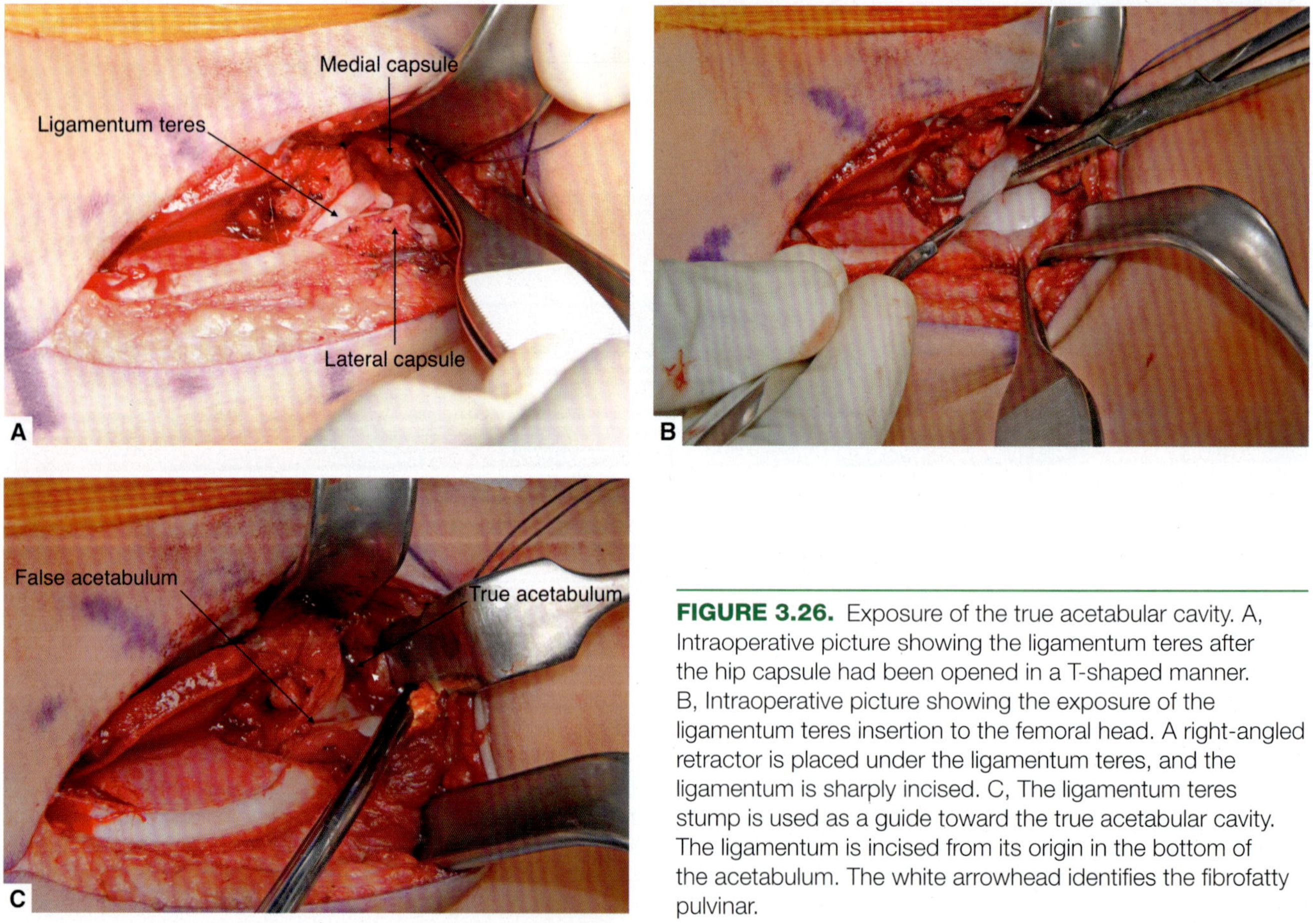

FIGURE 3.26. Exposure of the true acetabular cavity. A, Intraoperative picture showing the ligamentum teres after the hip capsule had been opened in a T-shaped manner. B, Intraoperative picture showing the exposure of the ligamentum teres insertion to the femoral head. A right-angled retractor is placed under the ligamentum teres, and the ligamentum is sharply incised. C, The ligamentum teres stump is used as a guide toward the true acetabular cavity. The ligamentum is incised from its origin in the bottom of the acetabulum. The white arrowhead identifies the fibrofatty pulvinar.

the hip is lost with external rotation or if excessive internal rotation is needed to keep the hip stable, then a femoral derotational osteotomy may be performed to reduce anteversion. If the hip becomes unstable with adduction, then anterolateral insufficiency can be partially corrected with the capsulorrhaphy, but this is often an indication that a pelvic osteotomy should be performed. Although lateral stability could be potentially corrected by a varus osteotomy, we rarely use varization when performing a femoral shortening osteotomy because the neck shaft angle is not typically abnormal in DDH.

If the femoral head cannot be reduced or if excessive traction is required for reduction, then a femoral shortening osteotomy should be performed. Evaluating how much tension is required for the reduction is subjective, and, to date, specific objective criteria are lacking. Most surgeons judge the force that is required to pull the femur distally to achieve the reduction. Others assess whether the knee can be easily flexed and extended with the hip in the reduced position. If the reduction is too tight, then extension of the knee from a flexed position may be more difficult because of the tight hamstrings. The surgeon should know that tension increases when a pelvic osteotomy is performed. As a general rule, we consider a femoral shortening osteotomy in patients after walking age who have a high (IHDI grade IV) dislocation. We routinely perform a shortening osteotomy for those older than 2 years.

In the described clinical scenario, there is a high dislocation. Intraoperatively, the force required to pull the femur distally to reduce the hip was determined to be excessive, and a femoral shortening derotation was recommended. When performing a femoral shortening osteotomy in combination with open reduction, the pelvic wound should be packed with a moist sponge. The femoral osteotomy is performed through a direct lateral approach to the femur. Briefly, a straight lateral incision is performed just distal to the greater trochanter in line with the lateral aspect of the femur (Figure 3.27). The subcutaneous tissue is dissected exposing the fascia lata. The fascia lata is open in line with the skin incision. The vastus lateralis is identified, and an incision is made in the posterior aspect of the vastus lateralis fascia exposing the muscle belly. The vastus lateralis muscle belly is retracted anteriorly, allowing for exposure of the femur extraperiosteally. We do not detach the vastus proximally like we typically would when performing an intertrochanteric osteotomy. The periosteum is incised in line with the longitudinal axis of the femur, and circumferential subperiosteal dissection is performed using a specific curved elevator (Crego elevator).

The femoral shaft can be exposed up to the level of the greater trochanter (Figure 3.28). We then introduce a 4-hole small fragment locking compression plate–dynamic compression plate (LCP–DCP) in the lateral aspect of the femur just distal to the greater trochanter. The two most proximal screws are inserted through the plate, and the level of the osteotomy is marked with an electric cautery. Using an oscillating saw, a straight line is created anteriorly to the plate from 1 cm proximal to the level of the osteotomy to about 2 to 1/2 cm distal. It is important to mark the reference line as distal as possible to avoid losing the reference of rotation once the shortening is performed. The plate is then removed along with the two proximal screws, and a subperiosteal retractor (Crego elevator) is placed at the level of the osteotomy. A straight osteotomy is performed perpendicular to the long axis of the femur. The amount of shortening is often difficult to determine precisely, but in general, it is between 1 and 2 cm depending on the patient's age and severity of the dislocation. A very popular technique is to reduce the femoral head and then leave the femur to overlap and measure how much overlap is present. However, we do not find

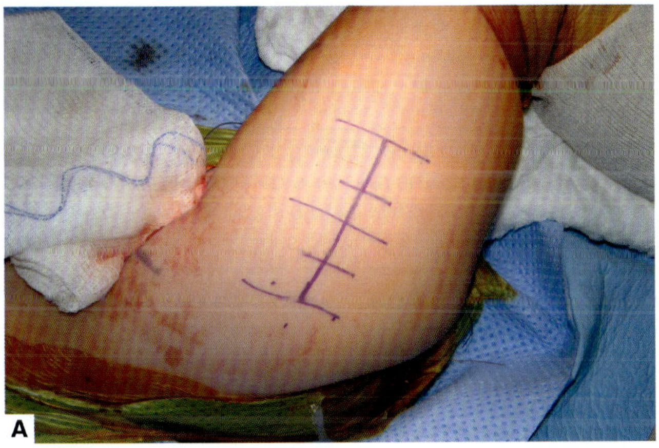
A

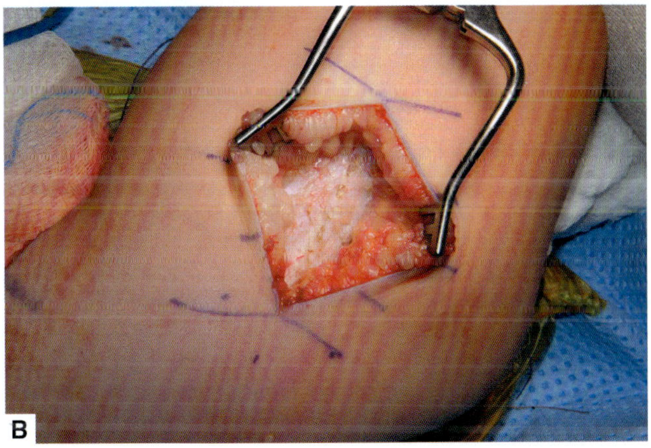
B

FIGURE 3.27. Lateral approach to the femur for femoral shortening osteotomy. A, Intraoperative picture showing a longitudinal incision is performed in the lateral aspect of the thigh just distal to the greater trochanter aiming toward the distal lateral femoral condyle. B, Intraoperative picture showing the superficial dissection had been performed allowing for full exposure of the fascia lata. The fascia should be split longitudinally in line with the skin incision.

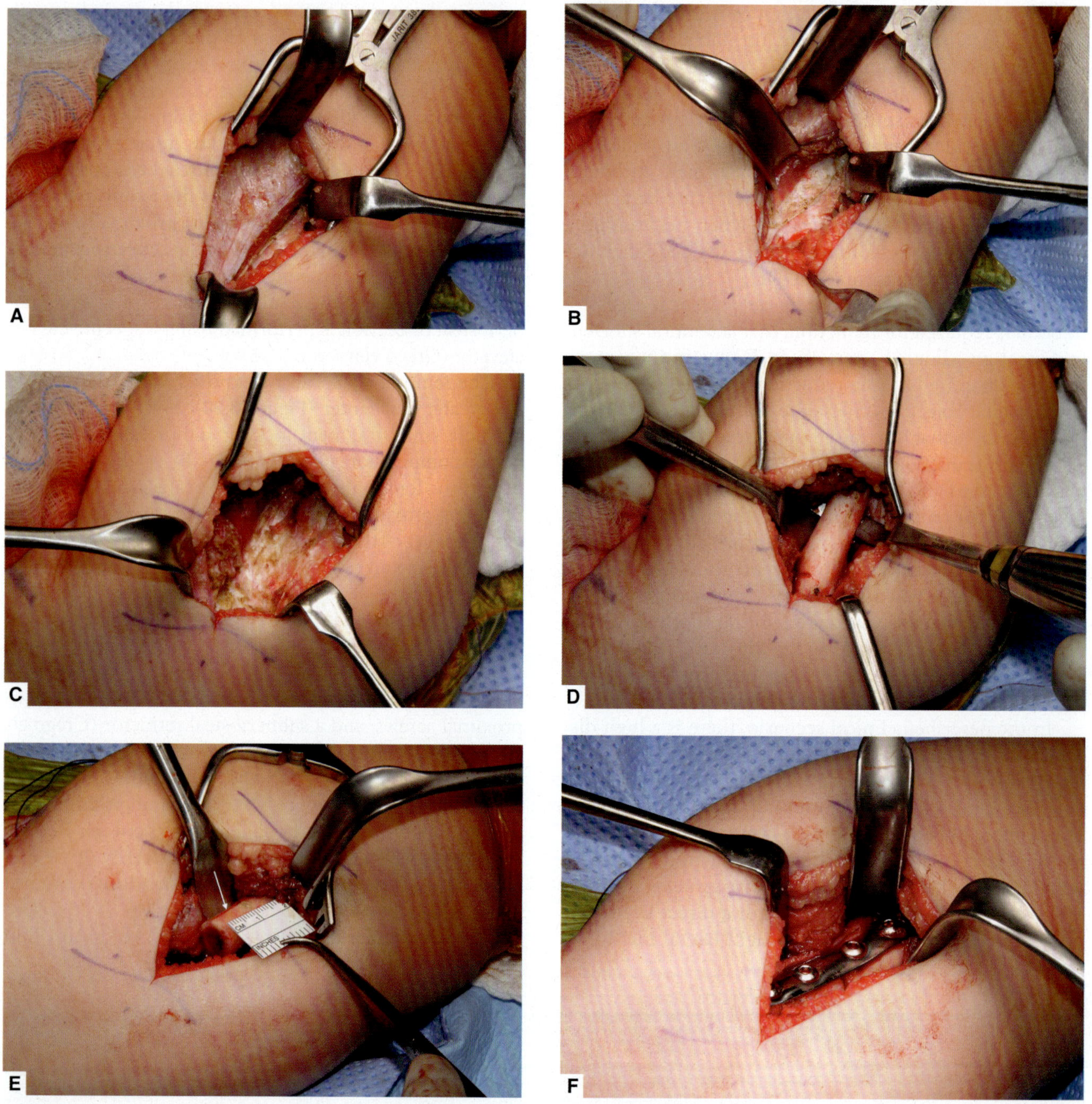

FIGURE 3.28. Deep dissection and femoral shortening osteotomy. A, Intraoperative picture showing the vastus lateralis muscle. An incision is performed in the posterior aspect of the vastus lateralis fascia. B, The muscle is detached from its insertion into the fascia and retracted medially, preserving the periosteum of the femur. C, Intraoperative picture showing full exposure of the proximal aspect of the femur with the periosteum preserved. D, Intraoperative picture showing subperiosteal placement of a medial and a lateral Crego retractor. In preparation for the femoral osteotomy, a longitudinal line had been marked in the anterior aspect of the femur with an oscillating saw. E, Intraoperative picture showing measurement of resection for the femoral shortening. Resection is performed from the distal fragment and measures between 1 and 2 cm. The anterior aspect of the femur had been marked with an oscillating saw (white arrow). F, Final intraoperative aspect of the femoral shortening with slight derotational osteotomy to correct the excessive femoral anteversion.

this helpful at all because the amount of overlap depends on the position of the leg, and any traction or axial push can change the assessment. The measured segment of the femur is resected with an oscillating saw in a transverse manner. The plate is then reapplied proximally with the two screws that had been previously used, and it can be fixed to the bone. At this point, we determine whether an external rotation of the distal fragment is needed to reduce excessive femoral anteversion. Femoral anteversion is commonly higher in DDH, but the degree of anteversion is variable; therefore, it should be measured. Femoral anteversion is measured in every patient in the beginning of the case by positioning the hip in flexion and abduction. Under C-arm fluoroscopy, the hip is then externally rotated until the femoral shaft lines with the ossific nucleus of the femoral head. The amount of external rotation (degrees) in this position is subtracted from 90°, and the difference is the degree of femoral anteversion.[9] As a general rule, we add derotation to the femoral shortening if excessive anteversion (>45°) is present with final goal of 25° to 30° of femoral anteversion. The plate is then fixed to the distal fragment with slight compression.

After the femoral osteotomy is finished and fixed with the 4-hole plate, the reduction of the hip is checked again. The reduction should not be tense after the femoral shortening osteotomy. However, excessive shortening is not beneficial; rather, it may be detrimental and may lead to instability. The surgeon can always resect more bone if needed, and a conservative femoral shortening is recommended when in doubt. A C-arm fluoroscopy image is obtained to confirm the adequate position of the plate and reduction of the hip. The vastus lateralis is sutured back, and the fascia lata is closed, followed by the subcutaneous tissue and the skin.

Attention is shifted back to the pelvic wound. At this point, the iliopsoas muscular tendinous junction is identified at the pelvic brim (**Figure 3.29**). A right-angled clamp is passed under the iliopsoas, and the tendon is pulled toward the surface. The tendinous sheet is opened longitudinally, and a tenotomy is performed with an electric cautery. Before incising the tendon, we recommend applying a cautery stimulus to avoid inadvertent injury to the femoral nerve.

The final step of the open reduction is the capsulorrhaphy. In preparation for the capsulorrhaphy, the hip should be dislocated, and a retractor pulls the iliopsoas as medial as possible. A nonresorbable suture (2-0 Fiber wire) is passed through the proximal edge of the capsule into the periosteum of the superior pubic ramus. Two to three additional sutures are passed more laterally. There are basically two ways to perform the capsulorrhaphy. First, in the technique described by Salter,[10] the superolateral and posterior segment of the capsule is excised. The hip is reduced, and the capsule is internally rotated, so the distal portion of the capsular "T"-shaped cut is sutured under the AIIS (**Figure 3.30**). Another option, which is the option we prefer, is to suture the corner of the lateral portion of the capsule as medial as possible and then suture the medial portion of the capsule on top like a vest-over-pants closure (**Figure 3.31**).

After the capsulorrhaphy is performed, the hip is injected with 1 mL of a 50% solution of ioversol and sterile saline for an arthrogram that should confirm the femoral head is deep and concentrically reduced in the acetabulum. The rectus femoris is repaired, and the iliac crest apophysis is sutured back in an anatomic manner. The aponeurosis of the external oblique is repaired, and the wound is closed in layers. The patient is transferred to a spica cast table after dressings are applied.

Spica cast application following an anterolateral open reduction: a spica cast is applied with the hips in 30° of flexion and 30° of abduction with neutral or slight internal

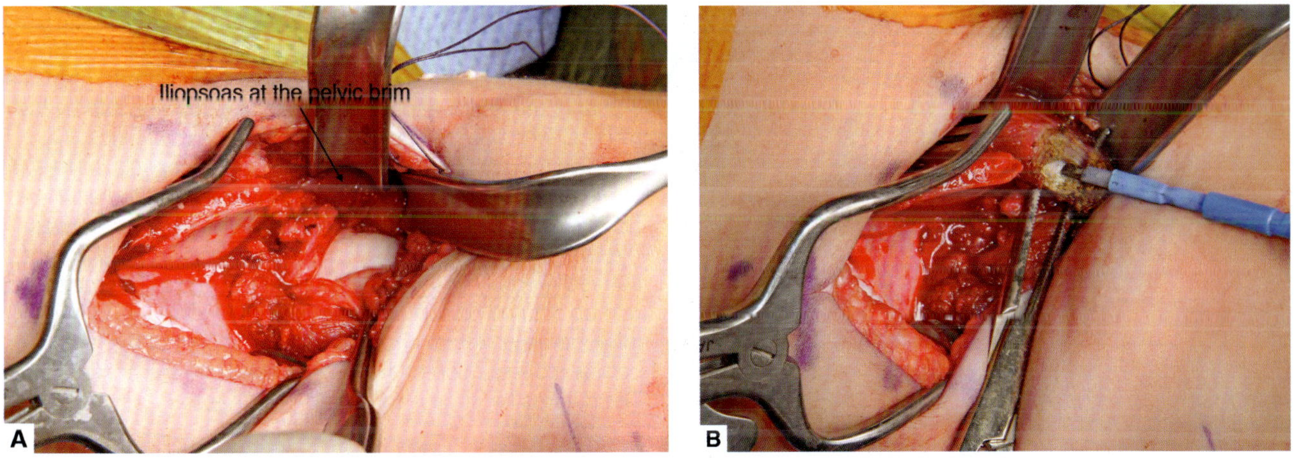

FIGURE 3.29. Tenotomy of the iliopsoas at the pelvic brim. A, Intraoperative picture showing the iliopsoas muscle–tendon junction identified at the level of the pelvic brim. B, Using a right-angled clamp, the iliopsoas tendon is pulled toward the surface, and muscle tendinous junction is incised with a cautery.

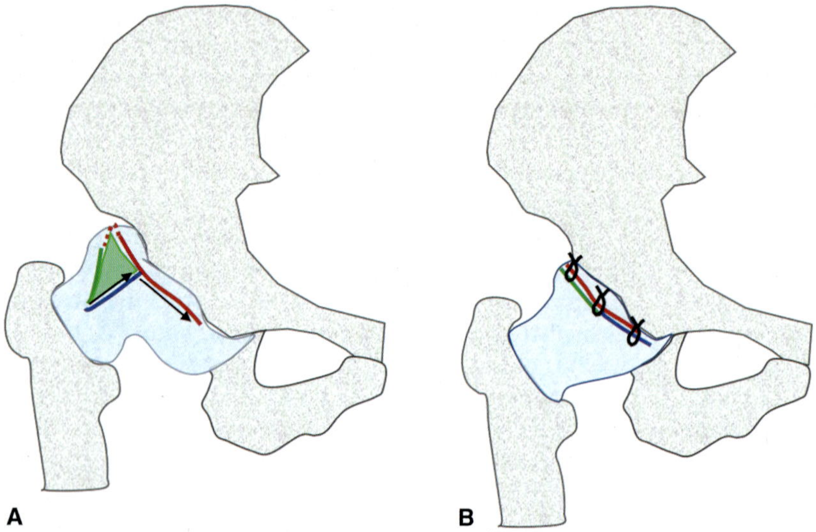

FIGURE 3.30. The Salter technique for capsulorrhaphy. A, Diagram showing the capsulotomy is performed in a T manner with an incision parallel to the acetabular rim (red line) and another incision in line with the femoral neck (blue line). The superior and lateral aspect of the capsule is redundant and should be excised (green line and triangle). B, The capsule is internally rotated after the hip is reduced, and the distal point between the excised capsule (green line) and the transverse T incision (blue line) is sutured under the anterior inferior iliac spine. The medial corner of the capsule (between the blue line and the red line) is brought medially and sutured to the periosteum of the pubis.

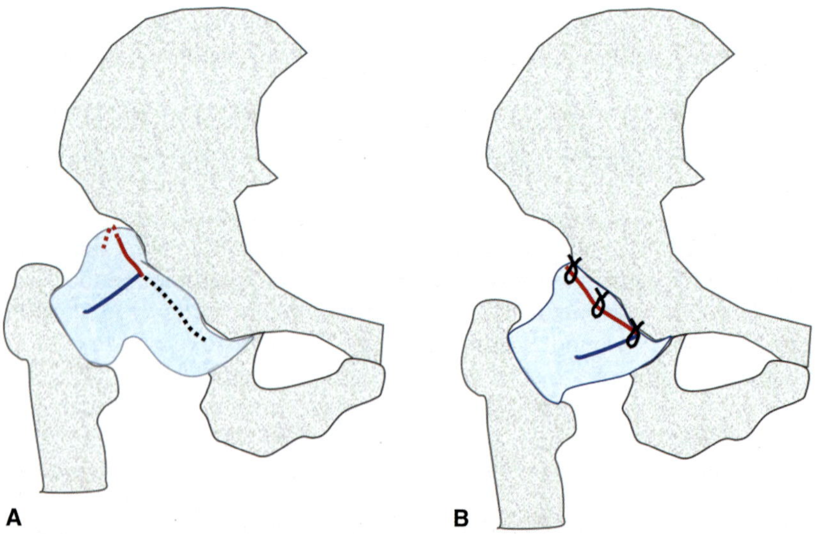

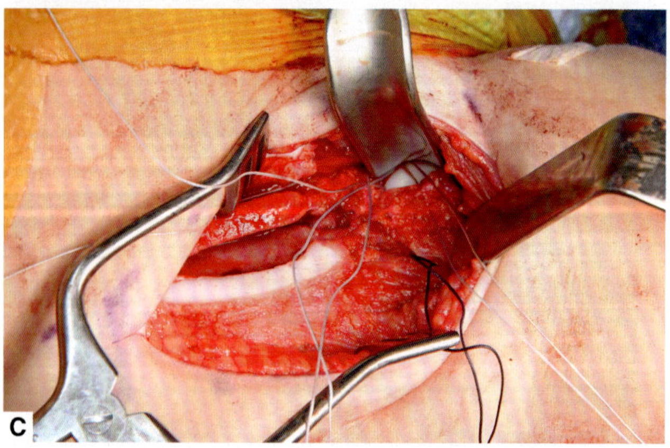

FIGURE 3.31. The vest-over-pants technique for capsulorrhaphy. A, The capsulotomy is similarly performed in a T shape: the lateral aspect of the shape is represented by the red line, whereas the medial aspect by a dashed black line. A blue line represents the distal incision of the capsule in line with the femoral neck. B, The capsule is internally rotated after the hip is reduced, and the lateral corner of the capsule (between the lateral [red line] and the transverse T incision [blue line]) is sutured medially to the periosteum of the pubis. The medial flap can be sutured on top, creating the vest-over-pants closure. C, Intraoperative picture showing the final aspect of the hip after concentric reduction of the femoral head into the acetabulum. The sutures for capsulotomy had been passed, but not yet completely tied.

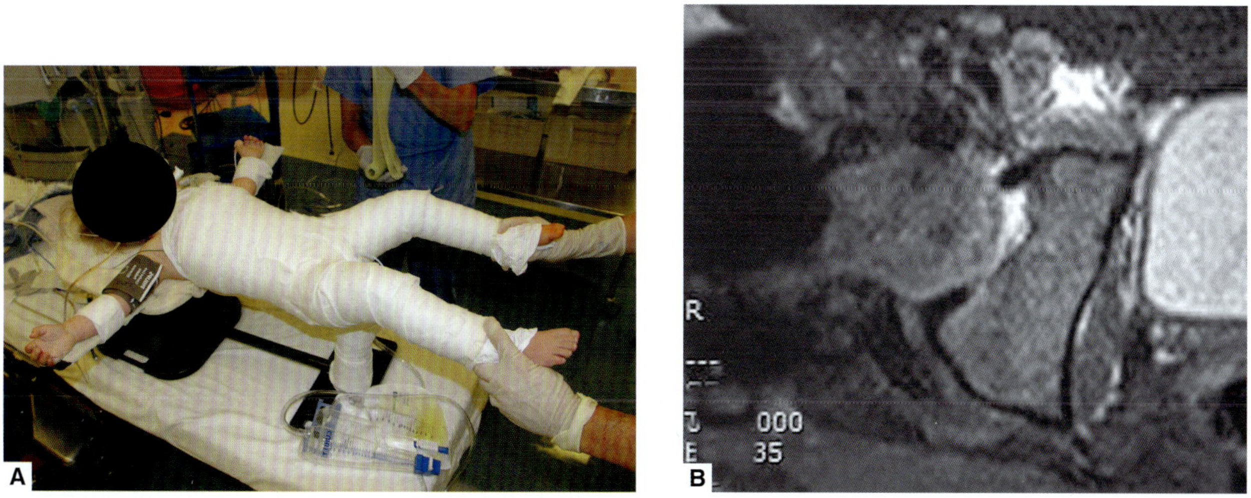

FIGURE 3.32. A, Intraoperative picture showing the application of the spica cast after an anterolateral open reduction in the so-called human position. The hip is flexed to 30° and abducted to 30° and kept in neutral or slight internal rotation. B, Postoperative axial magnetic resonance imaging showing concentric reduction of the right hip.

rotation (**Figure 3.32**). We highly recommend that fluoroscopy imaging is obtained after the cast is applied. After the spica cast is applied, an MRI is obtained to confirm the concentric reduction of the hip; unless osteotomies are performed with hardware, in which case, CT scan is performed. Based on surgeon preference, we bring the patient for a postoperative follow-up visit at 2 weeks after surgery. The purpose of this visit is to troubleshoot any potential issues or problems with the spica cast and to confirm the integrity of the skin. An anteroposterior (AP) pelvis radiograph in the spica cast is obtained during this visit. At around 6 weeks after surgery, the patient is brought back to the operating room for removal of the spica cast and for repeat arthrogram to assess the concentricity of the reduction. A bilateral half spica cast is applied and used for additional 6 weeks. The cast is removed in clinic, and an abduction brace is applied to be used at night time. We commonly recommend a night-time abduction brace until the patient is 2 years old following closed reduction or open reduction without an osteotomy. Although strong evidence supporting the use of an abduction brace after an open reduction of the hip is lacking, we favor the use of the brace while the acetabular is remodeling during the first 2 years after surgery (**Figure 3.33**).

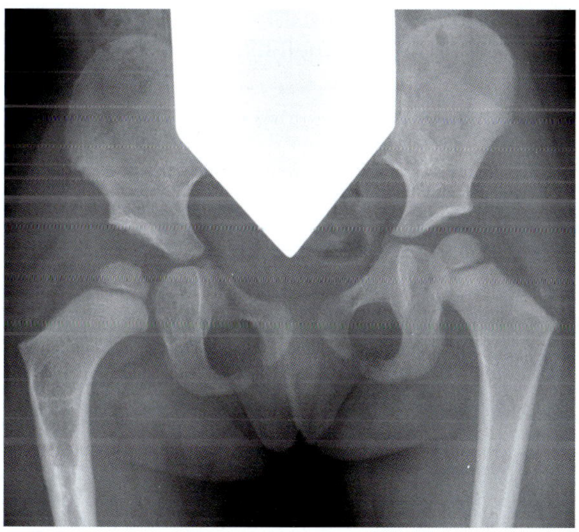

FIGURE 3.33. Postoperative anteroposterior pelvis radiograph at 2 years following open reduction of the right hip.

OPEN REDUCTION WITH FEMORAL SHORTENING OSTEOTOMY AND SALTER PELVIC OSTEOTOMY FOR OLDER CHILDREN

Open reduction in children older than 3 years is usually performed through the anterior approach combined with a femoral shortening (with possible derotational) osteotomy and a pelvic osteotomy. We recommend treatment of a dislocated hip secondary to DDH up to 8 years of age, especially for those patients with unilateral dislocations. The surgical technique is similar to the previous description with the addition of the pelvic osteotomy. Although controversy surrounds the best choice for pelvic osteotomy, the most common procedures are the Salter osteotomy[10] and the Pemberton[11] osteotomy. The Salter is a redirectional osteotomy that corrects the abnormal direction of the acetabular coverage without changing the congruency or reducing the acetabular capacity. The fulcrum of rotation of the Salter osteotomy is through the symphysis pubic. The Pemberton osteotomy hinges through the triradiate cartilage and changes the shape of the acetabulum. It is usually recommended when the shape of the acetabulum is oblong and capacious.

The indications to perform a Salter osteotomy combined with open reduction included instability of the hip anteriorly or anterior laterally determined intraoperatively. As a routine, a pelvic osteotomy is performed in patients older than 3 years. The surgical technique was similar to the one described for the previous clinical scenario. The prerequisites for a Salter osteotomy have been described and include complete and concentric reduction of the head into the true acetabulum, release of the contracture of the iliopsoas and the adductor longus, and reasonable congruity of the joint and good range of motion.[12]

Clinical Scenario

A 5-year-old girl presented to clinic for evaluation of right DDH. Her radiographs showed severe high dislocation of the right hip, and an open reduction of the hip was recommended along with a femoral shortening osteotomy and a Salter osteotomy of the pelvis (**Figure 3.34**).

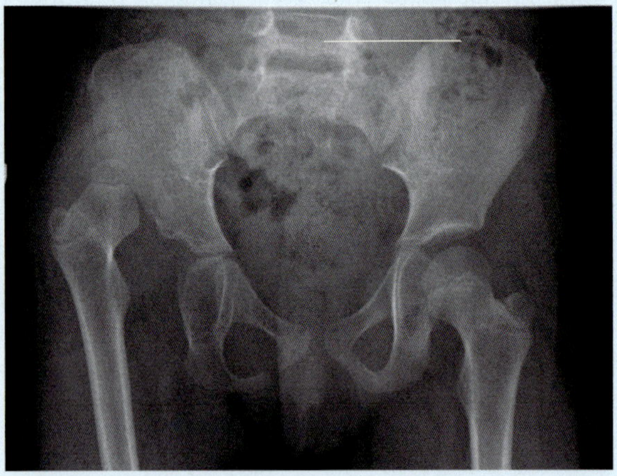

FIGURE 3.34. Preoperative anteroposterior pelvic radiograph of a 5-year-old female with severe high dislocation of the right hip.

The patient is position supine with a bump under the ipsilateral scapula up to the iliac crest, but not under the buttock to tilt the patient about 30° (**Figure 3.35**). An oblique incision is performed 1 cm distal to the iliac crest, aiming medially about a finger breath from the ASIS and toward the inguinal crease. Subcutaneous dissection is performed proximally, and the external oblique is carefully released from the iliac crest apophysis. The apophysis is split in its midline, and subperiosteal dissection of the inner and outer table of the ilium is performed to the level of the sciatic notch. Distally, the fascia of the tensor fascia lata is opened and the muscle retracted laterally, whereas the sartorius is retracted medially. The rectus femoris is exposed, and the indirect and the direct heads of the rectus are incised, and the muscle is retracted medially, allowing for full exposure of the anterior aspect of the hip capsule. The hip capsule should be exposed posteriorly and laterally by dissection of the gluteus minimus insertion and by releasing the periosteum of the outer table of the ilium (**Figure 3.36**). The iliopsoas is very tight in older patients, and it should be released before the capsulotomy to facilitate exposure of the anteromedial capsule.

Once the capsule is completely exposed from medial to lateral, a capsulotomy is performed. After capsulotomy, the femoral head can be seen articulating with the false acetabulum laterally (**Figure 3.37**). The true acetabular cavity is deep medially and commonly very small in older patients. If present, the ligamentum teres is excised from the femoral head and is traced down medially, guiding the exposure of the true acetabulum. The transverse acetabular ligament is usually very tight, and it limits the opening of the acetabular cavity (**Figure 3.38**). The true acetabular cavity is prepared by an incision through the transverse acetabular ligament and the insertion of the ligamentum teres, resection of the fibrofatty pulvinar and the pelvic wound is packed. The femoral shortening osteotomy is performed as previously described. In high dislocations in patients older

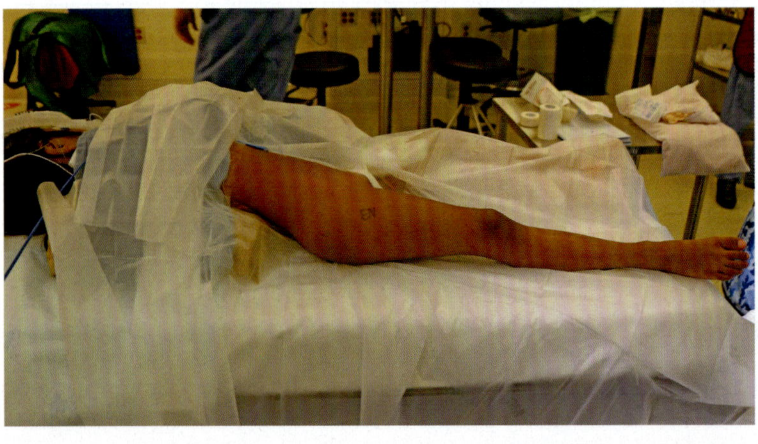

FIGURE 3.35. Intraoperative picture showing the patient position in preparation for an adductor tenotomy, open reduction through an anterolateral approach, and femoral shortening osteotomy and Salter osteotomy. The patient is tilted about 30° by a gel pad placed under the ipsilateral scapula.

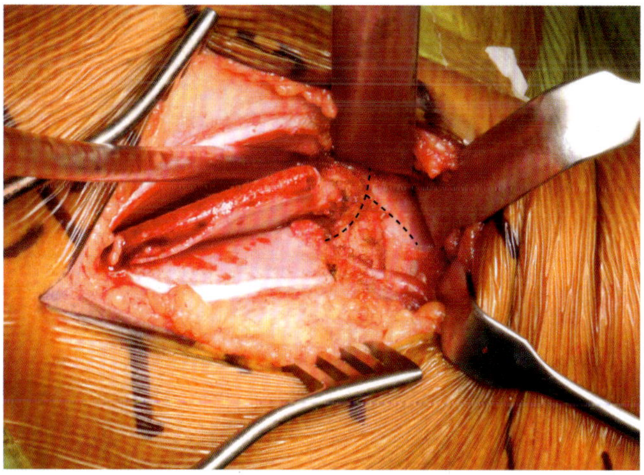

FIGURE 3.36. Intraoperative picture showing the complete exposure of the hip capsule prior to capsulotomy. The iliac crest apophysis has been split, and the rectus femoris tendon has been excised from the anterior inferior iliac spine and retracted medially. The dashed black lines mark the incision of the T-shaped capsulotomy.

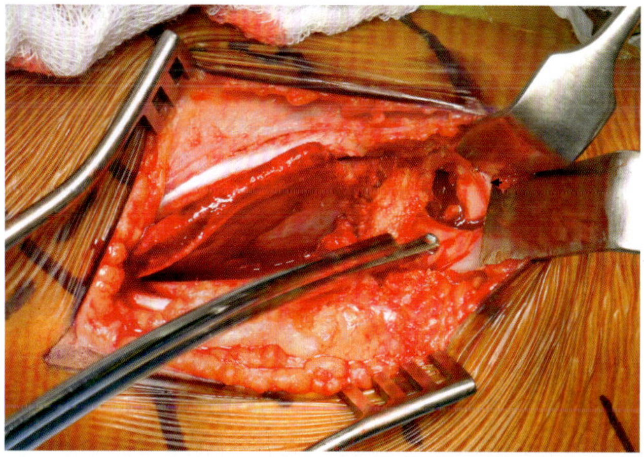

FIGURE 3.38. Intraoperative picture showing the exposure of the true acetabulum, which is facilitated after the iliopsoas is released at the pelvic brim. A black arrowhead marks the transverse acetabular ligament that is hypertrophic and tight limiting the introitus of the acetabular cavity.

than 3 years, shortening of the femur may be as much as 3 cm or more. Following the femoral shortening osteotomy, the acetabulum is prepared for the capsulorrhaphy. A nonabsorbable suture (2-0 Fiber wire) is passed through the proximal stump of the capsule and the periosteum of the pubic ramus as medial as possible. Two or three additional sutures are passed laterally (**Figure 3.39**). After the stitches are passed proximally, the attention is shifted to the pelvic osteotomy. During osteotomy, the hip remains dislocated.

Subperiosteal dissection of the inner and outer table of the ilium is complete to the level of the sciatic notch with a sharp periosteal elevator. Using a curved periosteal elevator facilitates the complete subperiosteal dissection of the sciatic notch. Careful dissection is recommended to avoid damage to the sciatic nerve and the superior gluteal artery (**Figure 3.40**). A pair of Rang retractors (Jantek Engineering, USA) is inserted from medial and lateral through the sciatic notch. These elevators are extremely helpful for the safe performance of

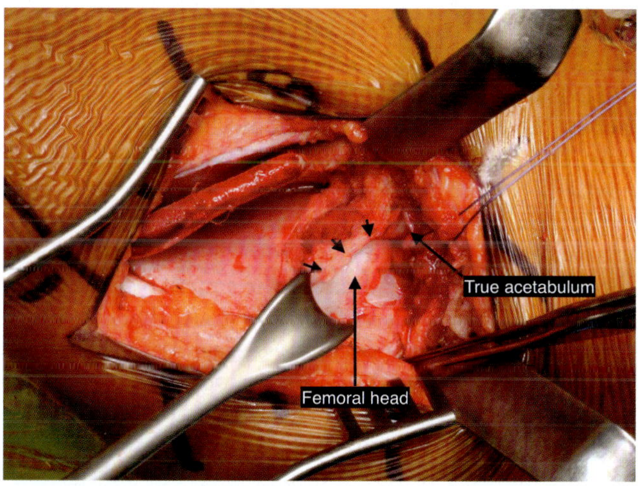

FIGURE 3.37. Intraoperative picture showing the capsulotomy is extended all the way posterior and lateral around the femoral head, allowing for full exposure of the head of the femur that typically articulates in the false acetabulum (black arrowheads).

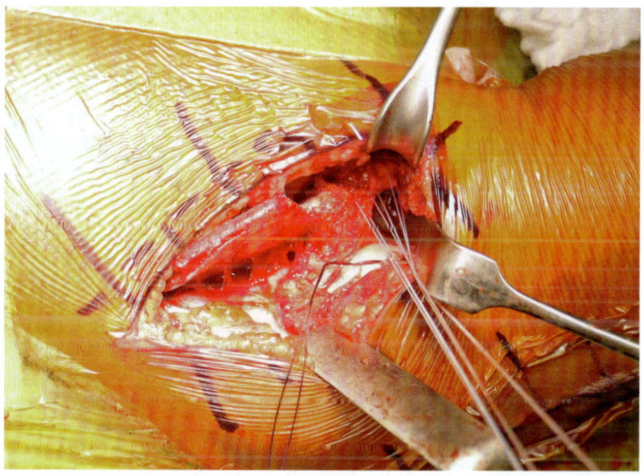

FIGURE 3.39. Intraoperative picture showing the passage of the nonabsorbable sutures (2-0 Fiber wire) from medial to lateral. It is crucial to place the first suture as medial as possible through the edge of the proximal aspect of the capsule and the periosteum of the superior pubic ramus. Two or three additional sutures are passed just lateral to the first. One of the sutures should be placed distal to the anterior inferior iliac spine as a reference landmark.

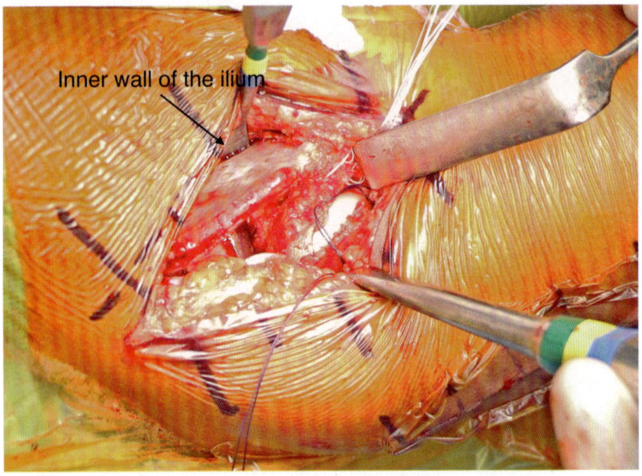

FIGURE 3.40. Intraoperative picture showing dissection of the inner wall of the ileum toward the sciatic notch as well as dissection of the outer table of the ilium toward the sciatic notch. Penetration of the sciatic notch should be done carefully with preservation of the periosteal sleeve to avoid damage of the superior gluteal artery and the sciatic nerve.

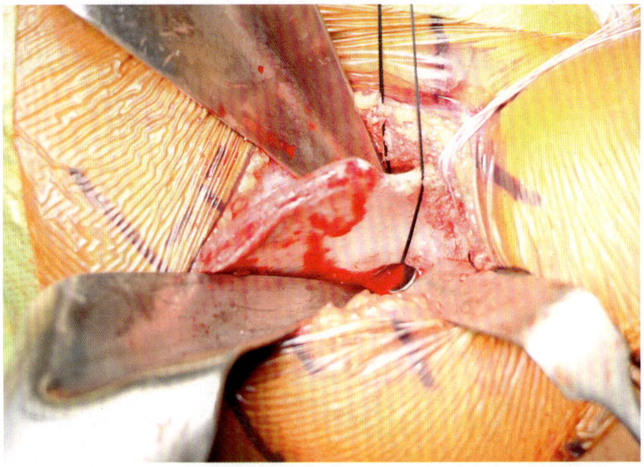

FIGURE 3.42. Intraoperative picture showing that in preparation for passage of the Gigli saw, a #1 silk tie has passed through the sciatic notch on top of the retractors from medial to lateral.

the Salter osteotomy because of the overlapping concave tips that facilitate passage of the Gigli saw (**Figure 3.41**). Once the two retractors are in place, a silk tie can be easily passed from medial to lateral through the sciatic notch (**Figure 3.42**). Then, a Gigli saw is tied to the lateral end of the silk tie, and the silk tie is retrieved medially, allowing for safe passage of the Gigli saw through the sciatic notch medially. The Gigli saw handles are attached in preparation to the osteotomy that should be performed with the surgeon holding the two ends of the saw with continuous tension and as far apart as possible

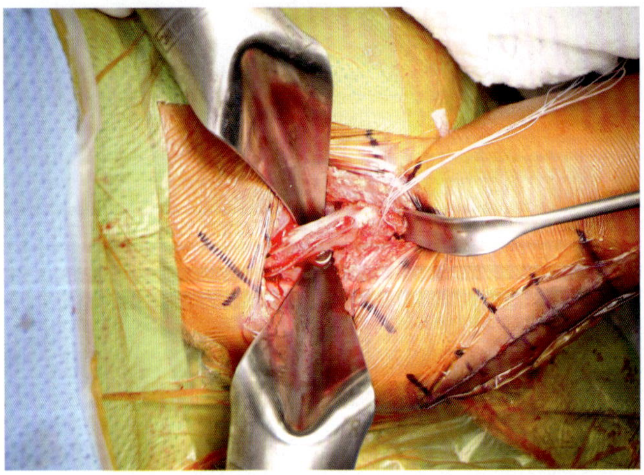

FIGURE 3.41. Intraoperative picture showing placement of two special retractors designed for the Salter osteotomy. These retractors are placed inside the sciatic notch from medial and lateral. The specific design of the Rang retractors allow for the tip of the retractors to engage facilitating passage of the Gigli saw.

to avoid getting the saw caught and stuck in the bone during the cut (**Figure 3.43**). The orientation of the Salter osteotomy is very important: it should be performed from the sciatic notch to 1 to 2 mm proximal to the AIIS.

Once the osteotomy is completed, the proximal and distal fragments are held with a pointed towel clamp. The proximal fragment is held only for stabilization, and no attempt is made to pull the proximal fragment cranially. The distal fragment should be pulled distally to allow for anterior and caudal rotation of the acetabulum through the symphysis. We cannot emphasize enough the importance of simply pulling the fragment distally while keeping the proximal fragment stable without pulling it proximally (**Figure 3.44**). Similarly, it is very important to avoid the temptation of using a laminar spreader to separate the osteotomy because this can cause translation and opening of the osteotomy posteriorly. The Salter osteotomy should be open anteriorly only, and displacement of the osteotomy posteriorly or medially is to be avoided.

Although the original Salter technique uses a triangular-shaped bone graft from the ilium, we do not recommend using the ilium as the source of bone graft. When the ilium is used for bone graft, there is a risk of a rather unpleasant cosmetic deformity of the pelvis. Furthermore, if a patient requires a periacetabular osteotomy in the future for correction of residual acetabular dysplasia, this procedure will be much more technically demanding if the ilium had been cut and used as a source of bone graft. We favor using the segment resected from the femur as the source of bone graft. Alternatively, an angled iliac cut can be made using an oscillating saw and a Gigli saw that is similar to an iliac cut used in the Bernese periacetabular osteotomy

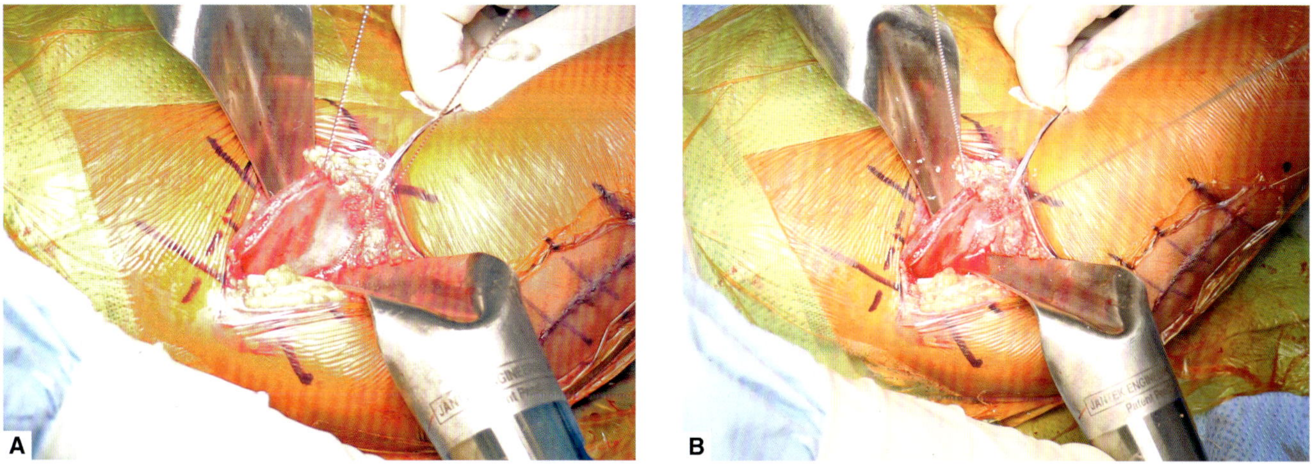

FIGURE 3.43. A, Intraoperative picture showing the Gigli saw is tied to the ends of the silk thigh and then it is pulled through the sciatic notch. The two handles of the saw are held and spread apart keeping symmetric tension to avoid incarceration of the saw in the middle of the bone. B, The osteotomy is performed from the sciatic notch in a straight line toward just above the anterior inferior iliac spine.

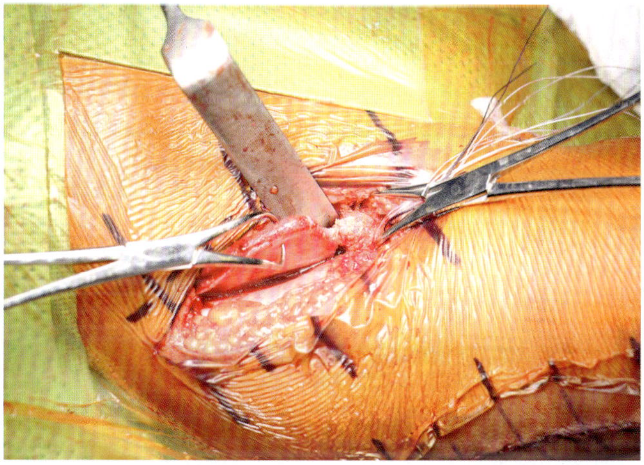

FIGURE 3.44. Intraoperative picture showing the two towel clamps used to hold the ileum proximally and the anterior inferior iliac spine distally. There should be no tension or pulling the proximal fragment. Proximally, the clamp is used to merely stabilize the ilium. The distal fragment is held with a towel clamp and mobilized anteriorly and distally. The maneuver is a simple distal pull of the fragment that will open the osteotomy anteriorly without losing contact posteriorly. It is very important to keep the posterior aspect of the osteotomy in contact and to avoid posterior or medial displacement of the osteotomy.

(**Figure 3.45**). If needed, a fibular allograft can be used if a femoral osteotomy is not performed. The bone graft should be cut in a triangular shape, and it should be inserted between the two fragments of the osteotomy after the distal fragment is pulled distally and anteriorly. Once the bone graft is placed, two threaded Kirschner wires are introduced from proximal to distal to fix the osteotomy (**Figure 3.46**). The wires should be placed posteriorly and medial to the acetabulum. The acetabular cavity should be palpated to confirm that no wires have penetrated the joint. This iliac cut configuration allows stable fixation of the osteotomy without the use of structural bone grafts.

Commonly, hip stability is improved after a Salter osteotomy. If residual instability is present anteriorly, the size of the bone graft can be increased. However, we recommend careful assessment of the range of motion of the hip after the Salter osteotomy and also recommend against excessive correction of anterior coverage because of the risk of femoral acetabular impingement later in life associated with overcorrection and acetabular retroversion. We recommend that the hip should have a minimum of 90° of flexion and at least 30° of internal rotation. The capsulorrhaphy is performed according to the technique previously described. After capsulorrhaphy, a hip arthrogram confirms the concentric reduction of the femoral head in the true acetabulum (**Figure 3.47**). The two threaded Kirschner wires are cut but left a little bit proud to facilitate future removal. The iliac apophysis is closed, and closure of the wound follows as previously described. Following a Salter osteotomy in association with an open reduction, the child should be immobilized in a spica cast in the human position with a hip flexed to no more than 20° or 30° and abducted to about 30°. The cast is removed in the operating room after 6 weeks and then a short spica cast is applied for additional 4 to 6 weeks. The threaded Kirschner wires and the femoral plate and screws are removed at around 1 or 2 years after surgery (**Figure 3.48**).

In summary, open reduction is the recommended treatment for a child with DDH who has not responded appropriately to bracing or if arthrogram reveals the hip is not suitable to closed reduction. Open reduction can be

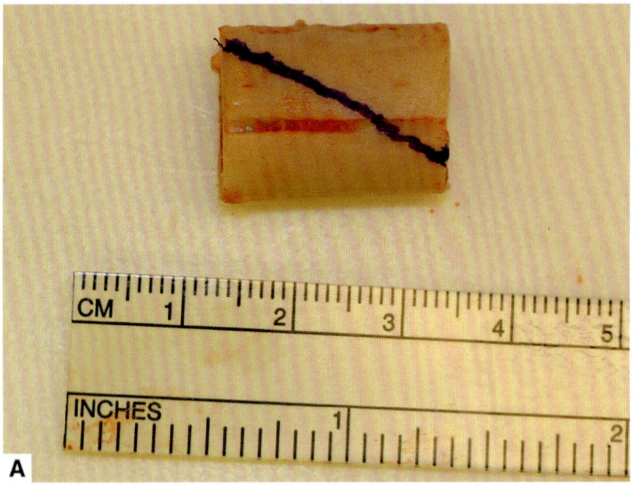

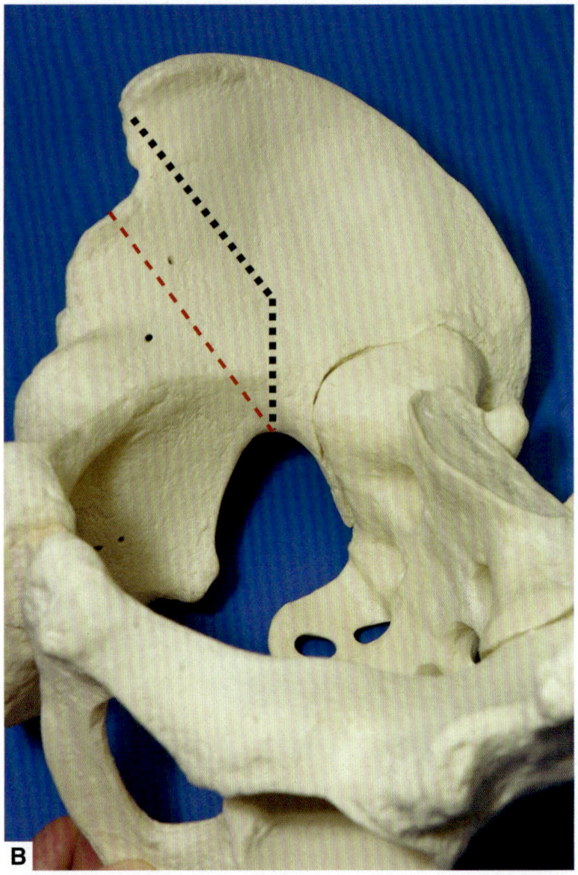

FIGURE 3.45. A, Intraoperative picture showing preparation of the segment resected from the femur to be used as the bone graft for the Salter osteotomy. The segment of the femur was large enough to allow for the creation of two triangles, which were carefully planned to be inserted to the osteotomy site. B, Picture of a pelvic model showing the angled cut of a modified Salter osteotomy: The red dashed line represents the classic Salter osteotomy. The black dashed line represents the double-angled osteotomy that will allow stable fixation of osteotomy without the need for a structural bone graft.

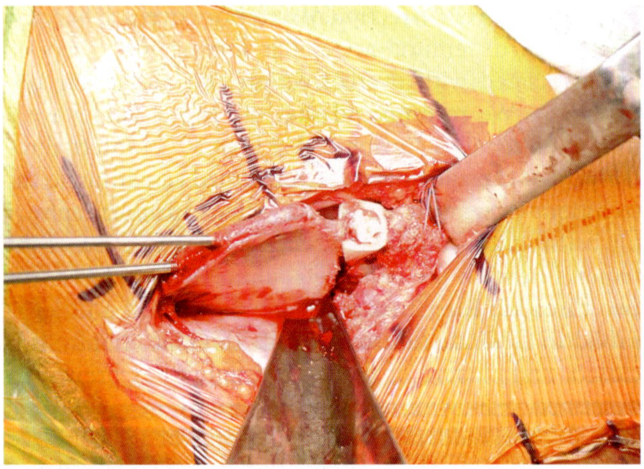

FIGURE 3.46. Intraoperative picture showing the final aspect of the osteotomy after insertion of the graft and fixation with two threaded Kirschner wires inserted from the proximal ilium through the osteotomy and the distal fragment.

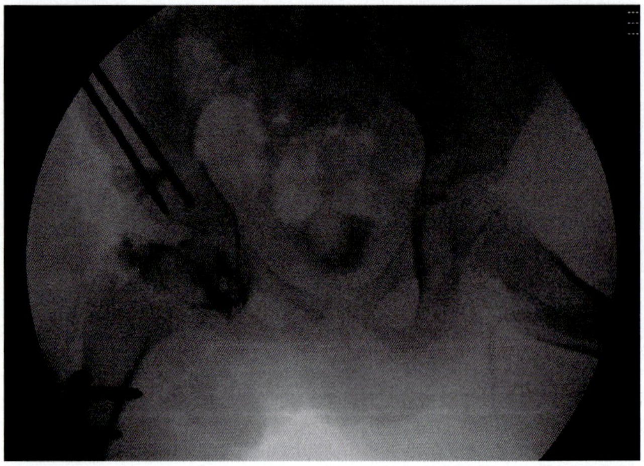

FIGURE 3.47. Intraoperative C-arm fluoroscopy after arthrogram was performed, which confirmed concentric reduction of the femoral head into the acetabulum.

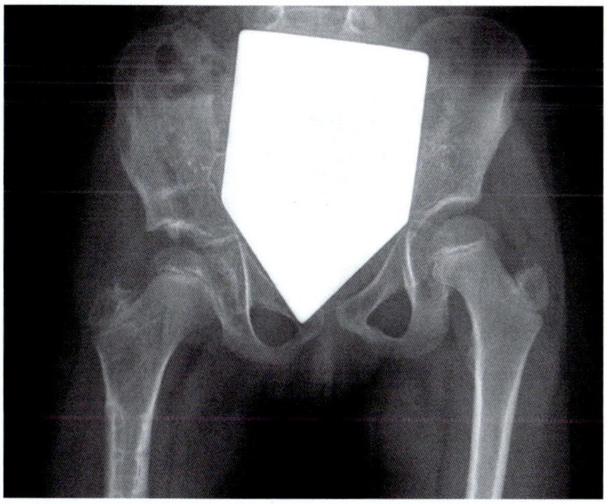

FIGURE 3.48. Postoperative radiograph at 2 years following surgery showing remodeling of the acetabulum and a well-seated femoral head concentrically reduced.

performed through a medial or an anterolateral approach. Although it remains controversial whether the medial versus the anterolateral approach provides better outcome for the patient, a recent systematic review of the literature showed no difference in the proportion of patients who developed growth disturbance to the proximal femur following each procedure.[13] The indications for medial and anterolateral approach overlap during the first year; however after the first year of life, we prefer to perform an open reduction through the anterolateral approach, which allows a good capsulorrhaphy to be performed in the same setting along with additional femoral or pelvic osteotomies when needed. The most common complications associated with an open reduction of the hip include residual instability with redislocation or subluxation, residual acetabular dysplasia with further growth and development, and proximal femoral growth disturbance or osteonecrosis. Management of such complications is discussed in the next chapter.

REFERENCES

1. Narayanan U, Mulpuri K, Sankar WN, et al. Reliability of a new radiographic classification for developmental dysplasia of the hip. *J Pediatr Orthop.* 2015;35(5):478-484.
2. Ludloff L. The open reduction of the congenital hip dislocation by an anterior incision. *Am J Orthop Surg.* 1913;10:438-454.
3. Ferguson AB Jr. Primary open reduction of congenital dislocation of the hip using a median adductor approach. *J Bone Joint Surg Am.* 1973;55(4):671-689.
4. Mau H, Dorr WM, Henkel L, Lutsche J. Open reduction of congenital dislocation of the hip by Ludloff's method. *J Bone Joint Surg Am.* 1971;53(7):1281-1288.
5. Weinstein SL, Ponseti IV. Congenital dislocation of the hip. *J Bone Joint Surg Am.* 1979;61(1):119-124.
6. Konigsberg DE, Karol LA, Colby S, O'Brien S. Results of medial open reduction of the hip in infants with developmental dislocation of the hip. *J Pediatr Orthop.* 2003;23(1):1-9.
7. Bache CE, Graham HK, Dickens DR, et al. Ligamentum teres tenodesis in medial approach open reduction for developmental dislocation of the hip. *J Pediatr Orthop.* 2008;28(6):607-613.
8. Wenger DR, Mubarak SJ, Henderson PC, Miyanji F. Ligamentum teres maintenance and transfer as a stabilizer in open reduction for pediatric hip dislocation: surgical technique and early clinical results. *J Child Orthop.* 2008;2(3):177-185.
9. Sankar WN, Neubuerger CO, Moseley CF. Femoral anteversion in developmental dysplasia of the hip. *J Pediatr Orthop.* 2009;29(8):885-888.
10. Salter RB. Role of innominate osteotomy in the treatment of congenital dislocation and subluxation of the hip in the older child. *J Bone Joint Surg Am.* 1966;48(7):1413-1439.
11. Pemberton PA. Pericapsular osteotomy of the ilium for treatment of congenital subluxation and dislocation of the hip. *J Bone Joint Surg Am.* 1965;47:65-86.
12. Salter RB, Dubos JP. The first fifteen year's personal experience with innominate osteotomy in the treatment of congenital dislocation and subluxation of the hip. *Clin Orthop Relat Res.* 1974(98):72-103.
13. Novais EN, Hill MK, Carry PM, Heyn PC. Is age or surgical approach associated with osteonecrosis in patients with developmental dysplasia of the hip? A meta-analysis. *Clin Orthop Relat Res.* 2016;474(5):1166-1177.

CHAPTER

4

Infant Hip Dysplasia: Residual Acetabular Dysplasia During Childhood

FUNDAMENTALS

The goals for treatment of a dislocated hip secondary to developmental dysplasia of the hip (DDH) are concentric reduction of the hip and maintenance of the reduction, allowing for acetabular and femoral remodeling. Although the hip may be reduced either by closed or open means, the remodeling of the acetabulum is not always complete, and residual acetabular dysplasia may persist. The management of residual acetabular dysplasia after closed or open reduction is highly controversial because there are limited data about the natural history of acetabular remodeling throughout infancy. Moreover, specific information about limits of acetabular morphology to accept during remodeling and the most appropriate age to intervene is lacking.

Therefore, the dilemma of whether and when to correct residual acetabular dysplasia during childhood remains. On one side of the debate are those who favor early intervention because it allows for correction of the hip mechanics and it may give the best chance of the hip to further develop as close to normal as possible. On the other hand, others may argue that early surgery will lead to some unnecessary surgery because of the capacity of remodeling with further growth and the authors' inability to precisely predict which patient will not sufficiently remodel. These surgeons favor waiting until an age close to skeletal maturity to determine whether or not reorientation of the acetabulum should be performed by a more powerful osteotomy of the pelvis, such as Bernese periacetabular osteotomy (PAO).

To plan better for the treatment of residual acetabular dysplasia, it is essential that one understands the natural development of a normal acetabulum during childhood, the remodeling of the acetabulum after closed or open reduction, and the available techniques to correct the dysplastic acetabulum. Classically, most surgeons use a reference of acetabular development based on the acetabular index (AI) measurements performed by Tönnis in the 1970s.[1] Recently, one study[2] evaluated 1152 normal anteroposterior pelvic radiographs to measure the AI and the acetabular depth–width ratio in children from 1 month to 14 years of age and reported a graph with the *Z*-score distribution of the AI for age (**Figure 4.1**). Therefore, assessment of acetabular remodeling should not be done by following only the raw values of AI. Instead, the authors recommend using *Z* scores and the percentile curves to evaluate whether the acetabulum is indeed remodeling over time. The authors consider true acetabular remodeling if the *Z* scores improve over time. In other words, at each visit, the values of AI are plotted against the normal graph, and true remodeling presents when the values are getting closer to the mean and changing categories for the percentile distribution. Simple decrease in the values of AI remaining in the same zone is not considered true remodeling and warrants close follow-up.

The appropriate age and AI thresholds to perform a corrective pelvic osteotomy after closed or open reduction of the hip remain controversial. Kim and colleagues recommended considering a pelvic osteotomy in hips with an upward acetabular sourcil and lateral displacement of the femoral head greater than 6% around 4 to 5 years of age.[3] Shin and colleagues showed that among hips with AI greater than or equal to 32° at the age of 3 years and those who have undergone an osteotomy, there was a higher proportion of satisfactory outcomes compared to those not treated.[4] Albinana and colleagues published the most valuable paper about acetabular remodeling after closed or open reduction.[5] These authors showed that the major improvement of AI after reduction occurred after the first year, but remodeling would continue up to 6 years of age if concentric reduction was present by 1 year postreduction. They confirmed that the severity of acetabular dysplasia at skeletal maturity was a predictor of the risk of a total hip arthroplasty because of joint arthritis later in life with a mean follow-up of 30 years. Moreover, age at reduction was highly correlated with residual acetabular dysplasia. Finally, the authors established thresholds for AI values and the sensitivity and specificity for residual acetabular dysplasia.

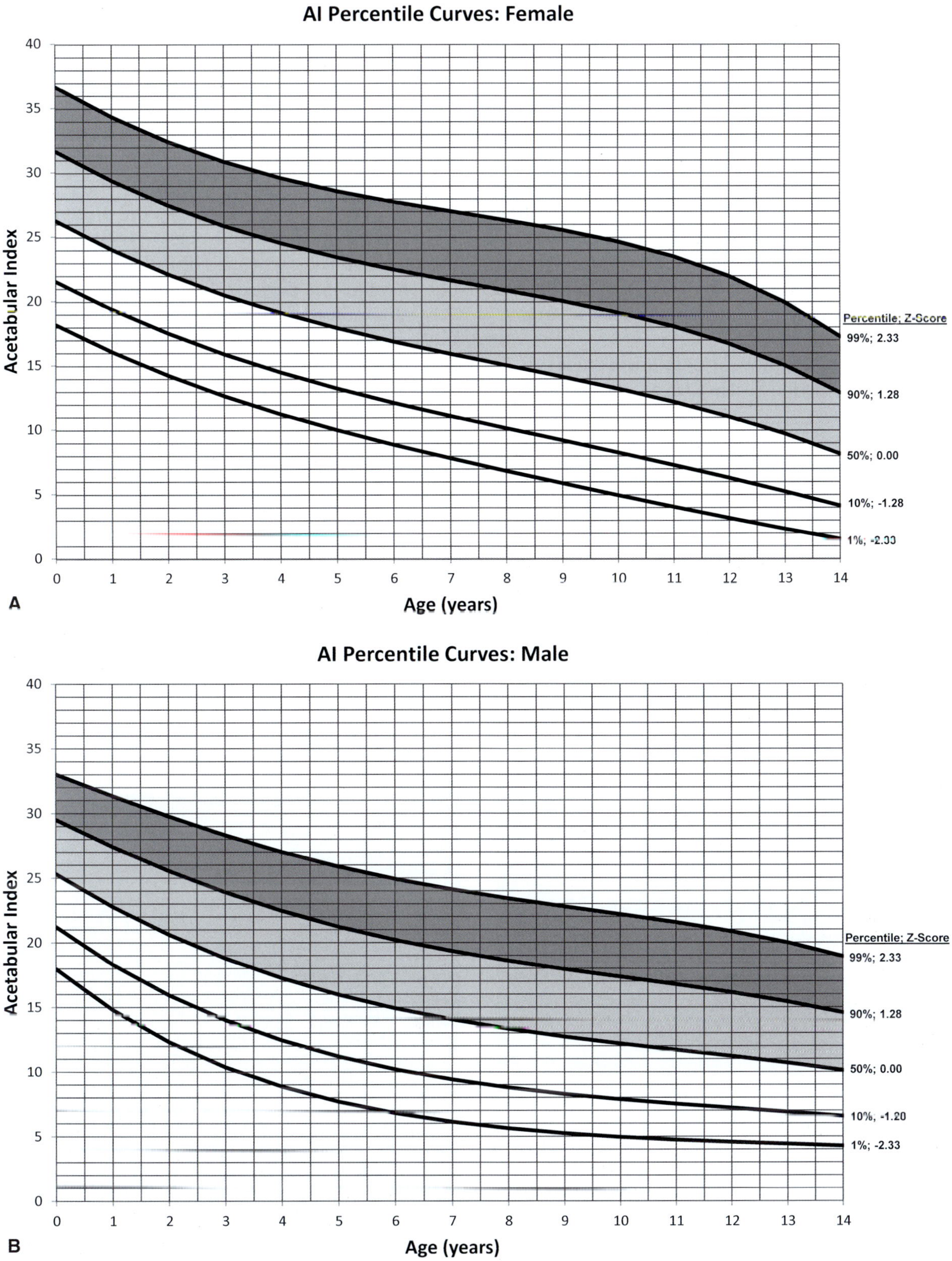

FIGURE 4.1. Graph describing the acetabular index according to age on a normal population of children and adolescents. The dark gray area represents values above the 90th percentile, and the light gray area represents values between the 50th and 90th percentile. A, Females. B, Males. Adapted from Novais et al.[2]

Another useful tool for the assessment of the quality of the acetabular cartilage during the remodeling phase is magnetic resonance imaging (MRI). Wakabayashi and colleagues showed that the presence of a high-signal-intensity area within the weight-bearing portion of the acetabular cartilage on T2-weighted MR coronal section images was associated with poor acetabular growth.[6] Therefore, MRI is currently used to assess the morphology of the acetabulum and femur and, most importantly, the quality of the cartilage in the acetabular weight-bearing area. The presence of high-signal-intensity area within the weight-bearing portion of the acetabular cartilage is not normal and is another relative indication for surgical correction.

The authors' preference is to follow patients after closed or open reduction yearly with an anteroposterior (AP) pelvis radiograph to assess the morphology of the acetabulum including measurement of the AI and depth–width ratio and assessment of the teardrop figure. The values of AI are plotted against the normal percentile curves, and the lack of significant improvement is a relative indication for a pelvic osteotomy. At around 4 years postreduction, the AI should be less than 22°. A pelvic osteotomy may be considered if the AI is higher than 22°, especially if MRI shows the presence of high-signal-intensity area within the weight-bearing portion of the acetabular cartilage. Hip subluxation with a broken Shenton line during follow-up after reduction is an absolute indication for surgical intervention because those hips do not remodel and are associated with poor Severin classification at skeletally mature age and development of osteoarthritis later in life.

Clinical Scenario

A 5-year-old girl presents to clinic for evaluation following treatment of a dislocated left hip performed elsewhere. When she was 20 months old, she underwent a closed reduction of the left hip at another hospital followed by immobilization in a spica cast for about 4 months (**Figure 4.2**). She was then subsequently seen at the authors' clinic at age 5 years (**Figure 4.3**). Although she had a large improvement in the AI from preoperative to 1 year after reduction, the values of AI remained high over the years following the closed reduction (**Figure 4.4**). Lack of improvement of the AI after closed reduction is a relative indication that the hip is not going to completely remodel with additional growth. MRI was obtained to search for changes in the weight-bearing portion of the acetabular cartilage in the affected left side. Notably, there was a high-signal-intensity area within the weight-bearing portion of the acetabular cartilage on T2-weighted coronal section images (**Figure 4.5**). The patient was then subsequently treated with a Dega pelvic osteotomy (see description later).

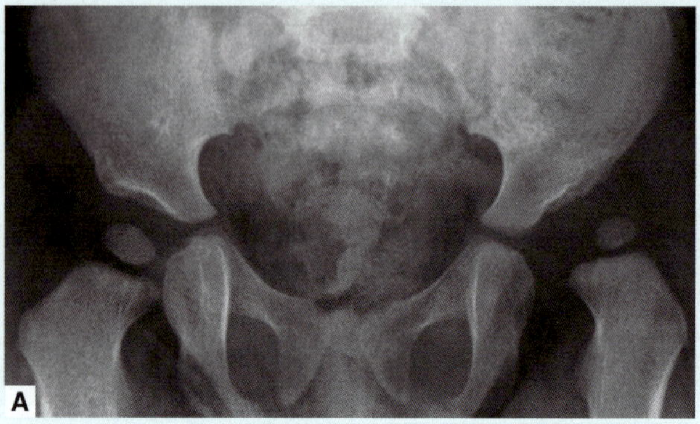

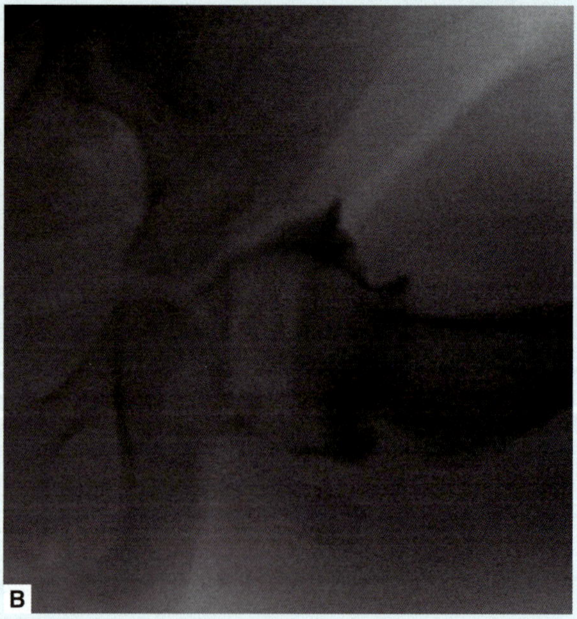

FIGURE 4.2. A 20-month-old female presented to an outside clinic with a left dislocated hip. A, Preoperative anteroposterior pelvic radiograph shows a complete dislocated left hip. B, Intraoperative arthrogram after closed reduction shows complete coverage of the femoral head by the acetabular labrum. The patient was subsequently placed in a spica cast.

Clinical Scenario (*continued*)

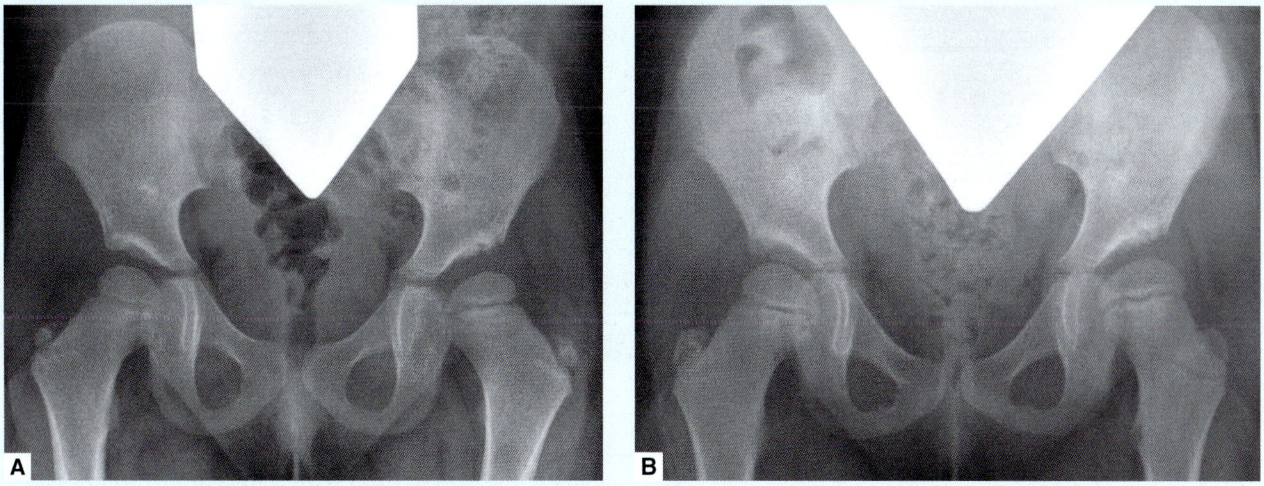

FIGURE 4.3. Postoperative anteroposterior pelvic radiograph obtained at (A) age 3 years and at (B) 5 years following closed reduction shows persistent acetabular dysplasia of the left hip.

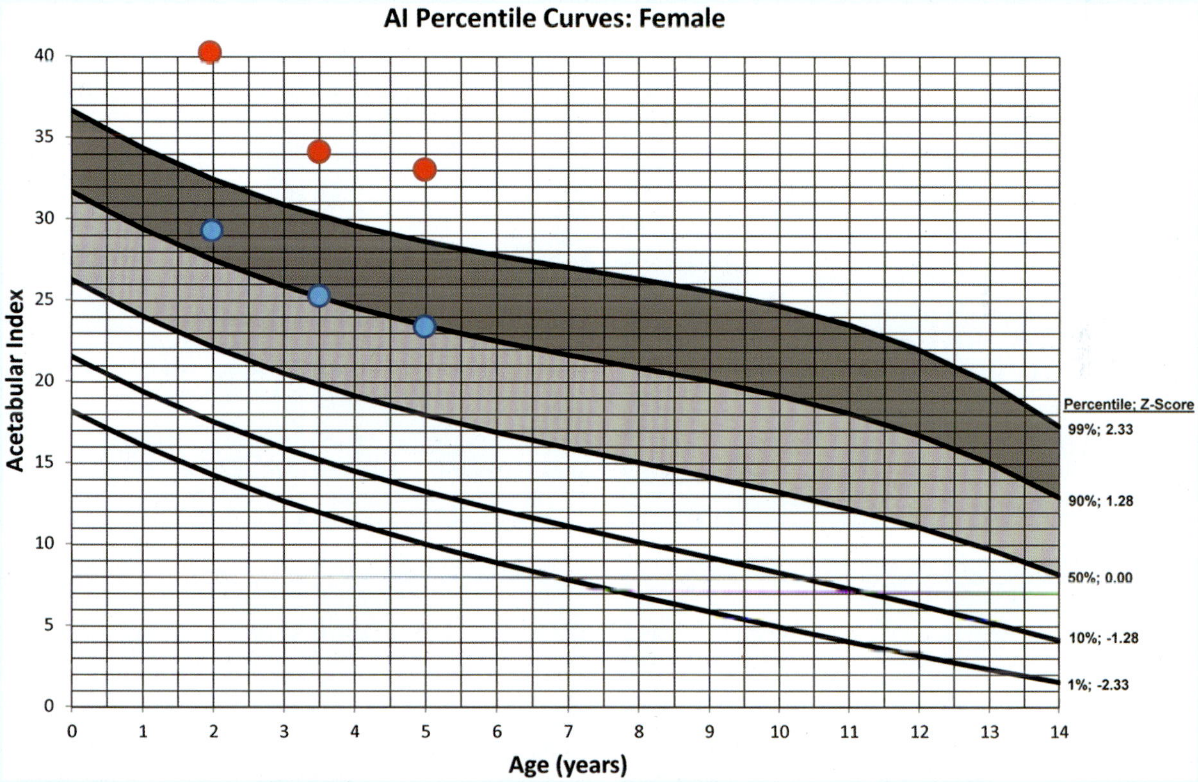

FIGURE 4.4. Patient-specific graph with the acetabular index (AI) measured over time since the closed reduction. Blue dots represent the values of AI measured for the right uninvolved hip, whereas red dots represent the left involved hip. The values of the left hip are consistently higher in the abnormal range without significant improvement at 3 years postreduction.

(*continued*)

Clinical Scenario (*continued*)

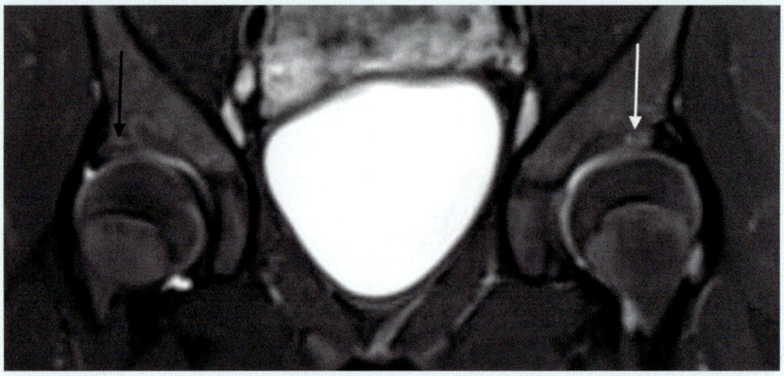

FIGURE 4.5. T2-weighted magnetic resonance coronal section image shows the presence of a high-signal-intensity area within the weight-bearing portion of the acetabular cartilage on the left hip (white arrow) with normal cartilage signal on the right hip (black arrow).

SURGICAL PROCEDURES TO TREAT RESIDUAL ACETABULAR DYSPLASIA DURING CHILDHOOD

Once the diagnosis of residual acetabular dysplasia with or without subluxation is made and a decision is in place for a corrective pelvic osteotomy, the next step is to determine the type of osteotomy to be performed. Osteotomies that reshape the acetabulum with a fulcrum of rotation at the triradiate cartilage include the Pemberton,[7] the Dega, and the San Diego osteotomies. Osteotomies that reorient the acetabulum include the Salter[8] and the double and triple pelvic osteotomies (**Figure 4.6**). Once the triradiate cartilage is closing, a complete redirectional osteotomy of the

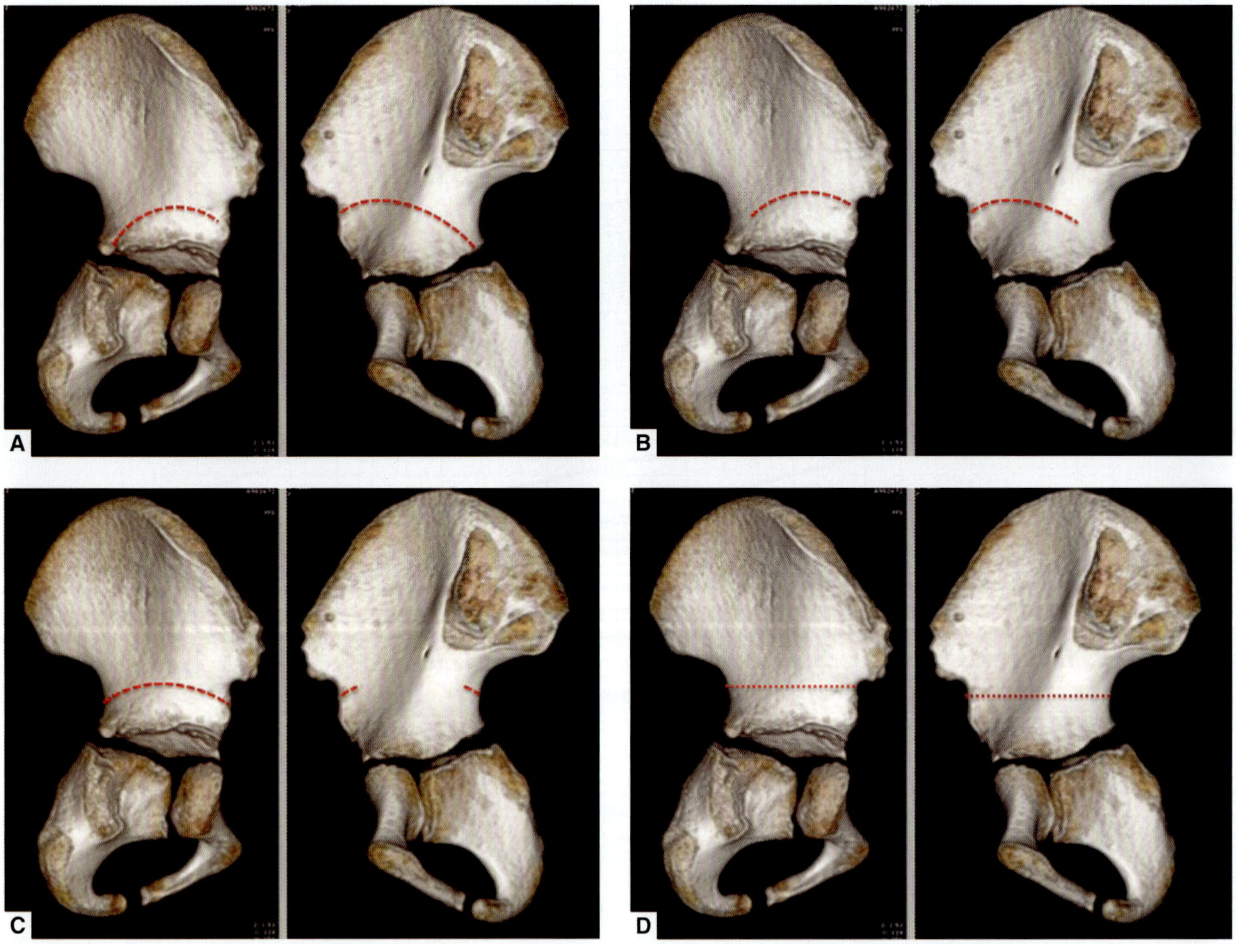

FIGURE 4.6. Computed tomography of the pelvis from a 6-year-old patient with acetabular dysplasia after closed reduction of the hip showing the outer (left hand) and inner (right hand) side of the pelvis and the line (traced red line) of each specific pelvic osteotomy. A, Pemberton osteotomy. B, Dega osteotomy. C, San Diego osteotomy. D, Salter osteotomy.

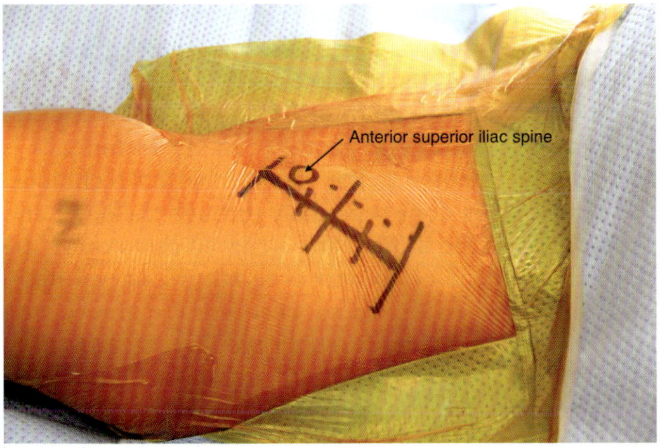

FIGURE 4.7. Intraoperative photograph showing the incision for the surgical approach for a pediatric pelvic osteotomy (left hip). The incision is performed distal to the iliac crest and in an oblique fashion, which yields a more cosmetic scar.

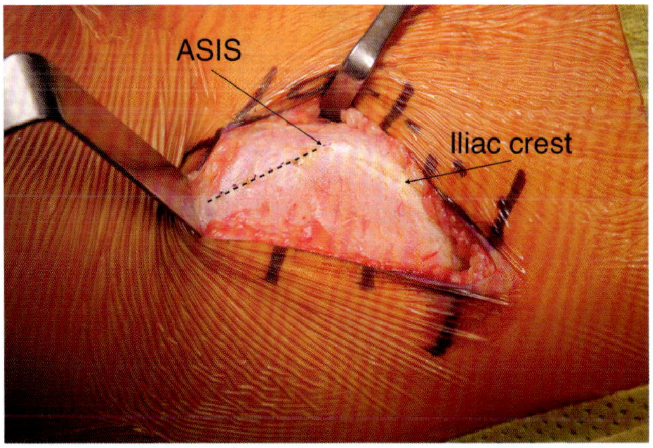

FIGURE 4.9. Intraoperative photograph shows the exposure of the distal aspect of the wound in preparation for opening the tensor fascia lata muscle. The superficial fascial layer is opened toward a lateral direction over the tensor muscle not in line with the tensor-sartorius interval. Note that instead of opening the superficial layer in line with the iliac crest and anterior superior iliac spine, the opening is drawn with about 30° of angulation laterally.

pelvis can be performed and the authors' preferred technique is the Bernese PAO,[9] which is described completely in Chapter 5.

Independent of the osteotomy performed, the surgical approach is done through the Smith-Petersen interval. The authors use a modified anterior approach to the hip joint through an oblique bikini-like incision (**Figure 4.7**). After skin incision, the subcutaneous tissue is dissected. The aponeurosis of the external oblique muscle is exposed and is carefully detached from the iliac crest (**Figure 4.8**). Next, the fascia of the tensor fascia lata is opened distally to the anterior superior iliac spine (ASIS) in about 30° of angulation (**Figure 4.9**). It is crucial to note that there are two layers of tissue covering the tensor fascia lata muscle: the most superficial layer corresponds to the fascia of the anterior compartment of the thigh and the deep fascia layer corresponds to the fascia covering the tensor fascia muscle. The deep fascia of the tensor fascia lata should be opened rather than the classical description of dissecting the interval between the tensor fascia lata and the sartorius to avoid damage to the lateral femoral cutaneous nerve (**Figure 4.10**). After opening the fascia of the tensor fascia lata, the muscle fibers are retracted laterally allowing for exposure of the rectus femoris. The rectus femoris direct head is followed to its origin at the anterior inferior iliac spine (AIIS) (**Figure 4.11**). The next step is sharp

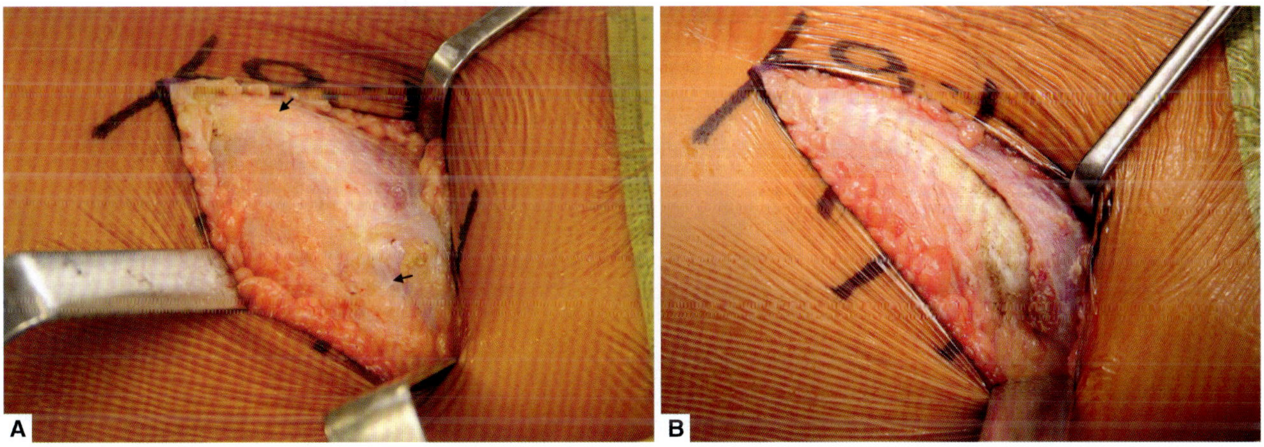

FIGURE 4.8. Exposure and dissection of the aponeurosis of the external oblique muscle. A, Intraoperative photograph shows the subcutaneous tissue dissection and exposure of the aponeurosis of the external oblique muscle at the level of the anterior superior iliac spine from distal to proximal (black arrows). B, The aponeurosis of the external oblique muscle is detached from the iliac crest and retracted medially and proximally for exposure of the crest apophysis.

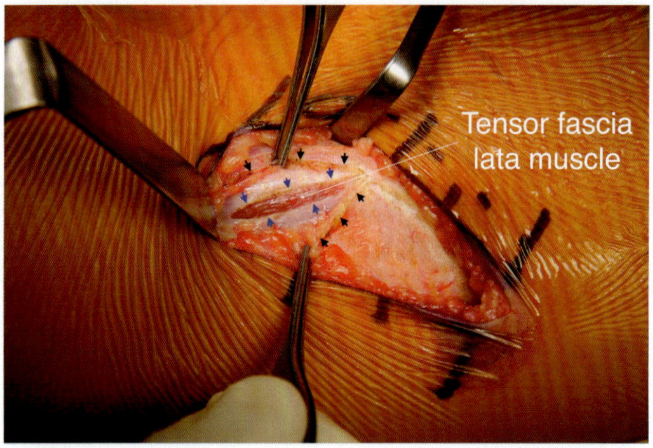

FIGURE 4.10. Intraoperative picture showing the two different layers of fascia that should be opened to expose the tensor fascia lata muscle belly. The most superficial layer (black arrowheads) is opened and then the deep fascia layer (blue arrowheads) should be open to expose the muscle.

division of the iliac crest apophysis (**Figure 4.12**). There are several variations including division of the lateral border only, but the authors' preference is to split the apophysis completely in and dissect subperiosteally the outer and the inner tables of the ilium. The iliac crest is split down to the level of the AIIS and as much proximally as possible. Subperiosteal dissection should be performed carefully to the level of the sciatic notch (**Figure 4.13**). The authors use a special design retractor called the Rang retractor to completely dissect the sciatic notch medially and laterally (**Figure 4.14**).

After complete exposure of the pelvis, there are variations in the technique used for the different osteotomies designed for correction of acetabular dysplasia of the pediatric pelvis. If a Salter osteotomy is selected, then a #1 silk suture is passed through the sciatic notch and a Gigli saw is attached to one of its ends and pulled through the notch (**Figure 4.15**). Complete description of the classic Salter and modified Salter techniques is available in Chapter 3. For the Pemberton technique, the osteotomy is done separately through the outer and inner tables of the ilium using a curved osteotome. The initial part of the osteotomy is to cut the lateral ilium just above the AIIS aiming posteriorly, parallel, and about 1 cm above the joint capsule (**Figure 4.16**). The osteotomy is performed toward the ilioischial limb of the triradiate cartilage and should not violate the sciatic notch. It ends between the notch and the posterior portion of the acetabulum. Then, the inner table of the ilium is cut in a similar fashion toward the triradiate cartilage. The direction of displacement of the osteotomy can be relatively controlled by adjusting the level of the outer and inner table cuts: if purely anterior correction is desired, then both osteotomies should be at the same level. If lateral coverage is to be corrected, then the inner table osteotomy should be relatively lower and relatively shifted forward toward the iliopubic junction of the triradiate cartilage to make the fragment tilt laterally as it is displaced. Finally, a curved large osteotome is inserted from anterior to posterior in the center of the ilium to finish the osteotomy. Although Pemberton recommended displacing the osteotomy *as much as possible* or to 1 to 1.5 inches, the authors caution that in most cases such correction is excessive, and it may lead to future femoroacetabular impingement.

The Dega osteotomy is a transiliac incomplete osteotomy that penetrates the anterior and the middle portions of the inner table of the ilium, preserving the most posterior and medial aspect of the inner table cortex

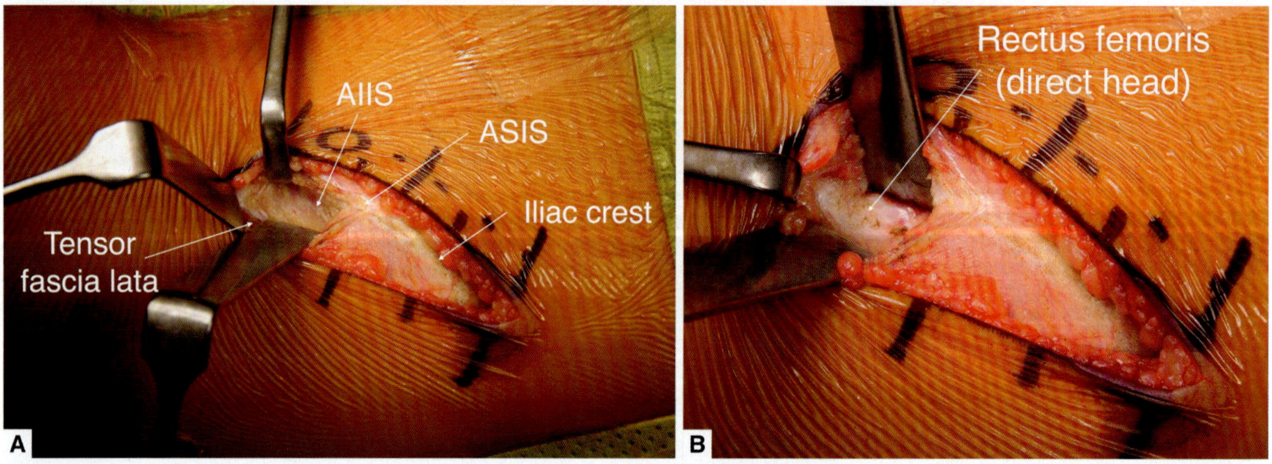

FIGURE 4.11. Exposure of the direct head of the rectus femoris. A, Intraoperative picture showing the tensor fascia lata is retracted laterally allowing for exposure of the anterior inferior iliac spine (AIIS). B, The direct head of the rectus femoris tendon is exposed at its origin at the AIIS.

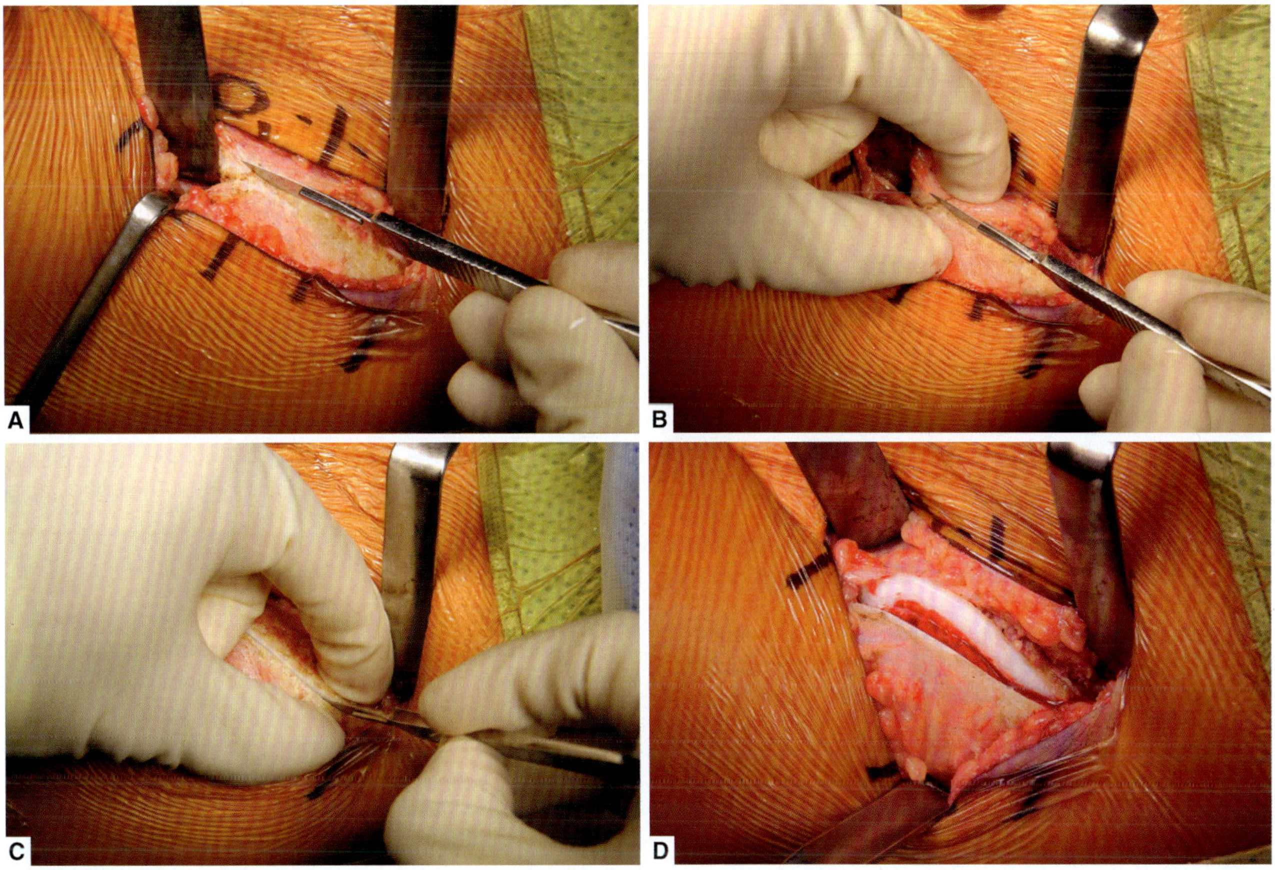

FIGURE 4.12. Sequence of intraoperative pictures showing the split of the crest apophysis. A, Retractors are placed distally to expose the anterior inferior iliac spine (AIIS) and proximally to expose the iliac crest. The apophysis should be split open sharply from the iliac crest distally to the AIIS. B, The iliac crest is held with the thumb and index finger to orient the surgeon to open the apophysis in the center. C, The apophysis of the iliac crest is sharply split all the way proximally. D, The apophysis splits easily if correct technique is used.

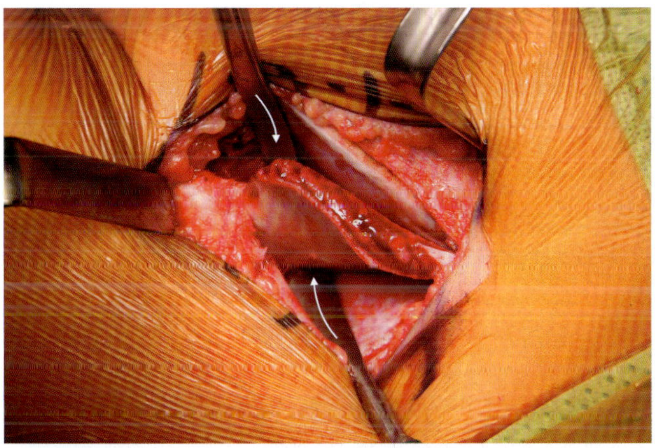

FIGURE 4.13. Intraoperative picture showing the complete subperiosteal dissection to the level of the sciatic notch laterally and medially (white arrows).

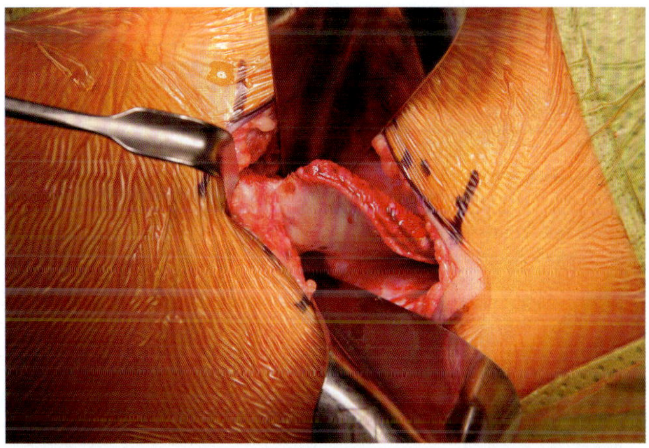

FIGURE 4.14. Intraoperative picture showing the application of the Rang retractor, which is a pair of two retractors designed to facilitate subperiosteal dissection and exposure of the sciatic notch and to protect the contents of the notch during osteotomy.

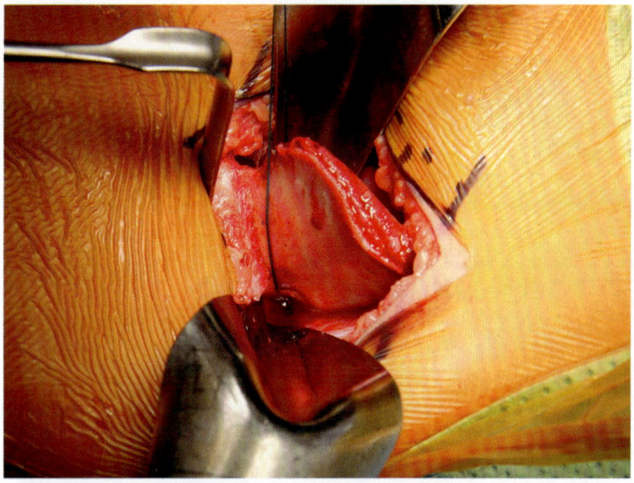

FIGURE 4.15. The Salter osteotomy: intraoperative picture showing the passage of a #1 silk suture through the sciatic notch that is protected by the Rang retractors. The suture is held simulating the orientation of a Gigli saw for the performance of a Salter osteotomy; the osteotomy extends in a straight line from the sciatic notch to the anterior inferior iliac spine (AIIS) and is perpendicular to the vertical axis of the ilium.

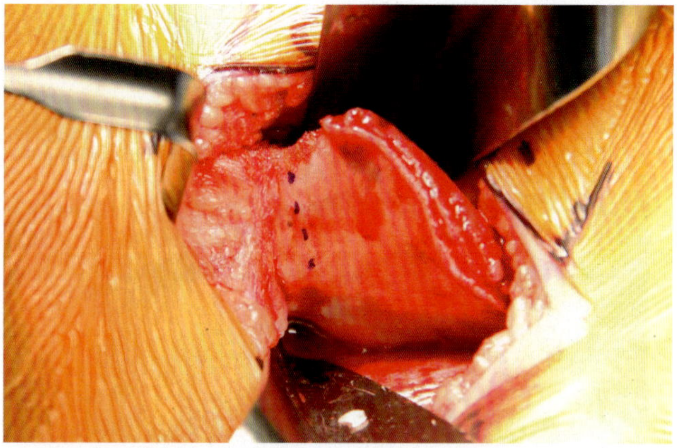

FIGURE 4.17. The Dega osteotomy: Intraoperative picture showing marking for the Dega osteotomy in the lateral table of the ilium.

(**Figure 4.17**). The osteotomy is performed from the lateral aspect of the ilium using straight and curved osteotomes (**Figure 4.18**). For all reshaping osteotomies, the Rang retractors are exchanged for a radiolucent retractor to allow for fluoroscopic guidance. Anteriorly, the Dega osteotomy starts just above the AIIS and is completed through the inner table of the ilium (**Figure 4.19**). The osteotomy should be slightly curved, with the most cephalad portion of the osteotomy corresponding to the middle of the acetabulum. Under fluoroscopy, the middle and posterior portions of the osteotomy are performed with the osteotome penetrating the inner table just above the iliopubic and ilioischial limbs of the triradiate cartilage but leaving the posterior third of the inner cortex intact to serve as a hinge correction of the deformity (**Figure 4.20**). The osteotomy continues posteriorly toward the sciatic notch but stops about 1 cm short of the notch (**Figure 4.21**). Once the osteotomy is complete, an osteotome is used to lever the acetabular fragment down. A laminar spreader is also used to hold the osteotomy open while the bone graft is prepared (**Figure 4.22**). Although for all pelvic osteotomies a bone graft is recommended to be taken from the ilium, it is the authors' preference to use a fibular allograft that is cut into the

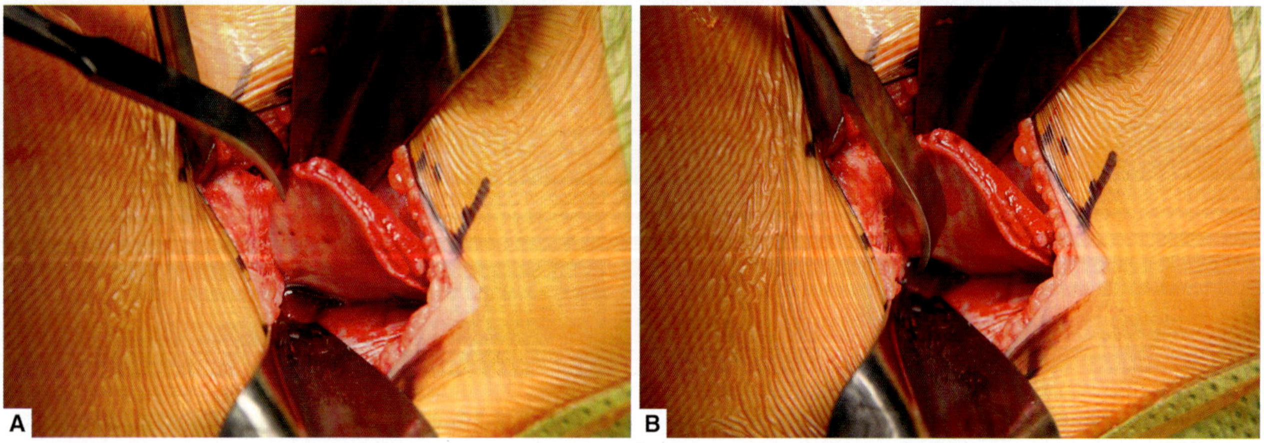

A B

FIGURE 4.16. The Pemberton osteotomy. A, Intraoperative picture showing the first step, which is an osteotomy of the anterior portion of the ilium just above the anterior inferior iliac spine (AIIS). B, Next, the lateral table of the ilium is cut with a curved osteotomy just above the AIIS aiming posteriorly, parallel, and about 1 cm above the joint capsule.

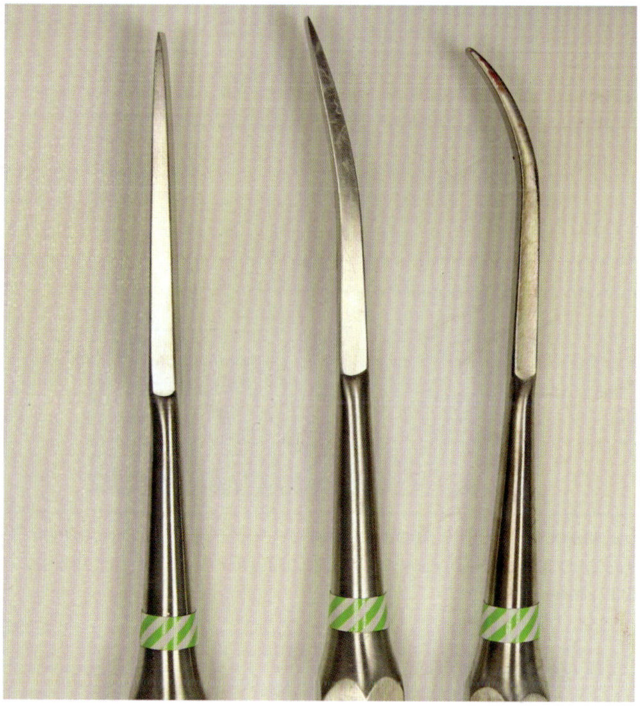

FIGURE 4.18. Intraoperative picture showing the three osteotomes used for the Dega osteotomy depending on the format and inclination of the acetabular sourcil.

small triangles (**Figure 4.23**). The bone grafts are placed typically lateral and anterior depending on the size of the osteotomy cleft to be filled (**Figure 4.24**). The advantage of an allograft is that the ilium is not deformed. After opening the osteotomy with a laminal spreader and inserting a bone graft, the authors highly recommend that the hip motion should be checked and an arthrogram should be performed to guarantee that the hip has a minimal of 90° of flexion and the labrum is not abutted with flexion and internal rotation (**Figure 4.25**).

In summary, the acetabulum has the potential to remodel after closed or open reduction of the hip for DDH. Treatment of residual acetabular dysplasia after DDH requires an understanding about the normal acetabular growth and the maximal potential for remodeling after reduction. Although monitoring with radiographs is the mainstay for surveillance, MRI of the hip may identify areas of high signal intensity within the weight-bearing portion of the acetabular cartilage on T2-weighted MR coronal section images that are associated with poor acetabular remodeling and growth. Several osteotomies have been described for the treatment of residual acetabular dysplasia in children. Although the choice for osteotomy is mostly based on surgeon's preference, the principles of correction described herein should be followed.

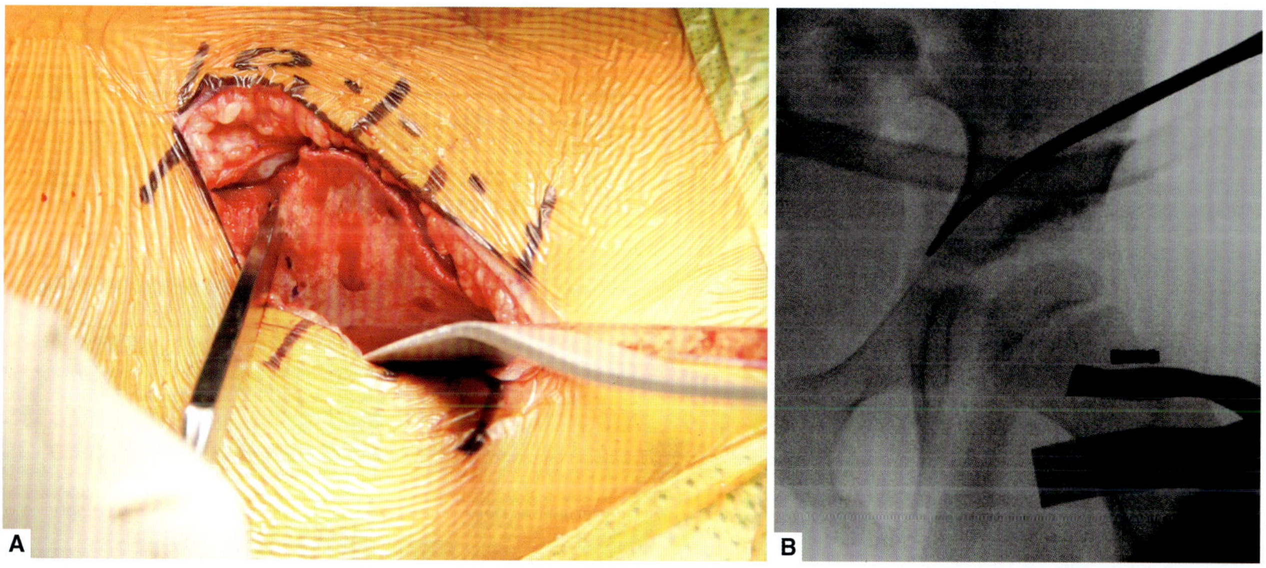

FIGURE 4.19. The anterior aspect of the Dega osteotomy: the osteotomy should go through the outer and inner table of the ilium. Note that the Dega osteotomy is performed from the lateral table of the ilium just above the anterior inferior iliac spine. The osteotome should be complete anteriorly and at the middle of the inner table of the ilium, penetrating the medial cortex just above the iliopubic and ilioischial limbs of the triradiate cartilage.

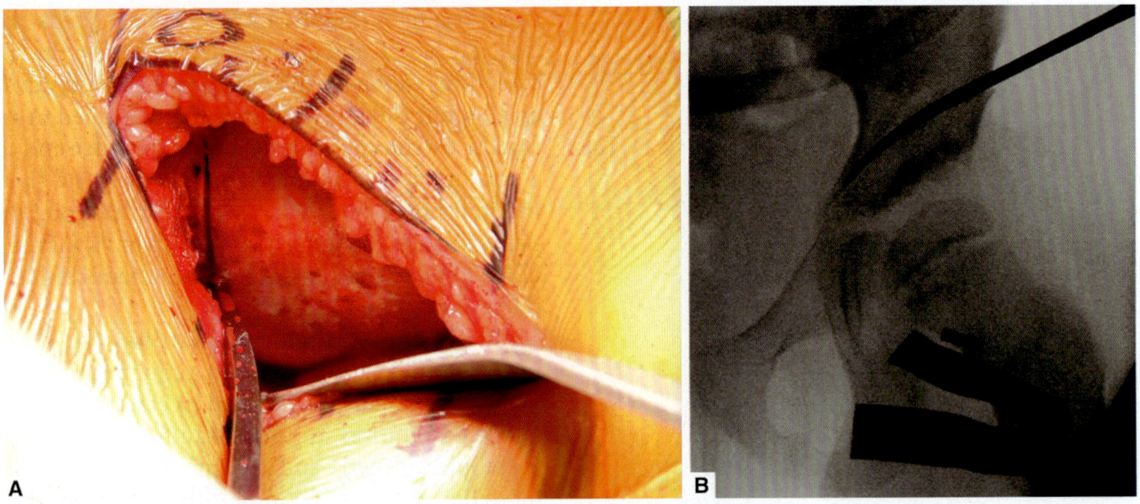

FIGURE 4.20. The posterior aspect of the Dega osteotomy. A, Intraoperative picture showing the osteotome is advanced posteriorly toward the sciatic notch but not through the notch. B, Fluoroscopy imaging showing the osteotome does not violate the inner table of the ilium posteriorly to leave an intact posteromedial hinge.

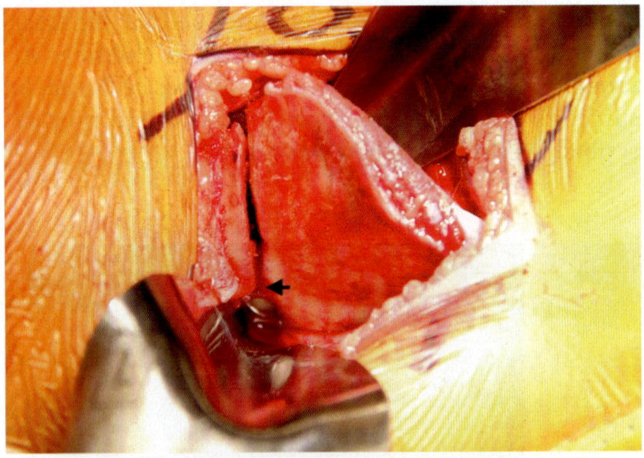

FIGURE 4.21. Intraoperative picture showing the osteotomy stops about 1 cm short from the sciatic notch posteriorly in the lateral cortex. Medially, the osteotomy should preserve about one-third of the posterior inner cortex.

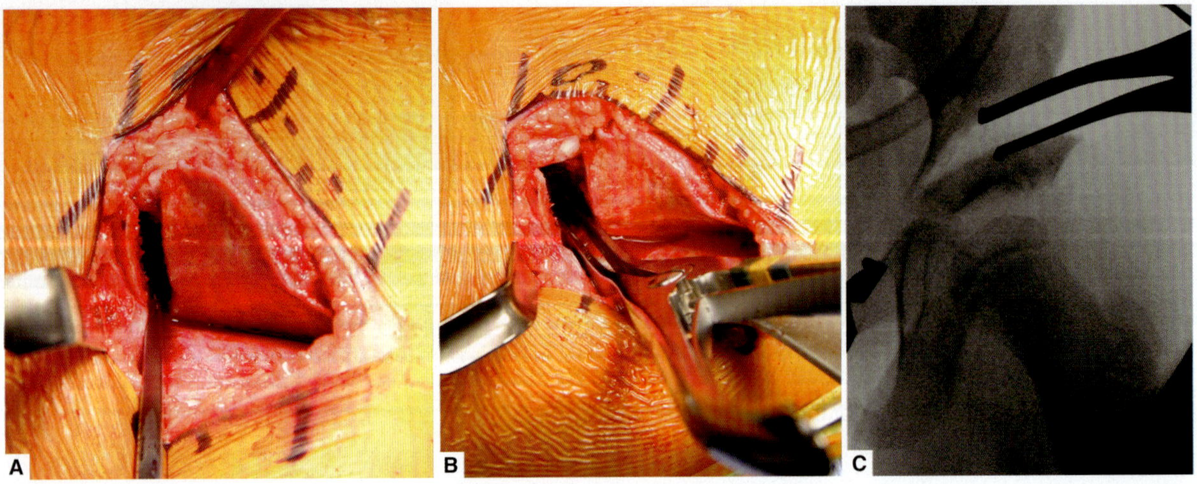

FIGURE 4.22. Opening of the Dega osteotomy. A, Intraoperative picture showing the osteotomy is initially opened by levering down the acetabular portion with the straight osteotome. B, A laminar spreader is useful to help open the osteotomy and to hold it open while the graft is prepared and placed in the osteotomy cleft. C, Fluoroscopy imaging showing the osteotomy has been opened and held by a laminar spreader.

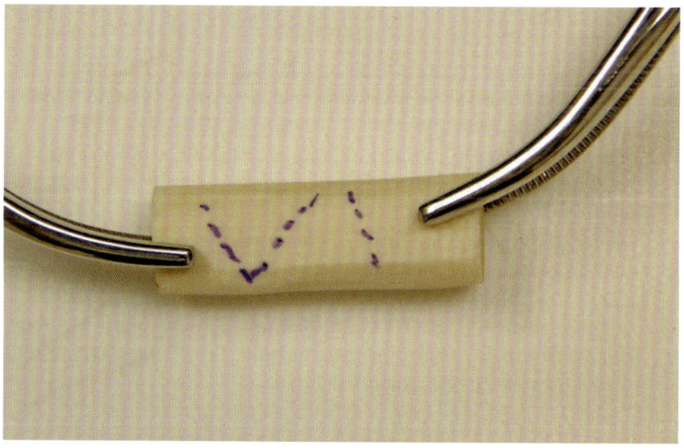

FIGURE 4.23. Preparation of a fibular allograft: two or three small triangles are cut from the fibular allograft depending on the amount of correction that is planned.

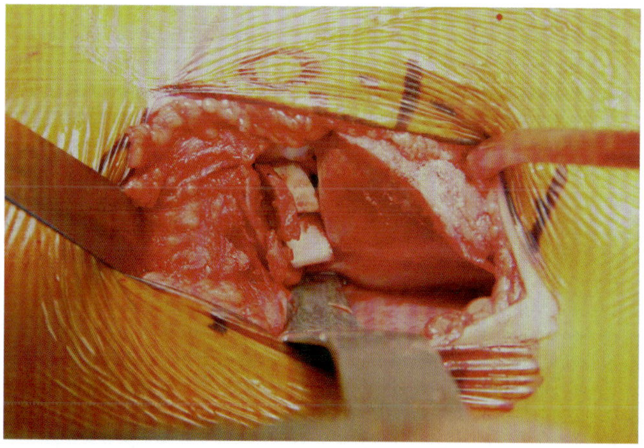

FIGURE 4.24. The allografts are placed in the lateral and anterior aspect of the osteotomy.

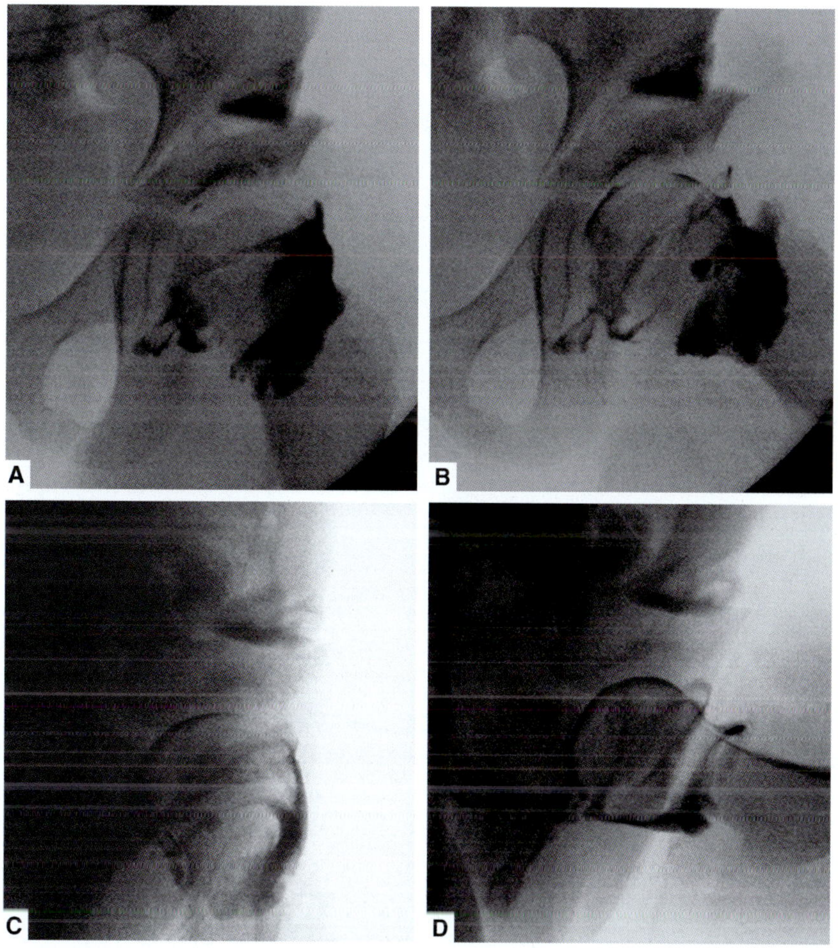

FIGURE 4.25. Arthrogram after Dega osteotomy. A, Anteroposterior (AP) view showing normalized coverage of the femoral head with normal osseous and cartilaginous acetabular index for age. B, AP view with the hip in maximum abduction showing no deformation of the labrum, confirming that coverage is adequate and not excessive. C, False profile view of the hip showing the anterior coverage of the femoral head has been normalized. D, False profile view in 90° of flexion showing absent deformation of the labrum without impingement.

REFERENCES

1. Tönnis D. Normal values of the hip joint for the evaluation of X-rays in children and adults. *Clin Orthop Relat Res.* 1976;(119):39-47.
2. Novais EN, Pan Z, Autruong PT, Meyers ML, Chang FM. Normal percentile reference curves and correlation of acetabular index and acetabular depth ratio in children. *J Pediatr Orthop.* 2018;38(3):163-169.
3. Kim HT, Kim JI, Yoo CI. Acetabular development after closed reduction of developmental dislocation of the hip. *J Pediatr Orthop.* 2000;20(6):701-708.
4. Shin CH, Yoo WJ, Park MS, Kim JH, Choi IH, Cho TJ. Acetabular remodeling and role of osteotomy after closed reduction of developmental dysplasia of the hip. *J Bone Joint Surg Am.* 2016;98(11):952-957.
5. Albinana J, Dolan LA, Spratt KF, Morcuende J, Meyer MD, Weinstein SL. Acetabular dysplasia after treatment for developmental dysplasia of the hip. Implications for secondary procedures. *J Bone Joint Surg Br.* 2004;86(6):876-886.
6. Wakabayashi K, Wada I, Horiuchi O, Mizutani J, Tsuchiya D, Otsuka T. MRI findings in residual hip dysplasia. *J Pediatr Orthop.* 2011;31(4):381-387.
7. Pemberton PA. Pericapsular osteotomy of the ilium for treatment of congenital subluxation and dislocation of the hip. *J Bone Joint Surg Am.* 1965;47(1):65-86.
8. Salter RB. Role of innominate osteotomy in the treatment of congenital dislocation and subluxation of the hip in the older child. *J Bone Joint Surg Am.* 1966;48(7):1413-1439.
9. Ganz R, Klaue K, Vinh TS, Mast JW. A new periacetabular osteotomy for the treatment of hip dysplasias. Technique and preliminary results. *Clin Orthop Relat Res.* 1988(232):26-36.

CHAPTER 5 Classic Adolescent and Adult Acetabular Dysplasia

INTRODUCTION

Acetabular dysplasia presenting in adolescence or young adulthood can result from unresolved or undiagnosed congenital/childhood developmental dysplasia of the hip (DDH) or it can occur in hips that were anatomically normal until adolescence. Normal acetabular development continues through adolescence, and late presenting acetabular dysplasia could be a result of deficient growth just prior to skeletal maturity.[1] This is postulated to be due to delayed ossification of the triradiate cartilage and insufficient development of the lateral secondary ossification centers at the acetabular rim that usually ossify between the ages of 12 and 18 years.[2] Acetabular dysplasia, characterized by a shallow and oblique acetabular weight-bearing zone, leads to unfavorable mechanics and increased cartilage contact stresses, which ultimately cause early cartilage degeneration and osteoarthritis. The incidence of hip dysplasia ranges from 1.7% to 20% in the general population, with females having an increased relative risk of hip dysplasia.[3] A recent US-based study of 950 patients, undergoing periacetabular osteotomy (PAO) for symptomatic acetabular dysplasia, reported 83% of the patients being females and 87.2% patients being Caucasians, with most patients being symptomatic for 1 to 3 years.[4]

CLINICAL ASSESSMENT

The commonest presenting complaint of patients seeking medical attention is activity-related pain around the hip.[5] Patients commonly localize the pain to the groin or the greater trochanter or both. Some patients have been misdiagnosed as having primary trochanteric bursitis and have undergone prolonged prior intervention for the same, often in the form of steroid injections.

It is very uncommon for patients with dysplasia to have buttock pain unless they have associated femoroacetabular impingement (FAI). The pain associated with hip dysplasia is usually related to abnormal mechanical loading of the involved hip. In due course of time, it becomes more persistent and frequent. This pain typically improves with rest and by weight-bearing activities of the involved hip. Catching and/or popping are frequent nonspecific hip symptoms and are usually due to extra-articular causes—iliopsoas riding over the iliopectineal eminence or the iliotibial (IT) band over the trochanter. Patients often seek physical therapy regimens and/or injections in and around the hip for pain relief in the absence of a specific mechanical diagnosis.

A thorough general medical, surgical, and social history is important. The history taking should also screen for neuromuscular causes of dysplasia (e.g., myelomeningocele, Charcot-Marie-Tooth disease, hypertonia). Hip dysplasia may have a genetic component, so family history of hip dysplasia and/or of early total hip replacement (THR) in the family is also pertinent. We recommend collecting a validated hip-specific patient function instrument, such as Western Ontario and McMaster Universities Osteoarthritis Index (WOMAC) or International Hip Outcome Tool (iHOT). In addition to documenting the patient's functional status, expectations should also be discussed during the patient interview.

Physical Examination

A brief general physical examination and a neurologic examination assessing motor power, bulk, reflexes, and sensation should precede the specific orthopedic evaluation.

Because many patients with hip dysplasia have ligamentous laxity, a screening tool like Beighton score is helpful. Beighton score is a nine-point scale that assesses joint hypermobility (**Table 5.1**).

A complete and accurate physical examination is facilitated if the patient wears shorts or tights. A thorough examination should include visual gait analysis followed by examination in standing, supine, prone, and side-lying position.

Focused hip examination begins with the assessment of gait, specifically looking for any limp, abductor lurch, or antalgic gait. Standing alignment in coronal and sagittal planes provides important clues, such as pelvic obliquity, scoliosis, or limb deformity. Range of motion of the

TABLE 5.1 Beighton Score

Joint	Side	Finding	Point
Little finger	Right	Passive dorsiflexion beyond 90°	1
	Left		1
Thumb	Right	Passive dorsiflexion to the flexor aspect of the forearm	1
	Left		1
Elbow	Right	Active hyperextension beyond 10°	1
	Left		1
Knee	Right	Active hyperextension beyond 10°	1
	Left		1
Forward flexion of the trunk with knees fully extended		Palms touch the floor	1
		Palms do not rest on the floor	0
Total			9

hips should be documented, as should strength of pertinent muscles and positions of discomfort or pain. Special tests are used to look for impingement and/or dysplasia. A suggested examination pattern is given in **Table 5.2** and **Figure 5.1**.

RADIOGRAPHIC ASSESSMENT

Patients presenting with hip symptoms due to underlying hip dysplasia may benefit from joint preserving surgery. Undiagnosed acetabular dysplasia usually leads to osteoarthritis, which may require otherwise-avoidable hip replacement. Hence, prompt diagnosis of dysplasia is important. Appropriate imaging is needed to assess acetabular dysplasia and to plan out further treatment. Plain radiographs, advanced cross-sectional imaging (computed tomography [CT] scans and magnetic resonance imaging [MRI]), and dynamic ultrasound assessment are important tools and have specific roles in the diagnosis and treatment of acetabular dysplasia. In addition to getting the appropriate projections, it is also important to have strict criteria to assess the quality of the images.[6]

The radiograph remains the gold standard for assessing structural hip abnormalities, including hip dysplasia. The minimum radiographic data set that are generally

TABLE 5.2 Hip Examination

Patient Position	Assessment	Note
Standing/walking	Visual gait examination	Limp/abductor lurch.
	Stance	Pelvic obliquity, limb length discrepancy, spine deformity.
	Trendelenburg test	
Supine	Hip range of motion with special mention of hip rotations with hip flexed and extended.	
	Apprehension test	Anterior hip pain or apprehension noticed when the contralateral hip is hyperflexed to the chest and the index hip is extended and internally rotated in slight adduction. This is indicative of possible rim damage or instability.
	Anterior impingement sign	Pain, localized to the groin region, with compression of anterior rim structures on flexion, adduction, and internal rotation of the involved hip. Usually positive if there is labral or acetabular rim most likely secondary to abnormal femoral head–neck anatomy.
Side-lying	Hip abductor power	
	Trochanteric tenderness	

Height **Weight** **Temp:**

Age: ____

Referred by: ______________ **Chief Complaint:** ______________

Symptoms: ________________________________

(Circle all that apply) Locking/Giveway/Catching/Limp/Crutch-cane/other ____________

Duration of Sx: ______________________

Associated Trauma: ______________________

Ever have any problems before? ______________________

What makes it better? ______________________

What makes it worse? Specific painful positions? Activity restrictions?

PMHx:
(esp. dysplasias, Down's CMT, SCFE. AVN) **Meds:** **Allergy**

Birth Hx: **#___ of ___ Children** **Vertex/Breech?** **Birth Wt: ______ (lbs/oz)**

Age when started walking: ___

Hx: DDH as infant? **Y/N What Rx DDH?** **Pavlik/Rhino/Cast/Closed/Open Reduction**
Other remote hip problems? **Other Hip Surgery:** ______________
ROS:

Family Hx of Hip Problems/other ortho? **Neuromuscular Problems?** ______________

Soc Hx (Smoke/EtOH?) ______________

PHYSICAL EXAM

Beighton Palms-floor 1 Knees 2 Elbows 2 fingers 2 thumbs 2
Total= ___

Stance: ______________

Gait: ______________

Spine: ______________

Assistive Devices: ______________

	Right Hip	**Left Hip**
Flexion/extension:	____	____
ER *Flex:*	____	____
IR *Flex:*	____	____
ER *Ext:*	____	____
IR *Ext:*	____	____
Abduction:	____	____
Adduction:	____	____
Patrick Test	____	____

	Right	**Left**
SLR/Lasegue	____	____
Lengths:	____	____
Thigh Circ:	____	____

Ant. Impingement Sign?	**Y / N**	**Y / N**
Ant Aprehension Sign?	**Y / N**	**Y / N**
Post Impgt sign	**Y / N**	**Y / N**
Bicycle sign	**Y N**	**Y N**
Piriformis tender	**Y N**	**Y N**
Greater troch tender	**Y N**	**Y N**
SI Joint tender	**Y N**	**Y N**
L-spine tender	**Y N**	**Y N**
Sciatic notch tender	**Y N**	**Y N**

FIGURE 5.1. Clinic visit summary outline. AVN, avascular necrosis; CMT, Charcot-Marie-Tooth; DDH, developmental dysplasia of the hip; ER, external rotation; Hx, history; IR, internal rotation; SCFE, slipped capital femoral epiphysis; SI, sacroiliac; wt, weight.

employed in assessing mature acetabular dysplasia include a well-centered anteroposterior (AP) radiograph of the entire pelvis (standing preferred in the United States; supine is preferred in Europe), faux profil views, and a modified Dunn lateral radiograph, taken in 45° of flexion, 30° of abduction, and neutral rotation, to show in profile that anterolateral neck area is the most common location of reduced offset. The AP radiograph is evaluated with measures of lateral and anterior coverage (lateral center-edge angle [LCEA], **Figures 5.2 to 5.4**, Shenton line intact or broken). The faux profil view predominantly assesses anterior coverage, quantitated by the anterior CE angle (**Figure 5.5**). The modified Dunn lateral helps in identification of a proximal femur cam

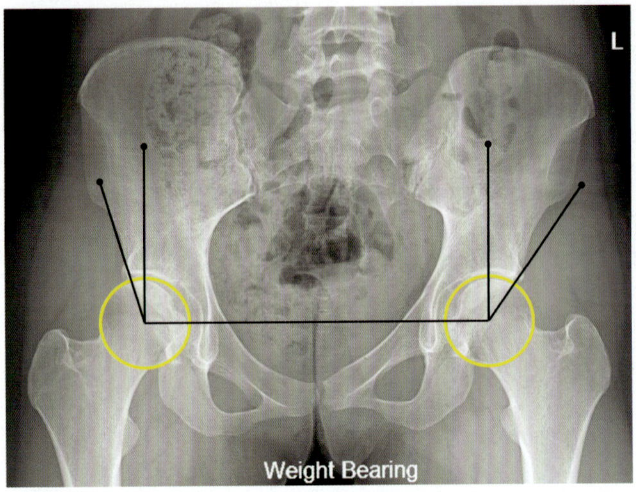

FIGURE 5.2. Lateral center-edge angle of Wiberg formed between the two lines passing through the center of the femoral head one of which extends to the lateral edge of sourcil and the line perpendicular to that joining the centers of the two femoral heads (of the two hips). The normal angle of an adult is greater than 25°. Beyond 40° may indicate pincer impingement.

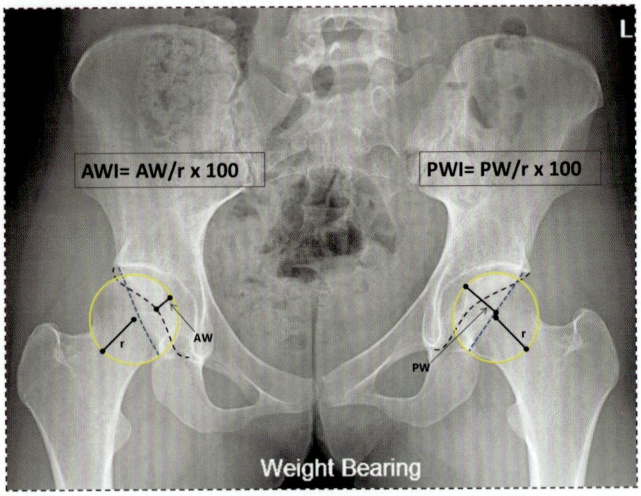

FIGURE 5.4. Anterior wall index (AWI) and posterior wall index (PWI). The AWI and PWI are calculated by dividing the distance of the anterior wall (AW) or posterior wall (PW) along the femoral neck line to the outer edge of the best fit sphere for femoral head by the radius (r) of the femoral head.

deformity (**Figure 5.6**). All radiographs should be scrutinized for changes indicative of osteoarthritis, including cartilage space width and appearance of the subchondral bone. **Table 5.3** presents the relevant measurements commonly made on these radiographs. For preoperative assessment of patients being considered for PAO, anticipated postoperative congruity is best confirmed by functional flexion, abduction, and internal rotation radiographs, simulating effect of the proposed redirection (**Figure 5.7**).

Additional imaging sometimes useful in assessing hip deformity and selecting treatment includes low-dose CT and MRI. CT in particular has improved our

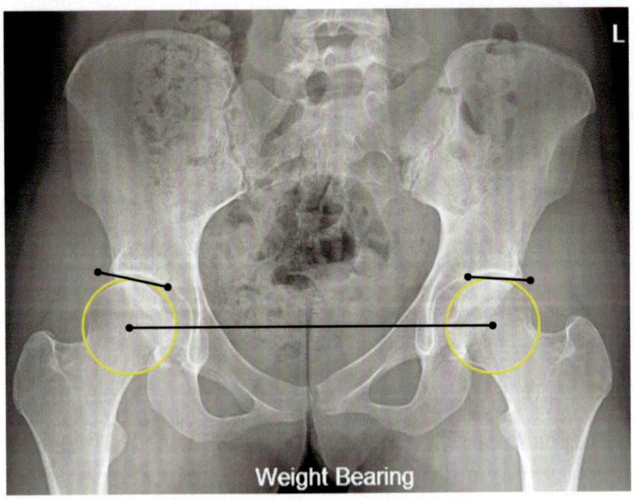

FIGURE 5.3. Tönnis angle. The angle formed by the intersection of horizontal line connecting the femoral head centers and the line that passes through medial edge of the sourcil. Tönnis angle greater than 10° is indicative of structural instability and less than 0° of pincer-type femoroacetabular impingement.

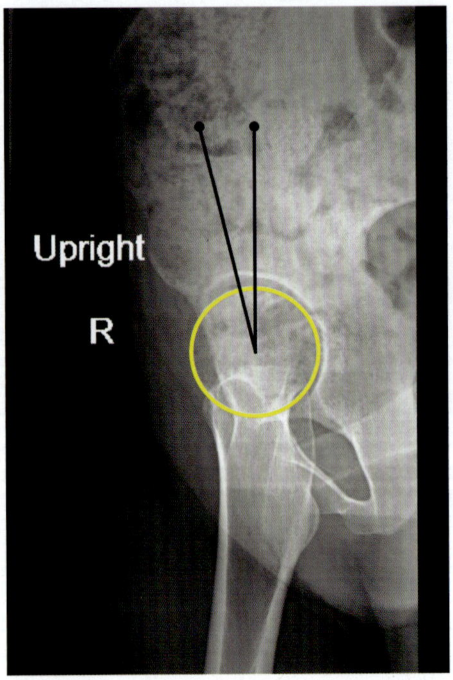

FIGURE 5.5. Anterior center-edge angle of Lequesne. A vertical line is drawn through the center of the femoral head intersecting another line drawn through the center of the femoral head, passing through the most anterior point of the acetabular sourcil. The angle created by the intersection of these two lines is measured.

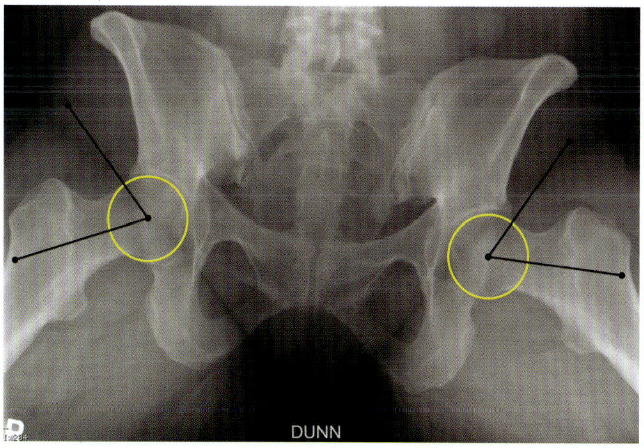

FIGURE 5.6. 45° Dunn view. An α angle is formed by intersection of lines drawn. 1. From the center of the femoral head through the center of the femoral neck. 2. From the center of the femoral head to the femoral head/neck junction, found by the point by which the femoral neck diverges from a circle drawn around the femoral head.

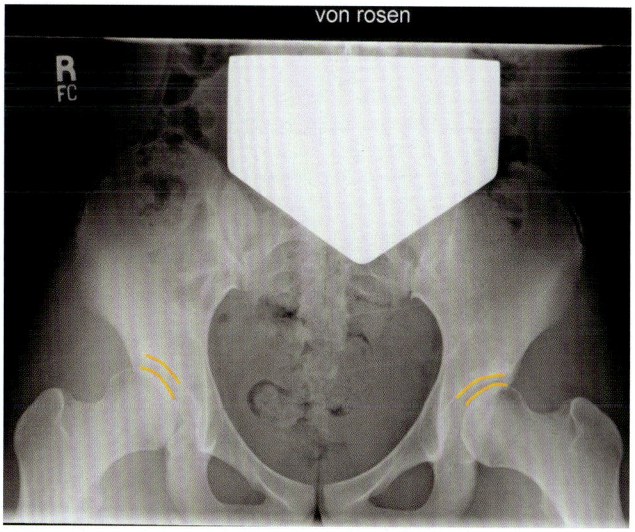

FIGURE 5.7. Von Rosen view. Anteroposterior radiograph done with both lower extremities in maximal abduction and internal rotation showing lateral coverage and joint congruity. The yellow curved lines demonstrate joint congruity and lateral coverage.

three-dimensional understanding of acetabular deformity in dysplasia. Acetabular dysplasia presents with three patterns of undercoverage: anterior, posterior, and global.[7,8] Recognition of the pattern of acetabular deficiency is critical in selecting the optimal acetabular reorientation. MRI allows evaluation of intra- and extra-articular soft-tissue structures of the hip affected by acetabular dysplasia. The acetabular labrum should be assessed for damage at the chondrolabral junction as well as global hypertrophy, both of which can remain symptomatic following PAO, if not addressed. In our institution, CT and MRI are also used to assess acetabular and femoral version. MR cartilage-specific sequences, such as delayed gadolinium-enhanced MRI (dGEMRIC), are invaluable in evaluating cartilage health (**Figure 5.8**) in hips with signs of early osteoarthritis. Preoperative dGEMRIC scores have been shown to have a predictive value in the survival of PAO[9] (**Figure 5.9**).

TABLE 5.3 Common Radiographic Measurements

	Normal	**Abnormal**
AP pelvis x-ray		
Lateral center-edge angle	Between 25° and 35°	<25° may indicate instability.
Tönnis angle	Between 0° and 10°.	>10° may indicate instability. <0° may subject to pincer impingement.
Anterior wall index	Between 15% and 30%	<15% dysplasia; >33% overcoverage.
Posterior wall index	Between 35% and 50%	<35% dysplasia; >50% overcoverage.
Shenton line	Smooth contour of the arc.	Disruption of more than 5 mm.
Neck shaft angle	Between 130° and 140°.	<120° coxa vara; >140° coxa valga.
Faux profil		
Anterior center-edge angle	Between 25° and 35°.	<20° considered dysplastic.
Modified Dunn view		
α Angle	<55°	>55° in females and >60° in males is indicative of a cam deformity causing femoroacetabular impingement.

AP, anteroposterior.

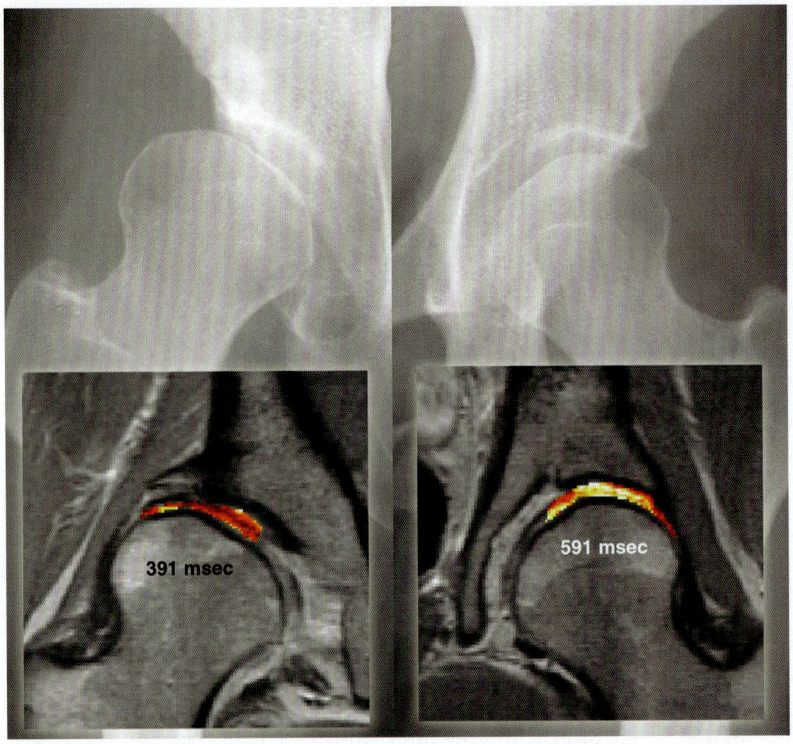

FIGURE 5.8. Delayed gadolinium-enhanced magnetic resonance imaging of cartilage (dGEMRIC). dGEMRIC is sensitive to the charge density of cartilage contributed by glycosaminoglycans (GAGs), which are lost early in the process of osteoarthritis. A higher number signifies healthier cartilage. Red color in the figure signifies lower dGEMRIC score and hence articular cartilage damage compared to yellow which signifies healthier cartilage.

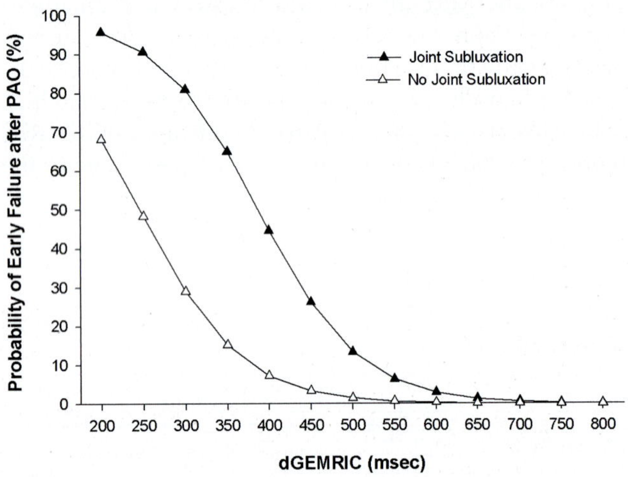

FIGURE 5.9. Delayed gadolinium-enhanced magnetic resonance imaging of cartilage values plotted against probability of early failure after a joint preserving periacetabular osteotomy (PAO). From Cunningham et al.[9]

Moving beyond static imaging, dynamic ultrasonography is being used at our center as a diagnostic tool in assessing both instability and impingement even in mature hips in which the mechanics are poorly understood.[10]

PATIENT SELECTION

The only multicenter prospective cohort study looking at outcomes after PAO, by the ANCHOR (Academic Network of Conservational Hip Outcomes Research) group, reported improved patient-reported outcomes, with a minimum follow-up of 2 years (mean = 2.6, 2-5.4 years) in 391 hips and a 99.2% hip survival rate and 93% early satisfaction rate. They reported improvements in pain, function, quality of life, overall health, and activity level. Increasing age and a body mass index status of overweight or obesity were predictive of improved results for certain outcome metrics. Male sex and mild acetabular dysplasia were predictive of lesser improvements in certain outcome measures. Three (0.8%) of the hips underwent early conversion to total hip arthroplasty, 12 (3%) required reoperation, and 26 (7%) experienced a major complication.[11]

Multiple retrospective studies report outcomes of PAO. The Bernese experience has the longest minimum follow-up of 30 years, noting conversion rate to total hip arthroplasty or arthrodesis of 12.4% at 10 years and 39.5% at 20 years. At 30-year follow-up, 30% of hips were asymptomatic without radiographic evidence of progression.[12-14]

Similar results from our center showed cumulative survival of 76% at 10-year follow-up and 74% at mean 18-year follow-up. At a mean of 18 years after PAO, 53% of patients were asymptomatic, and 26% were symptomatic based on WOMAC pain score greater than 10. In all, 21% of hips had been replaced, with a mean age of 9 years post-PAO.[15,16]

Troelsen et al described similar results from another high-volume PAO center, with 82% of hips surviving for a decade following surgery.[17-19]

Factors associated with poor outcome included older age, the severity of osteoarthritis, and evidence of labral pathology and poor acetabular index postoperatively.

Even though widely accepted, the use of conversion to THR as an end point is in some ways problematic. At the time of follow-up, more patients may have developed end-stage hip joint osteoarthritis or functionally compromising pain. These hip joints may also require THR in the near future; thus, the true failure rate may be underestimated. There is no commonly accepted definition of which secondary end points to consider. While the overall results among most studies looking at mid- to long-term outcomes were consistent, the characteristics of failed PAOs were also highly similar. Older patients, patients with severe preoperative dysfunction, radiographic osteoarthritis, and poor joint congruency prior to surgery were strong predictors of PAO failure in a number of studies.

What Is an Ideal Patient?

The patient subgroup with highest likelihood of good long-term result after PAO is less than 30 years of age, with good range of motion at the hip and absent impingement sign. There should be no limp and no or minimal radiographic arthrosis with good to excellent congruence on functional radiographs. Additionally, the ideal patient should have a good understanding of the demands of the procedure and reasonable postoperative functional expectations and should be willing to participate in a well-structured rehabilitation program.

Selection of Less Than Ideal Patients?

Many patients with symptomatic dysplasia who are not in the ideal subgroup may still benefit greatly from PAO. Inclusion of PAO in the treatment program for such patients may still be the best choice. There is no one-size-fits-all-approach when dealing with acetabular dysplasia. Following a well-defined scientific algorithm helps in providing the best treatment options for patients.

The successful outcome of a PAO is dependent on several factors:

- Improvement, and ideally normalization, of biomechanics of the hip joint. This can be ensured by:
  - Radiologic correction of the acetabular dysplasia and maintenance of congruence postoperatively (correctability confirmed by preoperative Von Rosen view)
  - Correction as needed of associated proximal femoral deformities (femoral head deformity, short femoral neck, version and rotational malalignment)
- Health of the existing articular cartilage. This can be ensured by:
  - Younger patients will tend to have healthier cartilage.
  - Presence of joint space on radiographs (>3 mm), which is maintained or improves on a functional radiograph
  - No radiographic evidence of osteoarthritis. Choosing patients with Tönnis grade 0 or 1 radiographic stage of arthrosis
  - Absence of labral and/or chondral damage on MRI
  - Absence of cartilage degeneration in older patients as determined by dGEMRIC study. (Ideally, a dGEMRIC index is > 400.)
- Avoiding/preventing complications
  - Surgeon factor is very important to avoid complications. Necessary hands-on training and familiarity with the surgical procedure as well as the anatomy are critical for a good outcome.
  - Optimal control of modifiable patient-related factors such as weight and other medical comorbidities (diabetes etc.) is also important to avoid wound-related complications.

BASIC PERIACETABULAR OSTEOTOMY TECHNIQUE WITH ANTERIOR ARTHROTOMY PEARLS

There are multiple techniques described in the literature to perform a PAO. We have been using a standard technique with a few modifications over the past 30 years.[20] We typically use an ipsilateral lumbar plexus block (**Figure 5.10**) for perioperative analgesia for 48 hours after surgery. A urinary catheter is inserted, and a cell saver is used intraoperatively. Preoperative antibiotic

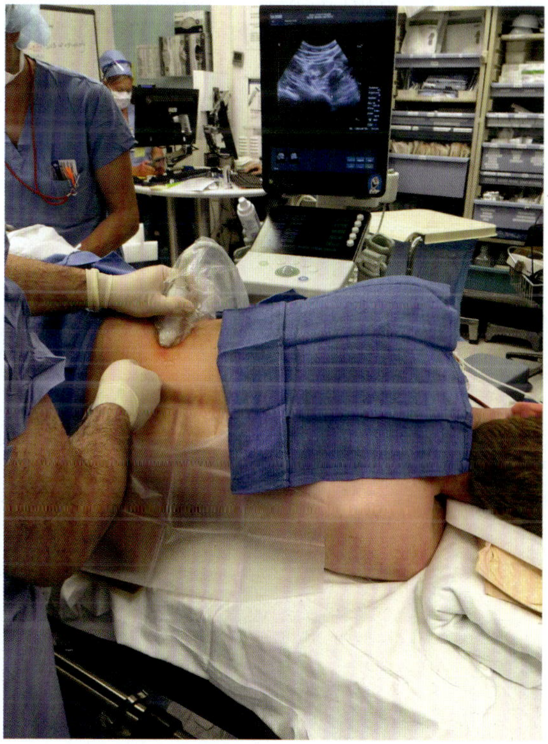

FIGURE 5.10. Placing the Lumbar plexus pain catheter.

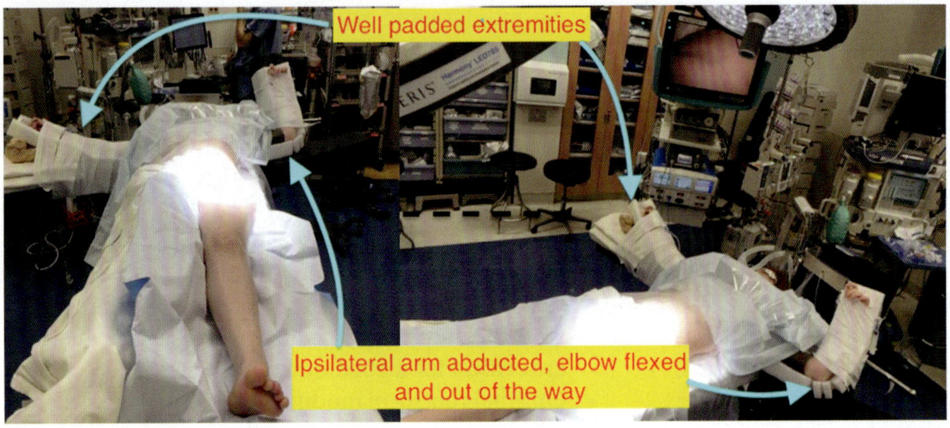

FIGURE 5.11. Patient positioning for the periacetabular osteotomy.

prophylaxis and tranexamic acid are also used. A large bump or a triangular leg positioner is typically useful for intraoperative leg positioning. Intraoperative anesthetic techniques using neuromuscular blockade are avoided during the period when intraoperative monitoring of motor nerve function may be useful, such as during the posterior column cut. This is important because the femoral, obturator, and sciatic nerves lie in proximity to the osteotomy cuts.

Positioning

- The patient is positioned supine on a well-padded radiolucent table (**Figures 5.11 and 5.12**).
- The arm on the operative side is set with elbow flexed, separate arm board behind the arm to keep the shoulder abducted and externally rotated to 90° (out of the way).
- The involved extremity is prepared and draped free to the costal margin, medially to the umbilicus, and posteriorly to the posterior third of the ilium.
- No bump under the buttock.

Skin Incision

- Modified ilioinguinal incision is roughly centered at the anterior superior iliac spine (ASIS) and about 1 to 2 cm below and parallel to the iliac crest (**Figure 5.13**).
- The entire length of the incision should be able to comfortably cover the anterior third of the crest, sartorius–tensor fascia lata (TFL) interval, anterior inferior iliac spine (AIIS), and the iliopectineal eminence.
- The incision should ideally not cross the groin crease for better wound healing and cosmesis. An alternative incision is the classic Smith-Petersen incision.

Careful attention to soft-tissue handling facilitates healing of not only soft tissues but of the underlying bone.

Superficial Dissection

- Incise through the Scarpa fascia and subcutaneous tissue until you reach the fascia overlying the external oblique (**Figure 5.14**).
- The fascia over the external oblique and gluteus medius is identified and incised posterior to the ASIS, and the

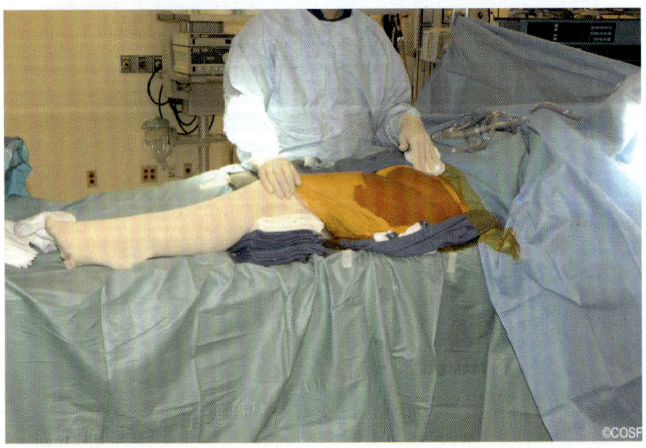

FIGURE 5.12. Draping.

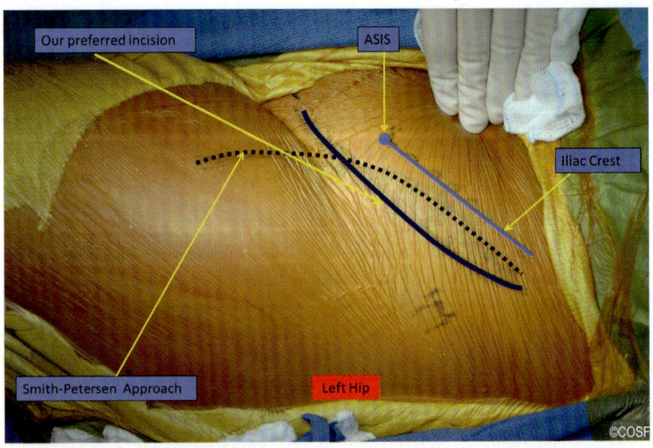

FIGURE 5.13. Incision for periacetabular osteotomy. ASIS, anterior superior iliac spine.

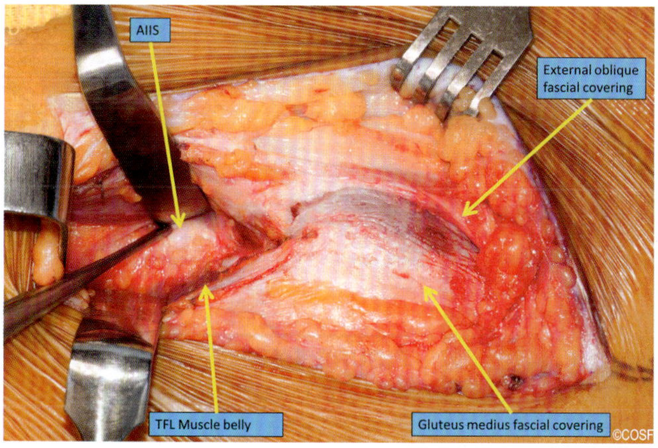

FIGURE 5.14. Superficial dissection. AIIS, anterior inferior iliac spine; TFL, tensor fascia lata.

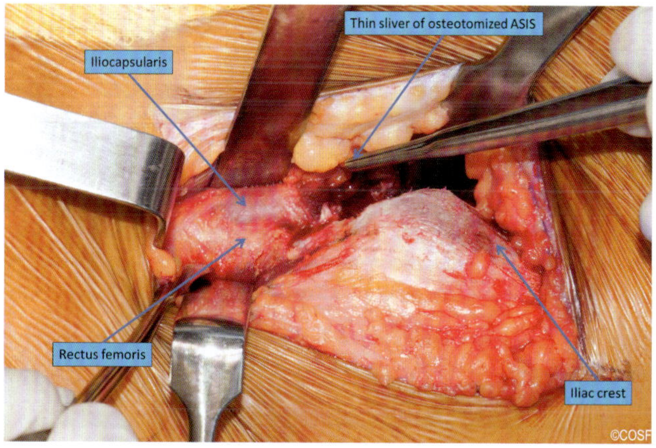

FIGURE 5.15. Deeper dissection.

plane between the two muscles is developed to expose the periosteum over the iliac crest.
  - A thin slice (~5 mm) of the anterior most portion of ASIS is then osteotomized from the ilium and retracted away medially with the sartorius and insertion of the inguinal ligament.
- A subperiosteal dissection of the inner table of the ilium is performed.
- More distally, the compartment of the TFL is entered (just lateral to the sartorius–TFL interval), and the muscle bluntly dissected off the medial fascia of the TFL.
  - The lateral femoral cutaneous nerve (LFCN) is not visualized directly but is carried medially, remaining just medial to the medial fascia of the TFL.
  - The floor of this compartment is identified and followed proximally until the anterior aspect of the ilium is palpated.

Deep Dissection

- The hip is now flexed and adducted to take tension off the anterior musculature of the hip. A large sterile pad or bump can be placed under the ipsilateral knee (**Figures 5.15 to 5.17**).
- The rectus tendon is then identified. The plane between the rectus and the iliocapsularis is then developed by detaching it away from the AIIS, anterior ilium, rectus, and the hip capsule.
- The psoas sheath is then retracted medially by subperiosteal release of its sheath from the pubic ramus proximally and then separating the sheath from the capsule distally.
- The interval between the medial joint capsule and the iliopsoas tendon is entered carefully.
- The tip of the Lane retractor is then used to palpate the anterior portion of the ischium at the infracotyloid groove. The appropriate level is distal to hip capsule but proximal to the obturator externus tendon. The proper placement is then confirmed with fluoroscopy. The medial and lateral borders of the ischium are felt with the Lane retractor.
- After confirmation that the tip of the Lane bone lever is at the right place, this interval is then sequentially dilated, leaving the tip of the instrument in constant contact with the infracotyloid groove.

Anterior Ischial Osteotomy

- The hip is flexed and adducted. With care, the special forked, angled/curved bone chisel (Mast chisel or a Ganz osteotome) is inserted through the previously created interval (**Figures 5.18 to 5.20**).
- The tip of the chisel lies in contact with the superior portion of the infracotyloid groove of the anterior portion of the ischium, just superior to the obturator externus tendon. Staying proximal to the obturator externus prevents injury to the nearby medial femoral circumflex artery.

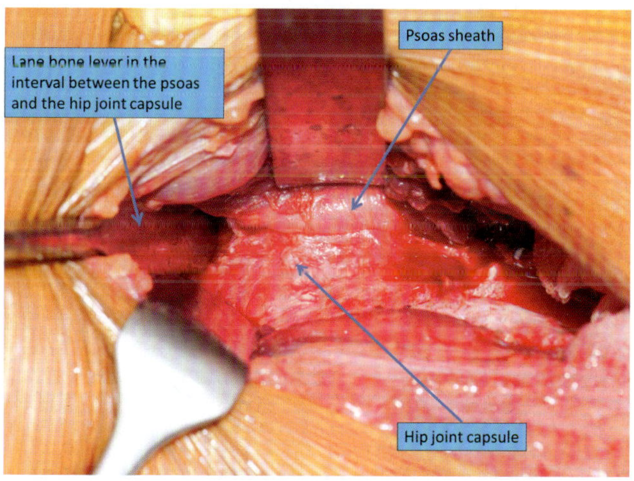

FIGURE 5.16. Lane bone lever positioned in the correct interval.

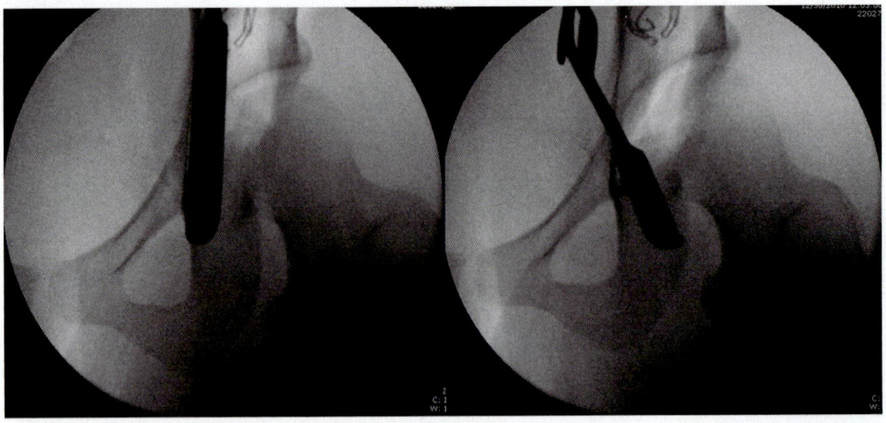

FIGURE 5.17. Confirmation of the Lane bone lever's position on fluoroscopy.

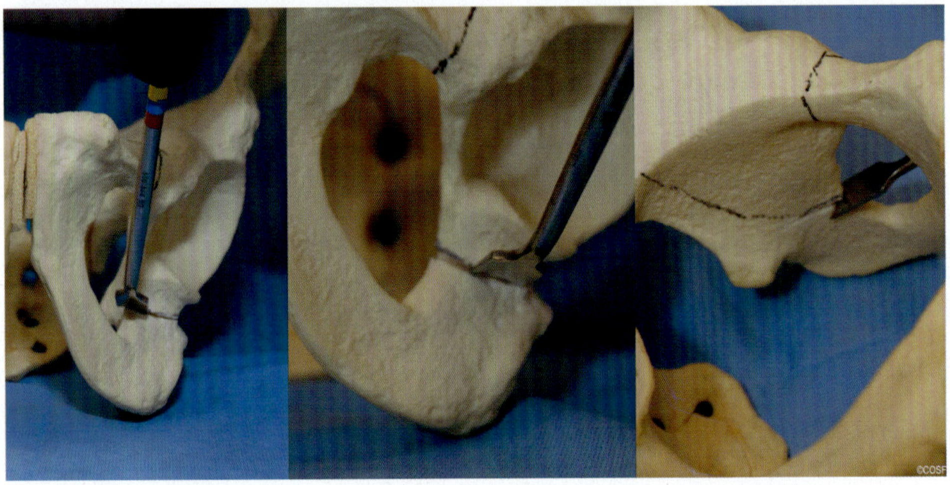

FIGURE 5.18. Bone model demonstration of the ischial cut.

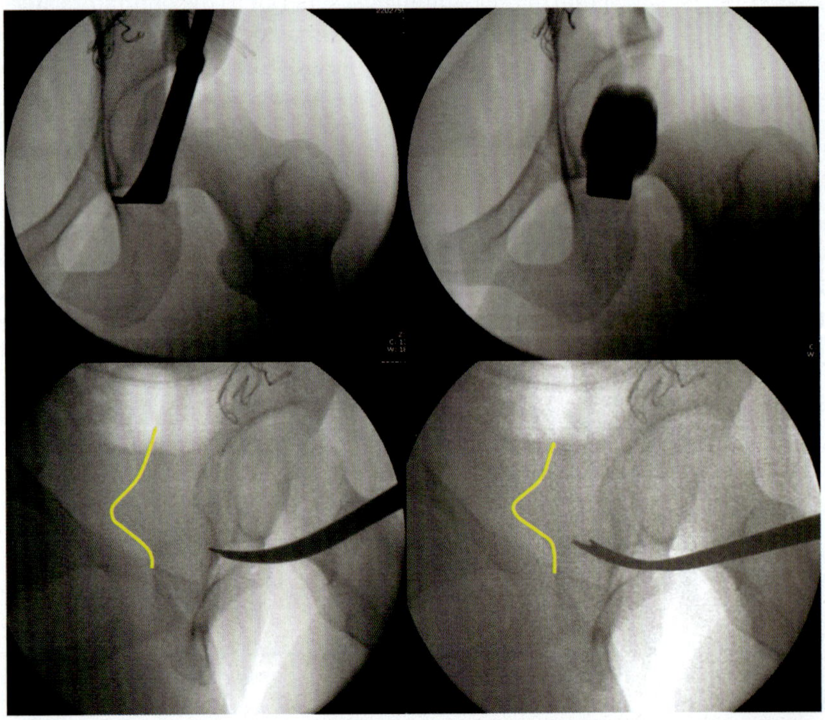

FIGURE 5.19. Fluoroscopic monitoring of the ischial cut. The curved yellow line defines the outline of the sciatic notch and ischial spine leading down towards the ischium.

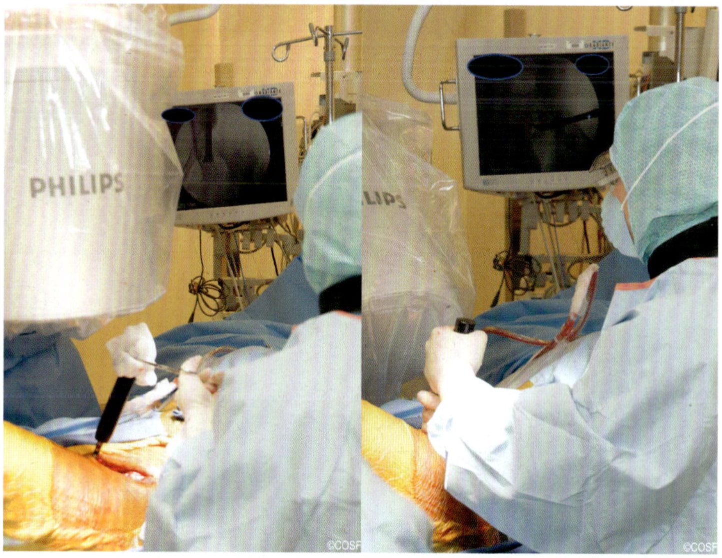

FIGURE 5.20. Surgeon assessing completeness of the ischial cut.

- The medial and lateral aspects of the anterior portion of the ischium are gently palpated with the chisel, the position of which is confirmed with image intensifier. The proper position of the chisel is approximately 1 cm below the inferior lip of the acetabulum with the tip of the chisel aimed at the ischial spine or at a point slightly above the ischial spine. The chisel is impacted to a depth of 15 to 20 mm through the medial cortex.
- The hip is extended, externally rotated, and abducted before the chisel cuts laterally, to move the nearby sciatic nerve away from the ischium.

Osteotomy of the Superior Pubic Ramus

- With the hip flexed and adducted, the psoas tendon and the medial structures are gently retracted medially and anteriorly to expose medially beyond the iliopectineal eminence (**Figures 5.21 and 5.22**).
- Careful circumferential subperiosteal dissection is performed around the superior ramus to avoid injury to the nearby obturator nerve and vessels.

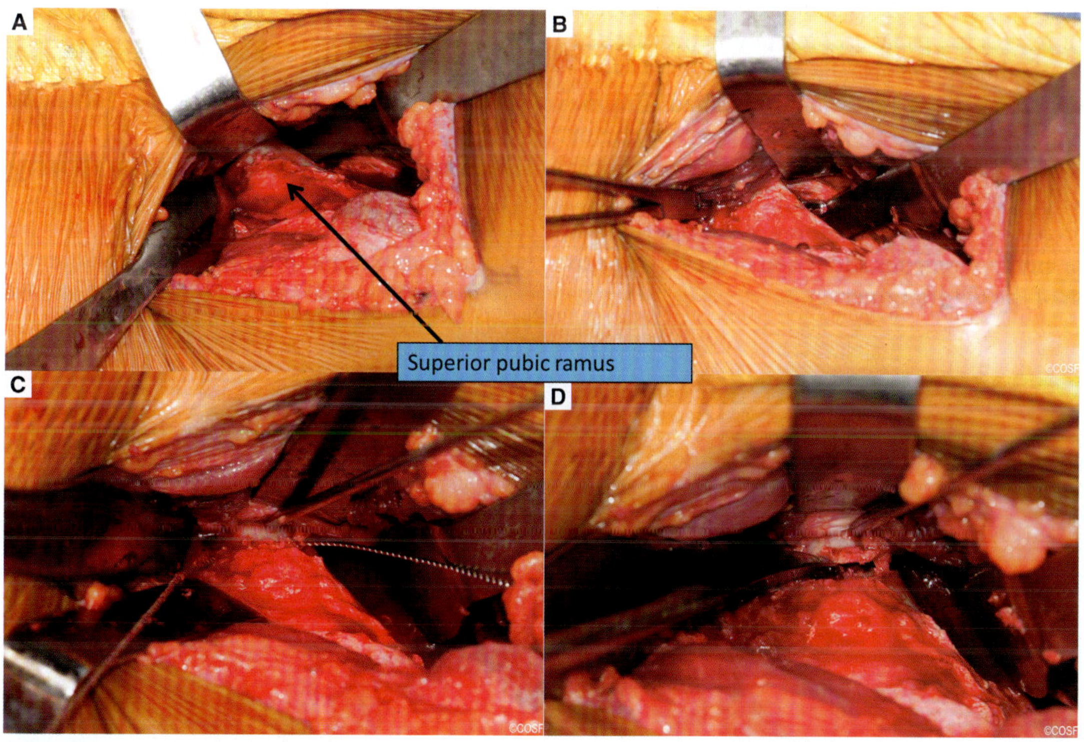

FIGURE 5.21. Pubic ramus osteotomy. A, circumferential subperiosteal exposure with appropriately placed Hohmann retractors. B, Satinsky clamp around the ramus. C, Gigli saw around the ramus. D, Completed osteotomy.

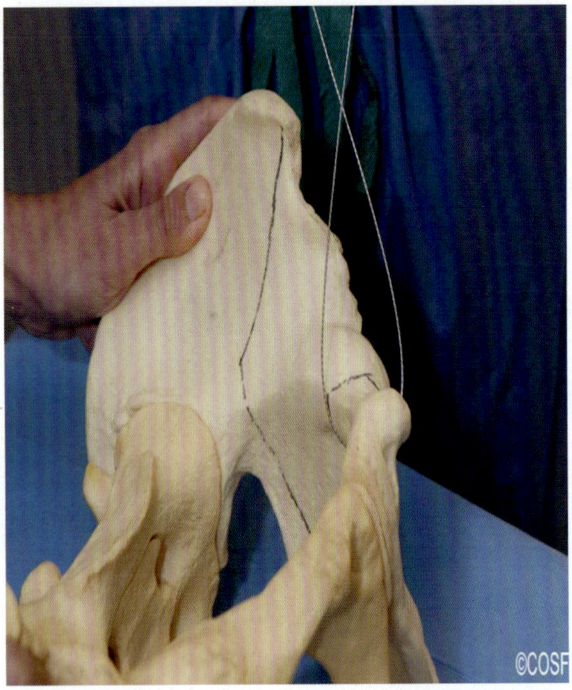

FIGURE 5.22. Gigli saw around the ramus (bone model).

- Lane bone retractors are placed anteriorly and posteriorly around the superior pubic ramus into the obturator foramen.
- Superior pubic ramus osteotomy is performed perpendicular to its long axis when viewed from above and oblique from proximal-lateral to distal-medial when viewed from the front. Maintaining the hip flexed and adducted relaxes the psoas and femoral neurovascular structures to allow good visualization.
- This osteotomy is to be performed (just medial to the iliopectineal eminence), using either an osteotome or a Gigli saw passed carefully under the superior pubic ramus with a Satinsky vascular clamp.
- While preparing for this osteotomy, it is important to watch for any spontaneous adduction of the hip (due to irritation of the obturator nerve).

Supra-Acetabular Iliac Osteotomy

- A small lateral subperiosteal window is created deep to the anterior abductors just close to the ASIS without disturbing the abductor origin, beginning anteriorly just distal to the ASIS. This window is deepened posteriorly as far as the greater sciatic notch (**Figure 5.23**).
- The hip is abducted and extended to relax the abductors. A narrow long Hohmann retractor is placed into the window with the tip pointing to the apex of the sciatic notch. The trajectory of this retractor is representative of the iliac osteotomy. The position of this retractor may be confirmed with the image intensifier to confirm the optimum level for the iliac osteotomy.
- A reverse Hohmann retractor is placed onto the quadrilateral surface to retract the iliacus medially. Its tip is placed on the ischial spine.
- Confirm that the abductor muscles laterally and the iliacus muscle medially are protected by retractors.
- Using an oscillating saw, under direct vision, the iliac osteotomy is performed, beginning anteriorly just distal to the ASIS and descending vertically in the direction of the apex of the sciatic notch. The end of this cut is approximately 1 cm above the iliopectineal line and 3 cm anterior to the sacroiliac (SI) joint. This represents the posterosuperior corner of the PAO and also the starting point of the posterior column osteotomy.
- Check to make sure that both the lateral and medial cortices are cut. A reliable method of doing this is to drive a chisel from anterior to posterior. The lateral retractor is removed.

Posterior Column Osteotomy

- With the hip flexed and adducted, the blunt reverse Hohmann retractor remains medially in place with the tip on the ischial spine (**Figures 5.24 and 5.25**).

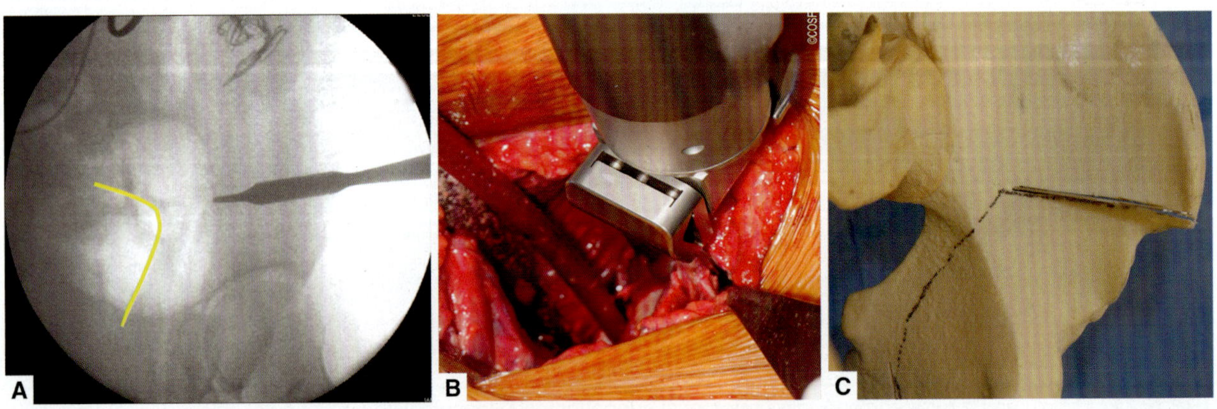

FIGURE 5.23. Supra-acetabular osteotomy. A, The level of the Hohmann retractor determines the level of the osteotomy. The yellow curved line defines the sciatic notch. B, Oscillating saw used for this step. C, Orientation of the cut on a bone model.

- To determine the angle and position of the posterior column osteotomy, a long straight osteotome is placed at the deep posterior end of the previous saw cut pointed toward the ischial spine.
  - The free medial edge of the osteotome should be rotated anteriorly about 15° away from the sciatic notch perpendicular to the lateral cortex of the posterior column. This is done to ensure that the osteotomy will ultimately be completed through the lateral cortex roughly midway between the posterior rim and the sciatic notch.
- Guided by the iliac oblique fluoroscopy, the osteotomy of the medial cortex is performed, directed toward the ischial spine. This extends from the posterior end of the iliac saw cut, then passes over the iliopectineal line, through the medial quadrilateral plate, and parallel to the anterior edge of the sciatic notch.
- Correct angulation and positioning are confirmed with the image intensifier.
- The posterior column osteotomy should extend at least 4 cm below the iliopectineal line (to insure that it is past the inferior edge of the acetabulum).
- The Ganz osteotome is used to connect the medial and lateral cortices, beginning at the proximal posterior column. This must be done very carefully so as not to injure the sciatic nerve and other structures that are exiting the sciatic notch.
- A bone spreader should be placed in the iliac osteotomy and slowly opened to confirm that the bone at the posterosuperior corner, at the junction between the iliac and posterior column osteotomies, has been completely divided. If not, then careful division of the lateral bone must be done with an osteotome. Opening the bone spreader in the iliac osteotomy further should demonstrate more mobility in the fragment.

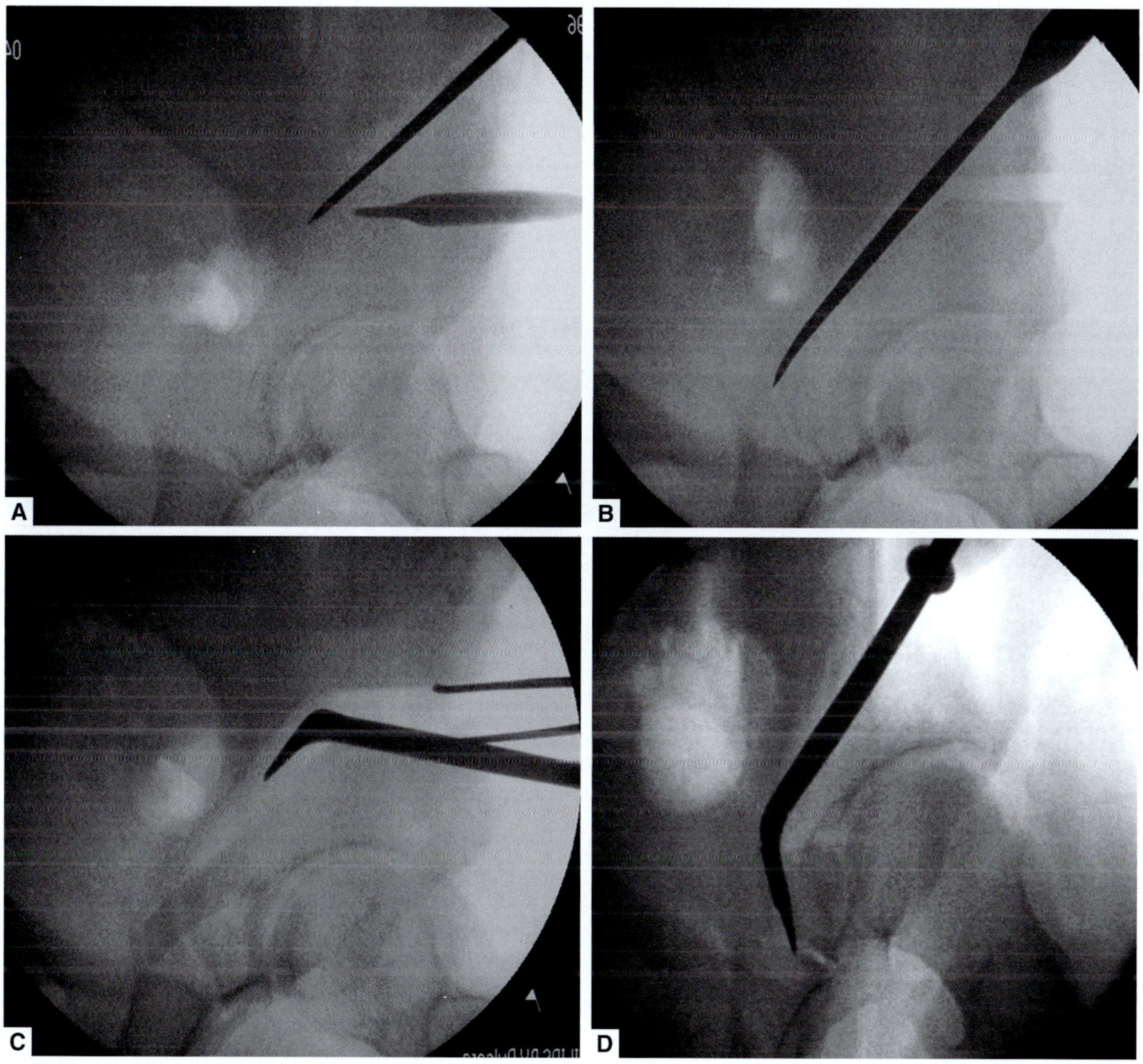

FIGURE 5.24. Various steps of the posterior column osteotomy (fluoroscopy). A, Beginning of the posterior column cut. B, Advancing the posterior column osteotomy with an osteotome. C, Connecting the medial and lateral cortices of the posterior column osteotomy with a Ganz osteotome. D, Final osteotomy of the posterior-inferior-medial corner of the quadrilateral plate.

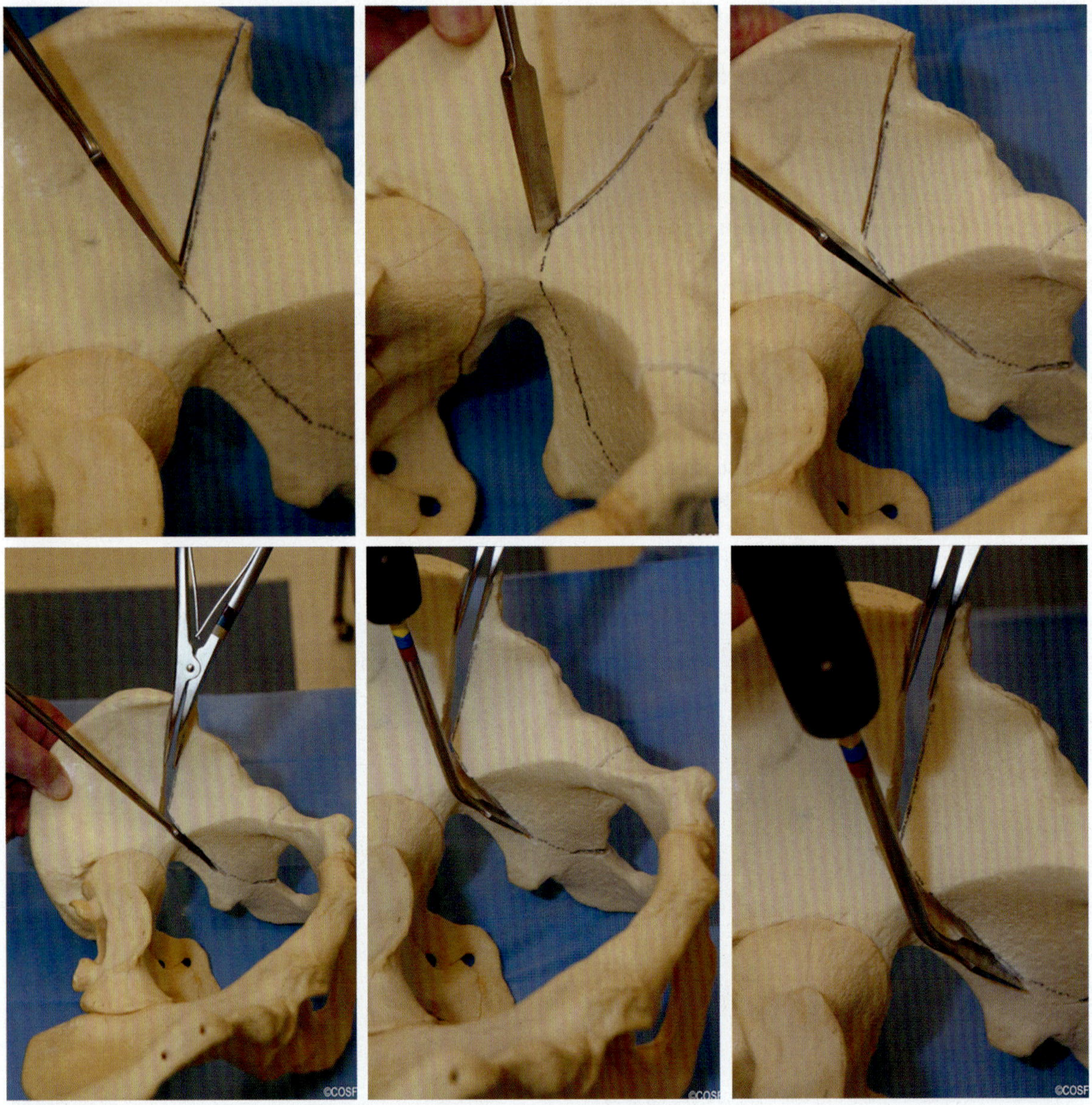

FIGURE 5.25. Various steps of the posterior column osteotomy (bone model).

Posterior Ischial Osteotomy

- The final osteotomy of the posterior-inferior-medial corner of the quadrilateral plate connects the anterior and posterior ischial cuts. This can be done directly using the Ganz chisel to connect these two prior osteotomies. This could, however, be done indirectly by controlled fracture.
- A single Schanz screw inserted from anterior to posterior into the acetabular fragment, distal and parallel to the iliac saw cut, is helpful in completion of the osteotomy and mobilizing the acetabular fragment (**Figure 5.26**).

Acetabular Positioning

- The tines of a Weber bone clamp are placed onto the superior pubic ramus portion of the acetabular fragment in such a way as to place its handle anterior and in contact with the Schanz screw (**Figures 5.27 and 5.28**).
- A bone spreader is placed into the iliac osteotomy between the posterior-superior portion of the intact ilium and the acetabular fragment anteriorly.
- With the help of the Schanz screw, Weber clamp, and the bone spreader, the acetabular fragment is gently mobilized.
- The fragment should be mobile and free of bony hinging. In case of any doubts, the osteotomy cuts can be revisited with the Ganz chisel again.
- Now the fragment can be positioned to obtain desired correction, not forgetting the desirability of maintaining bony contact at the superior ramus osteotomy.
- In general, improved anterior and lateral coverage is desired; therefore, the fragment is rotated anteriorly and laterally, maintaining or achieving appropriate acetabular version.

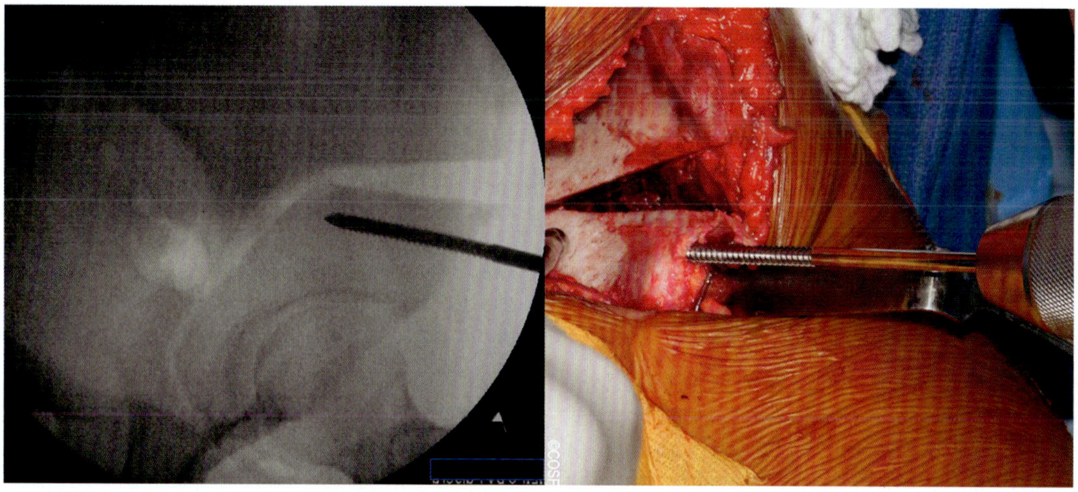

FIGURE 5.26. Schanz pin inserted into the mobile acetabular fragment.

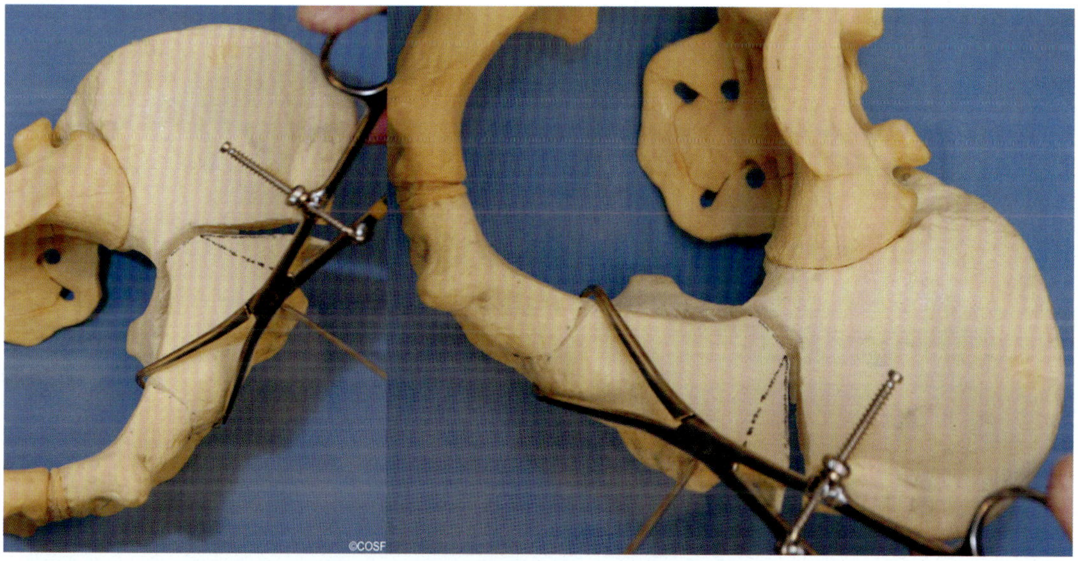

FIGURE 5.27. Application of the Weber bone clamp around the pubic ramus fragment.

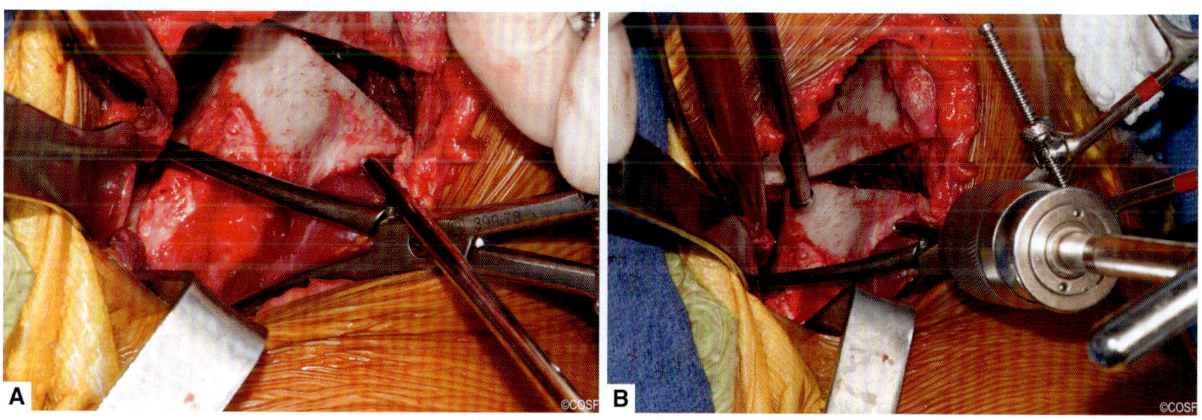

FIGURE 5.28. Manipulation of the fragment with the Weber clamp (A) and Schanz pin (B).

- The fragment is provisionally fixed with two to three smooth Kirschner wires, and imaging should be obtained.
- Optimal imaging technique is essential in accurately assessing the fragment position. Care must be taken to ensure that the tip of the coccyx is in perfect alignment with the pubic symphysis so that no artificial rotation is being projected, and subtle rotational adjustments of the imaging arm can be done to accomplish this.
- Once the appropriate acetabular correction is confirmed by imaging, passive hip range of motion, particularly internal rotation in 90° of hip flexion, is assessed to rule out iatrogenic impingement. This should be done by manual confirmation of freedom from anterior impingement, (placing a palpating finger over the anterior capsule as the hip is flexed), supplemented by imaging the hip in 90° of flexion in the faux profil projection. Any impingement should be corrected (**Figure 5.29**).
- Guidelines for optimal fragment positioning are as follows (**Figure 5.30**):
    - Shenton line should be intact.
    - No crossover sign.
    - No posterior wall sign.
    - Horizontal sourcil (few degrees of valgus is acceptable; any varus may indicate overcoverage)
- The wires are then sequentially exchanged for 3.5- or 4.5-mm cortical screws.

The stability of the fixed osteotomy is critically assessed. There should be impaction of the posterosuperior corner of the acetabular fragment into the iliac osteotomy site. There should be bony contact at the superior ramus osteotomy. Interposition bone grafting of this osteotomy may be necessary depending on the degree of correction and bony contact.

Optional Anterior Arthrotomy

Anterior arthrotomy is useful for correcting simple cam deformities and for debridement of small peripheral labral tears. This can be performed prior to the PAO or after. The direct head could be retracted laterally (our preference) or detached from the AIIS to expose the hip capsule. Usually, a T-shaped capsulotomy is performed, and stay sutures are inserted into the capsule. Using atraumatic retractors,

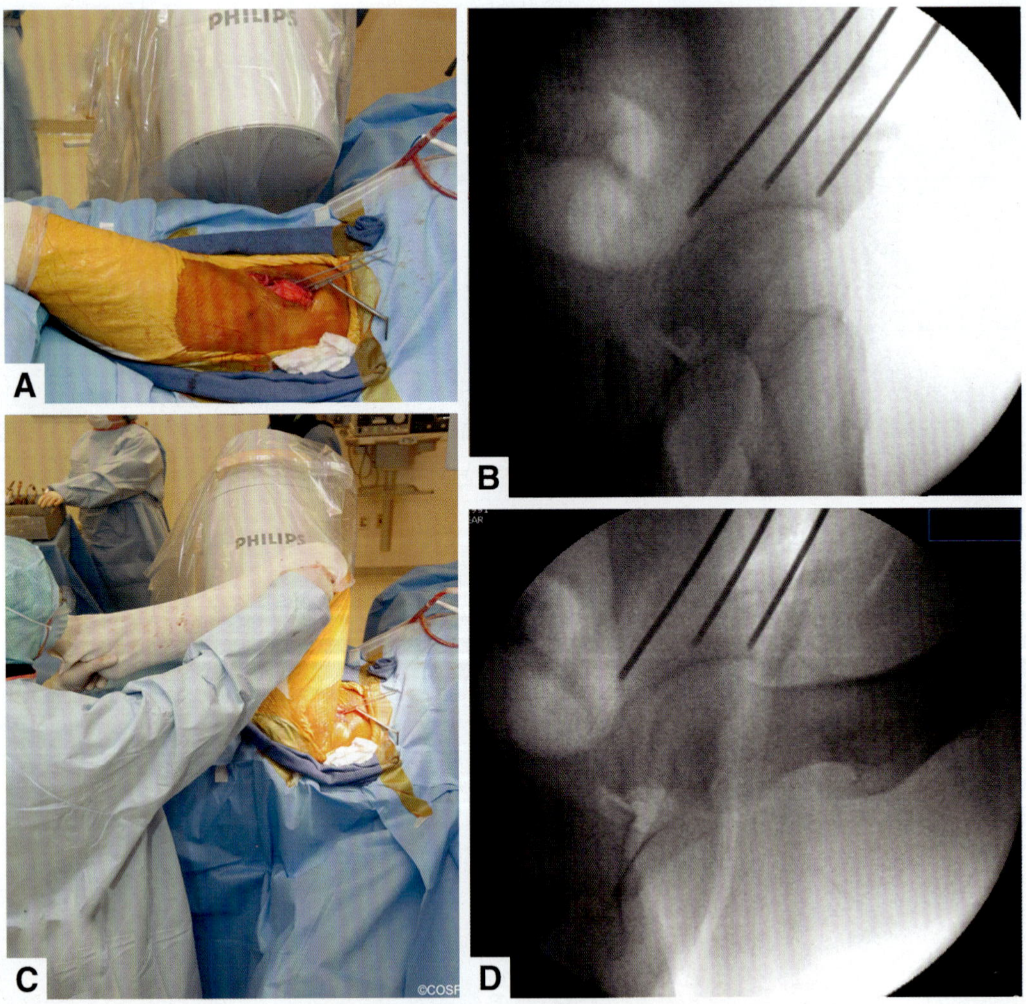

FIGURE 5.29. Provisional fixation and checking the correction and range of motion.

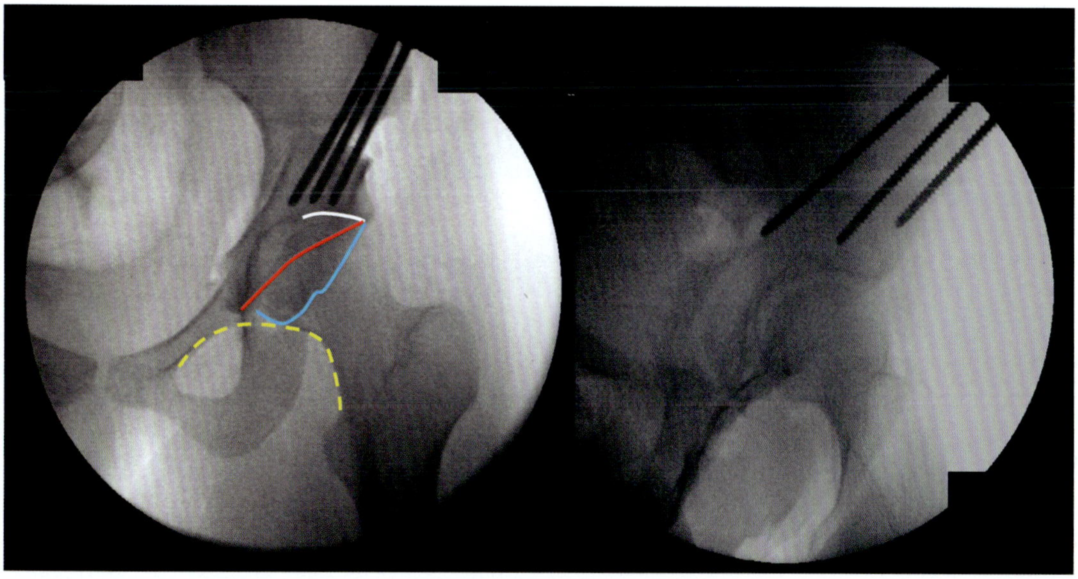

FIGURE 5.30. Assessing adequacy of correction. Intact Shenton line (yellow dotted line). Flat sourcil (white line). No crossover sign. Anterior wall (red line) and posterior wall (blue line) in the right position.

the inside of the hip joint is exposed. The central compartment is visually inspected for any labral or chondral pathology. A labral repair or debridement can then be performed if needed. A good suction seal is an indicator of a functionally intact labrum. The hip joint can be put through the entire range of motion to look for any impingement. If need be, an osteochondroplasty of the femoral head–neck area can be performed. The capsulotomy is then repaired (Figure 5.31).

Acetabulum cannot be visualized very well with the arthrotomy; therefore, extensive labral repairs and acetabular surgery cannot be performed well through this approach.

Closure and Soft-tissue Repair

Protruding bony edges are trimmed to reduce soft-tissue irritation, in particular the anterior ilium just distal to the iliac osteotomy, with the harvested bone graft subsequently packed into the osteotomy gaps (Figure 5.32).

Adequate hemostasis is usually present at this point in the procedure, though moderate bleeding always occurs from osteotomy surfaces while the fragment is being manipulated. Wound drains are not routinely used but may be indicated in rare cases.

Proper soft-tissue closure is imperative to allow early postoperative function.

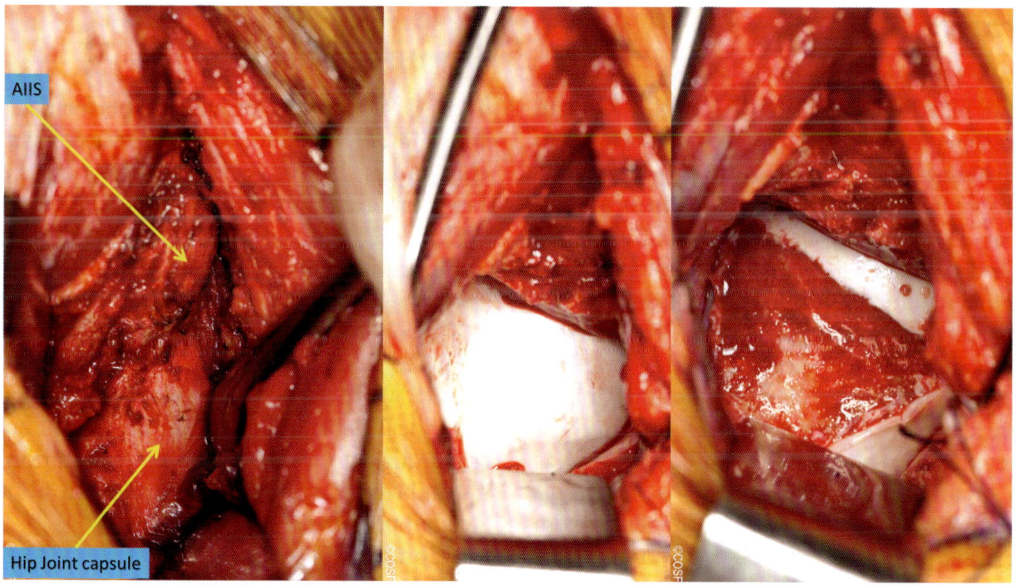

FIGURE 5.31. Concomitant arthrotomy and osteochondroplasty. AIIS, anterior inferior iliac spine.

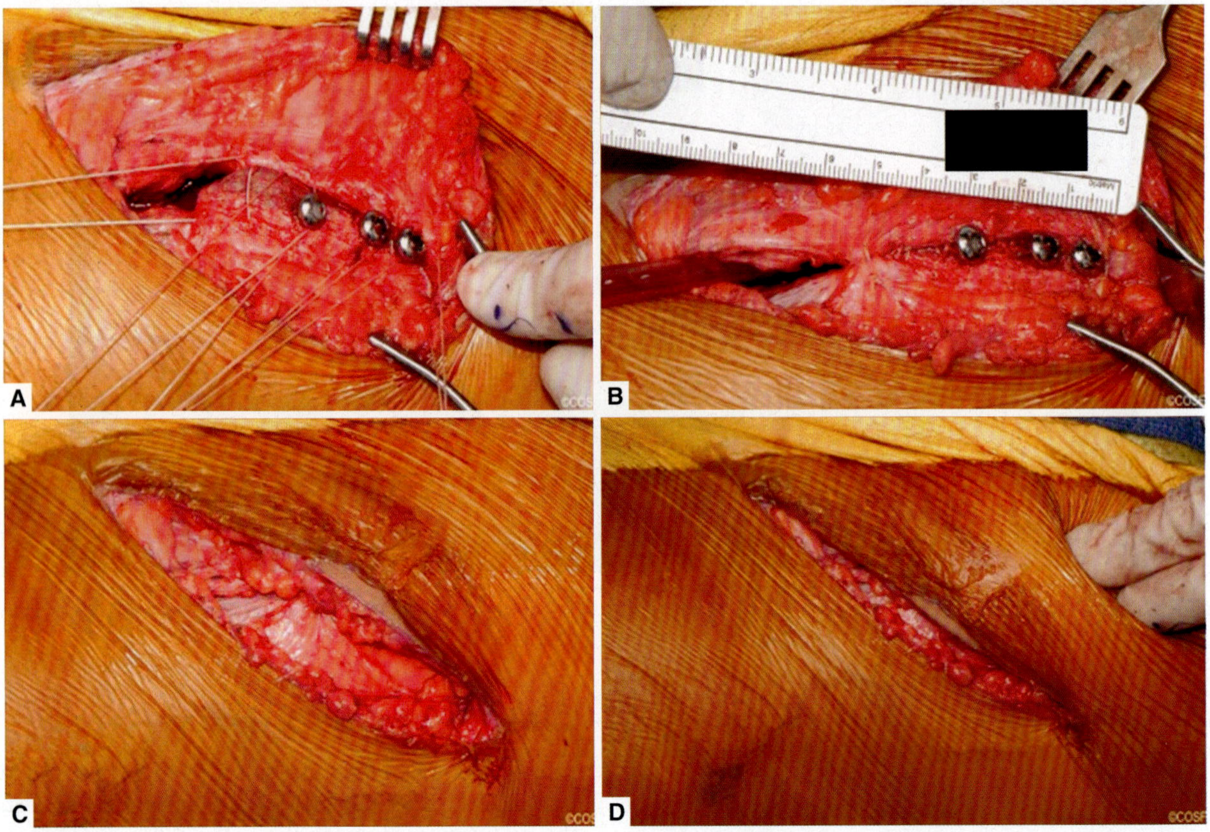

FIGURE 5.32. Good soft-tissue closure. A, Periosteal closure. B, Checking where the screws lie with respect to the ASIS. C, Approximation of the external oblique fascia to cover the screws. D, Just prior to skin closure.

We routinely use a cryo-cuff or ice packs over the surgical site.

A pillow under the ipsilateral knee in the immediate postoperative phase is very helpful to avoid any untoward stretch on the femoral and sciatic nerves.

Postoperative Care

After 24 hours of regional blockade by constant infusion into the lumbar plexus catheter, patients typically sit in a chair. By postoperative day 2, they are encouraged to begin a partial weight-bearing gait with crutches. Antithrombotic prophylaxis with low-dose aspirin is started the morning of postoperative day 1 and continued for 4 weeks. Prophylaxis against heterotopic ossification is done with naproxen, which is also used for 4 weeks. Discharge from hospital usually occurs after adequate pain control and able to carry out crutch walking on level ground and ascend and descend stairs. Resumption of full weight-bearing follows recovery of necessary muscle function and evidence of adequate osteotomy healing as confirmed by AP and faux profil radiographs. This typically occurs 8 to 12 weeks postoperatively, dependent on the patient's age and degree of correction required. Routine radiographs are taken at monthly intervals until complete osteotomy healing. Patients are followed annually with clinical examinations and radiographs, or more frequently if required (**Figure 5.33**). Full activity, including sport, is resumed according to individualized protocols, though, in general, at least 6 to 12 months is required before full return of maximum achievable function has taken place.

Complications

PAO is a complex procedure performed in the vicinity of multiple important neurovascular structures. Although the risk of serious complication is not very high, but there are many well-documented complications. The ANCHOR group in a prospective study reported a 15% complication rate within the first 10 weeks following surgery.[21] Seventy-seven percent of these complications were self-resolving or needed minimal intervention. These included LFCN neuropraxia (4%) and wound-related issues (5%). There were two deep infections (1%) requiring a surgical debridement and one case of acetabular fragment migration (0.5%) needing reoperation. Deep venous thrombosis was reported in three (1.5%) patients, which needed pharmacologic treatment.

Complications noted more than a year after surgery were about 24%. A majority of these (86%) did not need any treatment. Heterotopic ossification (HO) (24% patients),

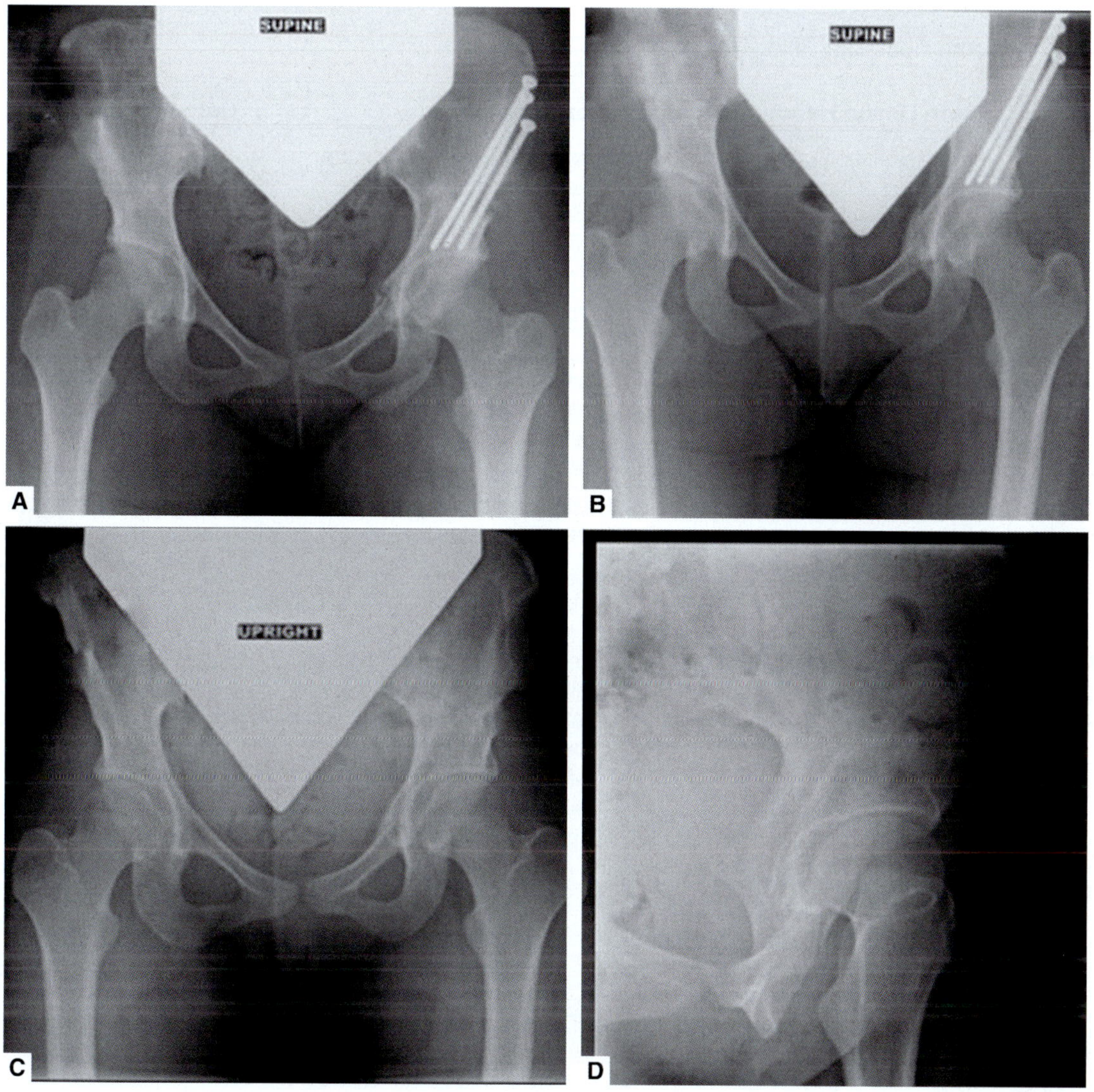

FIGURE 5.33: Follow-up x-rays. A, Supine anteroposterior (AP) pelvis x-ray at 4 weeks showing early signs of healing; hence, patient allowed progressively increased weight bearing. B, Supine AP at 3 months. Good healing started. Initiation of physical therapy. C, Standing AP pelvis and faux profil x-rays after 2 years and removal of screws.

nonunions (one in the pubic ramus and one in the posterior column), and stress fracture of the ischium formed most of the delayed complications. Five patients needed surgery for treating the delayed complications.[21]

One of the most dreaded complications of PAO is nerve injury. In the course of performing the PAO, the LFCN, sciatic, femoral, and obturator nerves are at risk of transient or permanent nerve injury. The reported incidence of nerve injury is around 2%, and almost half of these recover with time.[22] There are exposure techniques and ways of lower extremity positioning during different steps of the PAO, which may reduce the risk of any neurovascular injury[22-24] (**Table 5.4**).

Since PAO is a technically demanding surgery, appropriate mentoring with progressive surgical responsibility in a focused training program is desirable. Various studies have shown surgeon experience to be an important factor in reducing complications in PAO.[17,21,25-29]

CONCOMITANT ARTHROSCOPY WITH PERIACETABULAR OSTEOTOMY

Intra-articular pathology is very common in patients with acetabular dysplasia.[30-33] These can include proximal femoral cam deformity, labral tears and/or detachments, loose bodies, cartilage damage, and synovitis. Labral repair, femoral osteochondroplasty, microfracture, and removal of loose bodies are examples of procedures that are feasible through arthroscopic surgery in the setting of PAO.

TABLE 5.4 Avoiding Neurologic Injury

	Soft-Tissue Handling Tips	Positional Tips	Osteotomy Cuts
LFCN	Intrafascial mobilization of the TFL instead of dissecting within the tensor–sartorius interval.	Flexion of the hip to relax the nerve during initial deeper dissection.	
	Osteotomy of the ASIS with subperiosteal exposure of inner table of the pelvis to avoid undue manipulation.		
Obturator Nerve	Meticulous subperiosteal dissection on either side of the pubic ramus.	Flexion and adduction of the hip to make dissection easier while approaching the pubic ramus cut.	Using a Gigli saw or an osteotome with careful protection by retractors on either side of the ramus.
Femoral Nerve	Usually well protected by the iliopsoas muscle belly.	Flexion and slight adduction of the hip to relax the nerve.	If a large anterior and lateral correction attempted, the femoral nerve could be under stretch, which can be worsened by full hip extension.
Sciatic Nerve	Usually not at risk during soft-tissue dissection.	Extension and abduction of the hip with knee flexion helps relax the nerve. Important when performing the lateral part of the ischial cut as well the outer portion of the posterior column cut.	Lateral part of the ischial cut: Point the osteotome medially (toward contralateral shoulder) away from the nerve. Finishing the outer aspect of the posterior column cut: Avoid placing the chisel too far laterally (recognize the change in the pitch of the sound as the mallet strikes the osteotome). "Posterior column cut is more like splitting wood and less like sawing wood."

ASIS, anterior superior iliac spine; LFCN, lateral femoral cutaneous nerve; TFL, tensor fascia lata.

Advantages

1. Identify and treat intra-articular pathology.
2. Assess intra-articular cartilage. Rarely, if there is much more cartilage damage than expected, the planned PAO can be aborted.
3. Compared to arthrotomy, arthroscopy allows access to the entire central compartment and acetabular rim.

Disadvantages

1. Increased operative time
2. Potential for an increased risk of nerve injury due to traction followed by the osteotomy close to the sciatic nerve
3. Fluid extravasation into tissue planes prior to the PAO, which has the potential to make the soft-tissue dissection more difficult. There is also potential for more periarticular scarring postoperatively.

Technique

The hip arthroscopy is performed in the usual manner as described elsewhere in the book. Usually, two portals are used, anterolateral and the mid-anterior portal.

Pearls

- Minimizing the extent of capsulotomy will prevent fluid extravasation and allow easier anatomic dissection during the PAO.
- Keep the duration of the arthroscopic portion of the procedure to bare minimum to reduce fluid extravasation.
- Attempt to remove as much fluid as possible through the portals via suction.
- Performing only central compartment work on the labrum and acetabulum using the arthroscope, and doing any necessary peripheral compartment work through an arthrotomy minimizes traction time and fluid extravasation.
- The capsulotomy closure can be addressed better through the open anterior approach.

Pitfalls

- The dysplastic hip may not require as much traction as a nondysplastic hip, so care should be taken during setup for the hip arthroscopy using the traction table.
- The labrum in a dysplastic hip can be hypertrophic; hence, portal entry should be done carefully.
- Acetabular rim preparation for insertion of suture anchors for labral repair should be as minimal as possible and preferably be done using a shaver instead of a burr.

SUMMARY

Acetabular dysplasia can cause significant hip dysfunction and can be a hindrance to an active lifestyle in the adolescent and young adult population. Universal hip screening in infancy will definitely help in identifying hips at risk, but a certain proportion of young adults could have normal hips in infancy. Thus, prompt identification followed by adequate radiologic assessment and appropriate treatment is paramount not only in keeping this young population active but will also preserve the native hip for as long as possible. The use of a single cosmetic incision with the ability to achieve high degrees of correction in all planes and a very stable fragment fixation enabling early mobilization makes PAO a very attractive treatment option for acetabular dysplasia. However, it is important to remember that it is a technically complex procedure with a steep learning curve and a real risk of major complication.

REFERENCES

1. Lee CB, Mata-Fink A, Millis MB, Kim Y-J. Demographic differences in adolescent-diagnosed and adult-diagnosed acetabular dysplasia compared with infantile developmental dysplasia of the hip. *J Pediatr Orthop*. 2013;33(2):107-111. PMID: 23389561.
2. Tönnis D, Remus W. Development of hip dysplasia in puberty due to delayed ossification of femoral nucleus, growth plate and triradiate cartilage. *J Pediatr Orthop B*. 2004;13(5):287-292. PMID: 15552553.
3. Pun S. Hip dysplasia in the young adult caused by residual childhood and adolescent-onset dysplasia. *Curr Rev Musculoskelet Med*. 2016;9(4):427-434. PMCID: PMC5127949.
4. Sankar WN, Duncan ST, Baca GR, et al. Descriptive epidemiology of acetabular dysplasia: the Academic Network of Conservational Hip Outcomes Research (ANCHOR) periacetabular osteotomy. *J Am Acad Orthop Surg*. 2017;25(2):150-159. PMID: 28098707.
5. Nunley RM, Prather H, Hunt D, Schoenecker PL, Clohisy JC. Clinical presentation of symptomatic acetabular dysplasia in skeletally mature patients. *J Bone Joint Surg Am*. 2011 May;93(Suppl 2):17-21. PMID: 21543683.
6. Clohisy JC, Carlisle JC, Beaulé PE, et al. A systematic approach to the plain radiographic evaluation of the young adult hip. *J Bone Joint Surg Am*. 2008;90(Suppl 4):47-66. PMCID: PMC2682767.
7. Nepple JJ, Wells J, Ross JR, Bedi A, Schoenecker PL, Clohisy JC. Three patterns of acetabular deficiency are common in young adult patients with acetabular dysplasia. *Clin Orthop Relat Res*. 2017 Apr;475(4):1037-1044. PMCID: PMC5339139.
8. Wells J, Nepple JJ, Crook K, et al. Femoral morphology in the dysplastic hip: three-dimensional characterizations with CT. *Clin Orthop Relat Res*. 2017;475(4):1045-1054. PMCID: PMC5339134.
9. Cunningham T, Jessel R, Zurakowski D, Millis MB, Kim Y-J. Delayed gadolinium-enhanced magnetic resonance imaging of cartilage to predict early failure of Bernese periacetabular osteotomy for hip dysplasia. *J Bone Joint Surg Am*. 2006;88(7):1540-1548. PMID: 16818980.
10. d'Hemecourt PA, Sugimoto D, McKee-Proctor M, et al. Can dynamic ultrasonography of the hip reliably assess anterior femoral head translation? *Clin Orthop Relat Res*. 2019;477(5):1086-1098. PMID: 30531425.
11. Clohisy JC, Ackerman J, Baca G, et al. Patient-reported outcomes of periacetabular osteotomy from the prospective ANCHOR cohort study. *J Bone Joint Surg Am*. 2017;99(1):33-41. PMCID: PMC5198872.
12. Albers CE, Steppacher SD, Ganz R, Tannast M, Siebenrock KA. Impingement adversely affects 10-year survivorship after periacetabular osteotomy for DDH. *Clin Orthop Relat Res*. 2013;471(5):1602-1614. PMCID: PMC3613512.
13. Steppacher SD, Tannast M, Ganz R, Siebenrock KA. Mean 20-year follow-up of Bernese periacetabular osteotomy. *Clin Orthop Relat Res*. 2008;466(7):1633-1644. PMCID: PMC2505253.
14. Lerch TD, Steppacher SD, Liechti EF, Tannast M, Siebenrock KA. One-third of hips after periacetabular osteotomy survive 30 years with good clinical results, no progression of arthritis, or conversion to THA. *Clin Orthop Relat Res*. 2017;475(4):1154-1168. PMCID: PMC5339143.
15. Matheney T, Kim Y-J, Zurakowski D, Matero C, Millis M. Intermediate to long-term results following the Bernese periacetabular osteotomy and predictors of clinical outcome. *J Bone Joint Surg Am*. 2009;91(9):2113-2123. PMID: 19723987.
16. Wells J, Millis M, Kim Y-J, Bulat E, Miller P, Matheney T. Survivorship of the Bernese periacetabular osteotomy: what factors are associated with long-term failure? *Clin Orthop Relat Res*. 2017;475(2):396-405. PMCID: PMC5213921.
17. Troelsen A. Assessment of adult hip dysplasia and the outcome of surgical treatment. *Dan Med J*. 2012;59(6):B4450. PMID: 22677250.
18. Hartig-Andreasen C, Troelsen A, Thillemann TM, Søballe K. What factors predict failure 4 to 12 years after periacetabular osteotomy? *Clin Orthop Relat Res*. 2012;470(11):2978-2987. PMCID: PMC3462869.
19. Troelsen A, Elmengaard B, Søballe K. Medium-term outcome of periacetabular osteotomy and predictors of conversion to total hip replacement. *J Bone Joint Surg Am*. 2009;91(9):2169-2179. PMID: 19723994.
20. Matheney T, Kim Y-J, Zurakowski D, Matero C, Millis M. Intermediate to long-term results following the Bernese periacetabular osteotomy and predictors of clinical outcome: surgical technique. *J Bone Joint Surg Am*. 2010;92(Suppl 1 Pt 2):115-129. PMID: 20844169.
21. Zaltz I, Baca G, Kim Y-J, et al. Complications associated with the periacetabular osteotomy: a prospective multicenter study. *J Bone Joint Surg Am. 2014*;96(23):1967-1974. PMID: 25471911.
22. Sierra RJ, Beaule P, Zaltz I, et al. Prevention of nerve injury after periacetabular osteotomy. *Clin Orthop Relat Res*. 2012;470(8):2209-2219. PMCID: PMC3392380.
23. Kalhor M, Collado D, Leunig M, Rego P, Ganz R. Recommendations to reduce risk of nerve injury during Bernese Periacetabular Osteotomy (PAO*)*. *JBJS Essent Surg Tech*. 2017;7(4):e34. PMCID: PMC6132992.
24. Kalhor M, Gharehdaghi J, Schoeniger R, Ganz R. Reducing the risk of nerve injury during Bernese periacetabular osteotomy: a cadaveric study. *Bone Joint J*. 2015;97-B(5):636-641. PMID: 25922457.
25. Hussell JG, Rodriguez JA, Ganz R. Technical complications of the Bernese periacetabular osteotomy. *Clin Orthop Relat Res*. 1999;(363):81-92. PMID: 10379308.
26. Novais EN, Carry PM, Kestel LA, Ketterman B, Brusalis CM, Sankar WN. Does surgeon experience impact the risk of complications after Bernese periacetabular osteotomy? *Clin Orthop Relat Res*. 2017;475(4):1110-1117. PMCID: PMC5339113.

27. Thawrani D, Sucato DJ, Podeszwa DA, DeLaRocha A. Complications associated with the Bernese periacetabular osteotomy for hip dysplasia in adolescents. *J Bone Joint Surg Am*. 2010;92(8):1707-1714. PMID: 20660233.
28. Biedermann R, Donnan L, Gabriel A, Wachter R, Krismer M, Behensky H. Complications and patient satisfaction after periacetabular pelvic osteotomy. *Int Orthop*. 2008;32(5):611-617. PMCID: PMC2551712.
29. Howie DW, Beck M, Costi K, Pannach SM, Ganz R. Mentoring in complex surgery: minimising the learning curve complications from peri-acetabular osteotomy. *Int Orthop*. 2012;36(5):921-925. PMCID: PMC3337117.
30. Ross JR, Zaltz I, Nepple JJ, Schoenecker PL, Clohisy JC. Arthroscopic disease classification and interventions as an adjunct in the treatment of acetabular dysplasia. *Am J Sports Med*. 2011;39(Suppl):72S-78S. PMID: 21709035.
31. Goronzy J, Franken L, Hartmann A, et al. What are the results of surgical treatment of hip dysplasia with concomitant cam deformity? *Clin Orthop Relat Res*. 2017;475(4):1128-1137. PMCID: PMC5339118.
32. Kohno Y, Nakashima Y, Hatano T, et al. High prevalence of cam deformity in dysplastic hips: a three-dimensional CT study. *J Orthop Res*. 2016;34(9):1613-1619. PMID: 26713404.
33. Domb BG, Lareau JM, Baydoun H, Botser I, Millis MB, Yen Y-M. Is intraarticular pathology common in patients with hip dysplasia undergoing periacetabular osteotomy? *Clin Orthop Relat Res*. 2014;472(2):674-680. PMCID: PMC3890175.

CHAPTER

6 Stable Slipped Capital Femoral Epiphysis

FUNDAMENTAL PRINCIPLES OF SLIPPED CAPITAL FEMORAL EPIPHYSIS

Epidemiology and Etiology

Slipped capital femoral epiphysis (SCFE) is a disorder of the proximal femur in which the capital femoral epiphysis displaces in a posterior and inferior direction about the metaphysis. SCFE is the most common hip disorder affecting adolescents. The overall incidence of SCFE is 10.8 in 100 000, and it is more predominant in males.[1] The average age of presentation is 12 years for boys and 11 for girls.[2]

The etiology of SCFE is thought to be multifactorial with biologic, endocrine, and mechanical factors playing a role. Historically, SCFE is associated with obesity. However, only recently, one study confirmed a causal association between obesity and SCFE.[3] Another study showed that high levels of leptin, a polypeptide hormone secreted by adipocytes that has been shown to weaken the growth plate, are present in patients with SCFE independent of obesity.[4] The etiology of SCFE involves mechanical predisposition related to the morphology of the proximal femur. Femoral retroversion and increased posterior tilt of the capital femoral epiphysis are well-accepted factors associated with the etiology of SCFE.[5] Contemporary studies have proposed a rotational mechanism of SCFE, whereas the epiphysis rotates around the metaphysis with the epiphyseal tubercle serving as a fulcrum.[6]

Clinical Evaluation

The typical clinical presentation is of an adolescent with a history of knee, hip, or groin pain with a slight limp. The diagnosis may be delayed because patients can initially complain of knee or anterior thigh pain instead of actual hip pain. SCFE should be in the differential diagnosis in an adolescent who presents with unspecific thigh or knee pain, and, at minimum, a dedicated hip examination is recommended. Clinical evaluation includes assessment of patient's standing posture and gait pattern. Outward rotation of the involved lower extremity and a slight limp with the foot externally rotated can be observed at initial presentation. Direct examination of the hip may reveal abnormal range of motion. Flexion and internal rotation are the most commonly restricted and could elicit pain. Given the reduced femoral anteversion of the femur in SCFE, flexion of the hip requires external rotation, the so-called obligatory external rotation sign.

SCFE can be classified according to the timing of presentation, severity of the deformity, and stability of the capital femoral epiphysis. In regard to the time of presentation, SCFE is classified as acute if symptoms have been present for 3 weeks or less, chronic if symptoms have been present for more than 3 weeks, and acute on chronic when symptoms are present for more than 3 weeks but there is an acute exacerbation.[7] According to Loder and colleagues,[8] a slip is classified as unstable if the patient has such severe pain that walking is not possible even with crutches, regardless of the duration of the symptoms. The slip is classified as stable if walking and weight bearing are still possible with or without crutches. The severity of the slip displacement is classified using specific radiographic criteria.

The diagnosis of SCFE requires radiographic imaging, including an anteroposterior pelvic plain film and a lateral film of the femur. Although the frog-leg view is our preferred lateral radiograph, in acute and unstable slips, pain may limit the ability to obtain the adequate image, and a cross-table lateral view should be obtained to avoid pain and further epiphyseal displacement. Because of the high occurrence of bilateral SCFE, an anteroposterior pelvic film and bilateral lateral radiographs are recommended in the initial evaluation even in patients with unilateral symptoms. The radiographic appearance of SCFE varies according to the chronicity of the disease and the severity of the epiphyseal displacement. Radiographic classification of the displacement is performed by measuring the Southwick angle.[9] The Southwick angle measures the alignment of the femoral head in relation to the diaphysis. SCFE can, therefore, be classified as mild when the angle is less than 30°, moderate if the angle is between 30° and 60°, and severe when the Southwick angle is higher than 60° (**Figure 6.1**). Slight widening of the physis and lucency around the

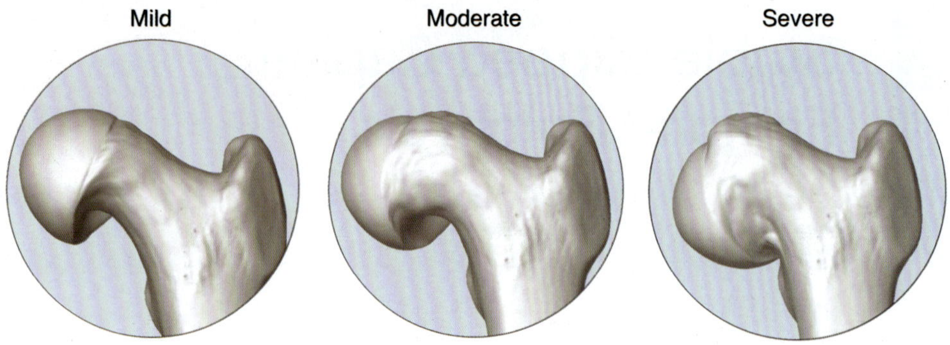

FIGURE 6.1. Diagram representing different severity of slipped capital femoral epiphysis displacement as mild, moderate, and severe. The epiphysis displaces in an inferior and posterior direction creating a retroversion deformity of the proximal femur, with the metaphysis being externally rotated about the epiphysis. Illustration by Nathan Billington.

epiphyseal tubercle (*peritubercle lucency sign*) are the early radiographic signs that may be present in the early preslip phase and in mild SCFE. With further displacement, the superior aspect of the femoral neck (Klein line) does not cross the epiphysis, and the alignment of the epiphysis assessed by the Southwick angle and the epiphyseal tilt or posterior slope becomes posteriorly oriented. Magnetic resonance imaging (MRI) and computed tomography (CT) are helpful to determine the extent of cartilage damage and the severity of deformity and to plan for femoral realignment osteotomy when indicated. Three-dimensional (3-D) printed modeling is a promising technique that improves the surgeon's ability to treat a severe SCFE deformity.

Treatment

Treatment of SCFE involves several controversies. Recommendations for treatment are based on the severity of displacement and instability of the epiphysis. Overall goals for treatment include stabilization of the epiphysis while avoiding the occurrence of complications, mainly osteonecrosis of the femoral head. A secondary goal for SCFE treatment is avoiding residual deformity of the femur that has been associated with femoroacetabular impingement (FAI) and articular cartilage degeneration and arthritis.[10-12]

Because treatment of a slip is guided by the stability and severity of displacement, we present principles of treatment of stable and unstable SCFE in different chapters of this book.

Treatment Algorithm for Stable Slipped Capital Femoral Epiphysis

For stable SCFE, the procedure performed most often is in situ fixation of the epiphysis (**Figure 6.2**). In situ pinning has been proven to allow for good long-term outcomes in mild SCFE; however in severe SCFE, there is a higher risk of deformity, causing FAI and long-term osteoarthritis.[13]

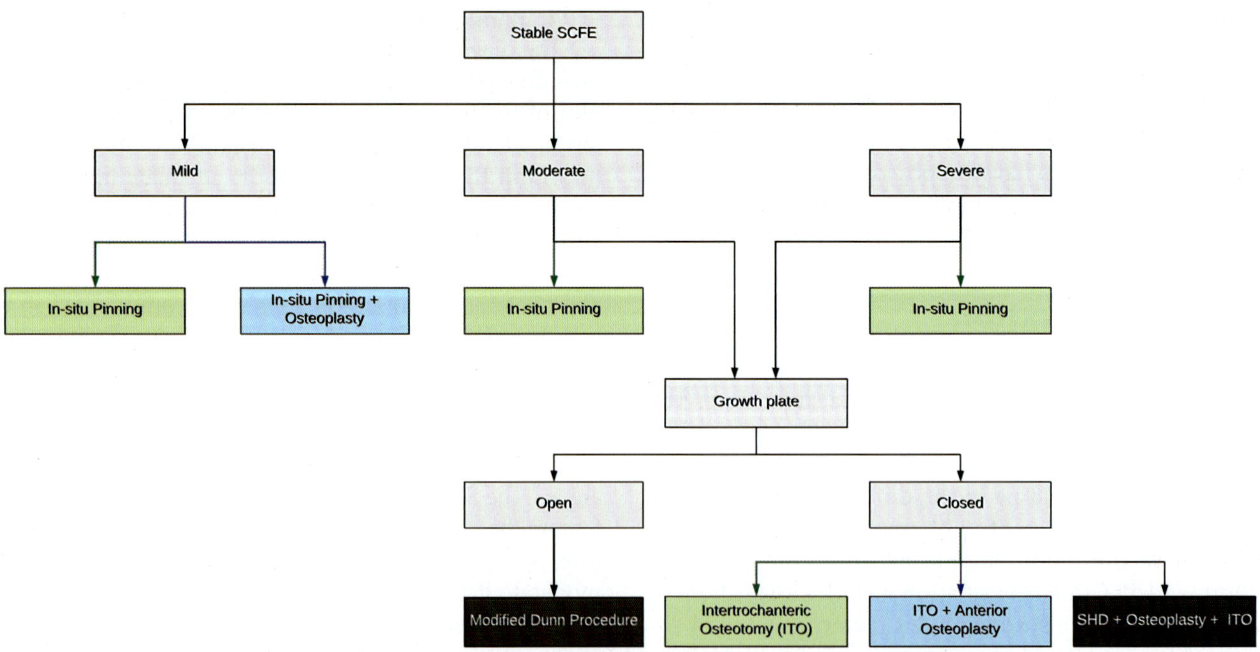

FIGURE 6.2. Treatment algorithm for stable slipped capital femoral epiphysis. The level of complexity is represented by the skiing categories: green (standard of care or easy techniques), blue (moderate level of difficulty), and black (high level of difficulty).

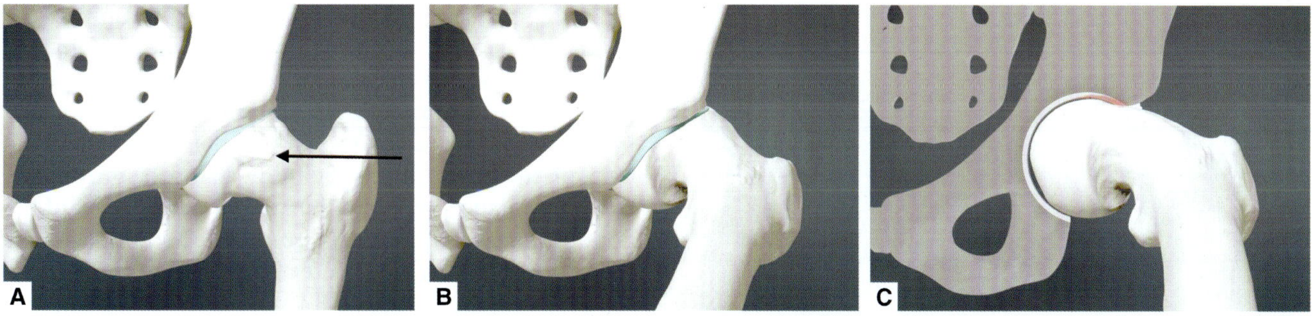

FIGURE 6.3. Diagram representing the mechanism of femoroacetabular impingement (FAI) in slipped capital femoral epiphysis. A, With progressive displacement of the epiphysis posteriorly and inferiorly, a metaphyseal prominence develops at the femoral head–neck junction (black arrow). B, Impaction type of impingement: the metaphyseal prominence abuts against the acetabular rim, deforming the acetabular labrum (in light blue). C, Inclusion type of impingement: with remodeling of the femoral head–neck junction, the metaphyseal prominence does not block motion. Instead, the metaphyseal bone enters the joint and impinges against the acetabular cartilage, causing damage represented in red. Illustration by Nathan Billington.

Historically, multiple pins have been used for the treatment of SCFE; however, contemporary fixation can be performed using guided fluoroscopy imaging and a cannulated screw system. In situ pinning is a universally applied surgical technique. Traditionally, the goal has been to provide stabilization of the epiphysis while allowing for closure of the growth plate. However, in situ pinning using nontransphyseal screw devices allows for femoral neck growth, increased remodeling of the deformity with an overall improvement of the femoral head–neck offset, and avoidance of FAI in mild SCFE.

In situ fixation has a long-term prognosis that is benign for patients with a mild deformity; however, with increasing deformity, there is a higher risk of degeneration changes of the hip and development of osteoarthritis secondary to cam-type FAI.[10-12] Even in mild SCFE at the early stages of the disease, cartilage damage can be present. Cartilage damage occurs because of impingement from the metaphysis into the acetabular rim. In SCFE, the impingement is thought to be an impact between the metaphyseal prominence into the acetabular rim, but with time and remodeling of the deformity, the metaphysis would enter the joint and damage the cartilage, which is called an inclusion type of impingement[14] (**Figure 6.3**). Because of the risk of cartilage damage associated even with mild SCFE, early resection of the metaphyseal prominence during in situ pinning may be of benefit. In moderate and severe unstable SCFE, in situ pinning may allow for resolution of symptoms in the short term with stabilization of the physis. However, the severity of the deformity is unlikely to allow for complete remodeling, and FAI would persist with a high likelihood of articular cartilage damage and osteoarthritis in the long term.[11-13] Treatment of moderate and severe SCFE, therefore, is often traditionally performed by in situ pinning alone with close monitoring for patients developing symptoms of FAI with further treatment by a proximal femoral realignment osteotomy. We, however, favor acute correction of the moderate and severe SCFE deformity. Realignment of severe SCFE can be performed at the subcapital level, base of the femoral neck, and intertrochanteric and subtrochanteric level. Although controversy surrounds the best level for deformity correction, most authors accept that close to anatomic realignment is only possible at the subcapital level. We favor subcapital realignment in moderate and severe SCFE using the modified Dunn technique through a surgical hip dislocation approach as in patients with wide-open growth plate. In skeletally mature patients with closed proximal femoral growth plates and moderate or severe SCFE deformity leading to FAI, our preferred technique is the surgical hip dislocation approach with osteochondroplasty of the femoral head–neck junction in association with an intertrochanteric flexion derotational osteotomy.

SURGICAL PROCEDURES

In Situ Pinning

Clinical Scenario

A 10-year-old boy presents with hip pain and a limp for several weeks, aggravated this past week after he tripped and fall at school. Radiographs obtained at presentation revealed a mild SCFE that was considered acute on chronic and stable (**Figure 6.4**).

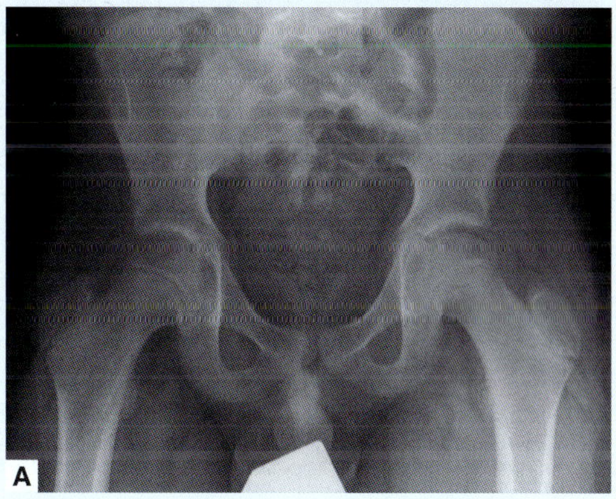

FIGURE 6.4. A, Anteroposterior pelvic radiograph showing slight widening of the right proximal femoral growth plate. B, Frog-leg lateral radiograph showing wide and irregular growth plate with mild posterior displacement of the epiphysis.

(continued)

Clinical Scenario (*continued*)

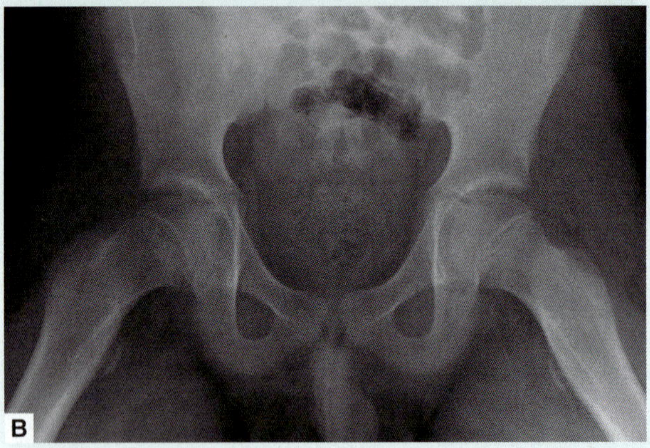

FIGURE 6.4. (*continued*)

Although in situ pinning can be performed with the patient on a fracture table, it is our preferred method to perform the surgery with the patient in a radiolucent flat table. A gel roll is placed under the patient's ipsilateral shoulder to allow for slightly trunk rotation, which aligns the lower extremity in neutral rotation with the patella pointing upward. The entire hemipelvis and the lower extremity are prepared and draped free.

Under C-arm fluoroscopy, the anteroposterior trajectory of the guidewire is marked aiming toward the center of the femoral head with an attempt to avoid the superior aspect of the femoral head to avoid the area corresponding to the epiphyseal tubercle and the penetration of the epiphyseal vessels. A line is drawn on the skin in line with the guidewire marking the trajectory of the pin in the anteroposterior view. The skin incision is performed in line with the guidewire mark in the anterolateral aspect of the thigh. Then, Schnidt clamp is introduced through the incision up to the anterolateral aspect of the bone at the level of the entry point. The Schnidt clamp is then spread, which would create a tunnel of the soft tissue (**Figure 6.5**). We use an 8-gauge bone marrow biopsy needle (Harvest Terumo BCT, Lakewood, Colorado) that is introduced to the desired point in the anterolateral aspect of the proximal femur. The needle is gently tapped into the desired entry point using C-arm fluoroscopy in the anteroposterior view (**Figure 6.6**). The hip is flexed up to about 45°, whereas the C-arm fluoroscopy view is moved into an oblique view to about 45°, which will allow for adequate visualization of a lateral view of the femur. By flexing the hip and rotating the C-arm, we avoid the popular maneuver to obtain the lateral view placing the hip in abduction and external rotation. Moving the hip in external rotation to allow for lateral view may cause bending of the guidewire. With the C-arm in the lateral view and with the hip flexed, the bone marrow biopsy needle can then be adjusted to aim toward the center of the femoral head (**Figure 6.7**). Typically, the surgeon's hand should move slightly posteriorly because the anterior entry point in the femur may create an excessively posterior path through the neck and end in the posterior quadrant of the epiphysis. The needle and later the screw should aim toward the center of the

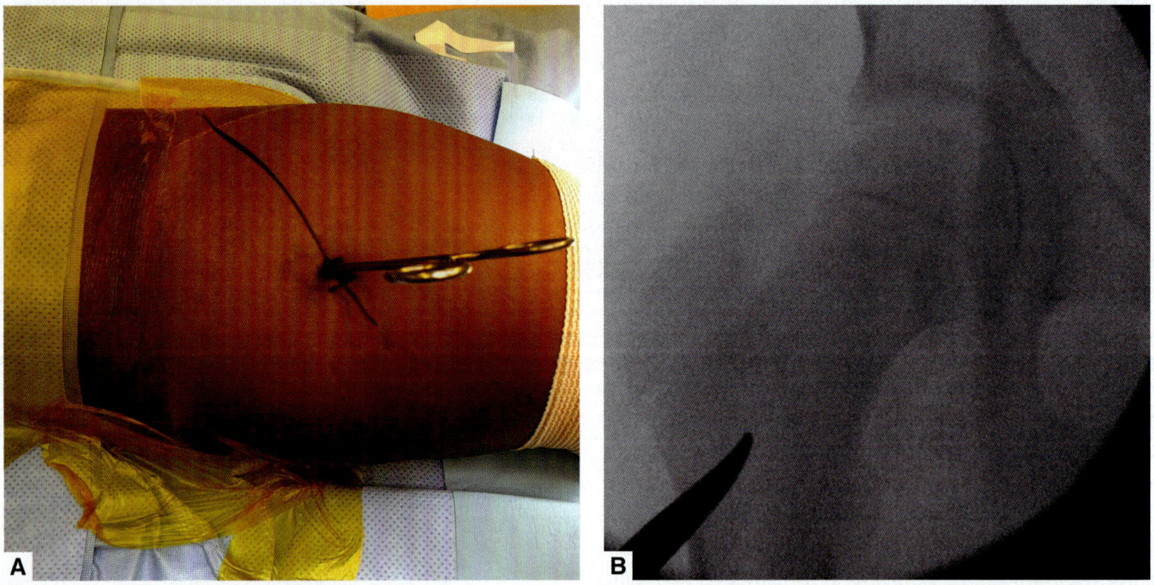

FIGURE 6.5. A, Intraoperative photography showing the insertion of a Schnidt clamp in the anterolateral aspect of the proximal femur in line with the femoral neck axis previously marked in the skin. B, Intraoperative fluoroscopy imaging corresponding to the placement of the Schnidt clamp in the anterolateral aspect of the femur.

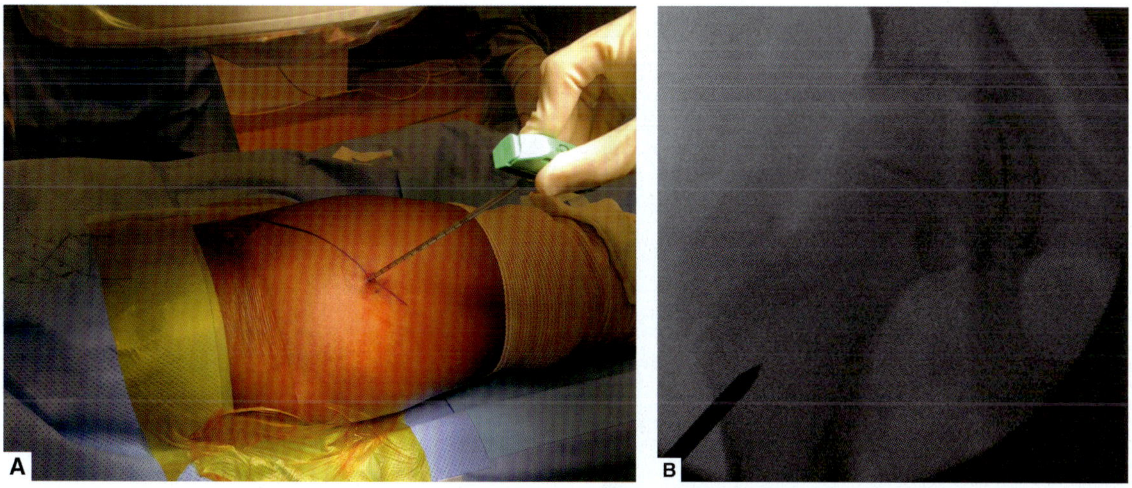

FIGURE 6.6. A, Intraoperative photography showing the insertion of an 8-gauge bone marrow biopsy needle (Harvest Terumo BCT, Lakewood, Colorado) in line with the skin mark. B, Intraoperative fluoroscopy imaging corresponding to the placement of the bone marrow biopsy needle in the anterolateral aspect of the femur.

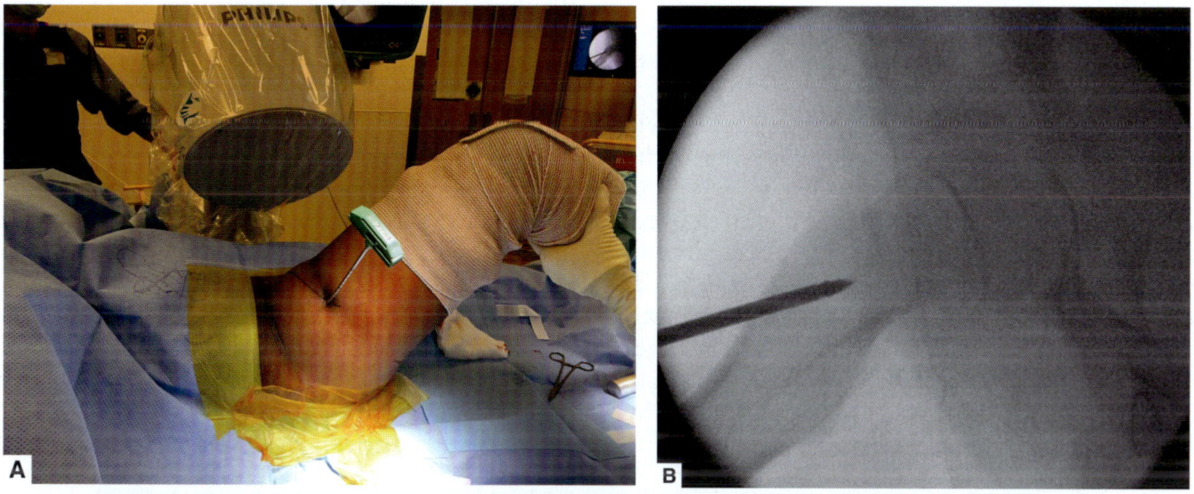

FIGURE 6.7. A, Intraoperative photography showing the position of the lower extremity for lateral radiograph. The hip is in neutral and flexed to about 45°, whereas the C-arm fluoroscopy is arched about 45°. As the bone marrow biopsy needle has been introduced in the femur, it does not disengage from the bone with simple flexion. B, Intraoperative fluoroscopy imaging in the lateral view showing the bone marrow biopsy needle adequately corrected to aim toward the center of the femoral head.

femoral head avoiding the posterior aspect of the epiphysis again to avoid penetration of the epiphyseal tubercle and the epiphyseal vessels. It is at this point during the procedure that the use of the bone marrow biopsy needle is very helpful. With gentle tapping, the bone marrow biopsy needle can be introduced into the anterolateral aspect of the metaphysis about 3 or 5 mm inside the bone. Slightly adjustments into varus or valgus or anterior or posterior direction are facilitated by the use of the bone marrow biopsy needle. Once the needle is placed in the adequate position, the internal trocar of the needle is removed and a long guidewire for the cannulated screw is introduced through the needle (**Figure 6.8**). An additional advantage of this technique is that the bone marrow biopsy needle allows for slightly adjustments in varus or valgus or anterior or posterior direction without bending of the guidewire. The wire is then advanced, while confirmation with the C-arm fluoroscopy is made with the anteroposterior view and the lateral view with the hip flex to about 45° and the C-arm machine in the oblique view at 45°. We cannot emphasize enough that to avoid bending of the wire, the hip is flexed up to 45° but is not brought into an external rotation or abduction in the typical figure-of-four or frog-leg lateral position, which is not necessary for perfect placement of the pin. It is our preference to advance the wire just

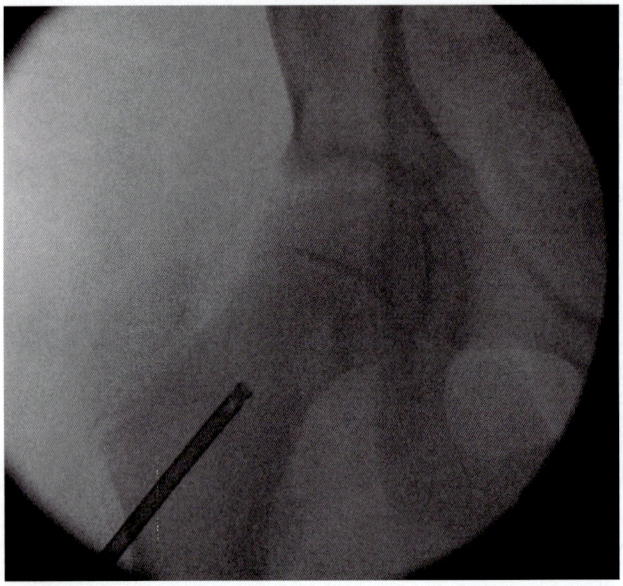

FIGURE 6.8. Intraoperative fluoroscopy in the anteroposterior view after the internal trocar of the bone marrow biopsy needle has been removed. The needle is confirmed to be pointing toward the center of the femoral head.

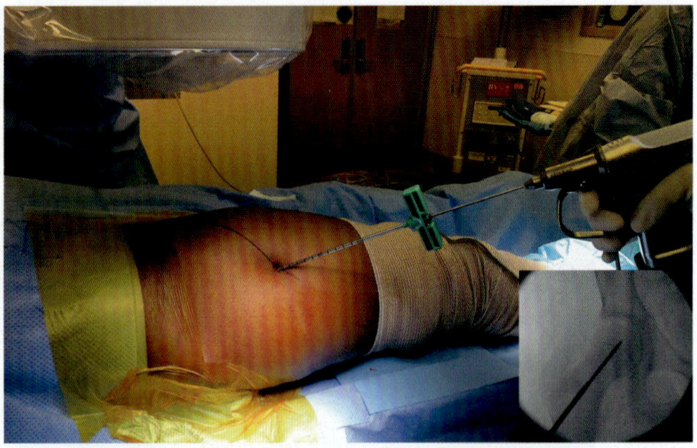

FIGURE 6.9. Intraoperative photography showing the introduction of the long guidewire through the bone marrow biopsy needle. In the bottom right corner, the correspondent fluoroscopy view shows the long guidewire introduced through the biopsy needle.

slightly passed the physis but not penetrating excessively the epiphysis to avoid any inadvertent penetration of the articular cartilage (**Figure 6.9**). Once the guidewire is in place, then the bone marrow biopsy needle is removed, and the regular soft-tissue protection is placed around the guidewire and the cannulated drill is inserted. It is our preference to drill just barely passed the growth plate into the epiphysis again to avoid inadvertent penetration of the femoral head cartilage while drilling and, more importantly, to avoid excessive heating caused by the drill, which has been identified as a potential cause of focal osteonecrosis of the femoral head (**Figure 6.10**). The guidewire is then measured, and we prefer to tap the screw path, even though the modern cannulated screws are self-tapping. Using the tap tool may protect from excessive heating while introducing the screw. It is our preference to use a fully threaded screw with a minimum of five threads placed across the growth plate into the epiphysis. For patients aged 10 years and younger, we use a 6.5-mm screw, whereas for patients older than 10 years, we prefer a larger screw of 7.3 mm. After the screw is introduced, a full inspection of the radiographic appearance is confirmed with an anteroposterior, frog-leg lateral, and a 45° Dunn view (**Figure 6.11**).

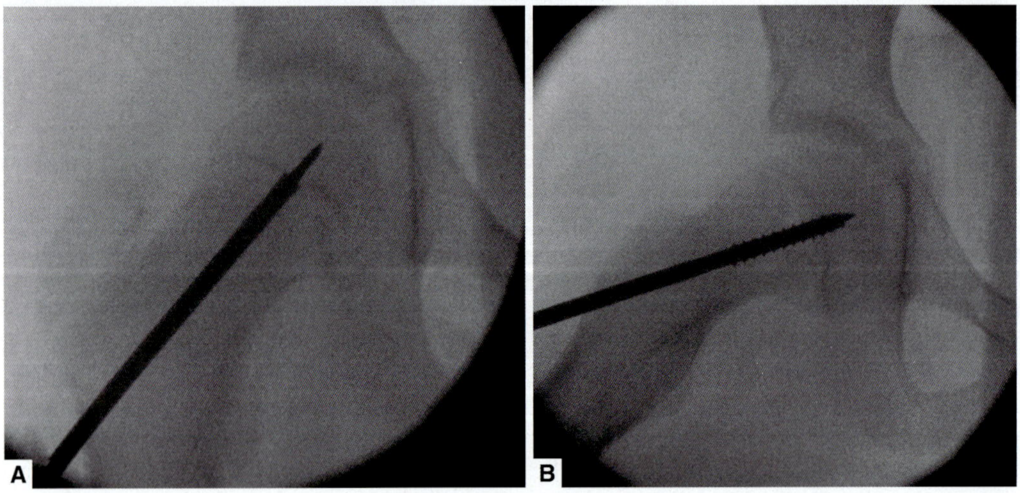

FIGURE 6.10. A, Intraoperative fluoroscopy in the anteroposterior view after the cannulated drill is introduced. Drill is placed just slightly past the physis to avoid excessive heating and inadvertent penetration of the femoral head. B, Intraoperative fluoroscopy imaging in the lateral view showing the tapping tool advanced past the physis into the femoral head.

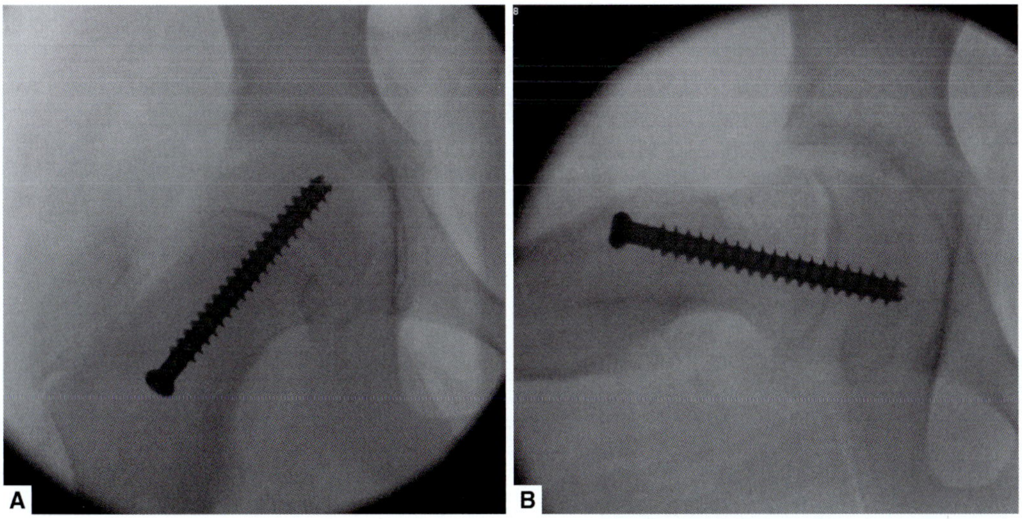

FIGURE 6.11. A, Final intraoperative anteroposterior view with the C-arm fluoroscopy revealing optimal position of the screw in center of the femoral head with five threads past the physis. B, Final intraoperative frog-leg lateral radiograph revealing optimal position of the screw in the center of the femoral head.

Postoperatively, patients are instructed to be toe-touch weight bearing with two crutches for 6 weeks. A wheelchair is provided for school use and for long distances. We see patients for postoperative check at 2, 6, and 12 weeks when physical therapy may be recommended. Additional follow-up is obtained at 6 and 12 months from surgery when we expect to observe signs of physeal closure. Return to full activities including sports is typically allowed after 12 months from surgery. We followed up patients with SCFE until they achieve skeletal maturity age to monitor for contralateral slip development in those not treated prophylactically. Prophylactic fixation is controversial; however, in general, we offer prophylactic fixation for patients aged 10 years or younger, those with endocrine disorders, and patients with a triradiate cartilage that is wide opened with an unreliable family/social situation to allow for close follow-up (**Figure 6.12**).

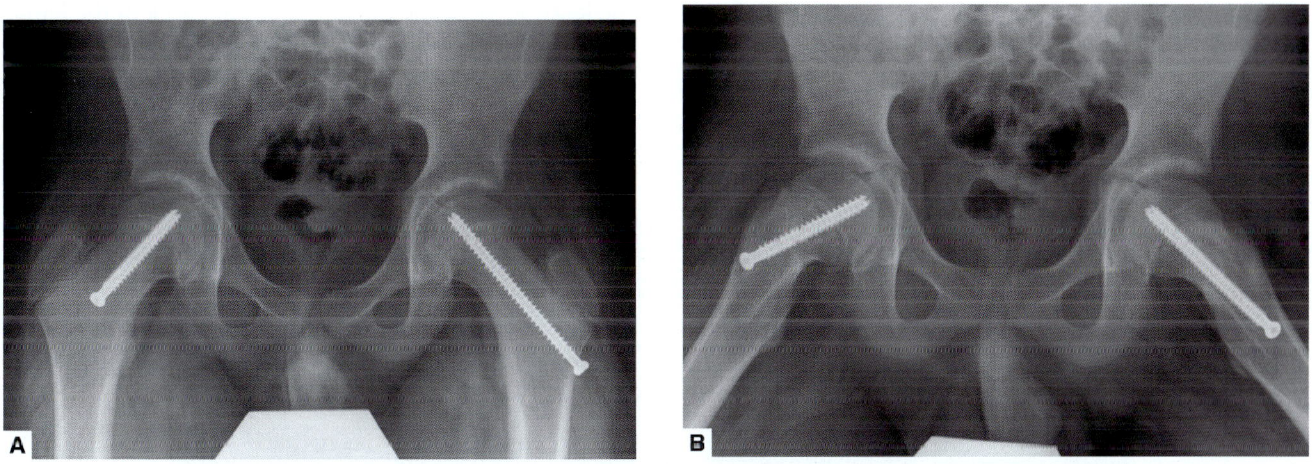

FIGURE 6.12. A, Anteroposterior pelvic radiograph obtained at 2 months postoperatively revealing correct placement of the screw for the right-sided slipped capital femoral epiphysis and for prophylactic fixation of the left hip. The indication for prophylactic fixation was based on age younger than or equal to 10 years. B, Postoperative bilateral frog-leg lateral radiograph revealing correct placement of the screws.

Clinical Scenario

A 13-year-old male presented with a limp and left hip pain and mildly displaced SCFE. Anteroposterior and frog-leg lateral radiographs revealed mild displacement of the capital femoral epiphysis (**Figure 6.13**).

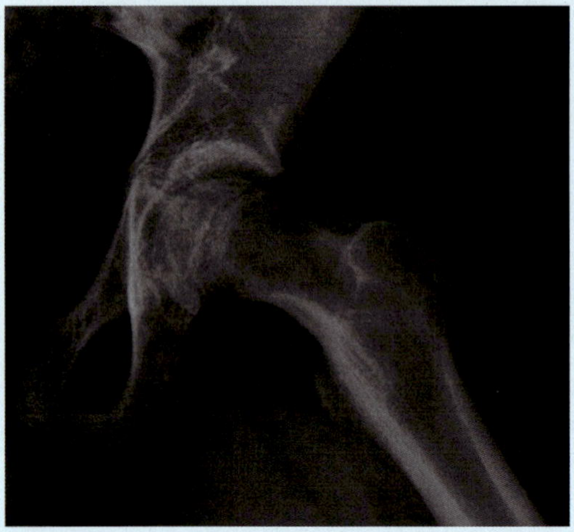

FIGURE 6.13. Preoperative frog-leg lateral radiograph of the hip revealing mild displacement of the epiphysis.

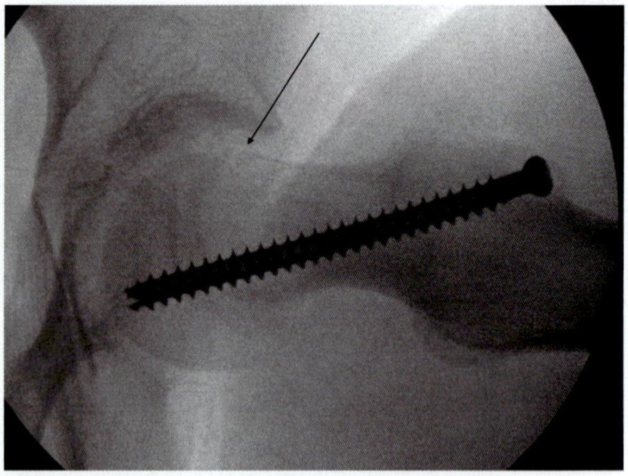

FIGURE 6.14. Intraoperative fluoroscopy revealing reduced femoral head and neck offset (black arrow) with the metaphysis of the femur inside the acetabulum.

In Situ Pinning + Osteochondroplasty of the Femoral Head–Neck Junction

We have performed osteochondroplasty using an arthroscopic approach that is described elsewhere in this book. We also have performed in situ pinning with an assisted mini-open approach using an anteriorly placed incision for a Smith-Petersen interval. Before the osteochondroplasty is performed, inclusion type of impingement with the metaphysis articulating with the cartilaginous surface of the acetabulum can be observed along with a reduced femoral head offset (**Figure 6.14**). For the anterior mini-open approach, a skin incision is performed 1 to 2 cm distal to the anterior superior iliac spine in an oblique manner aiming toward the fibular head and measuring about 8 to 10 cm. The subcutaneous tissue is dissected, and the fascia on top of the tensor fascia lata is open just laterally to the tensor fascia lata and sartorius interval to avoid damage to the lateral femoral cutaneous nerve. The tensor fascia lata is retracted laterally, and the rectus femoris is identified. The medial border of the rectus is identified, and an incision is made to expose the medial aspect of the rectus femoris tendon and muscle belly. The rectus is retracted laterally, and the iliocapsularis muscle can be elevated from the capsule medially with the iliopsoas. Once the capsule is exposed, a capsulotomy is performed in line with the femoral neck axis up to the level of the acetabular labrum. A T-shaped capsulotomy is then performed with a transverse limb parallel and distal to the labrum. With the capsule open, the neck of the femur is exposed, and the femoral head–neck junction can be trimmed using a combination of rongeur, curettes, and a high-speed bur. The osteochondroplasty is monitored with the C-arm fluoroscopy to avoid excessive or under-resection (**Figure 6.15**). The hip is tested dynamically and with

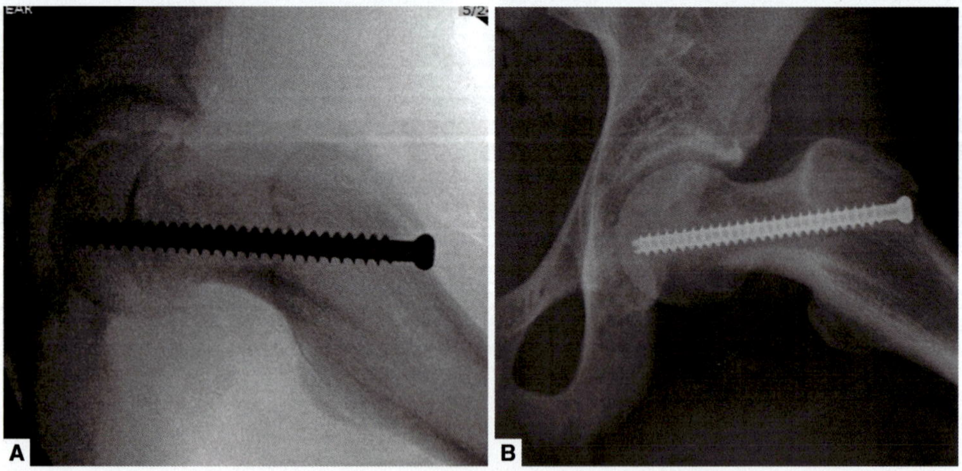

FIGURE 6.15. A, Intraoperative fluoroscopy after osteochondroplasty showing the femoral head and neck offset is restored to normal concavity. B, Postoperative frog-leg lateral radiographs of the left hip obtained 2 years after surgery revealing maintained normal femoral head–neck offset.

fluoroscopy to confirm no impingement is present with hip flexion and internal rotation. The hip capsule is closed, and the wound is closed layers. Postoperative protocol is similar to in situ pinning, but most patients undergoing and osteochondroplasty typically would require physical therapy starting at 6 weeks. The main advantage of performing the osteochondroplasty at the same setting is the acute treatment of the FAI morphology, which, in theory, may reduce the risk of cartilage damage.

Femoral Osteotomy for Slipped Capital Femoral Epiphysis and Postslip Deformity

Proximal femoral osteotomies for correction of SCFE or postslip deformity can be performed at the subcapital level,[15,16] through the femoral neck,[17] at the base of the femoral neck,[18,19] or at the intertrochanteric[20] or subtrochanteric level.[21] Our preferred technique is an intertrochanteric osteotomy for flexion and derotational osteotomy as described by Imhauser.[20] Although some authors recommend additional correction with valgus realignment during the osteotomy, the deformity associated with SCFE is retroversion of the proximal femur without true varus alignment, which can be corrected by the flexion component of the intertrochanteric osteotomy.

For the intertrochanteric osteotomy, the patient can be positioned supine close to the edge of the table with a blanket under the buttock to elevate the femur. However, it is our preferred technique to perform the osteotomy with the patient in the lateral decubitus, which facilitate control of the fragments, especially in obese teenagers (Figure 6.16). A longitudinal incision is placed on top of the greater trochanter for a direct lateral approach to the femur. Subcutaneous tissue dissection allows for exposure of the fascia lata. The fascia lata is opened in line with the skin incision, with careful exposure proximally to the greater trochanter between the gluteus maximus and the gluteus medius (Figure 6.17). The posterior fascia of the vastus lateralis is open longitudinally, and the vastus is elevated from the femur. Proximally, the insertion of the vastus lateralis is detached transversely up to the level of the vastus intermedius, allowing for full exposure of the greater trochanter and the metaphyseal diaphyseal junction (Figure 6.18). The periosteal of the femur can be opened circumferentially at the area of the planned osteotomy. Currently, choices for fixation of an intertrochanteric osteotomy include a blade plate or a proximal femoral locking plate. Surgery is performed using C-arm fluoroscopy. A guidewire is inserted through the base of the greater trochanter perpendicular to the long axis of the femoral shaft. The guidewire should be in the center of the femoral neck in the lateral view. For a large fragment blade plate, the typical distance from insertion to the osteotomy is around 2 or 2.5 cm depending on the plate manufacturer. A Kirschner (K) wire can be introduced at the level of the planned osteotomy parallel to the first wire. A cannulated chisel is inserted through the guidewire for the blade plate. Alternatively, the guiding block is placed into the bone for introduction of the two proximal screws if a locking plate is used. Angulation of the chisel is guided by the diaphyseal sleeve guide (Figure 6.19). If the sleeve

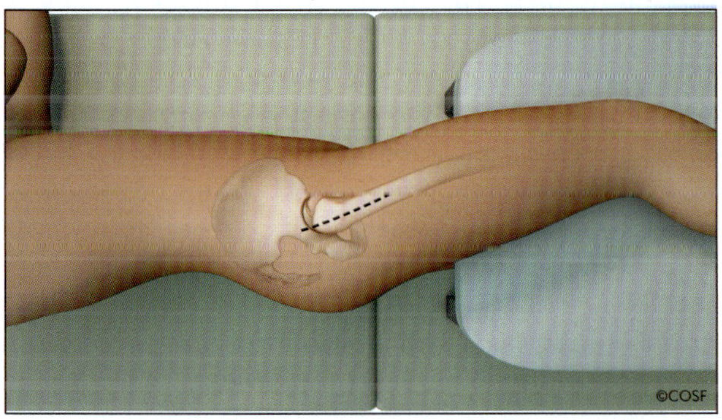

FIGURE 6.16. Illustration showing the patient positioned in the lateral decubitus and a longitudinal incision being placed on top of the greater trochanter for the intertrochanteric osteotomy technique for moderate or severe slipped capital femoral epiphysis. Black dashed line represents placement of the skin incision.

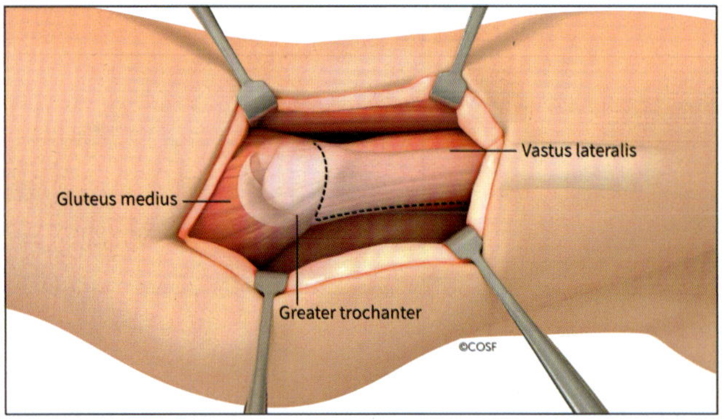

FIGURE 6.17. Illustration representing the fascia lata that has been opened in line with the skin incision with exposure proximally to the greater trochanter and identification of the gluteus maximus, gluteus medius, and vastus lateralis. A black dashed line marks the area of releasing the vastus lateralis from its insertion at the greater trochanter, leaving a small sleeve posteriorly for closure.

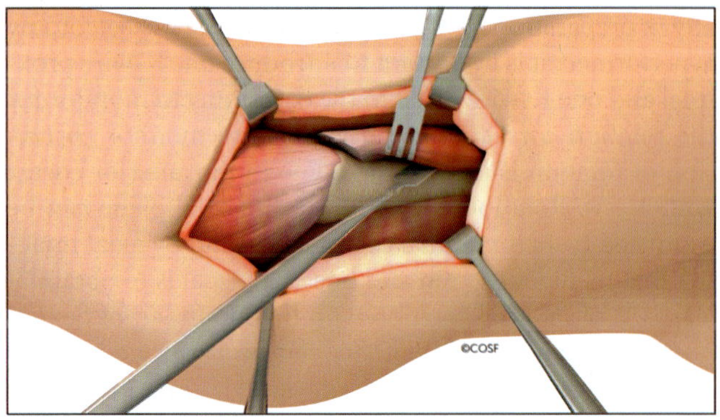

FIGURE 6.18. Illustration showing that proximally, the insertion of the vastus lateralis is detached transversely up to the level of the vastus intermedius. The posterior fascia of the vastus lateralis is open longitudinally, and the vastus is elevated from the femur.

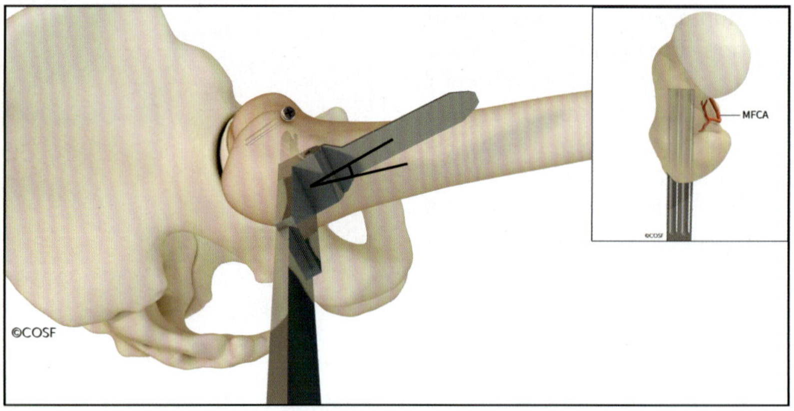

FIGURE 6.19. Illustration showing a guidewire inserted through the base of the greater trochanter perpendicular to the long axis of the femoral shaft. A cannulated chisel is inserted through the guidewire for the blade plate. The guidewire and the chisel should be in the center of the femoral neck in the lateral view but slightly anterior to the trochanter to avoid penetration of the posterior cortex of the femoral neck, which would risk damage to the deep branches of the medial femoral circumflex artery (MFCA) (top-right corner illustration). Angulation of the chisel is calculated by the diaphyseal sleeve guide. If the sleeve guide is aligned with the diaphysis, then no correction is obtained in the sagittal plane. Anterior angulation of the sleeve guide, as shown in this illustration (marked with a black line), creates an extension of the proximal fragment, whereas the distal fragment is flexed, which is the goal for slipped capital femoral epiphysis (SCFE) correction. The degree of angulation of the chisel in the sagittal plane is determined by the severity of the tilt between the femoral epiphysis and the femoral neck. The chisel is introduced into the greater trochanter with a mallet. We recommended introducing the chisel about 1 to 1.5 cm, then using the reverse tool or slotted fork to pull back the chisel about 5 mm before advancing the chisel further. C-arm fluoroscopy is used to guide the introduction of the chisel. After the chisel is introduced, the appropriate length of the blade component of the plate can be determined. If the femoral osteotomy is performed acutely at the time of SCFE presentation, then fixation of the epiphysis with a cannulated screw should be planned. The screw is placed anterior in the femoral neck, aiming toward the center of the femoral head and avoiding conflict with the blade or locking plate.

guide is aligned with the diaphysis, then no correction is obtained in the sagittal plane. Anterior displacement of the sleeve guide creates an extension of the proximal fragment while the distal fragment is flexed, which is the goal for SCFE correction. The degree of angulation of the chisel in the sagittal plane is determined by the severity of the tilt between the femoral epiphysis and the femoral neck. Another guide for correction is physical examination. Typically, the amount of correction is estimated by the lack of flexion with the hip in neutral. Often, the flexion correction is around 30°, and excessive correction beyond 45° should be avoided. After the chisel is introduced, the appropriate length of the blade component of the plate can be determined. Next, the osteotomy site is protected subperiosteally in preparation for the osteotomy. Before the osteotomy is performed, it is important to introduce one K-wire proximal and one K-wire distal to the osteotomy to monitor for the rotation correction. Another way to monitor correction of rotation is by creating a line in the anterior cortex with a saw. Rotation correction in the axial plane can be estimated by preoperative examination and by axial imaging that includes the hip and knee. The goal is to obtain at least 15° of internal rotation with the hip in 90° of flexion postoperatively. The osteotomy can be performed with a removal of an anterior wedge. However, it is our preference to perform a transverse osteotomy, which does not create shortening of the lower extremity and is relatively simpler (**Figure 6.20**). The osteotomy is then performed perpendicular to the long axis of the femoral diaphysis, whereas two Crigo or Hohmann retractors protect the femur subperiosteally. Once the osteotomy is performed, a large bone clamp is used to hold the proximal femur, and the chisel can be removed. A 90° blade plate is then inserted in the proximal femur in line with the cut created by the chisel, which is facilitated using a cannulated blade system. An additional screw can be inserted in the proximal femur just distal to the blade to augment the fixation. After fixation to the plate, the proximal fragment is brought into extension, and the plate will be aligned with the distal fragment. The distal fragment is then internally rotated following preoperative planning and reduced to the plate (**Figure 6.21**). The plate is then fixed to the distal fragment using the typical compression technique (**Figure 6.22**). The vastus lateralis is reattached, and the wound is further closed in layers. Postoperatively, the patient is encouraged to use a pair of crutches with a toe-touch weight bearing for the first 8 weeks after surgery. Gradual weight bearing is advanced for additional 4 weeks with crutches, and typically around 3 months after surgery, there is enough healing to allow for weight bearing to be advanced without crutches. Thromboprophylaxis with aspirin is recommended during the period of immobilization for 4 weeks following surgery. Complications of intertrochanteric osteotomy are associated with failure of hardware and delayed union and chondrolysis of the femoral head. In the long term, about 60% of patients with severe SCFE treated with an Imhauser osteotomy were found to have neither symptoms nor radiographic signs of osteoarthritis.[22]

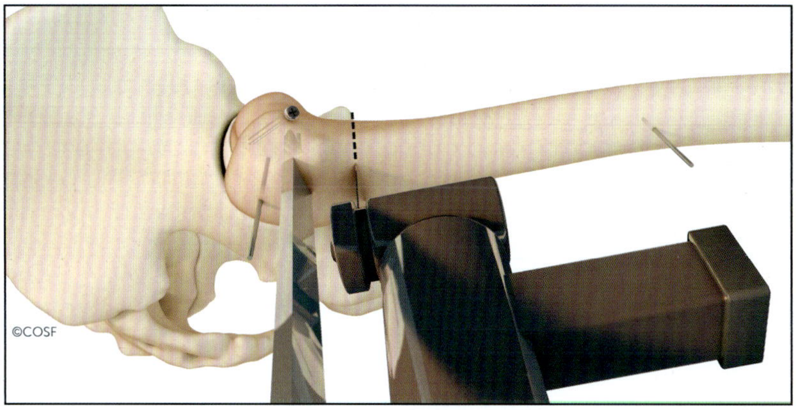

FIGURE 6.20. Illustration showing a transverse osteotomy perpendicular to the long axis of the femoral diaphysis and parallel to the blade being performed with an oscillating saw. Before the osteotomy is performed, it is important to introduce one K-wire proximal and one K-wire distal to the osteotomy to monitor for the rotation correction. Another way to monitor correction of rotation is by creating a line in the anterior cortex with a saw. Black dashed line marks the single osteotomy performed perpendicular to the long axis of the femur.

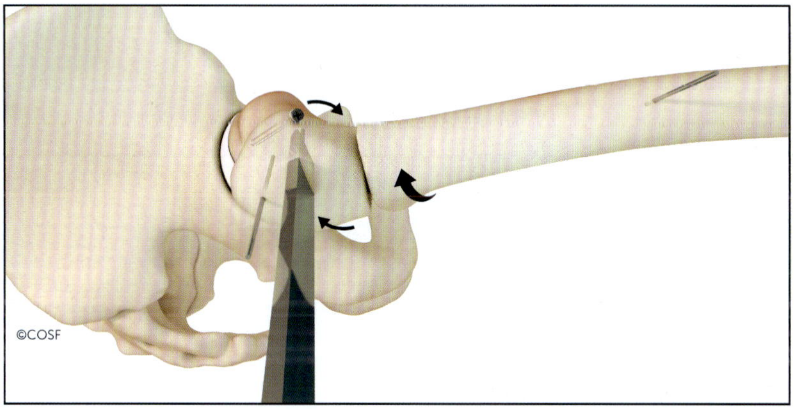

FIGURE 6.21. Illustration showing that after the osteotomy is performed, the bone fragments are aligned to obtain the planned correction. The proximal fragment is brought into extension (thin black arrows) and the plate will be in alignment with the distal fragment. The distal fragment is then internally rotated (thick black arrow), whereas the proximal fragment is externally rotated. Correction of rotation is measured by the angle formed between the proximal and distal K-wires.

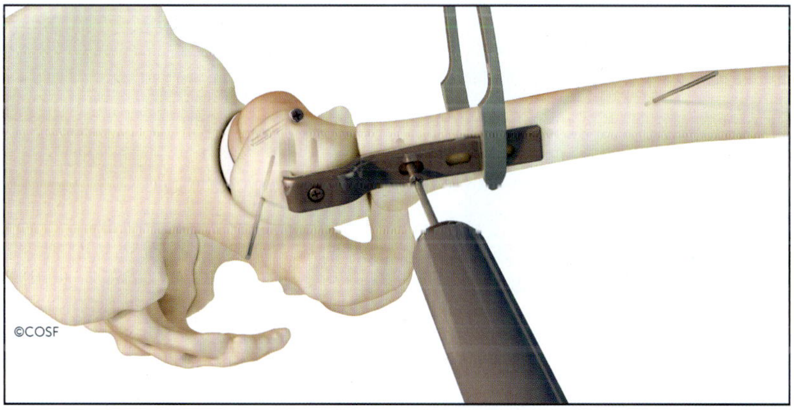

FIGURE 6.22. Illustration showing a 90° blade plate inserted in the proximal femur in line with the cut created by the chisel. An additional screw can be inserted in the proximal femur just distal to the blade to augment the fixation. After the plate is fixed to the proximal fragment, the plate is aligned with the distal fragment, and rotation is adjusted based on the reference K-wires. The plate is then fixed to the distal fragment using the typical compression technique.

Clinical Scenario

A 12-year-old female presents with a severe limp and hip pain that has been present for the past 18 months. She was previously seen at an outside facility where she was diagnosed with a stable, severe, chronic SCFE (**Figure 6.23**). She underwent in situ pinning, and during her 3-month follow-up, she was found to have persistent pain and she was sent to consultation. During physical examination, the patient was using a pair of crutches, and she was found to walk with the left foot severely rotated outward. If the hip was kept in external rotation to about 70°, it could be brought into flexion passively to about 80° or 90°. However, the hip in neutral rotation and extension flexion was limited to about 30° to 40° (**Figure 6.24**). A 3-D model of the proximal femur was produced and showed a very severe deformity (**Figure 6.25**). For the treatment of this patient, the intertrochanteric osteotomy was augmented by an anterior approach to the hip as described earlier for osteochondroplasty of the head–neck junction to allow for a clear range of motion and hip flexion without impingement (**Figure 6.26**).

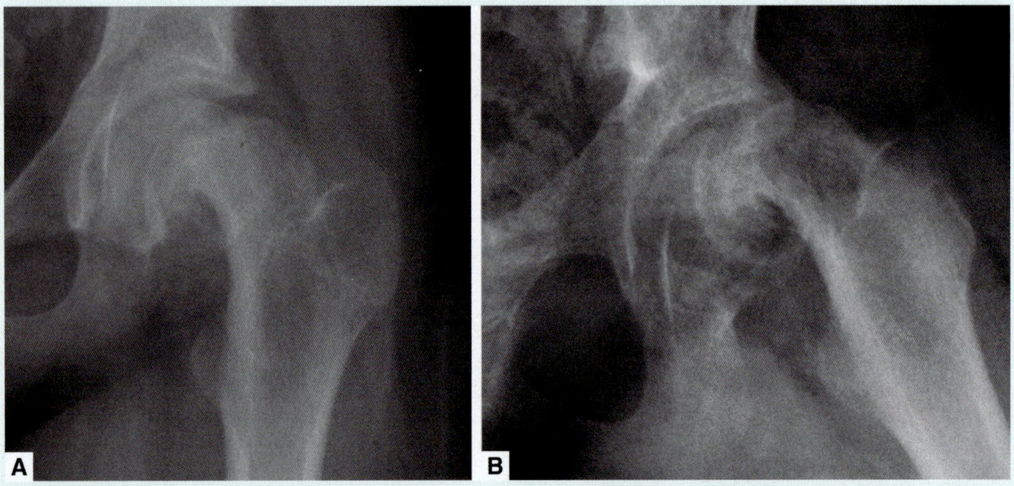

FIGURE 6.23. A, Anteroposterior and (B) frog-leg radiograph of the left hip demonstrating a severely displaced stable slipped capital femoral epiphysis.

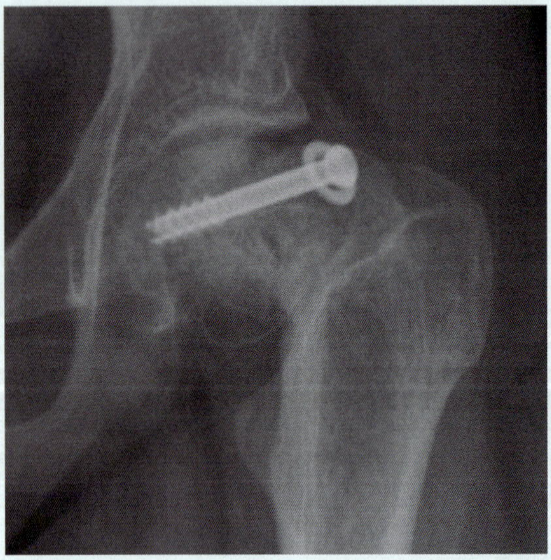

FIGURE 6.24. Preoperative radiograph showing a cannulated screw with a washer that is fixing the epiphysis of the left proximal femur. The screw was placed anteriorly in the femoral neck and too proximal to the point that it would impinge against the acetabular rim with hip flexion.

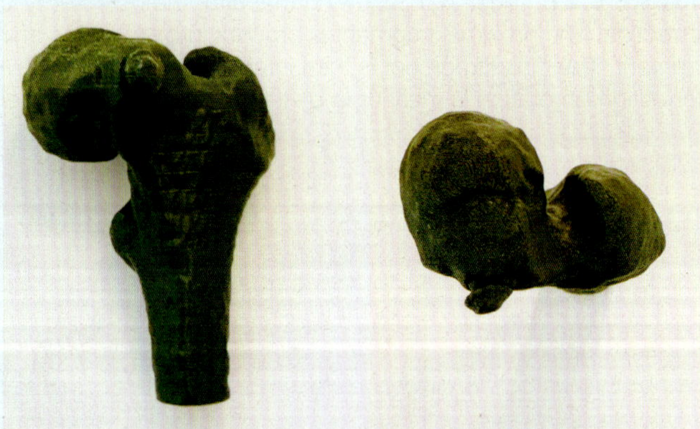

FIGURE 6.25. Picture of a three-dimensional printed model of the left hip used for preoperative planning. The severity of the deformity and early signs of healing with the epiphysis aligned in the posterior aspect of the neck was considered excessive for a realignment at the subcapital level, and a subtrochanteric flexion derotational osteotomy enhanced by an anterior open osteochondroplasty of the head–neck junction was planned.

Clinical Scenario (*continued*)

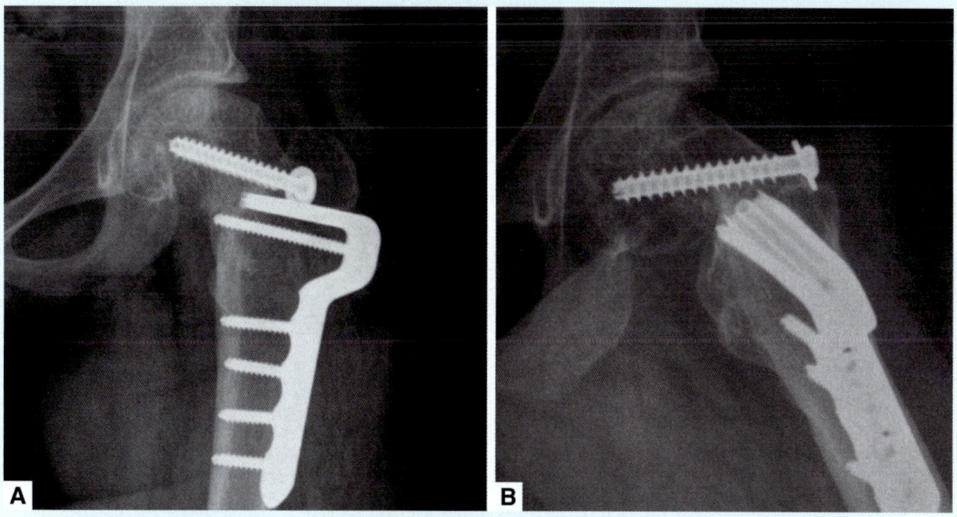

FIGURE 6.26. A, Postoperative anteroposterior and (B) lateral radiographs of the left hip revealing improvement of the femoral head and neck junction morphology along with the overall improvement in the anatomy of the proximal femur. The patient experienced improved hip flexion to about 90° with 10° of internal rotation.

Surgical Hip Dislocation With Osteochondroplasty and Femoral Osteotomy

For moderate and severe SCFE deformity patients with closed physis, our preferred method of treatment is to perform an osteochondroplasty of the femoral head–neck junction plus an intertrochanteric flexion and derotational osteotomy through a surgical hip dislocation approach. The full description of the surgical hip dislocation technique is presented in Chapter 13. Acetabular chondrolabral pathology is treated, and the femoral head–neck junction is reshaped through an osteochondroplasty. In moderate and severe SCFE, dynamic assessment of hip motion typically demonstrates residual impingement because of the retroversion positioned of the tilted femoral head in relation to the neck. An intertrochanteric osteotomy is performed after the hip capsule is closed in the usual manner. There are basically two techniques that we have used for the femoral osteotomy and fixation. The choice between the different techniques is based on the amount of flexion necessary to correct the proximal femoral anatomy. When the flexion component of the osteotomy is greater than 10° to 15°, which is often the case for severe SCFE, then our preferred method is to use an intertrochanteric osteotomy followed by fixation with a blade plate (**Figure 6.27**).

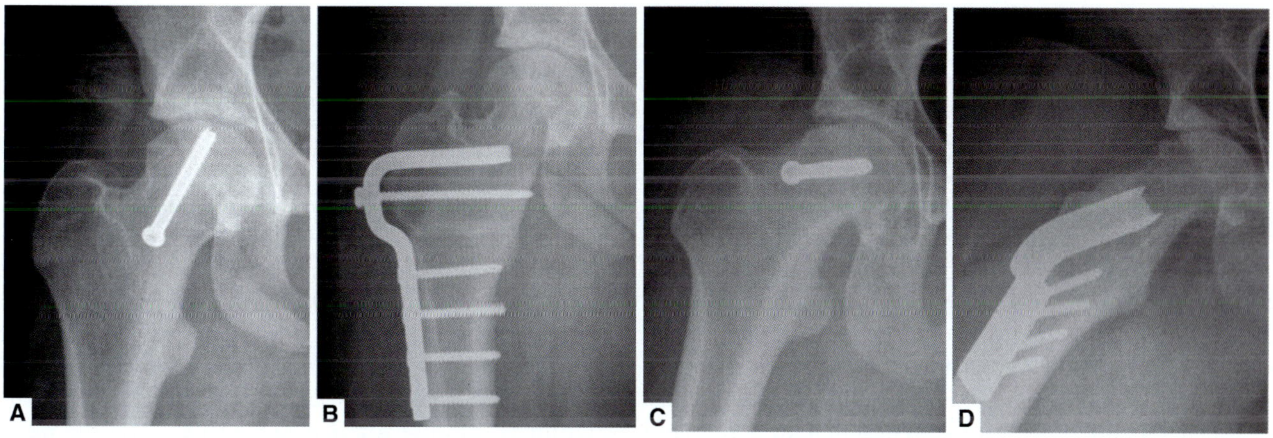

FIGURE 6.27. Surgical hip dislocation with osteochondroplasty of the femoral head and neck junction and an intertrochanteric osteotomy for the treatment of severe slipped capital femoral epiphysis (SCFE) deformity. A, Preoperative anteroposterior and (B) lateral radiographs of the right hip from a 15-year-old female previously treated with in situ fixation for a severe stable SCFE revealing abnormal morphology of the proximal femur. C, Postoperative anteroposterior and (D) lateral radiographs of the right hip revealing improvement of the femoral head and neck junction morphology along with the overall improvement in the anatomy of the proximal femur. For severe SCFE deformity, we recommend using a blade plate that provides better purchase of the proximal fragment, allowing for flexion correction.

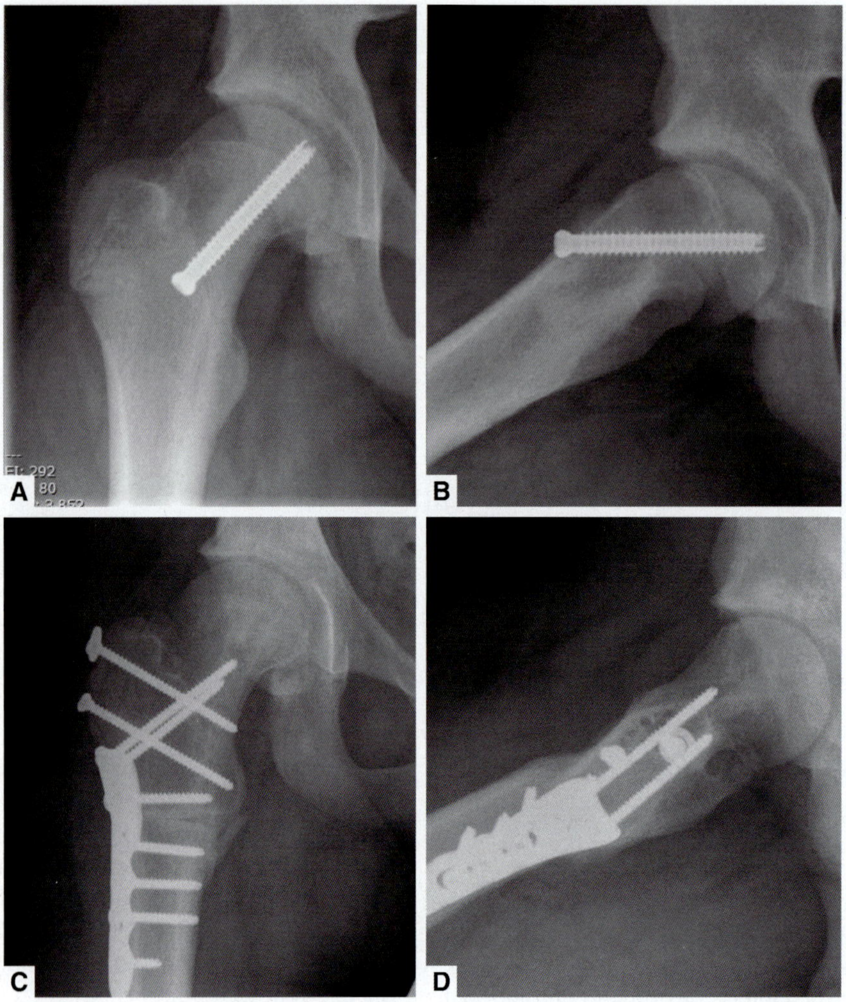

FIGURE 6.28. Surgical hip dislocation with osteochondroplasty of the femoral head and neck junction and an intertrochanteric osteotomy for the treatment for moderate slipped capital femoral epiphysis (SCFE) deformity. A, Preoperative anteroposterior and (B) lateral radiographs of the right hip from a 14-year-old boy with persistent hip pain due to femoroacetabular impingement following in situ fixation showing abnormal morphology of the proximal femur. C, Postoperative anteroposterior and (D) lateral radiographs of the right hip revealing improvement of the proximal femur anatomy. For moderate SCFE deformity, a proximal femoral locking plate can be used, as shown here.

In moderate SCFE deformity, major flexion correction may not be necessary to improve the range of motion of the hip. Instead, impingement-free motion can be achieved by the osteochondroplasty, about 10° to 15° of flexion and the derotational component of the osteotomy. Fixation can then be performed with a proximal femoral locking plate (**Figure 6.28**). Independent of the technique chose, patients are instructed to be on a toe-touch minimal weight-bearing protocol with a pair of crutches for minimum of 6 to 8 weeks when the trochanteric and intertrochanteric osteotomies should have signs of healing on radiographs. Advanced weight bearing and physical therapy follow, and patients should be able to resume weight bearing without crutches around 12 weeks after surgery. Complications with this technique include fracture of the greater trochanter or loss of fixation with hardware failure and need for revision surgery.

Modified Dunn Procedure for Stable Slipped Capital Femoral Epiphysis

For patients with stable moderate and severe SCFE with wide-open physis, the subcapital realignment using the modified Dunn procedure is the most powerful alternative for restoration of the proximal femoral anatomy. Preoperatively, CT or MRI imaging should be obtained to plan the osteotomy and to confirm the open status of the physis. We have been performing the modified Dunn technique for over a decade. Overall, we have had a positive experience with the procedure.[23,24] However, we have observed an inverse relationship between surgeon volume and patient outcomes, which has changed our institutional approach to SCFE.[25] We recommend that one of the two high-volume surgeons with most experience with this technique must be present during each modified Dunn to reduce the risk of complications. Several complications have been reported, including instability with dislocation after surgery and osteonecrosis. However, we believe that when performed by an experience surgeon in a high-volume center, the procedure has a low rate of complications.

Clinical Scenario

A 14-year-old female presents with a severe limp with the left lower extremity in outward rotation and hip pain. Symptoms were present for over 6 months. During physical examination, she was found to have severe limitation of the left hip motion. If the hip was kept in external rotation to about 60°, then it could be brought into 80° flexion, but with the hip in neutral rotation, flexion was limited to about 40°. Preoperative radiographs and CT imaging showed a severe SCFE, which was considered stable and chronic (**Figure 6.29**). A modified Dunn procedure was recommended to realign the capital femoral epiphysis.

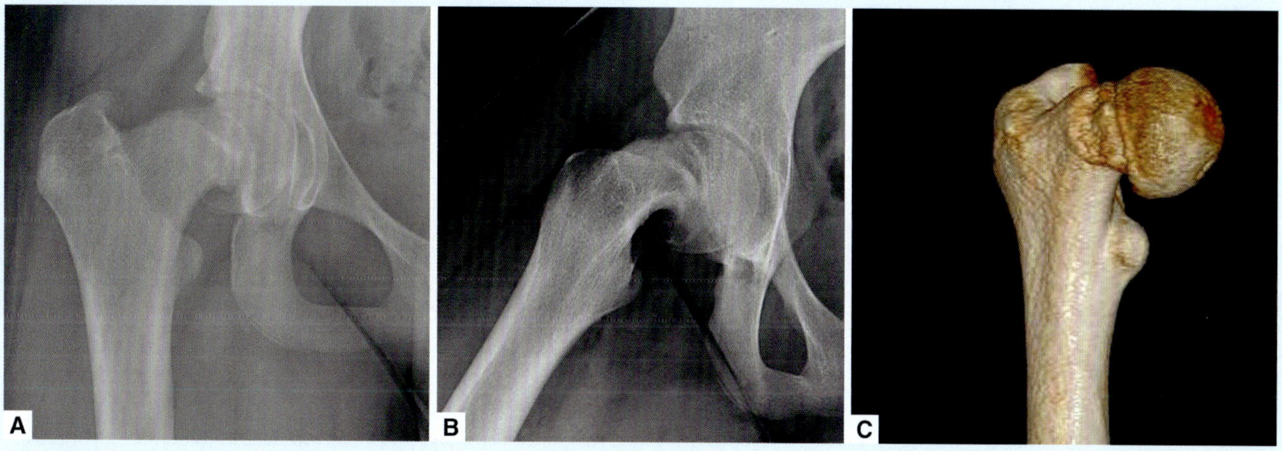

FIGURE 6.29. Preoperative imaging of a 14-year-old female with right severe, stable, chronic slipped capital femoral epiphysis. A, Anteroposterior radiograph of the right hip showing widening of the growth plate and severe displacement of the femoral head from the neck. B, Frog-leg lateral radiographs showing severe posterior tilt of the femoral head in relation to the femoral neck that is severely deformed with a typical posterior periosteal reaction (callus). C, Computed tomography image showing the severe displacement of the epiphysis with the neck almost completely dislodged from the epiphysis.

The modified Dunn procedure is performed through a surgical hip dislocation approach. Additional discussion about the surgical dislocation approach can be found in Chapter 13. The patient is positioned in a lateral decubitus on a radiolucent peg-board table with all bony prominences protected with gel pads. An axillary roll should be placed under the contralateral axilla to protect the brachial plexus. A lateral incision is performed longitudinally in the top of the greater trochanter, measuring approximately 20 cm (**Figure 6.30**). The subcutaneous tissue is dissected down

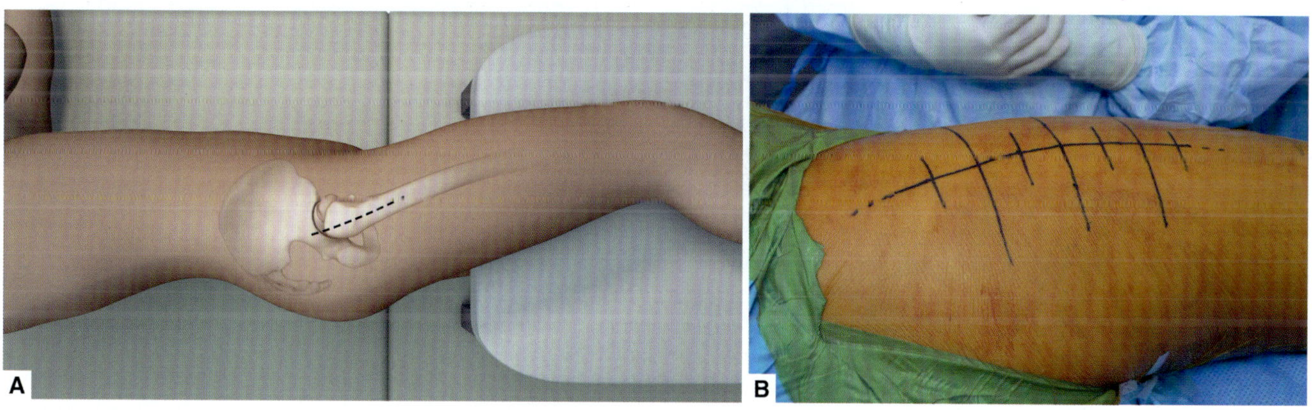

FIGURE 6.30. Position and incision for the modified Dunn procedure through a surgical hip dislocation approach. A, Illustration showing patient positioning in the lateral decubitus with the lower extremity to be operated on resting on a pillow. B, Intraoperative picture showing a straight lateral incision measuring about 20 cm that is performed on top of the greater trochanter.

to the fascia lata. The fascia lata is identified and split longitudinally in line with the skin incision. Proximally, the dissection should be performed following the Gibson approach between the gluteus maximus and the gluteus medius when possible (**Figure 6.31**). The anterior fibers of the gluteus maximus are retracted posteriorly, whereas the gluteus medius is retracted anteriorly, allowing for exposure of the greater trochanter. In obese patients, a gluteus maximus splitting approach may be necessary. In hips with severe SCFE, the anatomy of the proximal femur is abnormal, and the greater trochanter may be more posterior in close proximity to the pelvis. The piriformis tendon is identified, and the interval between the piriformis and the minimus is opened to expose the hip capsule proximally (**Figure 6.32**). Dissection of this interval at the beginning of the procedure is technically easier and associated with less bleeding.

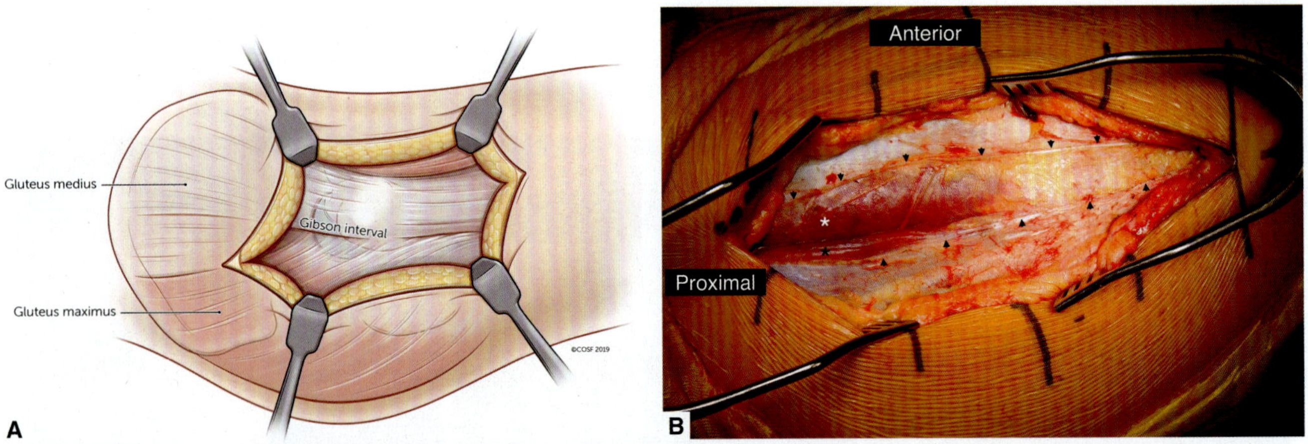

FIGURE 6.31. Superficial dissection through the Gibson approach between the gluteus maximus and the gluteus minimus without splitting the gluteus maximus like in a Kocher-Langenbeck posterior approach. A, Illustration showing the Gibson interval. The dissection follows the anterior margin of gluteus maximus where penetrating vessels should be identified as well as the posterior margin of the gluteus medius. B, Intraoperative picture showing that the incision of the fascia lata (black arrowheads) should be in line with the skin incision, but it extends proximally under the skin, allowing complete dissection of the intergluteal space. In the proximal aspect of the wound, the gluteus maximus is posterior (black asterisk), and the gluteus medius is anterior (white asterisk).

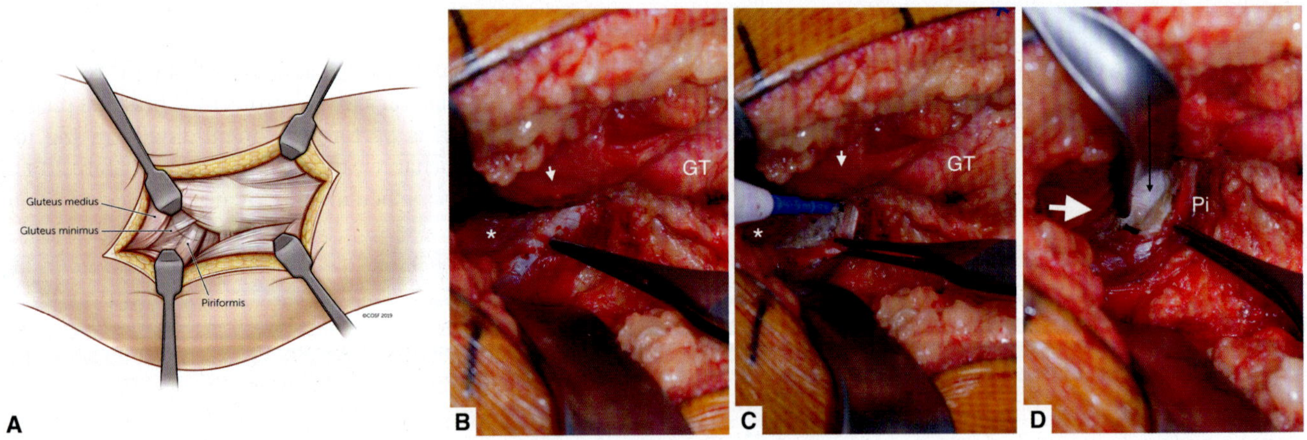

FIGURE 6.32. Deep dissection of the piriformis muscle and gluteus minimus interval in preparation for the trochanteric osteotomy. A, Illustration showing the gluteus medius has been retracted anteriorly, allowing for exposure and identification of the piriformis tendon and the gluteus minimus. B, Intraoperative picture showing the gluteus medius (white arrow) has been retracted anteriorly allowing for exposure of the gluteus minimum (white asterisk) and the piriformis muscle and tendon (on the tip of the forceps) underneath. C, Intraoperative picture showing the piriformis tendon is grasped with the forceps and pulled distally, allowing for exposure of the capsular insertion of the gluteus minimus (white asterisk). The gluteus minimus is dissected free from the capsule with an electric cautery. D, Intraoperative picture showing that the gluteus minimus has been retracted (black arrow marks the retractor), and the hip capsule can be exposed. The white arrow identifies the gluteus medius. GT, greater trochanter; Pi, piriformis muscle and tendon.

Any dissection distal and posterior to the piriformis is to be avoided because of the risk of damaging the branch of the inferior gluteal artery that runs along the inferior border of piriformis.

Distally, the vastus lateralis fascia is opened, and the muscle belly is dissected from the femur extraperiosteally in a posterior to anterior manner. A Hohmann retractor is placed under the vastus lateralis to facilitate the trochanteric osteotomy. A line between the posterior edge of the vastus lateralis origin and the insertion of the gluteus medius in the greater trochanter is marked in preparation for the trochanteric osteotomy (**Figure 6.33**). A trochanteric osteotomy is performed with an oscillating saw, creating a free trochanter piece that is approximately 15 to 20 mm in thickness (**Figure 6.34**). The piriformis tendon remains intact in the stable segment of the trochanter. The mobile fragment of the greater trochanter is flipped anteriorly, allowing full exposure of the hip capsule.

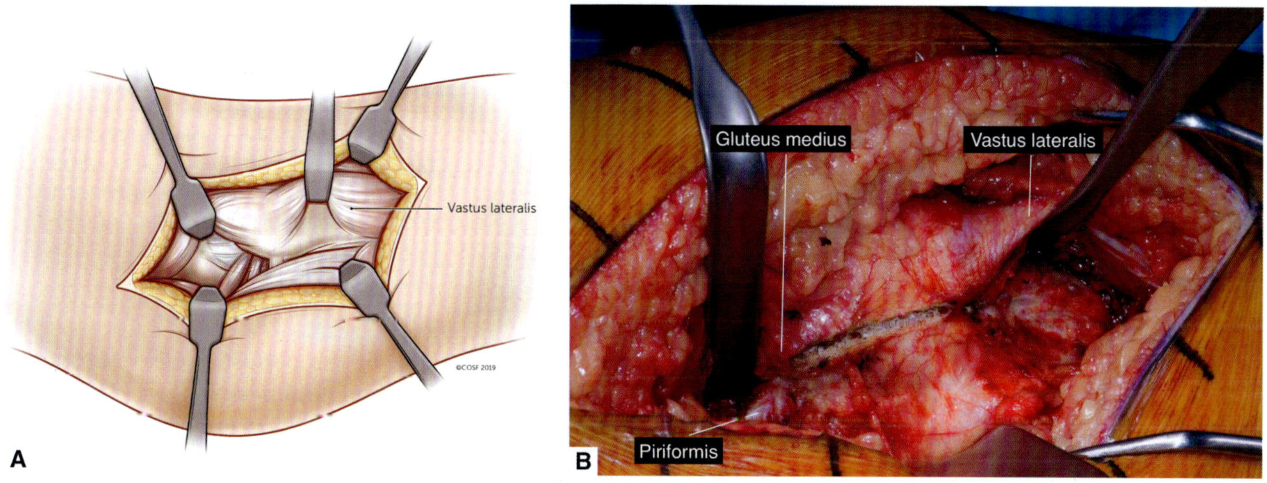

FIGURE 6.33. Dissection of the vastus lateralis from the femur before the trochanteric osteotomy. A, Illustration showing the vastus lateralis fascia is opened and the muscle belly is dissected from the femur extraperiosteally in a posterior to anterior manner. A Hohmann retractor is placed under the vastus lateralis, and a retractor is placed proximally under the gluteus minimus, exposing the piriformis tendon to guide the trochanteric osteotomy. B, Intraoperative picture showing a line marked in the trochanter in preparation for the osteotomy. Proximally, a 2- to 3-mm sleeve of the gluteus medius is left attached to the stable trochanter.

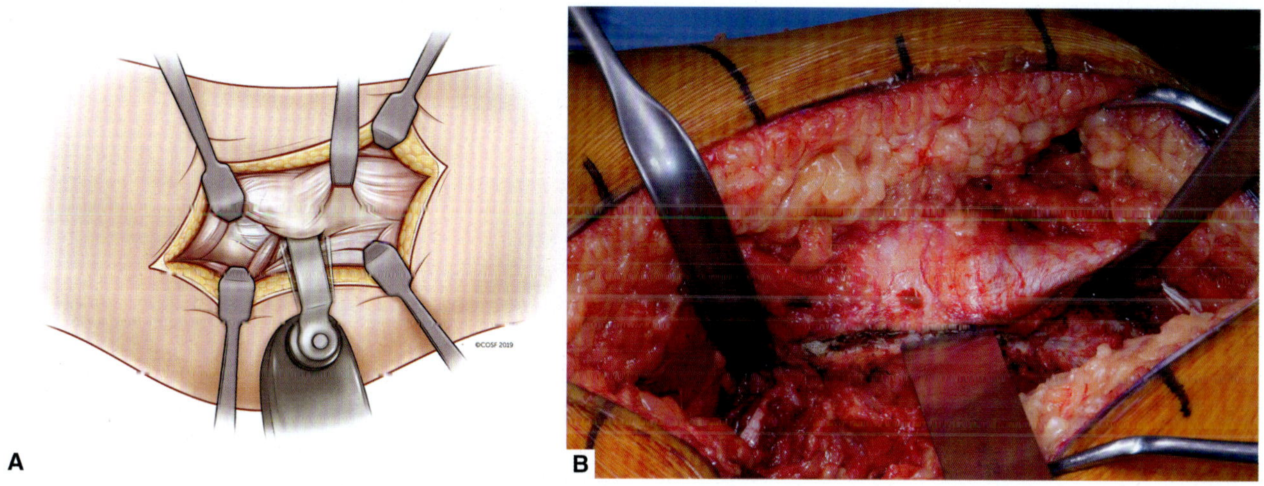

FIGURE 6.34. The digastric trochanteric osteotomy. A, Illustration showing the osteotomy being performed with exposure of the trochanter distally by placing a Hohmann retractor under the vastus lateralis and by retracting the gluteus minimus anteriorly in the proximal aspect of the wound to expose the piriformis tendon. The free fragment of the trochanteric osteotomy should be 15 to 20 mm because if it is too thin, it may fracture, and if it is too deep, it may include the insertion of the piriformis tendon, risking the vascular supply to the femoral head. B, Intraoperative picture showing that 2 to 3 mm of the insertion of the gluteus medius is left attached to the stable trochanter segment. Leaving a 2- to 3-mm sleeve of the gluteus medius is crucial to avoid cutting the piriformis tendon insertion to the trochanter. Exposing the piriformis tendon helps avoid damage as well.

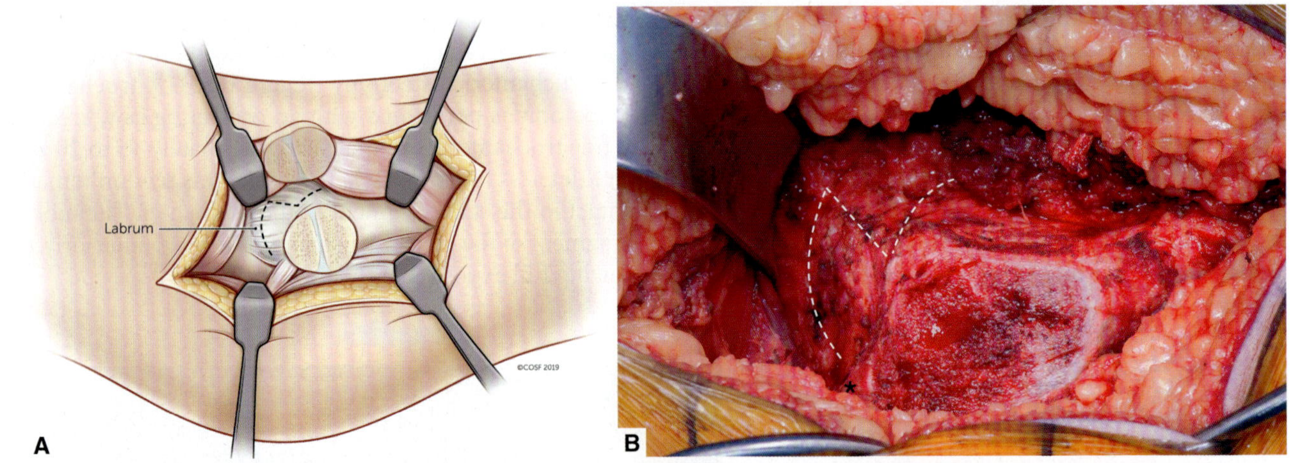

FIGURE 6.35. Capsulotomy. A, Illustration showing the lines for the capsulotomy. For the right hip, the capsulotomy has a Z shape: the initial capsulotomy cut is in line with the long axis of the femoral neck and starts at the anterosuperior corner of the stable trochanter. Using an inside-out technique, the anterior cut of the capsule is cut anteriorly and inferiorly toward the acetabular rim. The posterior cut of the capsule is performed along the acetabular rim toward the piriformis tendon. B, Intraoperative picture showing complete exposure of the hip capsule in preparation for the capsulotomy. The posterior limit of the capsulotomy is the piriformis tendon (black asterisk). White dashed line marks the incision of the hip capsule.

A capsulotomy is performed using an inside-out technique. The capsulotomy starts at the anterolateral corner of the stable trochanter along the femoral neck axis moving proximally until the labrum is identified. The capsulotomy is extended by cutting the capsule anteriorly and distally toward the anterior-inferior aspect of the acetabulum. Finally, a posterior limb of the capsulotomy is performed from the acetabular rim aiming posteriorly toward the piriformis tendon. The final capsulotomy has a Z shape for the right hip and an inverted Z shape for the left hip (**Figure 6.35**). The femoral head–neck junction is identified, and subtle instability of the epiphysis may be present even in hips classified as stable by the Loder[8] criteria. The anterior periosteum may be stretch or even torn, and its status should be recorded along the integrity of the retinaculum containing the vessels. If there is any instability of the epiphysis, or if the anterior periosteum is torn, then we recommend provisional fixation of the epiphysis with two threaded K-wires to prevent further displacement (**Figure 6.36**). The femur is partially dislocated from the acetabulum anteriorly by flexion and external rotation of the hip with the help of a bone hook placed anterior and inferior to the femoral neck, and the ligamentum teres is resected to allow for a complete dislocation (**Figure 6.37**). The acetabulum is inspected for assessment of chondral or labral injury.

The femoral head is reduced back in the acetabulum in preparation for the dissection of the retinacular flap containing the vessels from the medial circumflex artery, which is the main nutrient to the femoral head. A small smooth K-wire is used to create a hole in the femoral head to assess the blood supply to the femoral head (**Figure 6.38**). Femoral head perfusion can be monitored by observation of direct bleeding and by insertion of an intracranial pressure (ICP) probe that is connected to a monitor. Dissection of the periosteal sleeve around the stable trochanter and femoral neck follows (**Figure 6.39**). We start the dissection by the periosteum from the anterior aspect of the femoral neck moving proximally around the greater trochanter and distally in the lateral aspect of the femoral shaft. The periosteum is opened with a knife and dissected using a delicate periosteum elevator. The periosteum is dissected up to 4 cm distal to the greater trochanter laterally and posteriorly to the level of the lesser trochanter. The next step is resection of the stable

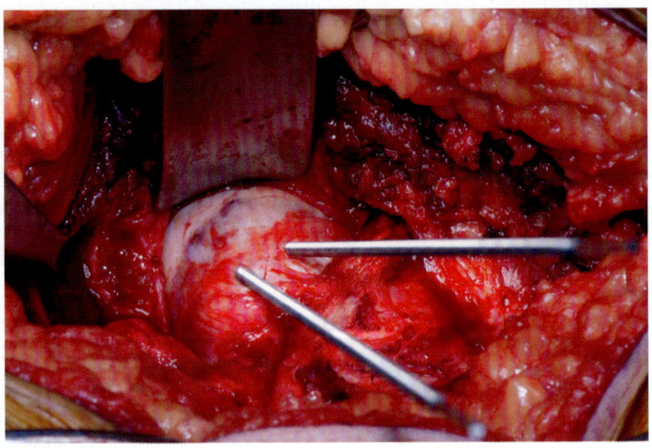

FIGURE 6.36. Intraoperative picture showing provisional fixation of the epiphysis with two 3/32 in threaded Kirschner wires introduced in the femoral neck to stabilize the epiphysis because epiphyseal instability may be present even in hips considered stable by the Loder criteria. We caution that these wires should be inserted carefully from the anterior aspect of the neck posteriorly under direct visualization and often C-arm fluoroscopy to avoid penetrating the acetabular cartilage.

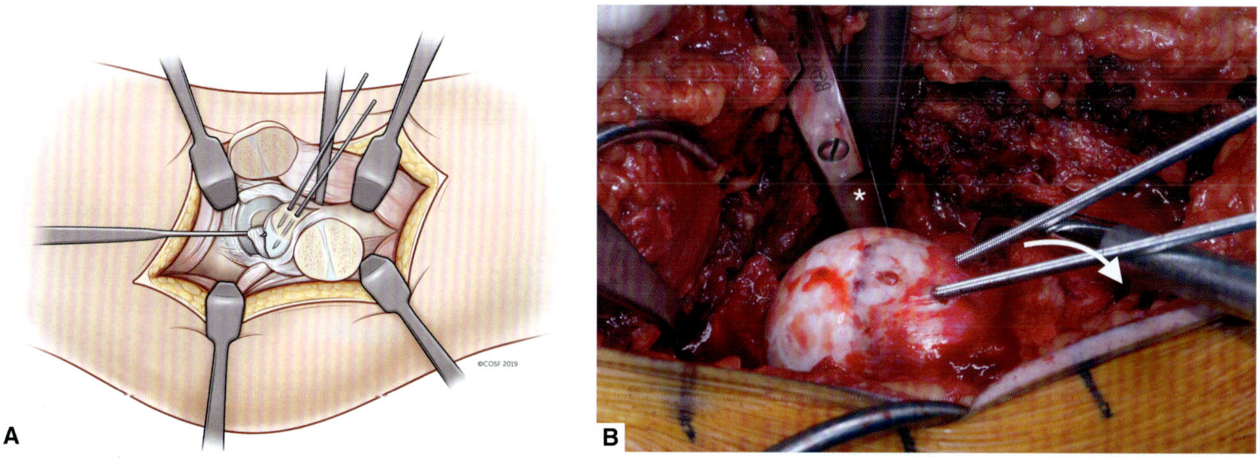

FIGURE 6.37. Resection of the ligamentum teres and dislocation of the hip. A, Illustration showing the hip is subluxated by positioning in flexion and external rotation, allowing for exposure of the ligamentum teres that should be transected. B, Intraoperative picture showing the hip in a subluxated position. A scissors (white asterisk) is placed in the acetabulum to cut the ligamentum teres, whereas a large blunt bone hook is placed under the femoral neck to pull the femur out of the acetabulum (white arrow).

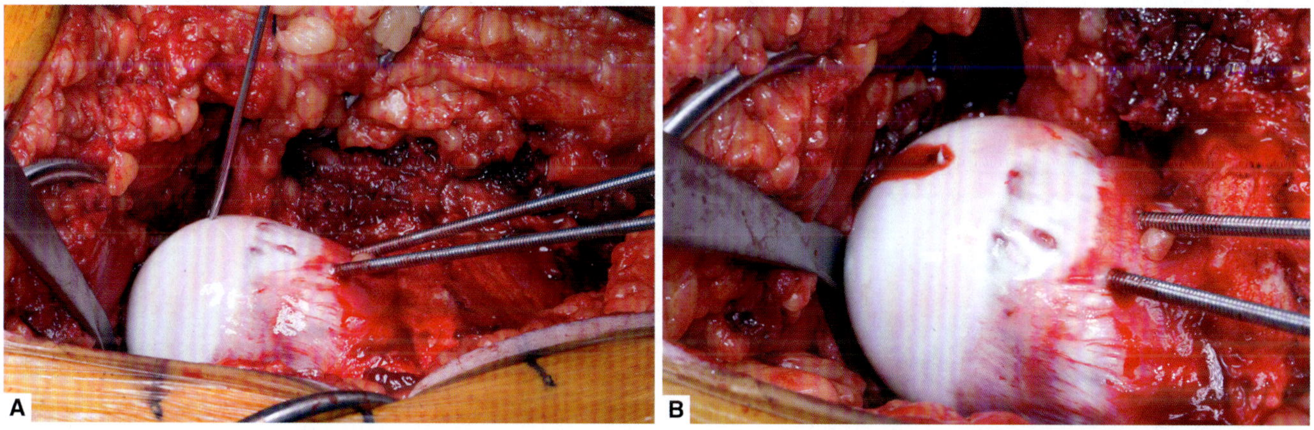

FIGURE 6.38. Monitor the blood flow to the femoral head. A, Intraoperative picture showing a small (1.6-mm) smooth K-wire introduced in the femoral head. B, Active bleeding should be observed through the K-wire hole after the wire is removed. The status of the femoral head perfusion (active bleeding present vs. absent bleeding) should be recorded. We recommend inserting an intracranial pressure monitor probe to determine the intraosseous pressure change in the femoral head.

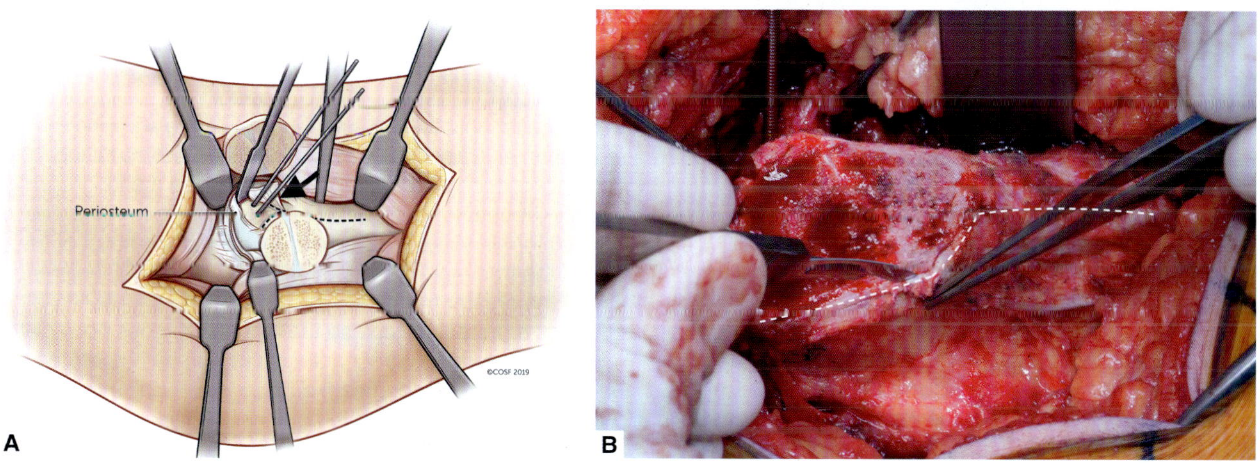

FIGURE 6.39. Dissection of the periosteal flap containing the retinacular vessels from the deep branch of the medial circumflex artery. A, Illustration showing the hip reduced in preparation for the dissection of the periosteal flap. Dissection of the periosteum is circumferential around the greater trochanter. The periosteum from the anterior aspect of the neck is sharply incised and partially elevated (black arrow). Black dashed line marks the incision of the periosteum. B, Intraoperative picture showing the greater trochanter. The white dashed line marks the line of incision of the periosteum that should extend distally to about 4 cm and come around the trochanter in a circumferential manner.

portion of the greater trochanter to free the retinaculum. In younger patients with a very thick periosteum, it is possible to remove the proximal aspect of the stable trochanter in one piece (**Figure 6.40**). In older adolescents, we prefer to remove the proximal piece of the trochanter using a rongeur and a piecemeal technique. This should be performed with caution to avoid penetrating the posterior periosteum. Independent of the technique used, the resection of the stable trochanter should be done until the resection surface levels the posterior and superior aspect of the femoral neck. Distally, the dissection of the subperiosteal flap extends to the posterior aspect of the lesser trochanter.

After removal of the stable trochanter, the femur is dislocated. A sponge is placed in the acetabulum to avoid inadvertent reduction of the femoral head into the acetabulum. The periosteum of the anterior and medial aspects of the femoral neck should be dissected to create a long flap. With adequate subperiosteal dissection, the neck is completely exposed, and a blunt retractor should be placed inferiorly to protect the soft tissues. The epiphysis is separated from the neck with a curved osteotome

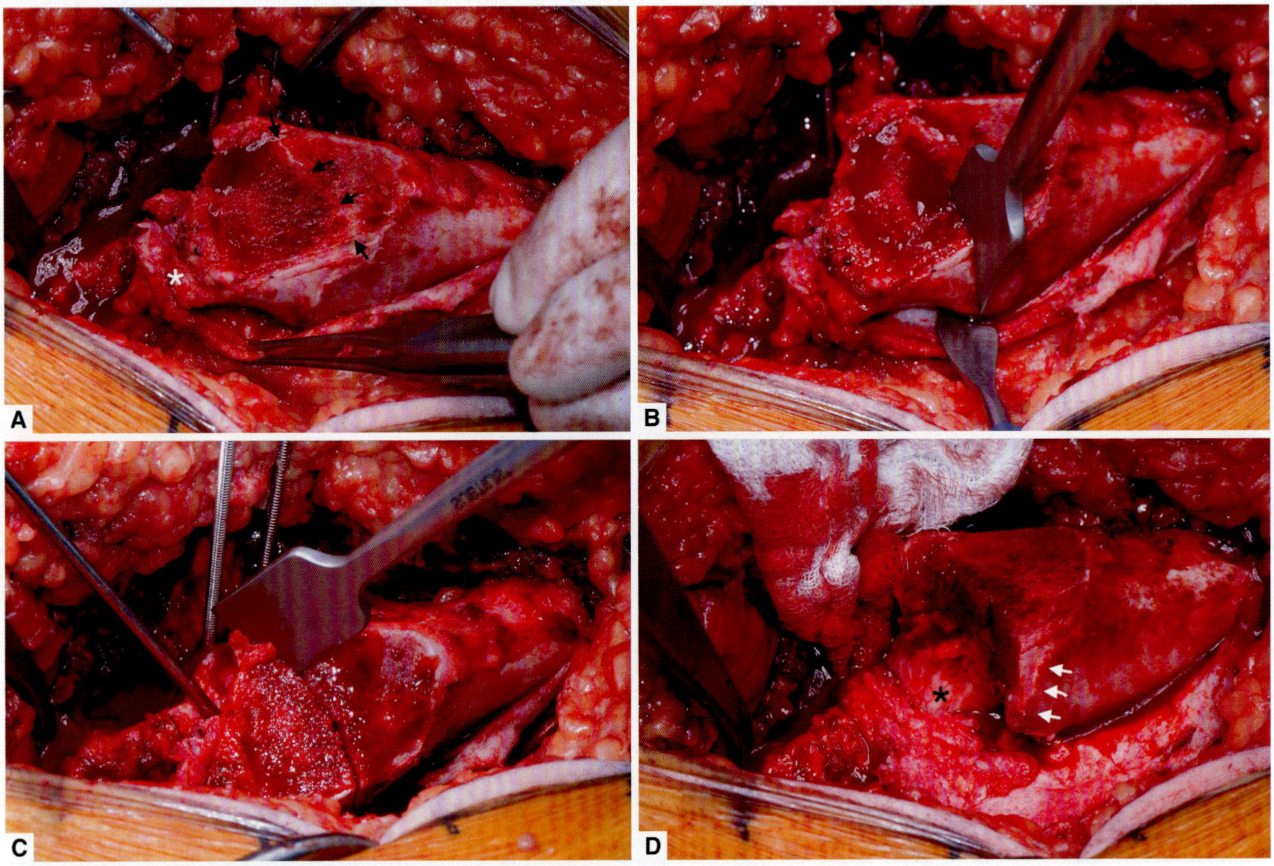

FIGURE 6.40. Resection of the stable greater trochanter—the *one-piece* technique. A, Intraoperative picture showing the posterior periosteum has been dissected around the stable greater trochanter. Dissection of the periosteum before taking down the stable greater trochanter is possible in young patients who have a thick periosteum, and it facilitates creating a long and intact retinacular flap. The periosteum is dissected around the stable trochanter to the level of the piriformis tendon. The piriformis fossa should not be dissected at this time. Dissection of the piriformis fossa is completely along with removal of the proximal portion of the stable trochanter. Black arrows mark the level of the trochanteric apophysis, which is used as reference for resection of the stable greater trochanter. B, The proximal portion of the greater trochanter (proximal to the apophysis) is carefully cut with an osteotome posteriorly. A periosteal elevator serves as a protective tool, so the osteotome does not violate the periosteum posteriorly. C, The anterior aspect of the proximal portion of the greater trochanter is cut with an osteotome. D, Then, the entire piece of the greater trochanter with the trochanteric fossa in the underneath surface is carefully mobilized and gradually released out of its periosteum, allowing for exposure of the posterior aspect of the femoral neck (black asterisk). White arrows mark the posterior aspect of the greater trochanter that should be trimmed down the level of the posterior neck to avoid tension of the retinaculum.

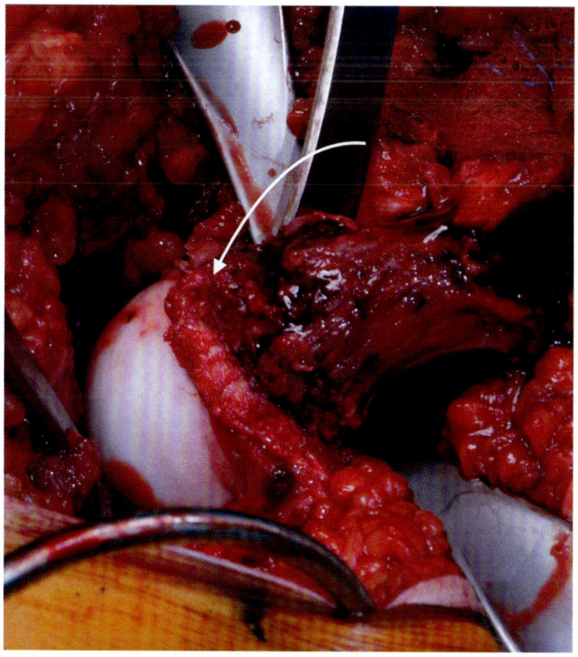

FIGURE 6.41. Mobilizing the epiphysis from the metaphysis. Intraoperative picture showing the metaphyseal portion of the femoral neck being completely exposed posteriorly. A curved chisel is used to help separate the epiphysis from the metaphysis (white arrow).

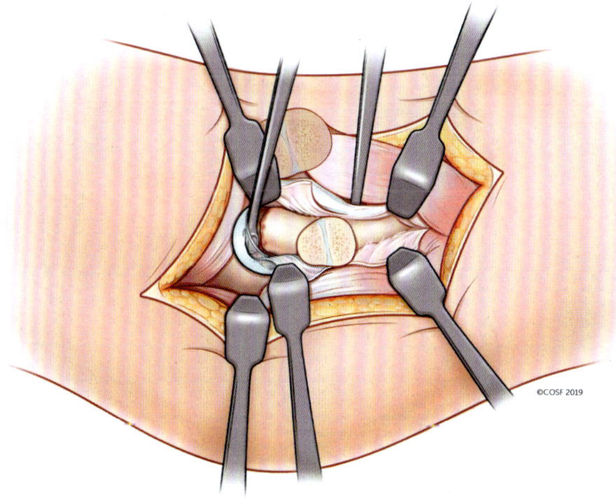

FIGURE 6.42. Preparation of the epiphysis for reduction. Illustration showing that once the metaphyseal portion of the femur is rounded and prepared, then a curette is used to resect the residual growth plate tissue from the femoral head with careful preservation of the retinaculum inserting in the posterior aspect of the femoral head.

using careful tapping with a mallet and levering motion to free the head from the neck (**Figure 6.41**). The posterior aspect of the neck is assessed, and the typical callus is removed using an osteotome, curate, and, eventually, a high-speed burr. The edge of the femoral neck should be rounded to receive the epiphysis. Although shortening of the femoral neck may theoretically reduce the tension on the retinaculum, the femoral neck should not be shortened more than 2 to 3 mm to avoid reducing the lever arm of the abductor musculature and potential instability postoperatively. The surgeon carefully holds the epiphysis exposing the inner aspect, allowing for curettage and resection of the remaining growth plate (**Figure 6.42**).

The femoral head is then reduced back over the neck under direct visualization to control the position and tension of the retinacular flap. During reduction, the femoral epiphysis in gently held and reduced on top of the femoral neck with constant attention to the retinacular flap to avoid excessive tension, kinking, and potential damage. Once the alignment of the epiphysis is deemed appropriate (which can be assessed by the position of the femoral fovea and the insertion of the retinaculum), a fully threated K-wire is inserted in a retrograde manner through the fovea. One or two additional threaded wires are then introduced in a regular manner from the lateral aspect of the femur, aiming toward the center or inferior portion of the femoral head. We avoid placing the wires on the superior and posterior region of the femoral head. The fixation is checked under C-arm guidance to allow adequate spread of the pins in the femoral head. Alternatively, two guidewires for cannulated screws can be introduced from lateral-distal to proximal-medial, and the epiphysis can be fixed with two 6.5-mm cannulated screws (**Figure 6.43**). The hip is then reduced, and the ICP monitor is again used to check the femoral head blood flow. If no blood flow is present and the retinaculum is intact, we free the retinaculum further distally, and, if needed, we shorten the neck 1 to 2 mm further. The periosteal sleeve should be approximated loosely. The hip capsule should be closed but not excessively tight to avoid tension over the periosteum flap. The trochanteric piece is fixed with slight advancement with two or three 3.5-mm screws (**Figure 6.44**).

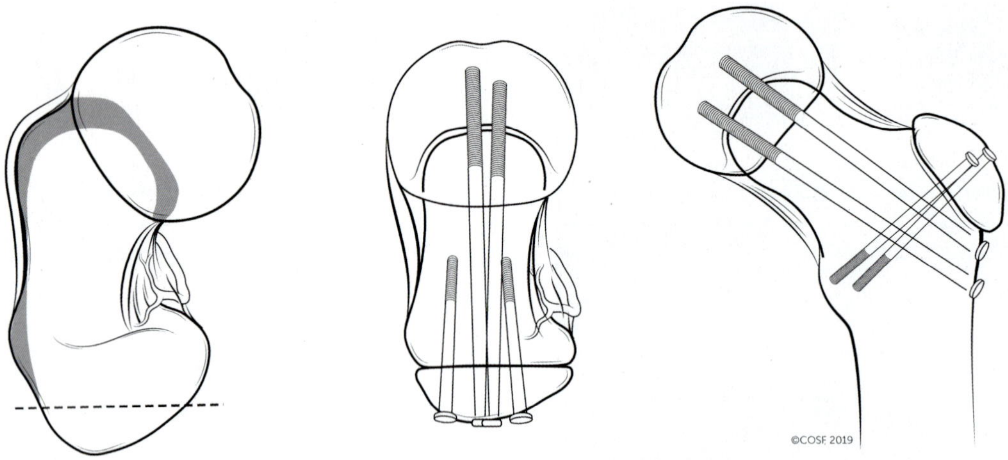

FIGURE 6.43. Realignment of the capital femoral epiphysis in severe slipped capital femoral epiphysis (SCFE). A, Illustration showing the relationship between the femoral head that is tilted posteriorly in relation to the femoral neck. The gray shaded areas represent the abnormal morphology of the femoral neck in severe SCFE in the area that should be trimmed during the modified Dunn procedure for realignment of the femoral head on the femoral neck. B, Illustration of the femoral neck and head relationship after the neck has been trimmed and rounded up to receive the femoral head after reduction. Note the posterior location of the epiphyseal vessels that should not be placed under tension at the time of reduction. C, Illustration showing the coronal alignment of the femoral head and neck and the fixation of the trochanter with slight advancement after modified Dunn procedure.

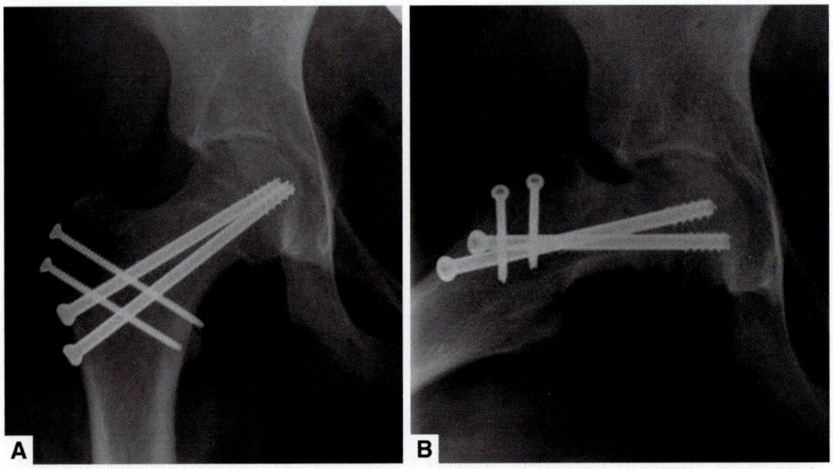

FIGURE 6.44. Postoperative images 15 months later when the patient resumed competitive volleyball. A, Anteroposterior radiograph of the right hip showing restoration of the normal anatomy with no signs of osteonecrosis. B, Frog-leg lateral radiographs showing improved anatomy of the proximal femur with normal femoral head–neck offset and normal tilt of the femoral head in relation to the neck.

REFERENCES

1. Lehmann CL, Arons RR, Loder RT, Vitale MG. The epidemiology of slipped capital femoral epiphysis: an update. *J Pediatr Orthop.* 2006;26(3):286-290.
2. Loder RT, Skopelja EN. The epidemiology and demographics of slipped capital femoral epiphysis. *ISRN Orthop.* 2011;2011:486512.
3. Perry DC, Metcalfe D, Lane S, Turner S. Childhood obesity and slipped capital femoral epiphysis. *Pediatrics.* 2018;142(5):1-10.
4. Halverson SJ, Warhoover T, Mencio GA, Lovejoy SA, Martus JE, Schoenecker JG. Leptin elevation as a risk factor for slipped capital femoral epiphysis independent of obesity status. *J Bone Joint Surg Am.* 2017;99(10):865-872.
5. Gelberman RH, Cohen MS, Shaw BA, Kasser JR, Griffin PP, Wilkinson RH. The association of femoral retroversion with slipped capital femoral epiphysis. *J Bone Joint Surg Am.* 1986;68(7):1000-1007.
6. Liu RW, Fraley SM, Morris WZ, Cooperman DR. Validity and clinical consequences of a rotational mechanism for slipped capital femoral epiphysis. *J Pediatr Orthop.* 2016;36(3):239-246.
7. Fahey JJ, O'Brien ET. Acute slipped capital femoral epiphysis: review of the literature and report of ten cases. *J Bone Joint Surg Am.* 1965;47:1105-1127.

8. Loder RT, Richards BS, Shapiro PS, Reznick LR, Aronson DD. Acute slipped capital femoral epiphysis: the importance of physeal stability. *J Bone Joint Surg Am.* 1993;75(8):1134-1140.
9. Southwick WO. Slipped capital femoral epiphysis. *J Bone Joint Surg Am.* 1984;66(8):1151-1152.
10. Dodds MK, McCormack D, Mulhall KJ. Femoroacetabular impingement after slipped capital femoral epiphysis: does slip severity predict clinical symptoms? *J Pediatr Orthop.* 2009; 29(6): 535-539.
11. Abraham E, Gonzalez MH, Pratap S, Amirouche F, Atluri P, Simon P. Clinical implications of anatomical wear characteristics in slipped capital femoral epiphysis and primary osteoarthritis. *J Pediatr Orthop.* 2007;27(7):788-795.
12. Helgesson L, Johansson PK, Aurell Y, Tiderius CJ, Karrholm J, Riad J. Early osteoarthritis after slipped capital femoral epiphysis. *Acta Orthop.* 2018;89(2):222-228.
13. Carney BT, Weinstein SL, Noble J. Long-term follow-up of slipped capital femoral epiphysis. *J Bone Joint Surg Am.* 1991;73(5):667-674.
14. Rab GT. The geometry of slipped capital femoral epiphysis: implications for movement, impingement, and corrective osteotomy. *J Pediatr Orthop.* 1999;19(4):419-424.
15. Dunn DM. The treatment of adolescent slipping of the upper femoral epiphysis. *J Bone Joint Surg Am.* 1964;46:621-629.
16. Leunig M, Slongo T, Kleinschmidt M, Ganz R. Subcapital correction osteotomy in slipped capital femoral epiphysis by means of surgical hip dislocation. *Oper Orthop Traumatol.* 2007;19(4):389-410.
17. Fish JB. Cuneiform osteotomy of the femoral neck in the treatment of slipped capital femoral epiphysis. *J Bone Joint Surg Am.* 1984;66(8):1153-1168.
18. Barmada R, Bruch RF, Gimbel JS, Ray RD. Base of the neck extracapsular osteotomy for correction of deformity in slipped capital femoral epiphysis. *Clin Orthop Relat Res.* 1978(132):98-101.
19. Kramer WG, Craig WA, Noel S. Compensating osteotomy at the base of the femoral neck for slipped capital femoral epiphysis. *J Bone Joint Surg Am.* 1976;58(6):796-800.
20. Imhauser G. [Late results of Imhauser's osteotomy for slipped capital femoral epiphysis (author's transl)]. *Z Orthop Ihre Grenzgeb.* 1977;115(5):716-725.
21. Southwick WO. Osteotomy through the lesser trochanter for slipped capital femoral epiphysis. *J Bone Joint Surg Am.* 1967;49(5):807-835.
22. Schai PA, Exner GU, Hansch O. Prevention of secondary coxarthrosis in slipped capital femoral epiphysis: a long-term follow-up study after corrective intertrochanteric osteotomy. *J Pediatr Orthop B.* 1996;5(3):135-143.
23. Ziebarth K, Zilkens C, Spencer S, Leunig M, Ganz R, Kim YJ. Capital realignment for moderate and severe SCFE using a modified Dunn procedure. *Clin Orthop Relat Res.* 2009;467(3):704-716.
24. Novais EN, Hill MK, Carry PM, Heare TC, Sink EL. Modified Dunn procedure is superior to in situ pinning for short-term clinical and radiographic improvement in severe stable SCFE. *Clin Orthop Relat Res.* 2015;473(6):2108-2117.
25. Upasani VV, Matheney TH, Spencer SA, Kim YJ, Millis MB, Kasser JR. Complications after modified Dunn osteotomy for the treatment of adolescent slipped capital femoral epiphysis. *J Pediatr Orthop.* 2014;34(7):661-667.

CHAPTER 7

Unstable Slipped Capital Femoral Epiphysis

FUNDAMENTAL PRINCIPLES OF SLIPPED CAPITAL FEMORAL EPIPHYSIS

A slipped capital femoral epiphysis (SCFE) is classified as unstable if the patient has such severe pain that walking is not possible even with crutches, regardless of the duration of the symptoms.[1] Treatment of unstable SCFE is more difficult than that of stable SCFE because of the risk of damage to the blood supply to the capital femoral epiphysis and subsequent development of osteonecrosis of the femoral head. There are several controversies surrounding the best strategy for the management of an acute, severely displaced, and unstable SCFE.

The etiology of osteonecrosis of the femoral head: The blood supply to the femoral head is provided by the terminal branches of the medial femoral circumflex artery. To date, the pathogenesis of osteonecrosis in acute severely displaced SCFE remains unclear. Damage to the ascending branches of the medial femoral circumflex artery can occur at the time of the injury, although most authors believe that this is a rare event. However, there are reports of surgical observation of a completely torn periosteum flap containing the vessels to the femoral head.[2] Kinking of the vessels has been shown to cause blood flow disruption in preoperative angiographic imaging of unstable SCFE.[3] Increased pressure from an intracapsular hematoma has also been reported as a factor in the increased risk for osteonecrosis, through a tamponade effect. One study reported that measured pressures from the hip joint with unstable SCFE were higher than those of the contralateral unaffected hip.[4] Another study showed that the blood supply, assessed by an intracranial pressure probe, can be restored after capsular decompression.[5] However, a systematic review of the literature did not find that capsular decompression was associated with decreased occurrence of osteonecrosis.[6] It is possible that the blood supply to the femoral head in patients that develop an acute and unstable SCFE is more tenuous.

If these proposed factors are the cause of osteonecrosis in unstable SCFE, timing of treatment may play a role in the development of osteonecrosis. Theoretically, an acute to severely displaced unstable SCFE functions as an intracapsular femoral neck fracture. In the adult literature, surgical intervention for intracapsular femoral neck fractures has been recommended to be performed as early as possible because of the lower risk of developing osteonecrosis of the femoral head. However, in SCFE, the issue of timing as a factor in the development of osteonecrosis also remains a controversial topic.

Ideally, surgical treatment of an acute, severely displaced, and unstable SCFE would allow for stabilization of the epiphysis with improvement of the deformity in order to avoid future problems related to femoral acetabular impingement. Treatment options for an acute, severely displaced, and unstable SCFE include in situ fixation, closed reduction and percutaneous fixation, and open reduction with realignment.

IN SITU FIXATION WITHOUT REDUCTION OR FOLLOWING AN INADVERTENT REDUCTION AFTER POSITIONING

In situ fixation without reduction or following an inadvertent reduction after positioning on the surgical table can be performed on a radiolucent table or a fracture table. Most authors favoring the use of a fracture table would argue that it allows for gentle positioning of the leg with the patella pointing upward to facilitate an inadvertent nonforced improvement of the epiphysis alignment. Unfortunately, treatment outcomes after in situ fixation for acute, severely displaced, and unstable SCFE are associated with high rates of osteonecrosis, varying from 3% to 60%.[7]

The number of screws used to fix the epiphysis in cases of unstable SCFE remains somewhat controversial. The placement of two cannulated screws instead of one single screw will add stability to the fixation and is our preferred method of fixation for an acute, severely displaced, and unstable SCFE. The technique for percutaneous fixation is similar to that described for stable SCFE, which has been discussed in the previous chapter.

PERCUTANEOUS FIXATION FOLLOWING CLOSED REDUCTION PLUS CAPSULAR DECOMPRESSION WITH MONITORING OF THE FEMORAL HEAD BLOOD FLOW

Clinical Scenario

A 12-year-old male presented with inability to walk or bear any weight in his right lower extremity owing to right hip pain aggravated after a tackle during football practice. He had a history of 1 to 2 weeks of mild discomfort in his right hip that did not stop him from playing football until he was tackled. Anteroposterior (AP) and frog-leg lateral radiographs showed complete severely displaced slip on the right (**Figure 7.1**). He was treated with in situ pinning after minimum traction with a percutaneous capsular decompression and fixation with a single screw.

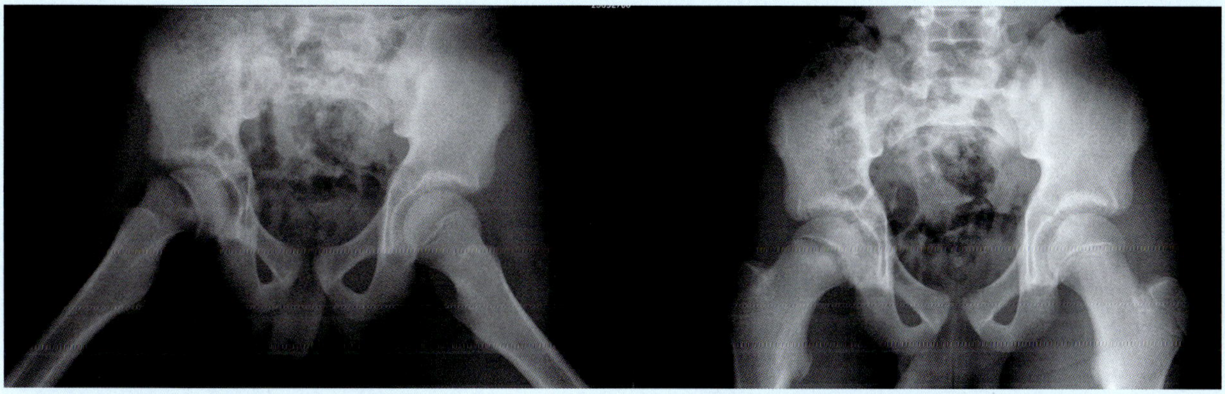

FIGURE 7.1. Frog-leg and anteroposterior pelvic radiographs reveal right moderate displaced slipped capital femoral epiphysis.

Percutaneous fixation following closed reduction and capsular decompression has recently been gaining popularity given its universal application and relatively easy technique.[5] In situ pinning has been the mainstay of SCFE treatment for decades, and our technique is described in Chapter 6. Briefly, the patient is positioned supine on a radiolucent table or on a fracture table. We prefer the radiolucent flat-top table, and we place a large gel roll under the patient's ipsilateral scapula to facilitate neutral positioning of the lower extremity with the patella pointing upward. Closed reduction of the SCFE can be performed with longitudinal traction followed by flexion and internal rotation; however, it is our preference to simply position the leg in neutral rotation and fix the epiphysis in situ without forceful reduction. Once the epiphyseal alignment is confirmed by fluoroscopy, a guide wire is inserted in the anterolateral aspect of the proximal femur distal to the intertrochanteric line. The guide wire is gradually advanced toward the center of the epiphysis in the AP and lateral projection (**Figure 7.2**). To obtain a lateral image, we strongly recommend rotation of the C-arm about 45° to 60° and simply flex the hip, avoiding external rotation and abduction that could displace the epiphysis and bend the guide wire. The screw length is determined, and a drill is advanced just past the physis to avoid penetration of the wire into the joint (**Figure 7.3**). During drilling, it is important to clear the flutes of bone to avoid heat necrosis of the bone, which can cause osteonecrosis. The screw is then inserted, and an intracranial pressure (ICP; Integra Camino; Integra Life Sciences) probe is introduced through the screw to monitor for pressure changes in the femoral head (**Figure 7.4**). In the case of absent waveform, a percutaneous capsulotomy is performed by introducing either a pair of scissors or a Cobb in the lateral aspect of the hip capsule. The surgeon then slides the Cobb medially to open the capsule while the intracapsular hematoma is expected to drain out of the wound (**Figure 7.5**). After decompression of the intracapsular hematoma, the changes in pressure and to the femoral head can be captured by the ICP monitor that should show a waveform that corresponds to the patient's heart rate.

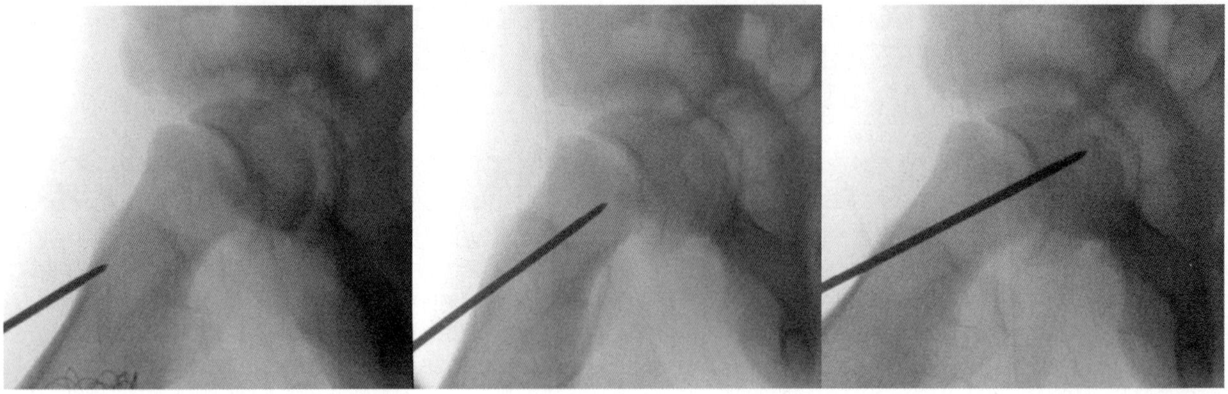

FIGURE 7.2. Intraoperative lateral fluoroscopy image shows gradual advancement of the guide wire for the cannulated 7.3-mm screw system. Note that the epiphysis remains with displacement, although it is slightly reduced after the patient is positioned on the radiolucent table in comparison with the preoperative imaging. The guide wire is typically introduced through the anterior cortex of the femoral metaphysis and should point toward the center of the femoral head.

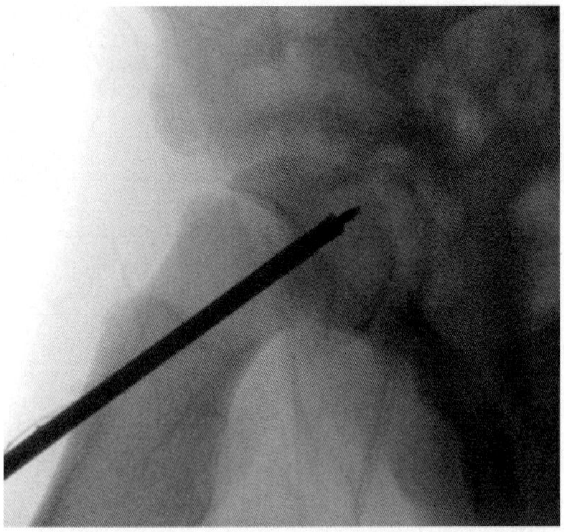

FIGURE 7.3. Intraoperative fluoroscopy image in the lateral projection showing a cannulated drill introduced over the guide wire and just past the physis. We attempt not to pass the drill too deep into the epiphysis to avoid penetration of the subchondral bone by the pin and perforation into the joint and also to avoid overheating the subchondral bone.

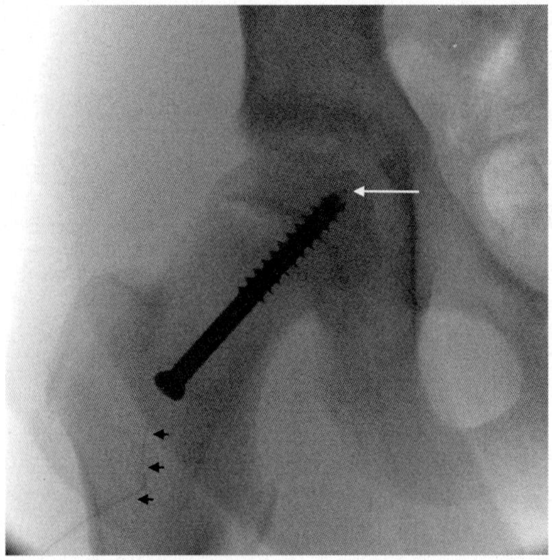

FIGURE 7.4. Intraoperative fluoroscopy image in the anteroposterior projection shows the screw is in good position. Note that there is an intracranial pressure probe introduced through the screw. (White arrow points to the tip of the probe in the femoral head; black arrowheads point to the tail of the intracranial pressure probe.) The probe did not read changes in the pressure of the femoral head.

In this particular case, the patient was discharged home the next day from surgery with instructions to be non–weight-bearing in the right lower extremity. He was seen 2 weeks following surgery when fixation of the epiphysis was confirmed to be adequate. However, about 4 weeks after surgery, he slipped and fell at home and presented to the emergency room with further displacement of the epiphysis and a broken screw (**Figure 7.6**). Given the presence of a bent/broken screw and further displacement of the epiphysis, we opted to address this complicated problem using a surgical hip dislocation and a subcapital realignment according to the modified Dunn technique. The bent screw was removed after the femoral neck was exposed following dissection of the retinacular flap (**Figure 7.7**). The femoral metaphysis was carefully exposed and the callus from the posterior aspect of the neck resected (**Figure 7.8**). The epiphysis was then reduced onto the metaphysis and fixed with two cannulated

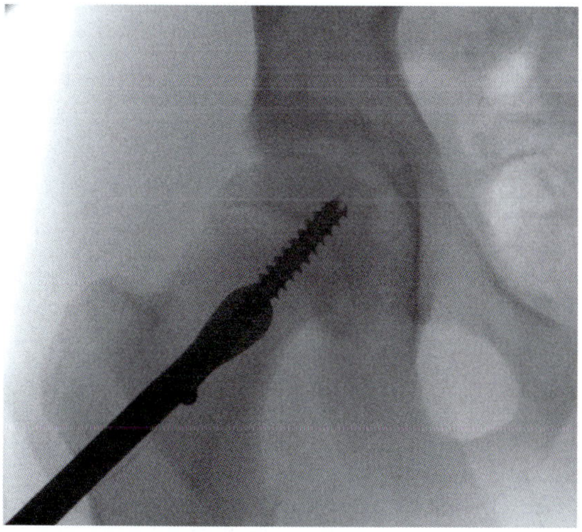

FIGURE 7.5. Intraoperative fluoroscopy image in the anteroposterior projection shows a Cobb elevator that was introduced percutaneously to open the anterolateral hip capsule. A hip capsulotomy is performed by pushing the Cobb medially. The indication for the capsulotomy was to evacuate the hematoma and decompress the joint. Following capsulotomy, the intracranial pressure monitor registered a waveform.

screws (Figure 7.9). Following the modified Dunn procedure, the patient was on a non–weight-bearing protocol for 8 weeks, before resuming ambulation with crutches followed by unrestricted activities. His most recent radiographs at 1.5 years after the modified Dunn procedure showed a completely healed SCFE, and he was released to full activities (Figure 7.10).

SUBCAPITAL REALIGNMENT USING THE MODIFIED DUNN PROCEDURE FOR UNSTABLE SLIPPED CAPITAL FEMORAL EPIPHYSIS

Treatment of unstable SCFE using the modified Dunn procedure has potential advantages, including the complete decompression of the intracapsular hematoma and the realignment of the capital femoral epiphysis, while protecting the retinacular flap containing the blood supply to the femoral head. The first study from our center, in collaboration with the University of Berne in Switzerland,

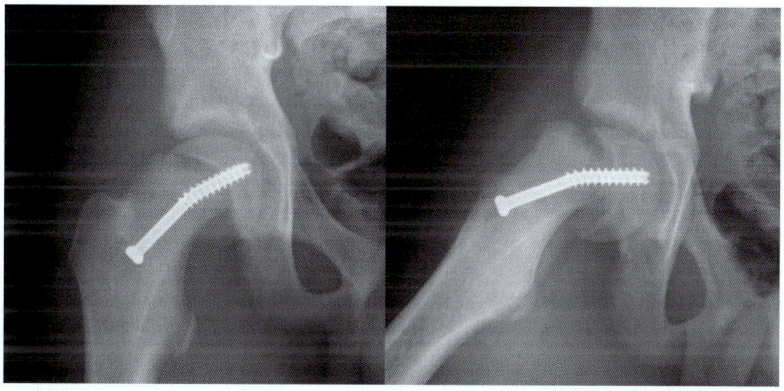

FIGURE 7.6. Anteroposterior and frog-leg lateral radiographs of the right hip about 4 weeks after in situ pinning following a fall at home showing the single screw is bent/broken.

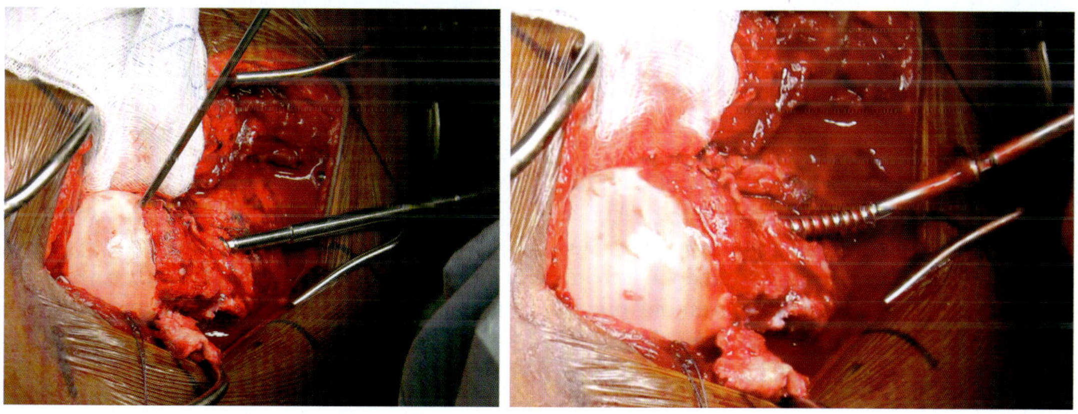

FIGURE 7.7. Intraoperative photograph shot during the modified Dunn procedure shows that removal of the bent screw is difficult but facilitated by the exposure.

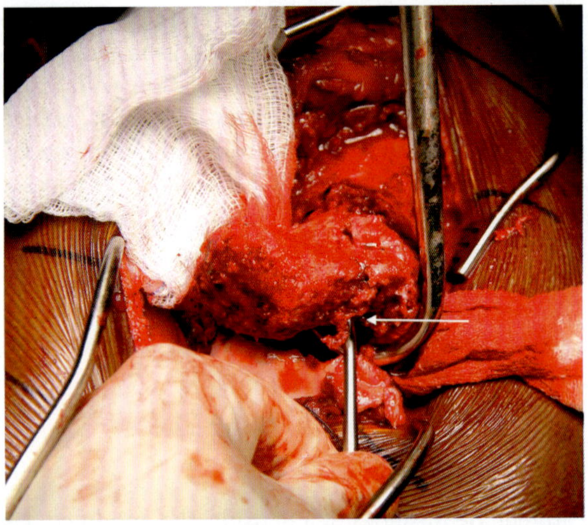

FIGURE 7.8. Intraoperative photograph taken after the epiphysis has been separated from the metaphyseal stump. A bone hook is placed in the posterior aspect of the femoral neck to lift the femur and to expose the posterior area of the metaphysis, facilitating removal of the abundant callus with a curette (white arrow).

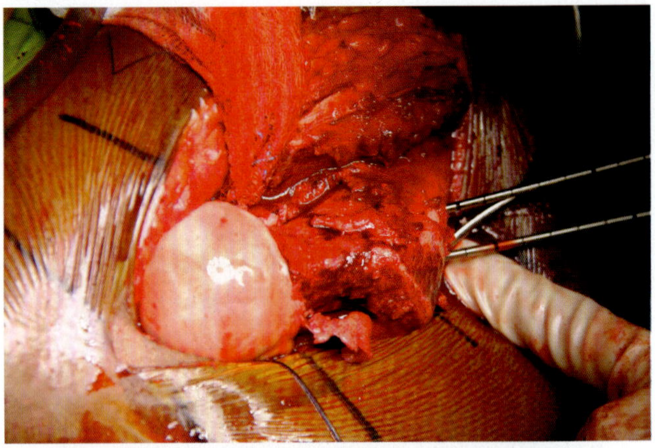

FIGURE 7.9. Intraoperative photograph showing the femoral head being reduced into the femoral neck after adequate resection of the posterior callus; it is fixed with two guide wires for the 7.3-mm cannulated screw system in a parallel fashion.

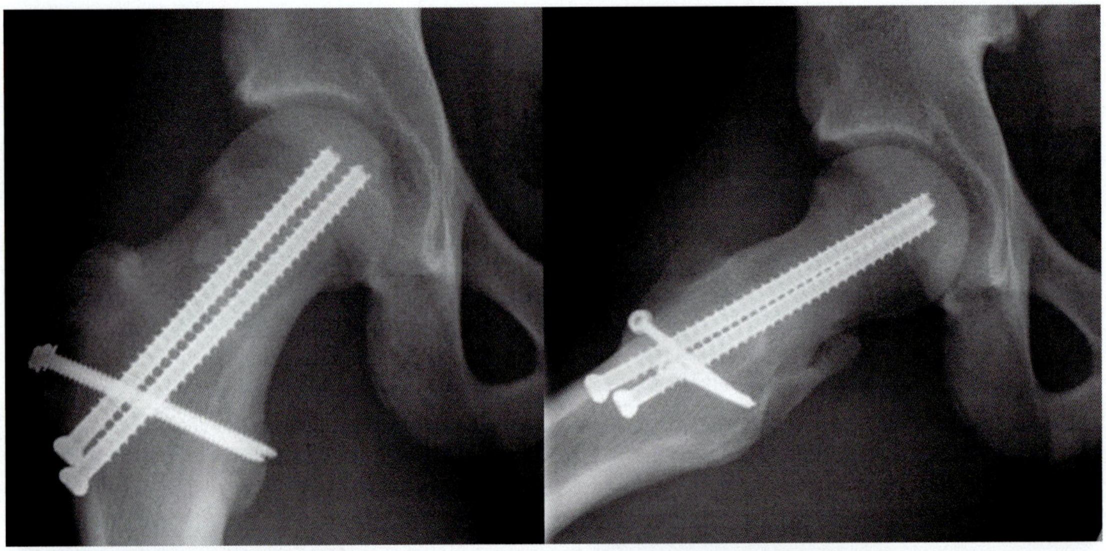

FIGURE 7.10. Postoperative anteroposterior and frog-leg lateral radiographs obtained at 18 months following surgery show completely healed slipped capital femoral epiphysis with normal concavity of the anterior femoral head and neck junction.

showed promising results with a minimal rate of complications.[8] However, recent series have reported an overall rate of 25% of osteonecrosis of the femoral head after the treatment of unstable SCFE with the modified Dunn in multiple centers across North America.[9] Given our previous reported experience,[8] we continue to favor the modified Dunn procedure for unstable SCFE if surgery is to be performed during the regular hospital hours when we can rely on the orthopedic nursing and scrub technician staff. The modified Dunn technique is performed using a surgical hip dislocation approach with dissection of the extended retinacular flap containing the nutrient vessels to the femoral head, as described by Professor Reynold Ganz.[8,10,11]

Clinical Scenario

A 13-year-old male presented with hip pain and inability to walk or bear any weight in his right lower extremity since a fall at school. AP radiograph showed complete severely displaced slip on the right (**Figure 7.11**). The patient was brought to the operating room the same day for a subcapital realignment using the modified Dunn procedure.

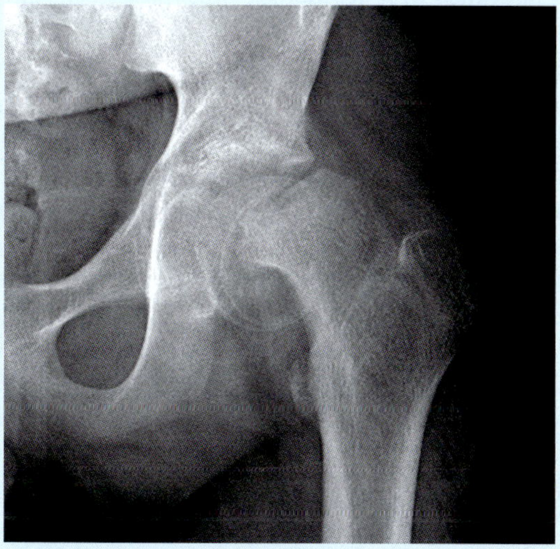

FIGURE 7.11. Preoperative anteroposterior radiograph of the right hip showing a severely displaced unstable slipped capital femoral epiphysis.

For acute severely displaced unstable SCFE, the patient should be carefully positioned in the lateral decubitus, avoiding internal rotation of the hip, which theoretically puts the retinacular vessels under increased tension as it tries to reduce the slip. The operated leg rests on a flat pillow, and the entire lower extremity and the hemipelvis are draped free (**Figure 7.12**). A straight incision on top of the greater trochanter slightly anterior to the tip of the trochanter is performed (**Figure 7.13**). At least two-fifths of the incision should be proximal to the trochanter. The subcutaneous tissue is dissected, exposing the fascia lata and the fascia covering the abductor muscles (**Figure 7.14**). Opening of the fascia lata can be performed from distal to proximal and from proximal to distal. If performed from distal to proximal, the fascia is opened, and at the tip of the greater trochanter, the surgeon places the index finger under the fascia to feel the interval between the gluteus maximus and the tensor fascia lata muscle. The fascia is then opened in the anterior aspect of the gluteus maximus musculature following the Gibson interval. Historically, this procedure was described through the posterior Kocher-Langenbeck, but currently it is preferred to be performed through the Gibson interval to avoid damage to the gluteus maximus muscle belly. Another option is to perform the split of the fascia from proximal to distal. To do so, the anterior border of the gluteus maximus is identified through the fascia and is opened at that level. Proximally, the fascia and the muscle belly of the gluteus medius can be easily identified, and the interval between the gluteus maximus and the gluteus medius is developed, whereas the fascia lata is split distally in line with the incision.

The trochanteric bursa and the gluteal bursa are open, allowing for exposure of the gluteus medius tendon and muscle belly, which should be retracted anteriorly to allow for exposure of the piriformis tendon. The piriformis tendon can be easily palpated, and the tendon is grasped with a pickup and pulled posteriorly to allow for identification of the most posterior aspect of the gluteus minimus inserting into the hip capsule. The interval between the gluteus minimus and the piriformis muscle is dissected to facilitate later identification of this interval for the trochanteric osteotomy. The gluteus minimus should be elevated from the posterior aspect of the capsule and the ileum up

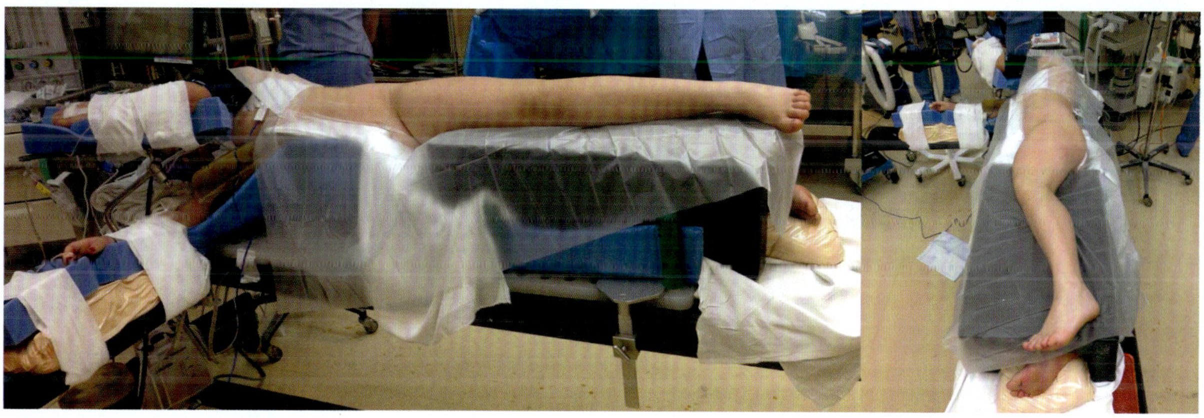

FIGURE 7.12. For the modified Dunn technique, the patient is positioned in a lateral decubitus position on a radiolucent flat table with a pegboard. A special leg support is used as a flat platform on which the operated leg rests during the initial part of the procedure and the contralateral limb positioned under the leg support. For positioning of the arms, a foam is used to avoid pressure over the bony prominences. The contralateral arm rests with slight elbow flexion to avoid tension of the median nerve.

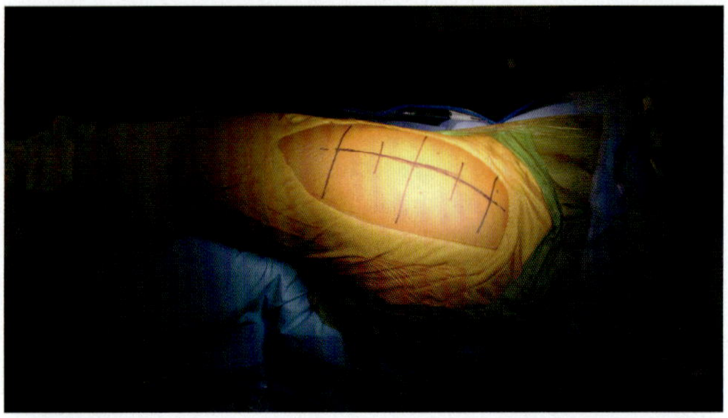

FIGURE 7.13. Intraoperative photograph showing the straight incision marked slightly anterior to the tip of the greater trochanter. The incision measures around 20 to 25 cm depending on the patient's size and thigh circumference.

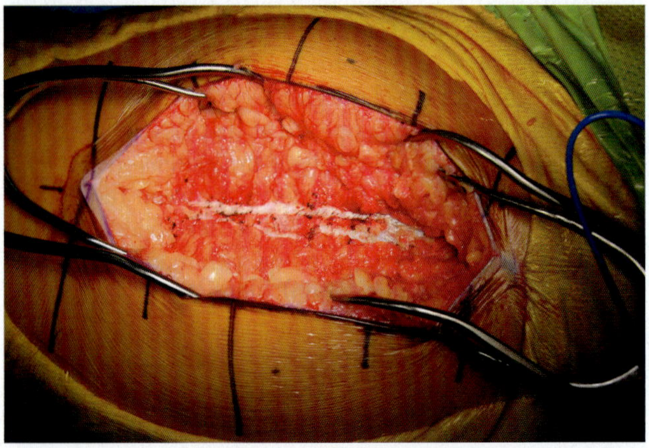

FIGURE 7.14. Intraoperative photograph showing the fascia lata and the fascia covering the abductor muscles exposed after the subcutaneous tissue is dissected. The incision of the fascia lata is marked and should follow the Gibson interval proximally.

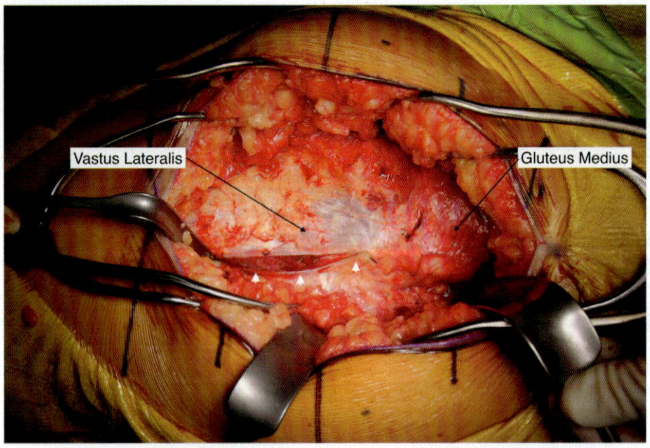

FIGURE 7.15. Intraoperative photograph showing the vastus lateralis and the gluteus medius after the fascia lata has been split longitudinally. An incision is performed at the most posterior aspect of the vastus lateralis muscle, and the muscle is dissected from the femur in a posterior to anterior fashion (white arrowheads).

to the level of the sciatic notch to reduce tension during the dislocation. Careful dissection is recommended, and dissection distal and posterior to the piriformis is not encouraged in view of the risk of damage to the branches from the inferior gluteal arteries that performed an anastomosis with the medial femoral circumflex artery. Next, the vastus lateralis and the sleeve of the tendinous insertion of the gluteus maximus are identified distally to the greater trochanter. A sleeve of the posterior aspect of the vastus lateralis fascia is opened, and the vastus lateralis is elevated from the femur while preserving the periosteum intact (**Figure 7.15**). A thin Hohmann retractor is placed in the anterior aspect of the femur just distal to the greater trochanter, facilitating exposure of the posterior aspect of the vastus lateralis insertion, which serves as a reference for the distal end of the trochanteric osteotomy that will follow. Proximally, the gluteus minimus is retracted anteriorly, allowing for exposure of the piriformis tendon to guide the trochanteric osteotomy.

The trochanteric osteotomy is performed with an oscillating saw (**Figure 7.16**). While performing the osteotomy, close attention should be paid to avoid an excessively deep osteotomy that would violate the trochanteric or piriformis fossa and potentially damage the deep branch of the medial circumflex artery. As a reference, the osteotomy should start proximally and about 3 to 5 mm medial to the insertion of the gluteus medius tendon into the trochanter. Distally, the reference point is the posterior aspect of origin of the vastus lateralis. Once the osteotomy is performed, it should be completely at its medial aspect with an osteotome. The trochanteric free fragment

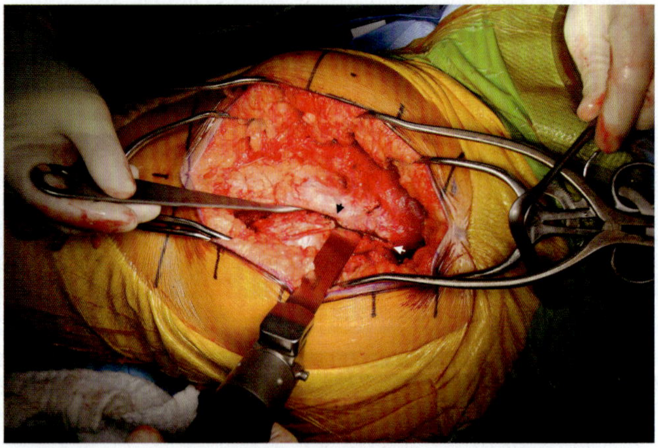

FIGURE 7.16. Intraoperative photograph showing a transverse straight digastric osteotomy of the greater trochanter performed with an oscillating saw. The reference points for the osteotomy are the posterior origin of the vastus lateralis (black arrowhead) at the trochanteric ridge and the insertion of the gluteus medius. About 3 mm of the most posterior fibers of the gluteus medius (white arrowhead) is left attached to the greater trochanter base to avoid creating an osteotomy that is excessively medial because this may cause damage to the deep branch of the medial femoral circumflex artery.

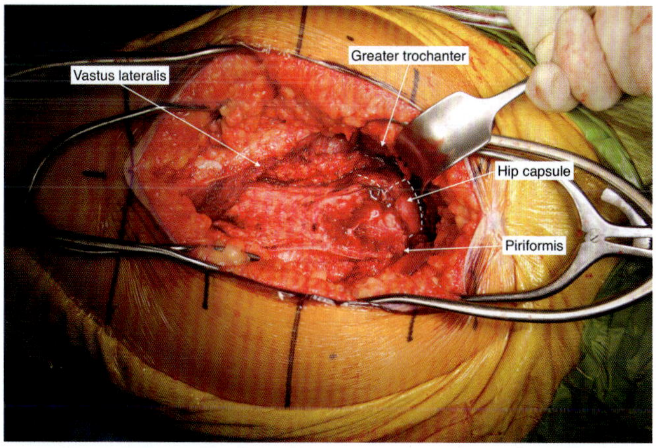

FIGURE 7.17. Intraoperative photograph showing the exposure of the hip capsule after the interval between the piriformis tendon and the gluteus minimus was dissected and the greater trochanter fragment had been mobilized anteriorly. Traced white lines mark the capsulotomy that is performed in three steps: first, the capsule is cut in line with the femoral neck, starting at the superior-medial corner of the trochanteric base; second, the capsule is cut from that corner toward the inferior aspect of the acetabulum. The third cut of the capsule is performed from the end of the first cut at the level of the acetabular rim in a posterior direction, parallel to the labrum and toward the piriformis tendon.

is then flipped anteriorly with insertion of the gluteus medius and the vastus lateralis, allowing exposure of the capsule (**Figure 7.17**). For capsular exposure, it is recommended that posteriorly, the interval between the gluteus minimus and the piriformis is fully developed and the gluteus minimus is retracted anteriorly and elevated from the hip capsule. Distally, the vastus intermedius should be elevated from its insertion to allow for complete exposure of the hip capsule. The indirect head of the rectus femoris can be identified, and it serves as a reference point that enough exposure of the capsule is achieved anteriorly. At this point, a thin Hohman retractor can be inserted into the superior and lateral aspect of the ilium above the acetabular rim for exposure.

Next, a capsulotomy is performed. The capsulotomy is performed with three limbs. For the right hip, it has the shape of the letter Z. The longitudinal limb of the capsulotomy is along the femoral neck axis, and it should start at the proximal and anterior corner of the trochanteric osteotomy and be performed in a retrograde fashion toward the acetabular rim. An inside-out capsulotomy is performed to avoid damage to the underlying periosteum and acetabular labrum. Next, the capsulotomy is continued with the inferior length of the Z shape. For that limb, the capsule is cut toward the inferior aspect of the acetabulum. Finally, the capsule is opened posteriorly in the superior limb of the Z shape toward the piriformis muscle. There is no need to pass the capsulotomy distal to the piriformis, and that should be avoided. Immediately after the capsulotomy is performed, acute hematoma extravasation can be observed from the joint.

After capsulotomy, the femoral neck can be visualized, but, typically, not the femoral head. Very carefully, slight traction can be applied, and this would allow for visualization of the femoral head to plan for provisional fixation. Once the femoral head is partially visualized, two 2.5-mm threaded Kirschner wires should be used to provisionally fix the femoral head to the neck (**Figure 7.18**). The pins are placed anteriorly in the neck ending toward the head very carefully to avoid penetrating through the femoral head into the acetabulum because this could damage the acetabular cartilage with any attempt to dislocate the hip. After provisional fixation, the hip can be brought into flexion and external rotation, thereby allowing a break in the suction seal and subluxation of the femoral head. The ligamentum teres should be cut at its base to allow complete dislocation of the femoral head with further flexion and external rotation of the hip. The leg should rest in a sterile bag placed at the opposite side of the surgical table. A 1.6-mm K-wire can be used to create a hole in the femoral head to monitor blood flow. Blood flow monitoring can be undertaken via assessment of active bleeding and be incremented by using an ICP monitor. Identification and recording of the retinacular flap insertion in the femoral head and the anterior periosteum are recommended. The anterior periosteum is typically always torn, but the retinacular flap insertion in the posterior aspect of the femoral head is typically preserved. Complete disruption of the retinaculum, however, has been reported and is a bad prognostic factor for osteonecrosis of the femoral head. The acetabular cavity should be inspected, and the severity of articular cartilage damage recorded. The

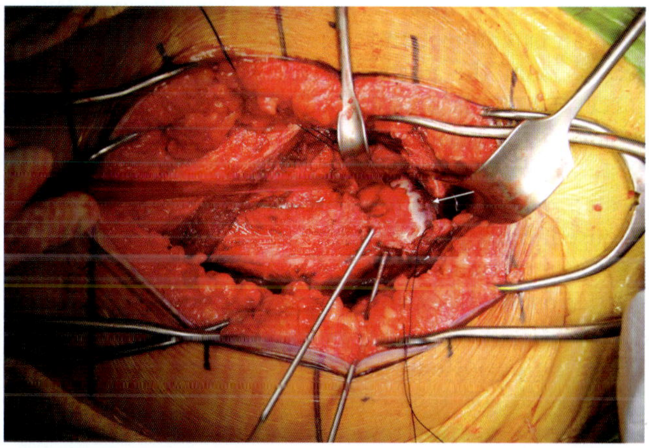

FIGURE 7.18. Intraoperative photograph showing the metaphysis of the proximal femur that is prominent anteriorly (white arrow). The hip capsule was opened, and the capsule segments were tagged with a number 0 Vicryl. Two threaded K-wires (2.5 mm) were inserted into the anterior aspect of the metaphysis, pointing toward the center of the epiphysis. Careful insertion is recommended to avoid penetration of the joint.

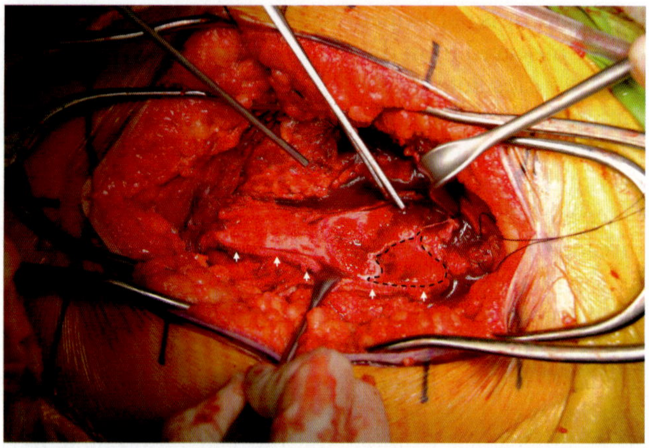

FIGURE 7.19. Intraoperative photograph showing the lateral aspect of the proximal femur. With the hip relocated in the acetabulum, the retinacular soft tissue is dissected, to allow for resection of the posterior/proximal aspect of the proximal trochanter (marked in dashed black lines). Dissection of the posterior aspect of the trochanter was started in a subperiosteal fashion from about 4 cm distally. A small periosteal elevator facilitates the posteriorly oriented dissection of the periosteum (white arrowheads).

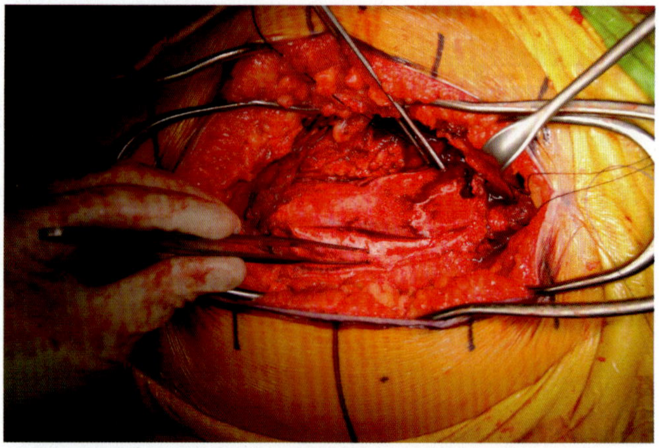

FIGURE 7.20. Intraoperative photograph showing the dissected thick periosteum (grasped by the forceps). Partial subperiosteal dissection around the greater trochanter base posteriorly and superiorly was performed before the trochanter was resected.

femoral head is then relocated back in the acetabulum for dissection of the retinacular soft tissue flap.

The retinacular soft tissue flap is dissected by resection of the proximal/posterior portion of the greater trochanter (**Figure 7.19**). The flap contains the deep branches of the medial circumflex artery and the short external rotators to the femoral head. Resection of the trochanter can be done using a piecemeal technique or by dissecting the posterior aspect of the periosteum and resecting the posterior trochanter as a unit. In older patients, the piecemeal technique is typically performed with an osteotome, and a small segment of bone is released from the posterior trochanter. The small free piece of bone is grasped with a rongeur and rotated, exposing the periosteum around it. Sharp periosteum dissection releases the free piece, and the process is repeated until the posterior aspect of the femoral neck is exposed. Most patients with SCFE, however, are young and have a rather thick periosteum, which facilitates subperiosteal dissection around the posterior aspect of the trochanter before any bone is resected (**Figure 7.20**). Once the periosteum is dissected posteriorly, the trochanter can be removed. The trochanteric apophysis is the reference for resection of the stable trochanter because it corresponds to the base of the femoral neck (**Figure 7.21**). The periosteum of the anterior aspect of the femoral neck is sharply incised with a scalpel, and the periosteum along with the soft tissue flap is freed proximally. Distally, dissection of the soft tissue flap is extended to the level of the lesser trochanter, creating a long flap without tension. After resection of the greater trochanter is completed and the posterior aspect of the femoral neck is exposed, the hip is dislocated with flexion and external rotation. A moist sponge should be placed in the acetabulum to prevent the femoral head from reducing back into the joint. The anterior periosteum is then dissected from the anterior and inferior aspects of the femoral neck, allowing complete exposure of the neck. The threaded K-wires that were provisionally fixing the epiphysis are removed, and the epiphysis can be easily separated from the metaphysis.

The femoral neck is completely exposed to the level of the lesser trochanter and protected with a blunt

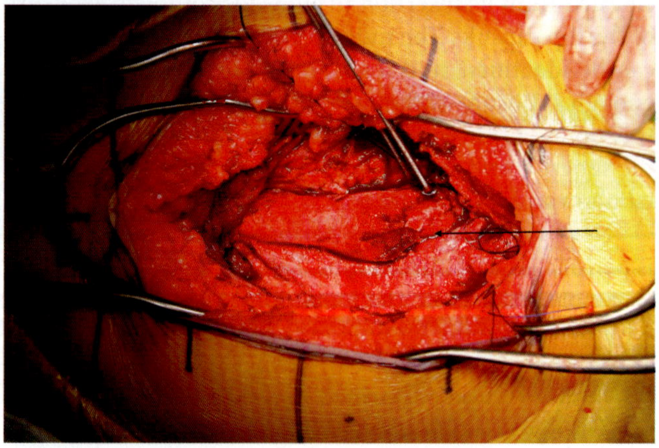

FIGURE 7.21. Intraoperative photograph after the trochanter was reduced by resection of the bone proximal to the greater trochanteric apophysis, allowing exposure of the posterior aspect of the femoral neck (black arrow). Note that the retinacular soft tissue flap is completely dissected from the stump of the metaphysis proximally and to the level of the lesser trochanter distally to decrease the tension on the flap once the epiphysis is reduced back into the metaphysis.

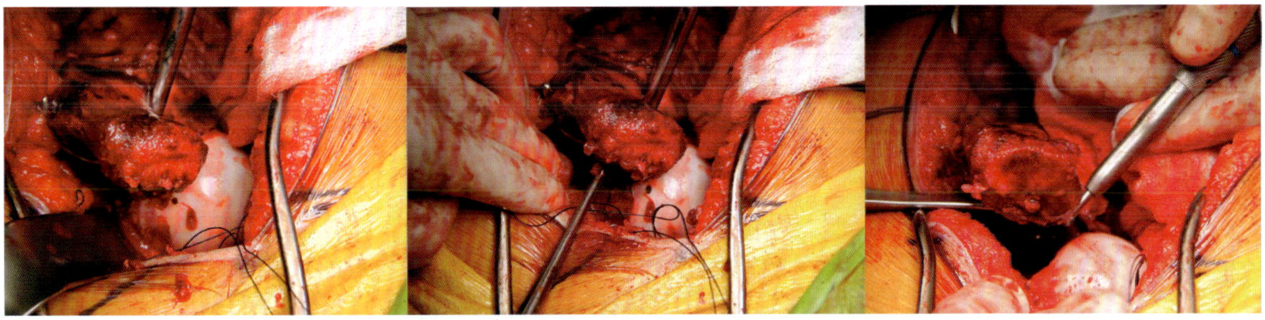

FIGURE 7.22. Intraoperative photograph showing the femoral neck that had been exposed by a blunt retractor placed underneath it. The metaphysis must be contoured before the epiphysis is reduced. The posterior callus formation is resected using a curette (middle image). A high-speed burr (left-sided image) facilitates contouring of the metaphysis stump into a round surface.

retractor. The neck stump is recontoured into a round shape by resection of the posterior callus, taking care to align it perpendicular to the axis of the neck. If needed, the femoral neck may be shortened slightly to facilitate reduction of the epiphysis. However, we rarely performed shortening more than 2 to 3 mm. Excessive femoral neck shortening is not recommended because of the potential risk of instability with the decreased offset of the proximal femur (**Figure 7.22**). The surgeon carefully grasps the epiphysis, exposing the undersurface so the residual physis can be removed with a curette. Once the epiphysis and the metaphysis are prepared, the leg is slightly internally rotated, and the epiphysis can be carefully reduced onto the femoral neck while the soft tissue retinacular flap is protected. The epiphysis should be reduced in correct alignment, and this can be assured by the position of the fovea and the retinaculum. Once the reduction is deemed adequate, the epiphysis can be fixed to the metaphysis (**Figure 7.23**). After fixation, the blood supply to the femoral head is rechecked both by observing the presence of active bleeding and by checking the ICP probe and checking for the waveform in the monitor. If the blood supply is reduced or not restored, careful assessment of the retinacular tension is recommended.

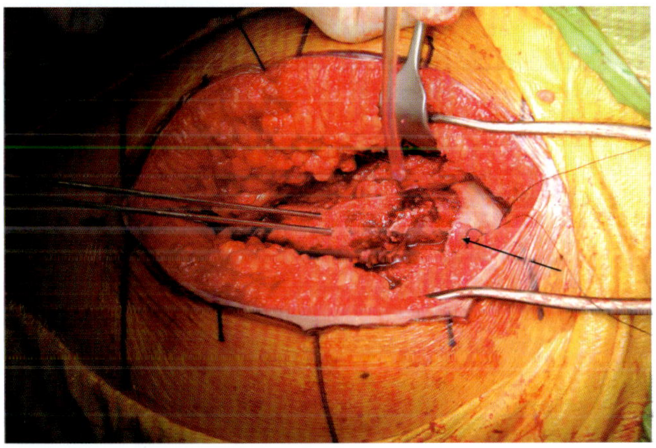

FIGURE 7.23. Intraoperative photograph showing that the epiphysis has been reduced onto the metaphysis and fixed with two guide wires for the 6.5-mm cannulated screw system. The retinacular flap containing the deep branches of the medial circumflex artery is intact in the posterior aspect of the femoral head (black arrow).

We have used two different techniques for epiphyseal fixation. The traditional fixation is performed in a retrograde fashion by a 3-mm fully threaded K-wire introduced through the fovea and exiting the lateral cortex just distal to the greater trochanter. Once the wire is completely introduced, the femoral head can be reduced back in the acetabulum and the varus-valgus alignment confirmed. One or preferably two additional threaded wires are added for fixation. Alternatively, the epiphysis can be fixed by two 6.5-mm cannulated screws placed in the usual fashion from the anterolateral aspect of the femur just distal to the trochanteric osteotomy onto the femoral epiphysis. The guide wires are placed initially, the femoral head reduced, and the fixation is finalized with the hip in a reduced position. After the epiphysis is fixed and C-arm fluoroscopy confirms the correct alignment and appropriate fixation, the periosteal flap can be loosely approximated and sutured with two or three 3.0 Vicryl stitches, avoiding any tension. The hip capsule is also closed and sutured with a 2.0 Vicryl in a loose fashion, avoiding excessive tension. The greater trochanter is reattached with two or three 3.5-mm screws, applied using standard compression technique.

Postoperatively, patients are placed on a foam abduction pillow for the first 2 to 3 weeks. We recommend a non–weight-bearing protocol with the use of a wheelchair and transfers only for the first 6 to 8 weeks while consolidation of the epiphysis and greater trochanter takes place. Partial weight-bearing with crutches is then recommended for 4 additional weeks, and the patient typically resumes ambulation without any aids thereafter. We monitor the femoral head healing with radiographs obtained at a 3-month interval (**Figure 7.24**).

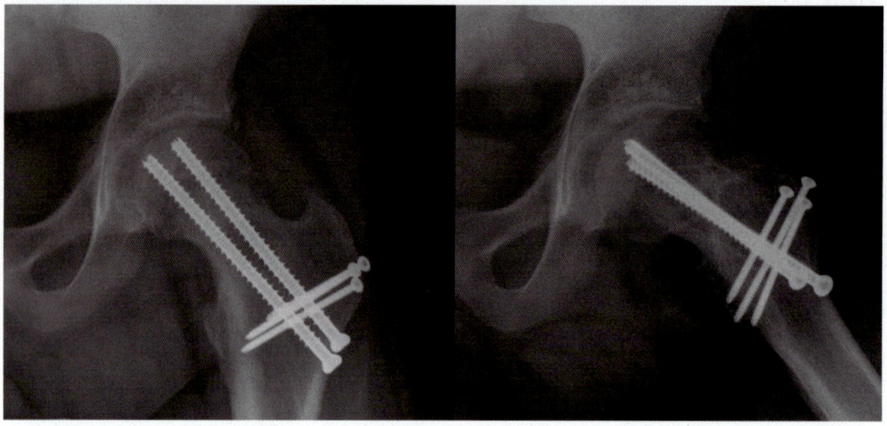

FIGURE 7.24. Postoperative anteroposterior and frog-leg lateral radiographs obtained 18 months after surgery demonstrating healed slipped capital femoral epiphysis with preserved concavity of the femoral head and neck junction.

OPEN REDUCTION THROUGH AN ANTEROLATERAL WATSON-JONES APPROACH—A STRATEGY FOR THE TREATMENT OF UNSTABLE SLIPPED CAPITAL FEMORAL EPIPHYSIS IN THE MIDDLE OF THE NIGHT

Often, the logistics of a busy operating room may forbid treatment to be done during regular hours. The ideal timing for an unstable SCFE to be treated remains controversial. However, we believe that an unstable SCFE should be treated as soon as the diagnosis is confirmed and, ideally, in the first 12 hours and no later than 24 hours after the onset of acute symptoms. If treatment needs to happen late in the day or during the night, when a dedicated orthopedic staff team is not available, performing a modified Dunn may be difficult. In those situations, we have been using the open reduction technique described by Parsch and colleagues.[12] In the original study, the authors reported an overall 5% proportion of osteonecrosis for the treatment of unstable SCFE.[12]

Clinical Scenario

A 15-year-old male presented with inability to walk or bear any weight in his left leg. He had had intermittent mild hip pain for the past 2 weeks but had been able to ambulate and play sports. He slipped and fell at home and felt immediate pain and was unable to ambulate. He was taken to the emergency department (ED) the next day, and at evaluation he was holding the left lower extremity in external rotation, and any attempt to move the hip led to severe pain. AP pelvic radiograph revealed severely displaced SCFE (**Figure 7.25**). Given the long evolution and the time of injury to presentation, we decided to bring him to the operating room that night for an open reduction using an anterolateral Watson-Jones approach.

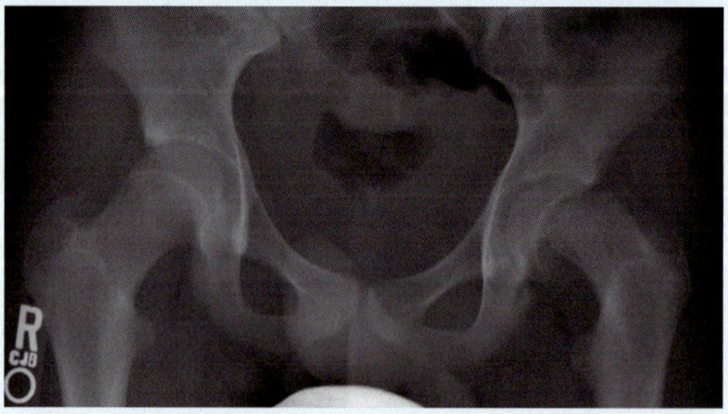

FIGURE 7.25. Preoperative anteroposterior radiograph of the pelvis showing a left severely displaced unstable slipped capital femoral epiphysis.

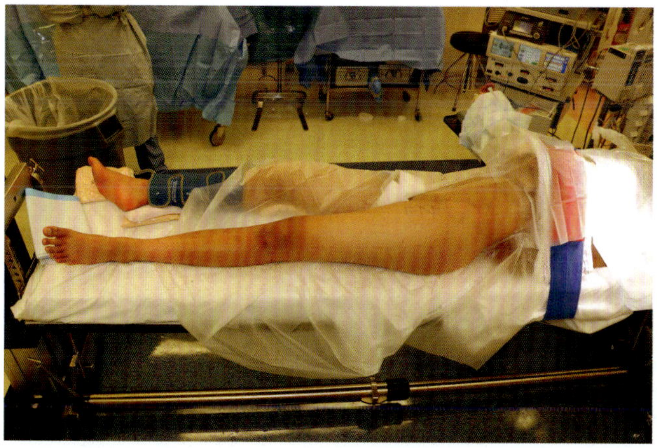

FIGURE 7.26. Intraoperative photograph showing the patient positioned supine on a radiolucent table with a bump under the ipsilateral shoulder. The ipsilateral arm is crossed over the chest. The entire hemipelvis and lower extremity should be prepared and draped free.

Although open reduction of SCFE can be performed using the Smith-Petersen approach, we favor the Watson-Jones anterolateral approach because it allows complete exposure of the epiphysis, metaphysis and greater trochanter and subtrochanteric area, allowing the surgeon to reduce the deformity while fixing with screws or pins using the same approach. Open reduction of SCFE through an anterolateral approach is performed with the patient on a radiolucent table placed in what we called a sloppy lateral position (Figure 7.26). The entire lower extremity is prepared and draped free. An incision is placed beginning about 1 to 1.5 cm distal and 1 to 1.5 cm lateral to the anterior superior iliac spine curved distally and posteriorly around the greater trochanter and then placed in line with the greater trochanter and femoral diaphysis (Figure 7.27).

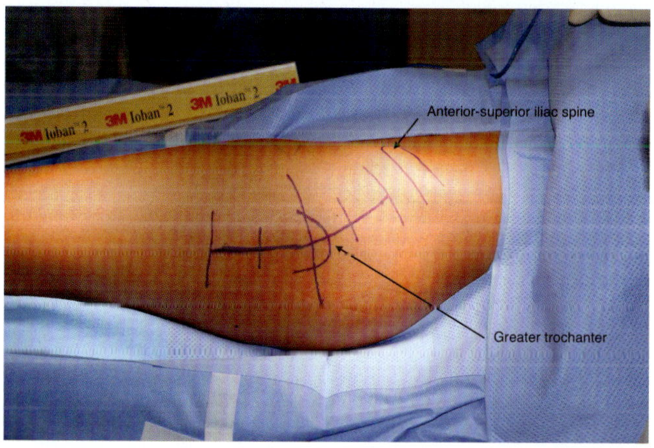

FIGURE 7.27. Intraoperative photograph showing the incision marked in the skin: it is placed about 2 to 3 cm distal and lateral to the anterior superior iliac spine and gently curved laterally toward the greater trochanter and then curved distally in line with the lateral aspect of the femoral shaft.

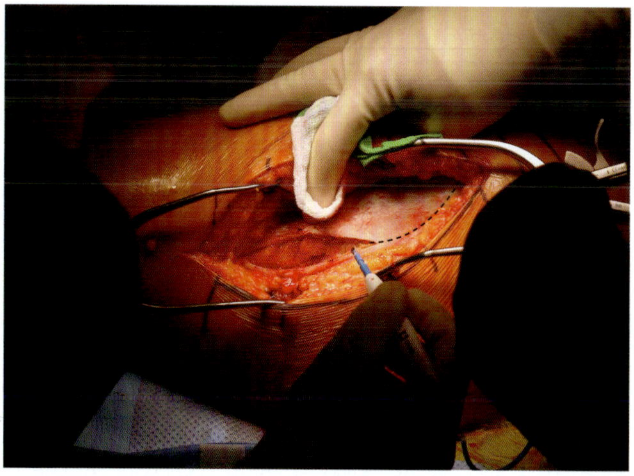

FIGURE 7.28. Intraoperative photograph showing the opening of the fascia lata in line with the skin incision. The fascia has been opened distally in line with the lateral aspect of the femur up to the greater trochanter, where it is curved proximally (dashed black lines) toward the anterior superior iliac spine.

After skin incision, the subcutaneous tissue is dissected, exposing the fascia lata (Figure 7.28). The fascia lata is open distally in line with the femur and proximally the fascia lata curved in line with the skin incision. We prefer to start by opening the fascia distally because it makes the identification of the tensor fascia lata and gluteus medius interval easier and more reliable. Identification of the interval between the gluteus medius and the vastus lateralis is the next step (Figure 7.29). The interval between the vastus lateralis along with the vastus intermedius and the most anterior fibers of the gluteus medius is dissected in a stepwise fashion (Figure 7.30). The vastus-gluteus medius interval is developed distally, whereas the gluteus medius is dissected free from the fascia lata proximally to develop the interval between the gluteus medius and the

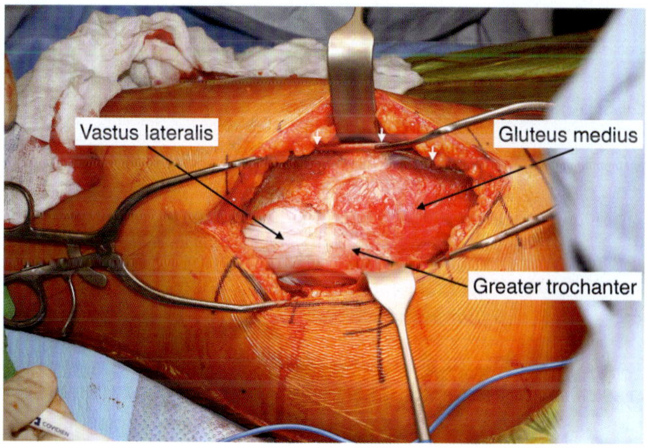

FIGURE 7.29. Intraoperative photograph taken after the fascia lata (small white arrows) has been opened, allowing extensive exposure of the vastus lateralis and gluteus medius.

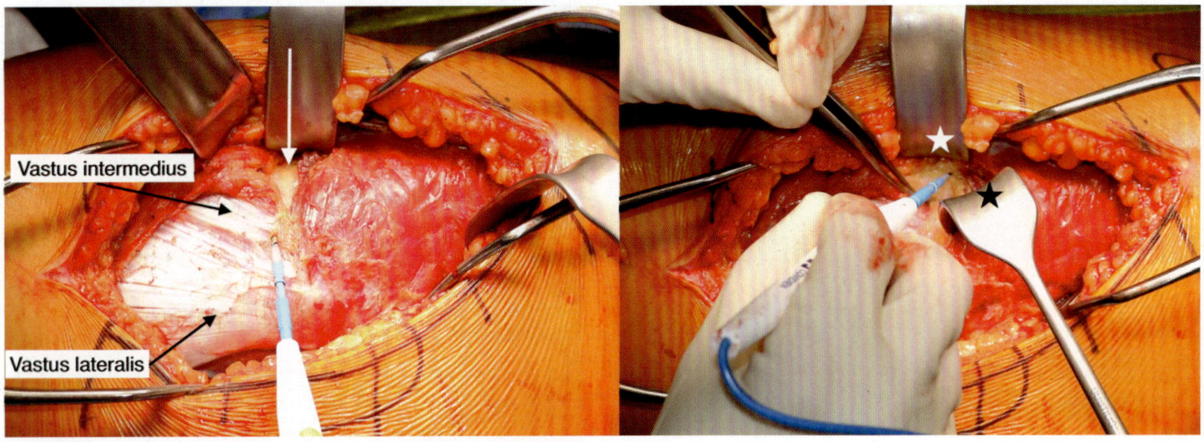

FIGURE 7.30. Intraoperative photograph showing, on the left-hand side, the interval (white arrow) between the anterior border of the gluteus medius and the vastus lateralis-intermedius complex. On the right-hand side, a photograph shows placement of one retractor (white star) posterior to the tensor fascia lata and one retractor (black star) anterior to the gluteus medius to facilitate the dissection of the interval between the two muscles.

tensor fascia lata muscle. The interval between the tensor fascia lata and the gluteus medius is exposed with careful protection of the branches from the superior gluteal vessels and nerve that innervates the tensor fascia lata muscle (**Figure 7.31**). With advanced dissection and proximal retraction of the gluteus medius, the hip capsule can be identified. Wide exposure of the hip capsule is achieved by detachment of the iliocapsularis muscle anteriorly and the capsular insertion of the gluteus minimus posteriorly (**Figure 7.32**). Before proceeding with capsulotomy, we expose the anterolateral aspect of the proximal femur in preparation for screw insertion. The vastus lateralis should be partially dissected free of its insertion in an L-fashion to expose the anterolateral cortex of the femur (**Figure 7.33**).

At this point in the operation, the entire anterior aspect of the capsule is exposed in preparation for the capsulotomy. The indirect head of the rectus femoris is typically identified proximally and serves as an anatomic reference that capsule exposure is adequate. Capsulotomy is performed in a T fashion, with the longitudinal arm of the capsulotomy in line with the femoral neck using an inside-out technique to avoid damage of the acetabular labrum proximally (**Figure 7.34**). As soon as the capsule is opened, extravasation of an intracapsular hematoma is routinely observed. The transverse opening of the capsule is performed just proximal to the indirect head of the rectus femoris. The capsule should be opened medially and laterally for an additional 1 cm in each direction parallel

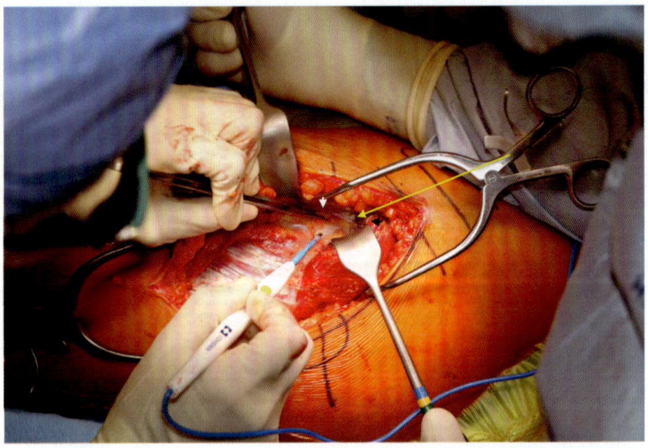

FIGURE 7.31. Intraoperative photograph showing advanced dissection of the tensor fascia lata (white arrowhead) and gluteus medius (black arrowhead) interval. With progressive dissection proximally, there will be small vessels and nerve branches (yellow arrow) from the superior gluteal nerve that should be dissected and preserved to avoid damage to the innervation of the tensor fascia lata muscle.

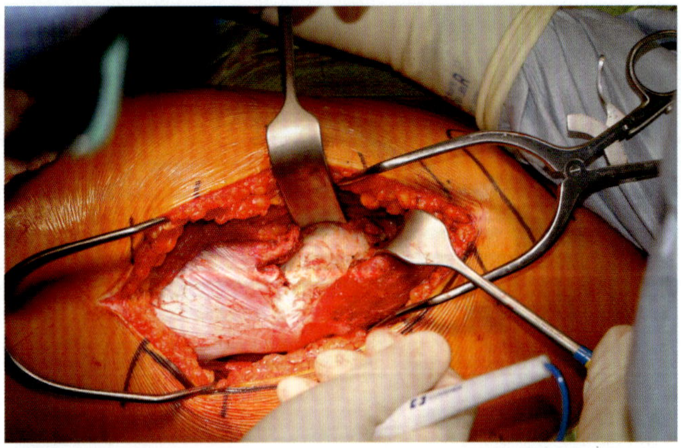

FIGURE 7.32. Intraoperative photograph showing ample exposure of the hip capsule after the iliocapsularis has been dissected from the capsule and retracted anteriorly and the gluteus minimus has been freed and dissected in line with the gluteus medius posteriorly.

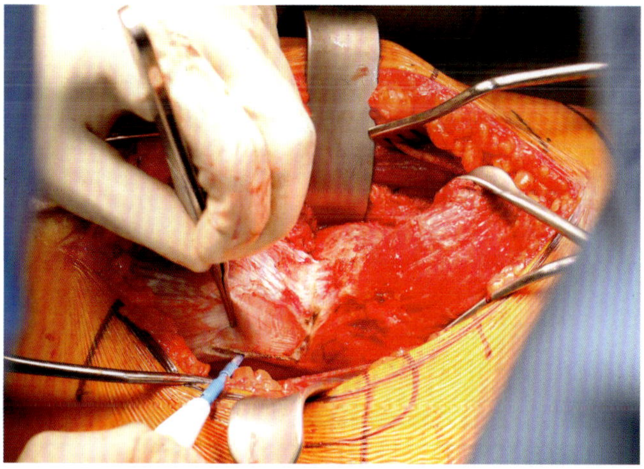

FIGURE 7.33. Intraoperative photograph showing the release of the vastus lateralis origin from the greater trochanter, allowing exposure of the anterolateral aspect of the femur for insertion of the guide wires and cannulated screws.

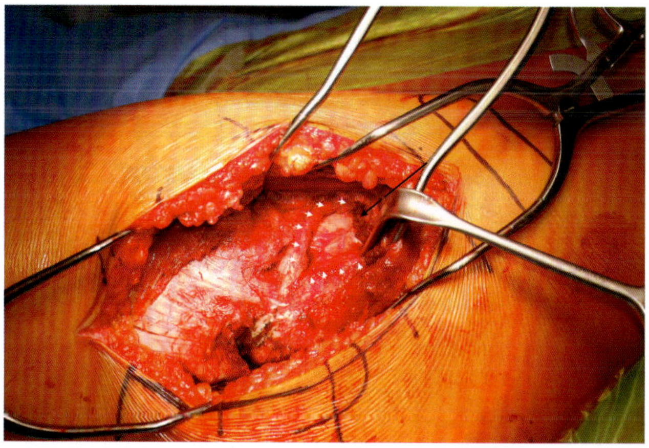

FIGURE 7.35. Intraoperative photograph taken after the capsulotomy (white arrowheads) has been completed showing the stump of the femoral neck metaphysis with a torn anterior periosteum (black arrow).

to the acetabular rim and labrum using an inside-out technique. Following completion of the capsulotomy, the metaphyseal stump of the femoral neck is identified (**Figure 7.35**). Once the femoral neck is identified, the epiphysis can be reduced. However, before the epiphysis is reduced, two guide wires for the cannulated screw system are introduced from the anterolateral aspect of the femur onto the neck under C-arm fluoroscopy. The two guide wires must stop short of the metaphyseal stump of the femoral neck (**Figure 7.36**).

One of the advantages of open reduction using the anterolateral approach is that it allows for gentle maneuver for reduction of the epiphysis. The reduction is performed with an assistant applying slight traction and flexion to about 45° or 60° with gradual gentle internal rotation. As a key step during the reduction, the surgeon's index fingertip should be placed in the anterior aspect of the metaphysis controlling the reduction. The surgeon places the index finger in the anterior and lateral aspect of the metaphysis and pushes the femoral neck guide while slight traction is provided by the assistant (**Figure 7.37**). Very importantly, the reduction maneuver should not be aimed toward an anatomic reduction of the femoral head. Rather, the reduction goal is to achieve alignment of the epiphysis with the metaphysis, reducing the acute component of the slip. In most, if not at all, cases of acute, severely displaced

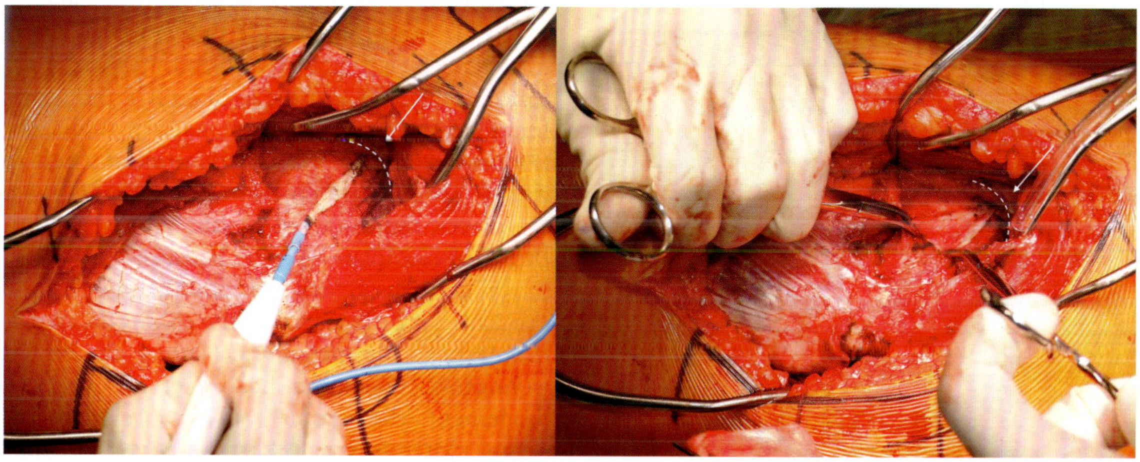

FIGURE 7.34. Intraoperative photograph showing the technique for the capsulotomy. On the left-hand side, a photograph showing the longitudinal limb of the capsulotomy has been marked to the level of the indirect head of the rectus femoris (white arrow). On the right-hand side, the capsule has been opened distally, and two clamps hold the capsule allowing for an inside-out cut of the capsule to the level of the indirect head of the rectus (white arrow). If needed, the indirect head can be released to facilitate exposure and repaired later at the time of wound closure.

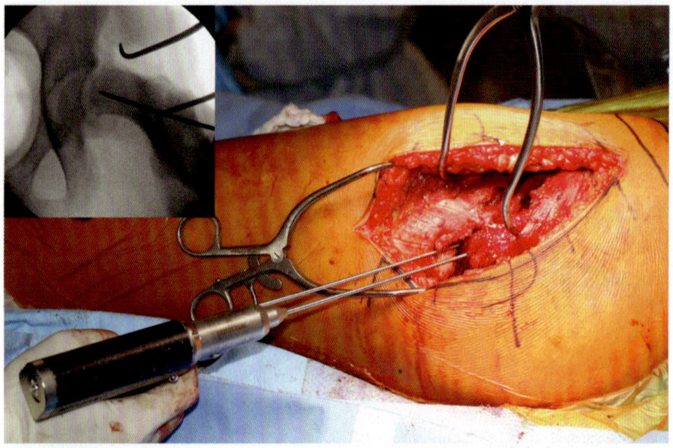

FIGURE 7.36. Intraoperative photograph showing provisional placement of the guide wires from the anterolateral aspect of the femur before the epiphysis is reduced. In the top-left corner, the corresponding fluoroscopy image shows the guide wire introduced in the center of the femoral neck that should stop short of the metaphyseal stump.

unstable SCFE, there is a spectrum of variation from a chronic process. In some cases, there is only mild remodeling of the femoral neck, whereas in most cases, remodeling of the neck and the presence of a posterior callus would make reduction to an anatomic position almost impossible. Therefore, we cannot emphasize enough that reduction through an open anterolateral approach should be performed to facilitate alignment of the epiphysis with the neck in the best position possible but should not aim toward anatomic alignment. Another major advantage of this procedure is that any residual metaphyseal bump that would remain in the anterolateral aspect of the metaphysis after reduction and fixation can be resected using a combination of a rongeur and a high-speed burr to allow for a better concavity of the head-neck junction.

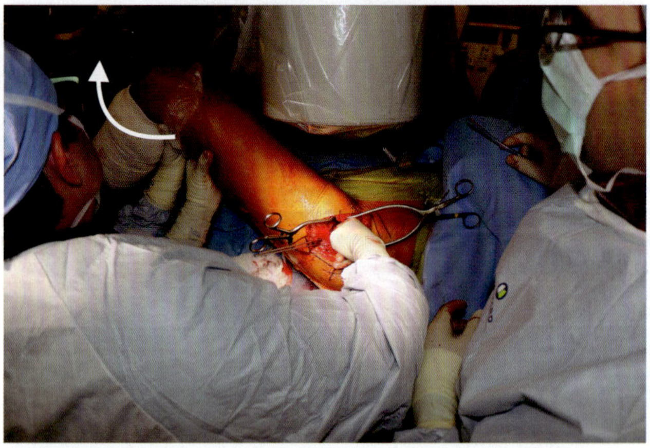

FIGURE 7.37. Intraoperative photograph showing the reduction maneuver. The assistant applies traction with the hip in 45° to 60° of flexion and slight internal rotation. The surgeon places the index finger in the metaphysis and controls the gentle reduction of the epiphysis.

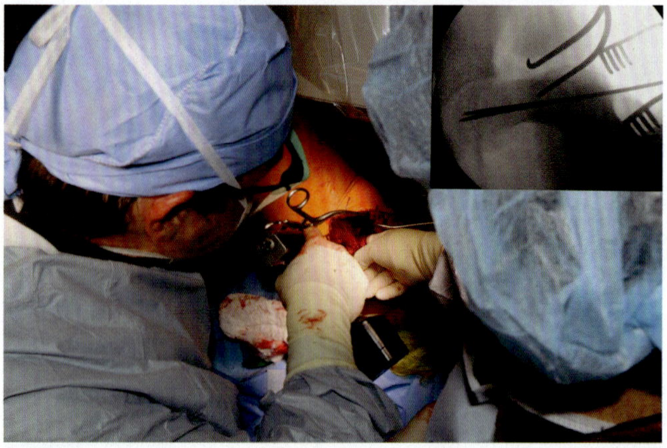

FIGURE 7.38. Intraoperative photograph showing fixation of the epiphysis. While keeping the index finger in the metaphysis controlling the reduction, the two previously placed guide wires are advanced under fluoroscopy guidance to provisionally fix the epiphysis. In the top right-hand corner, the corresponding fluoroscopy image shows the guide wire being introduced in the center of the femoral neck, which and should stop short of the subchondral bone to avoid intra-articular penetration.

After the surgeon confirms the reduction of the metaphysis on the epiphysis, the guide wire is advanced, allowing temporary fixation of the epiphysis (**Figure 7.38**). It is important for the surgeon to keep the index finger holding the reduction while the guide wires are advanced. Intraoperative fluoroscopy confirms the position of the guide wires advanced into the epiphysis. Further adjustment and modification of the orientation of the guide wires can be performed if needed. Once the epiphysis is fixed into the metaphysis using the two guide wires and assessment of the reduction using intraoperative fluoroscopy is deemed appropriate, a 1.6- mm K-wire is used to perforate the femoral head to monitor active bleeding. Active bleeding should be present through the hole, and we used an ICP monitor to assess for intraosseous pressure changes in the femoral head (**Figure 7.39**). If blood flow is present, the cannulated drill is used, and then two 6.5-mm cannulated screws are placed fixing the epiphysis. We prefer to use fully threaded cannulated screws because they allow easy removal compared with partially threaded screws. Once the screws are placed fixing the epiphysis, an osteochondroplasty of the metaphyseal bump can be performed to improve the femoral head-neck offset and avoid impingement. The capsule is then loosely closed, and the skin is closed in layers. Postoperative protocol includes no weight-bearing in the involved lower extremity for the first 6 or 8 weeks after surgery. Weight-bearing assisted by crutches follows for 4 additional weeks, and then weight-bearing as tolerated with physical therapy and rehabilitation follows (**Figure 7.40**).

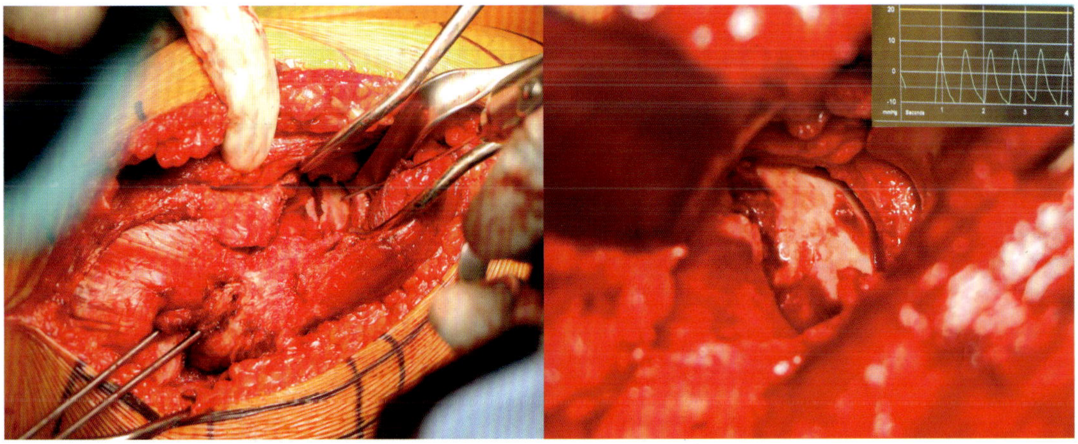

FIGURE 7.39. Intraoperative photograph showing monitoring of the blood flow of the femoral head. On the left-hand side, a photograph showing a K-wire introduced into the femoral head. On the right-hand side, the photograph shows active bleeding from the epiphysis. In the top right-hand corner, a picture of the intracranial pressure monitor screen shows a pulsatile waveform.

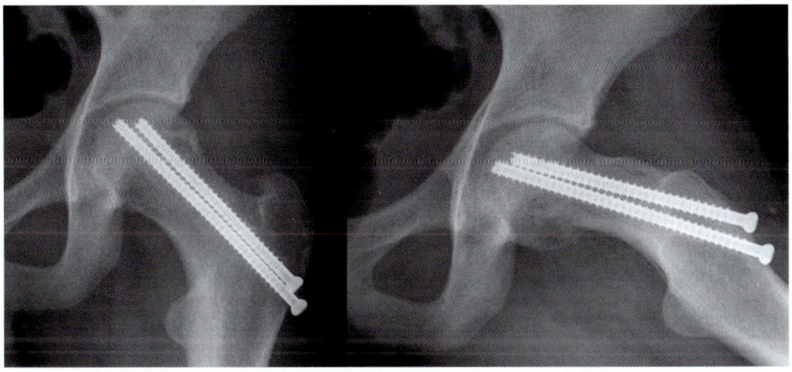

FIGURE 7.40. Postoperative anteroposterior and frog-leg lateral radiographs obtained 18 months after surgery demonstrating healed slipped capital femoral epiphysis with preserved concavity of the femoral head and neck junction.

REFERENCES

1. Loder RT, Richards BS, Shapiro PS, Reznick LR, Aronson DD. Acute slipped capital femoral epiphysis: the importance of physeal stability. *J Bone Joint Surg Am.* 1993;75(8):1134-1140.
2. Novais EN, Sink EL, Kestel LA, Carry PM, Abdo JC, Heare TC. Is assessment of femoral head perfusion during modified Dunn for unstable slipped capital femoral epiphysis an accurate indicator of osteonecrosis? *Clin Orthop Relat Res.* 2016;474(8):1837-1844.
3. Maeda S, Kita A, Funayama K, Kokubun S. Vascular supply to slipped capital femoral epiphysis. *J Pediatr Orthop.* 2001;21(5):664-667.
4. Herrera-Soto JA, Duffy MF, Birnbaum MA, Vander Have KL. Increased intracapsular pressures after unstable slipped capital femoral epiphysis. *J Pediatr Orthop.* 2008;28(7):723-728.
5. Schrader T, Jones CR, Kaufman AM, Herzog MM. Intraoperative monitoring of epiphyseal perfusion in slipped capital femoral epiphysis. *J Bone Joint Surg Am.* 2016;98(12):1030-1040.
6. Ibrahim T, Mahmoud S, Riaz M, Hegazy A, Little DG. Hip decompression of unstable slipped capital femoral epiphysis: a systematic review and meta-analysis. *J Child Orthop.* 2015;9(2):113-120.
7. Loder RT. What is the cause of avascular necrosis in unstable slipped capital femoral epiphysis and what can be done to lower the rate? *J Pediatr Orthop.* 2013;33(Suppl 1):S88-S91.
8. Ziebarth K, Zilkens C, Spencer S, Leunig M, Ganz R, Kim YJ. Capital realignment for moderate and severe SCFE using a modified Dunn procedure. *Clin Orthop Relat Res.* 2009;467(3):704-716.
9. Sankar WN, Vanderhave KL, Matheney T, Herrera-Soto JA, Karlen JW. The modified Dunn procedure for unstable slipped capital femoral epiphysis: a multicenter perspective. *J Bone Joint Surg Am.* 2013;95(7):585-591.
10. Leunig M, Slongo T, Kleinschmidt M, Ganz R. Subcapital correction osteotomy in slipped capital femoral epiphysis by means of surgical hip dislocation. *Oper Orthop Traumatol.* 2007;19(4):389-410.
11. Ganz R, Huff TW, Leunig M. Extended retinacular soft-tissue flap for intra-articular hip surgery: surgical technique, indications, and results of application. *Instr Course Lect.* 2009;58:241-255.
12. Parsch K, Weller S, Parsch D. Open reduction and smooth Kirschner wire fixation for unstable slipped capital femoral epiphysis. *J Pediatr Orthop.* 2009;29(1):1-8.

CHAPTER 8

Legg-Calve-Perthes Disease: Containment Principles

INTRODUCTION

Legg-Calve-Perthes disease (LCPD) is a self-limited childhood hip disorder of unknown etiology that can produce permanent deformity of the femoral head. Legg, of the United States; Calve, of France; and Perthes, of Germany, independently described the disease in 1910.[1] The onset of LCPD is between 2 and 15 years of age, with a peak between 4 and 9 years. Sundt, in 1920, reported that boys were four times more likely to have the disease than girls and that 10% of patients developed bilateral disease.[2] Molloy and MacMahon, in 1966,[3] and Catterall, in 1981,[4] reported similar findings, with bilateral disease occurring in 10% to 15% of patients and a male-to-female ratio of 4-5:1. The diagnosis of LCPD requires either plain radiography or magnetic resonance imaging along with a careful history and physical examination. Symptoms and physical findings with early LCPD are nonspecific, and the diagnosis can often be one of exclusion. Other pediatric conditions that produce femoral head osteonecrosis or LCPD-like changes on radiography must be ruled out by performing a thorough history, physical examination, and radiographic assessment.

LCPD is a challenging condition to treat, with a wide age range of presentation and both variability in stage and severity of disease. Despite more than a century of research and treatment directed at LCPD, there is currently no consensus on the optimal treatment for it. However, there is agreement that the primary goal of treatment is to prevent further femoral head deformity and maintain hip sphericity. Femoral head deformity, although tolerated best in younger children, will lead to arthritis, pain, and dysfunction over time.[5,6]

STAGES OF DISEASE

Plain radiography remains the primary diagnostic assessment tool for LCPD. An anteroposterior (AP) and frog-lateral radiograph of the pelvis are used to determine the radiographic stage of the disease, the extent of head involvement, and serial progression of the disease. Catterall[4,7] described a series of classic head-at-risk signs during the progression of the disease including lateral subluxation, Gage sign (V-shaped radiolucency in the lateral portion of the epiphysis and/or adjacent metaphysis), calcification lateral to the epiphysis, and horizontal alignment of the growth plate. These are late radiographic signs of a "head at risk" for having a poor prognosis. More recently, research effort has been focused on using earlier radiographic features to determine the prognosis and long-term outcome.

Waldenstrom[8] described four radiographic stages of disease progression: the initial or avascular necrosis stage (stage I), fragmentation or resorptive stage (stage II), reossification or healing stage (stage III), and healed stage (stage IV). Herring et al[9] found that the time from first radiographic evidence of disease to start of fragmentation had a mean of 6 months (range, 1 to 14 months), with the fragmentation stage lasting 8 months (range, 2 to 35 months) and the reossification stage lasting 51 months (range, 2 to 122 months).

In 2003, Joseph et al[10] reported their modification of the Waldenstrom staging described in 1972 by Canale et al[11] The modified staging is referred to as the Elizabethtown classification. Each of the first original three stages described by Waldenstrom was further subdivided into two substages as stages Ia, Ib, IIa, IIb, IIIa, IIIb, and IV (**Figure 8.1**). Stage Ia is the initial stage of the disease, characterized by sclerosis of the epiphysis without any loss of epiphyseal height. In stage Ib, the epiphysis is sclerotic, and there is loss of epiphyseal height. There has not yet been fragmentation of the epiphysis, and the epiphysis remains as a single piece. In stage IIa, the epiphysis begins to fragment with bone resorption, which is seen on radiograph as radiolucent perpendicular lines relative to the epiphysis on either the AP or frog-lateral view of the hip. Stage IIb represents further fragmentation and collapse, with maximal flattening

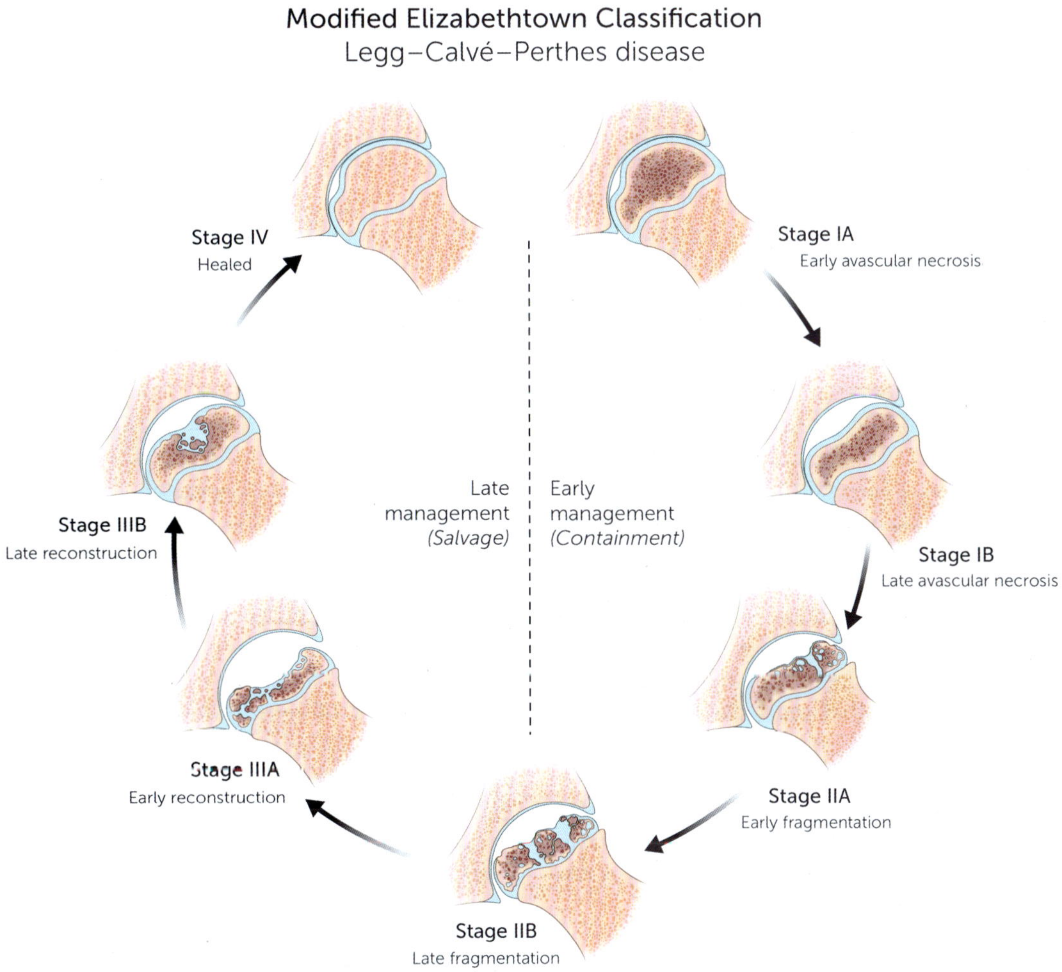

FIGURE 8.1. Modified Elizabethtown Classification. Adapted from Joseph et al.[10]

and multiple perpendicular lucencies representing severe fragmentation. Stage IIIa represents the beginning of the healing stage, with new bone formation seen at the lateral epiphysis. This reossification occurs at the periphery of the necrotic fragment, and the new bone is not of the same radiodensity and covers less than one-third of the circumference of the epiphysis. In stage IIIb, the new bone of normal radiodensity now covers more than one-third of the circumference of the epiphysis. Finally, stage IV represents completion of healing, and there is no radiographically identifiable avascular bone. These modifications to the original classification demonstrated good inter- and intraobserver reliability. Joseph et al[10] calculated the duration of the initial four stages (Ia to IIb) to be approximately 4 months for each stage and the duration of stages IIIa and IIIb twice and thrice that of the preceding stages, respectively. It appears that the greatest amount of epiphyseal extrusion and flattening occurs in late fragmentation, leading to the recommendation of attempting to "contain the hip" or prevent further deformity by placing the hip in the socket for protection prior to stage IIb.

THE PRINCIPLE OF CONTAINMENT

The concept of containment was first described by Harrison and Menon in 1966 as follows[12]: "[I]f the head is contained within the acetabular cup, then like the jelly poured into a mold, the head should be the same shape as the cup when it is allowed to come out after reconstruction." Containment is the term used to describe interventions that place the anterolateral part of the femoral epiphysis within the acetabulum, thereby protecting the epiphysis from being subjected to deforming stresses. This concept was further advanced by the work of Robert Salter, who, using a piglet model, created a Perthes-like condition by ligating the arterial supply of the femoral head.[13,14] In his studies, he demonstrated that the outcomes were optimal in the pigs treated with abduction, regardless of weight-bearing status. Both operative and nonoperative treatments have been popularized to take advantage of the "plasticity" associated with the early stages of LCPD and relative femoral head fragility. The main overriding principle is that for containment to work, the goal is to intervene in the early stages (stage Ia-IIb) and contain the femoral head before extrusion of the lateral epiphysis, which can typically be seen in late fragmentation and early ossification.[15]

In children older than 8 years at onset of disease, extrusion of the lateral aspect of the femoral head can occur quickly in the course of the disease, and hence containment should be initiated as soon as the diagnosis is made.[10,16] In children younger than 8 years, the likelihood of extrusion developing is less certain, and close monitoring with conservative therapies can be a reasonable first line of therapy, provided that close monitoring with clinical and radiographic examination occurs every 3 months. Containment can be achieved by two different methods. The first involves positioning the femur in abduction/internal rotation or abduction/flexion, which can be achieved by casting, bracing, or surgery on the femur. Alternatively, containment can be achieved by an osteotomy of the pelvis that reorients the acetabulum such that it covers the anterolateral part of the femoral epiphysis (eg, Salter or triple pelvic osteotomy) or by creating a bony shelf over the extruded part of the epiphysis. For children under 8 years at onset, the outcomes of brace treatment and surgical containment are approximately equal.[17,18]

NONOPERATIVE CONTAINMENT TREATMENT

It is imperative that an adequate range of motion of the hip is present when containment treatment is instituted, as a stiff hip cannot be contained. In the early stages of LCPD, the hip is irritable and associated with synovitis, which can lead to inflammation and guarding of the hip with movement. This is typically manifested with a limp that can be insidious in onset and frequently present toward the end of a particularly active day in younger children. Older children tend to present more acutely with pain, dysfunction and ambulatory difficulty. First-line therapy for the early stages of nonoperative containment include rest, physical therapy, nonsteroidal anti-inflammatory drugs (NSAIDs), and restriction of weight-bearing. Depending on the age at presentation, restriction of weight-bearing may be achieved by using a wheelchair, walker, or crutches. In addition to the use of a short course of NSAIDs, an intra-articular steroid injection may be beneficial to help reduce inflammation and decrease pain in the early symptomatic phases of the disease. In most situations, restricting weight-bearing will decrease the hip pain. Children are able to participate in school in their wheelchair or with their crutches so as to avoid missing prolonged periods of school.

The early stages of LCPD can last between 1 and 2 years, depending on when the initial diagnosis is made. In addition to avoiding high-impact activities and restricting weight-bearing, consideration of a bracing program is also critical to facilitate nonoperative containment. The most effective position to decrease intra-articular pressure is a combination of slight flexion, abduction, and external rotation.[19-21] Positions associated with full extension can increase hip capsular pressure and lead to more symptoms associated with LCPD. Various abduction orthoses and casting have been shown to effectively "contain" a symptomatic hip nonsurgically. Petrie and Bitenc described a weight-bearing cast in abduction that allowed the child to be more active and functional within the family home.[22] The typical position described is close to 45° of abduction and 5° to 10° of internal rotation with about 10° to 15° of knee flexion held in two long leg casts with a bar holding the legs in the set position, which has come to be known as Petrie casts.

A number of more convenient weight-bearing orthoses have been subsequently described to emulate the position and function of the Petrie casts.[23-25] The initial results with abduction braces were positive; however, long-term follow-up has demonstrated inconsistent results.[26,27] The most recent report on 25-year experience with abduction A-frame orthosis has been positive.[24] To be successful, the authors describe a regime of wearing the brace for 20 hours per day for 13 months on average during the early stages of the disease (**Figure 8.2A-D**). In their cohort, the majority of hips at maturity were spherical without evidence of arthrosis or significant femoral head deformity. Abduction bracing can be seen as tedious and labor intensive and may not be attractive to parents looking for a "quick fix" for their child's disease. Occasionally, activity modification, physical therapy, and bracing are not enough to settle down an irritable hip, and additional measures are required to surgically "contain" the hip in the socket. These operative measures are described below.

OPERATIVE CONTAINMENT TREATMENTS

The primary limitation to nonoperative containment in the early stage of LCPD is from a lack of hip abduction, either from adductor spasm, contracture, or irritability. Examining under anesthesia is helpful to differentiate whether the child is suffering from spasm or true contracture of the adductor muscle. In addition, the utility of an arthrogram can demonstrate dynamic motion of the femoral head in the socket and identify whether the hip is

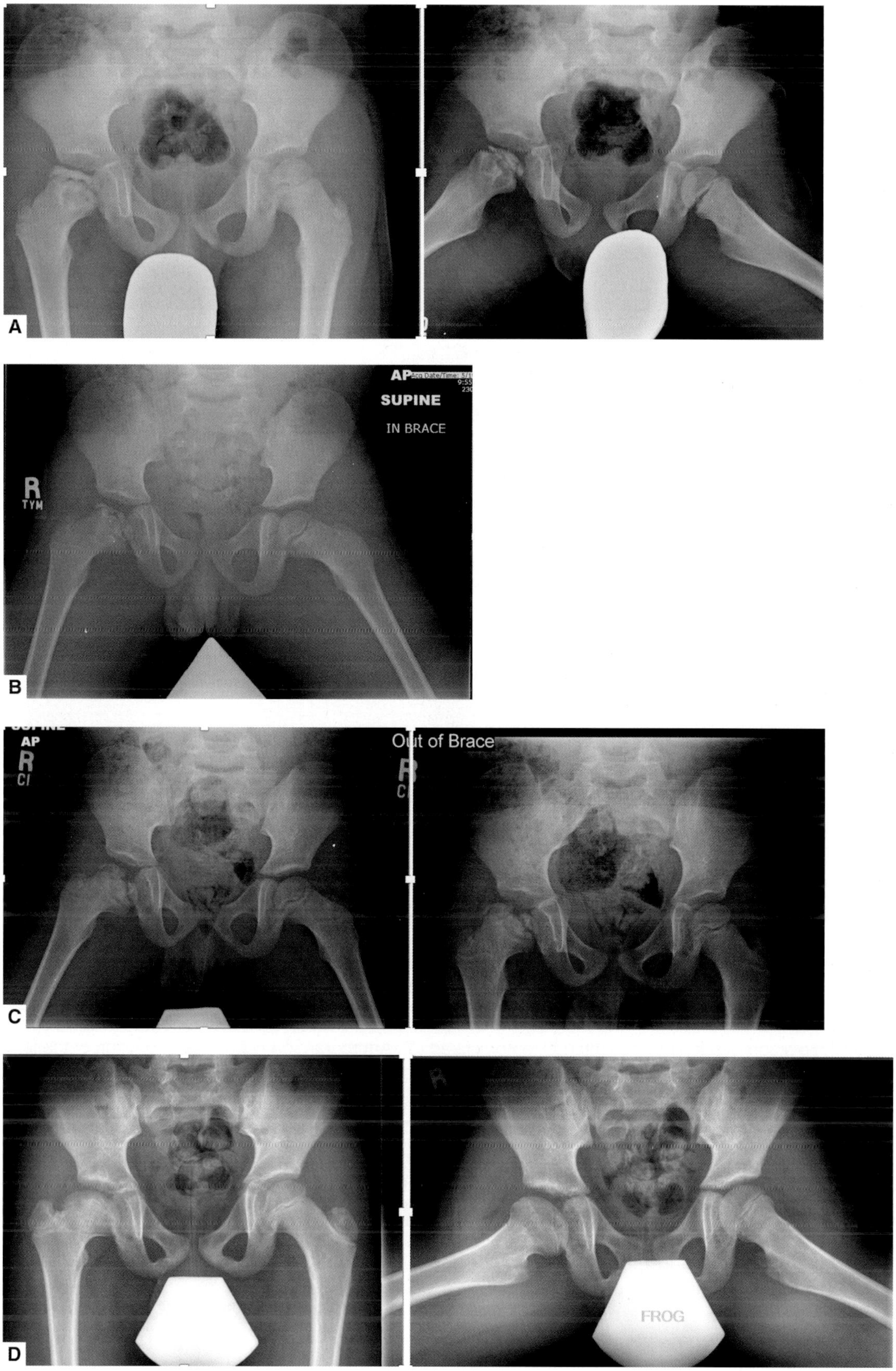

FIGURE 8.2. An example of nonoperative containment. A 5-year-old presented to clinic in early fragmentation with an irritable right hip (A). He was treated with activity restriction, abduction bracing (B, C), and therapy and healed with a Stulberg II hip at final follow-up (D).

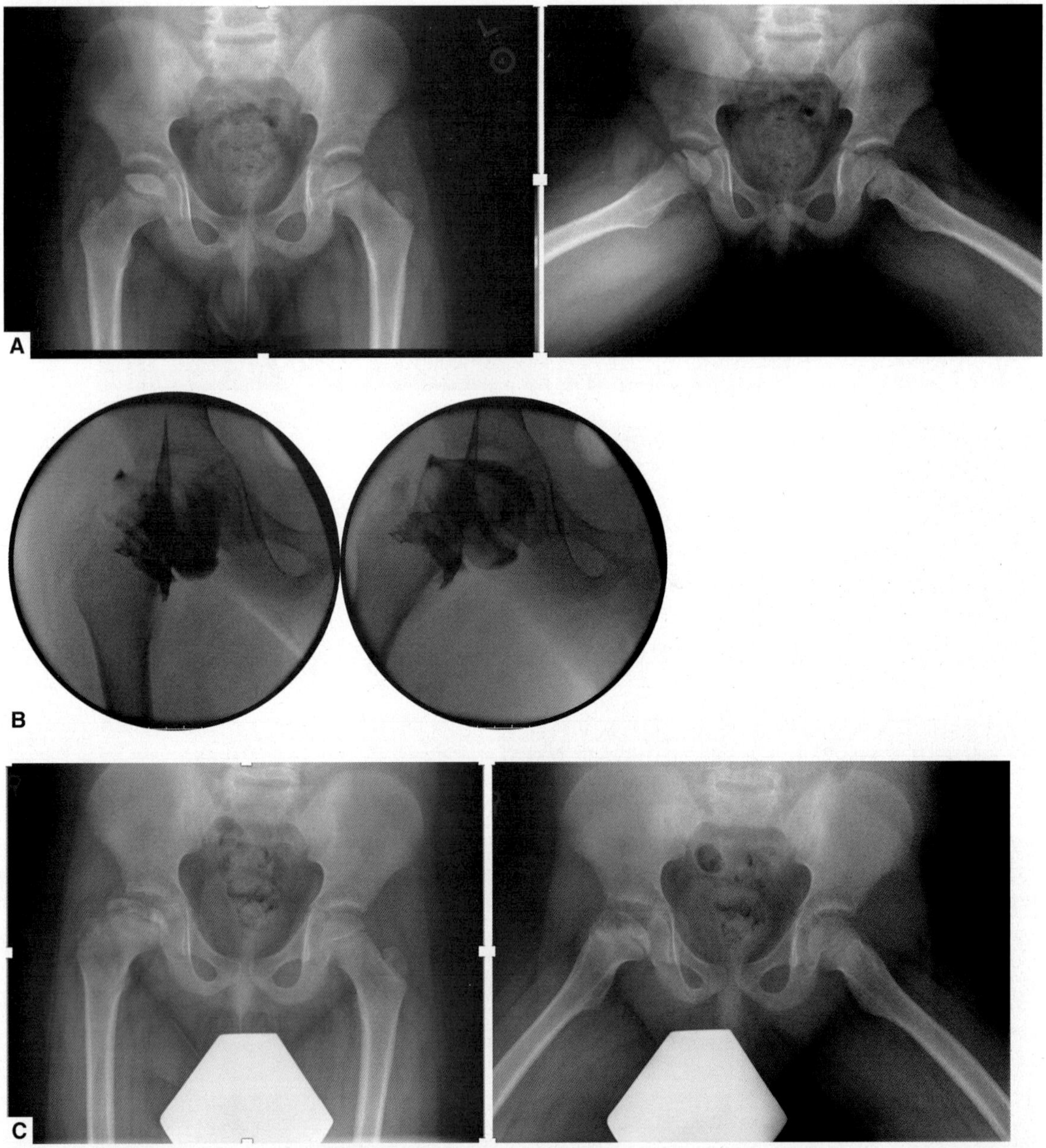

FIGURE 8.3. An example of operative containment with arthrogram and phenol injection to the obturator nerve. This 8-year-old male presented with a stage Ib sclerotic and flattened femoral head (A). Arthrogram demonstrates reduction of the femoral head under the labrum (B). One year post injection with Petrie bracing demonstrates a Stulberg II hip with a healing central area of necrosis (C).

truly containable (**Figure 8.3A-C**). In young children under 8 years of age, an isolated adductor tentotomy can be used to gain motion to facilitate "containment" and bracing. Moya-Angeler et al[28] investigated the efficacy of isolated adductor tenotomy and found minimal differences in those children who received adductor tenotomy, therapy, and bracing compared to those children who received isolated bracing and therapy; however, the two patient groups were asymmetric in terms of patient numbers.

There have been numerous reports of surgical containment by proximal femoral varus osteotomy since Axer reported this method in 1965.[29] The mechanism by which the varus osteotomy alters the natural history of LCPD is not clear. A potential benefit of performing a varus osteotomy in the initial stage of LCPD is that one can bypass the fragmentation stage and shorten the overall duration of the disease.[30] When compared with Salter and triple pelvic osteotomies, the functional outcomes are comparable.[17,31] Both procedures should be performed in the "early stage" of disease (stage Ia-IIb), and patients must have a full range of motion preoperatively to have successful outcomes. In older children (>9 years), the proximal femoral varus osteotomy may be less suitable because remodeling is unreliable.[32]

Proximal femoral osteotomy is a familiar procedure for most pediatric surgeons; however, several technical features must be considered in LCPD. (1) A child must demonstrate at least 30° of abduction in extension prior to considering a femoral osteotomy.[33] In situations where this is not present, a trial of casting, adductor lengthening, or even the use of botox/phenol to the adductor compartment to gain motion is reasonable. (2) In general, no more than 15° of varus is necessary to contain the femoral head, and more varus creates a significant abductor lurch that does not remodel.[34] (3) Be careful not to rotate the distal fragment externally because these children have lost some of their internal rotation preoperatively.[35] (4) Build in 15° of extension at the osteotomy to help reduce the flexion effect from the oblique plane osteotomy.[36] (5) Medialize the distal fragment to prevent subsequent genu valgum.[36] (6) If more than 20° of varus is necessary to contain a hip, then consider concomitant pelvic osteotomy for additional containment.[37] (7) Limit weight-bearing for a period of at least 6 weeks and longer if range of motion is decreased. (8) Consider trochanteric epiphysiodesis in younger children to prevent trochanteric overgrowth (**Figure 8.4A-C**). Femoral varus osteotomy is our preferred technique for containment in typical LCPD patient.

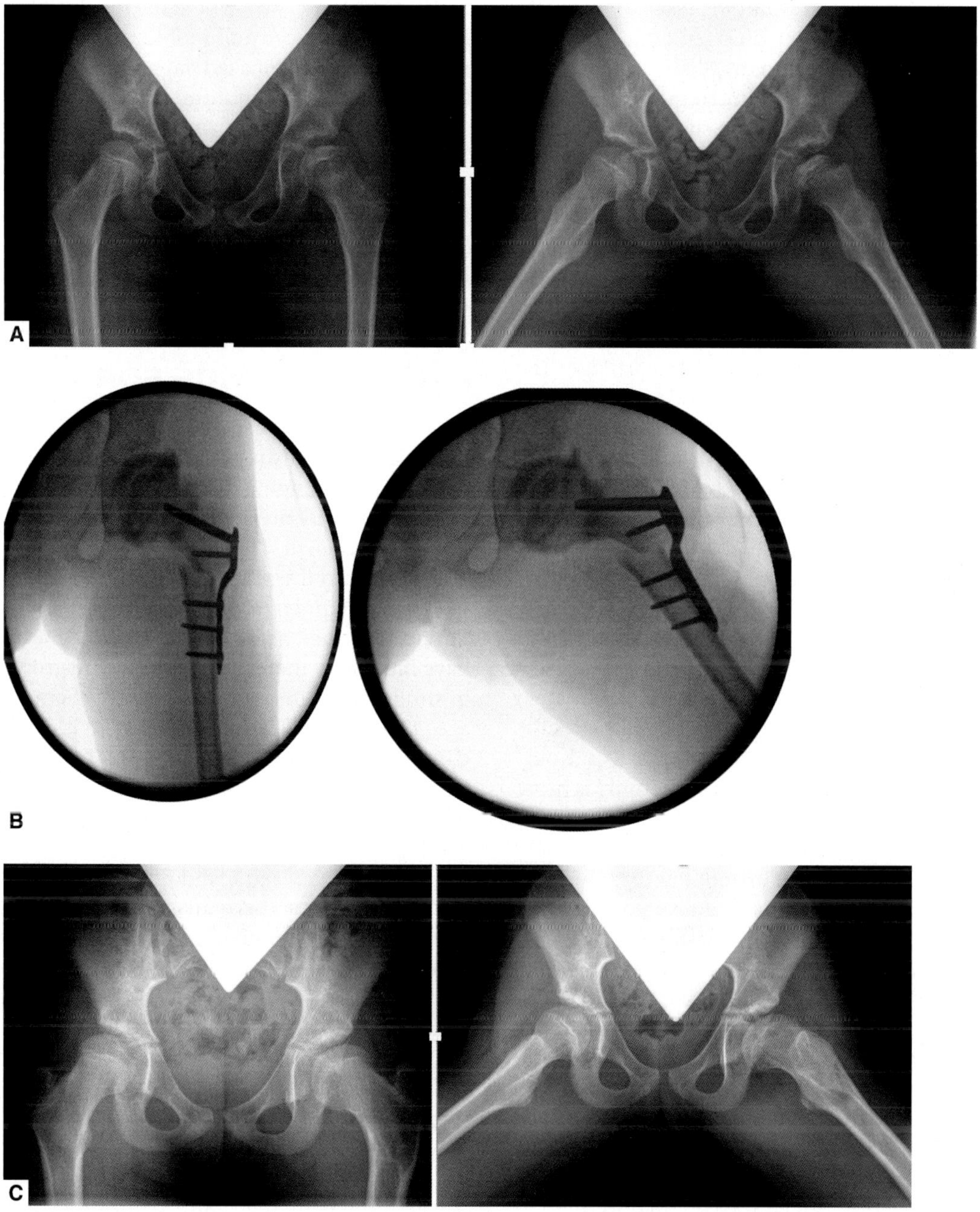

FIGURE 8.4. An example of containment with a femoral osteotomy. A 10-year-old female presented in early Perthes with sclerosis and minimal flattening (A). Based on her age of presentation, containment with femoral osteotomy was performed (B). Her end result was a Stulberg I hip (C).

The Salter osteotomy was initially described for the management of developmental hip dysplasia; however, over time it has been used to cover the extruded anterolateral femoral head in LCPD.[38] The osteotomy that is transverse from the sciatic notch to just above the anterior inferior iliac spine allows for rotation of the acetabulum laterally and anteriorly using the pubic symphysis as a hinge. Indications for this osteotomy in LCPD include a round femoral head with a full range of motion. The osteotomy is typically opened anteriorly about 1 to 1.5 cm. Typically, psoas over the brim must be released to help with rotation of the iliac segment. The osteotomy is fixated with threaded Steinmann pins to improve stability, and, typically, a spica cast is not necessary. For severe LCPD, a combination of Salter plus femoral osteotomy has been described and is preferred.[39,40] The merits of the combined procedure include minimizing the amount of femoral varus necessary to avoid limb shortening and abductor weakness. Additionally, there is a decreased risk of impingement from the Salter osteotomy owing to a smaller correction being necessary in combined scenarios.

The triple pelvic osteotomy combines the transverse osteotomy of Salter with complete osteotomies of the superior pubic ramus and ischium. The additional pelvic cuts allow greater mobility of the acetabulum without interfering with the growth of the triradiate cartilage. The triple pelvic osteotomy has been proposed as a method of containment for older patients with more severe disease.[41,42] Indications for the triple are similar to the Salter, with the hip demonstrating full range of motion and being containable without evidence of hinge abduction. In older children with more severe disease, the triple pelvic osteotomy can likely provide more coverage than the Salter osteotomy when the amount of femoral remodeling after femoral osteotomy is limited. In our center, both Salter and triple pelvic osteotomies are rarely used for LCPD.

Alternate osteotomies to consider would include a shelf acetabuloplasty. Huang and Huang[43] compared the results of shelf to triple pelvic osteotomy and found good outcomes in both groups. The triple pelvic osteotomy is more technically demanding, with additional complications compared to the shelf, but the shelf group had slightly less sphericity of the femoral head at final follow-up. The shelf acetabuloplasty may be a useful alternative containment method in older children (age >9 years), where femoral remodeling may not be reliable.

Treating providers must be aware of and scrutinize the preoperative arthrogram for the presence of hinge abduction. Hinge abduction is a clinical scenario where, owing to the shape of the femoral head or lack of hip motion, the femoral head is unable to be contained within the acetabulum. Essentially, with abduction, the femoral head does not pass underneath the labrum. The diagnosis and reliability of hinge abduction can be elusive,[44] but in the scenario of hinge abduction, it is contraindicated to attempt a containment procedure such as a femoral osteotomy or redirectional pelvic osteotomy.

The shelf acetabuloplasty is designed to provide additional acetabular coverage over the lateral uncovered femoral head. The shelf has been described as a salvage procedure for children with hinge abduction as well as an alternate containment procedure to a femoral or Salter osteotomy. The benefit of the shelf is that the labrum is protected and the lateral acetabular growth center is stimulated while preventing femoral head deformity. In addition, the shelf preserves limb length and avoids excessive trochanteric prominence. The goal, from a technical perspective, is to have the auto or allograft sit right against the capsule of the hip to facilitate the formation of true "supporting shelf". The author's preferred technique was described by Daly et al[45], where the reflected head is released from the direct head and mobilized on its capsular attachment. A proximally based flap of bone is elevated laterally from the outer table of ilium directly cranial to the lateral acetabular growth cartilage, where a slot is also created. Allograft or autograft bone is then placed under this flap of bone laterally into the new slots. The new bone is stabilized under the proximal flap of bone by the reflected head of rectus (**Figure 8.5A-D**). A postoperative spica is used to hold the bone in place, and protected weight-bearing is employed until the graft has been incorporated.

BEST EVIDENCE FOR TREATMENT

Despite over a 100 years of research on LCPD, we have yet to achieve consensus on the optimal treatment strategy. LCPD is a challenging disease that affects a wide age range of patients who present at various stages of disease. In general, treatment strategies should be based on age, stage of disease, and the amount of femoral head involvement.

Children under 6 years of age represent a large capacity to remodel their involved femoral head. Multiple studies have illustrated that surgery in this age group has resulted in similar outcomes to nonoperative therapy.[18,46,47] In this age group, nonoperative containment is offered with close clinical and radiographic follow-up (every 3 to 4 months). If activity restriction or pain cannot be controlled with physical therapy, then a course of cast or Petrie orthosis is utilized.

Children between 6 and 8 years represent a challenging age group for the management of LCPD with operative and nonoperative containment treatments being applied at our institution. With continued prospective multicenter study (*International Perthes Study Group*), we hope to identify the superior treatment strategy for this age group. In this age group, the principle of containment and activity modification is paramount. Children are restricted in their activities in a wheelchair and instructed to avoid jumping or running. If there is concern about a loss of hip range of motion or presence of early lateral extrusion of the hip, then a hip arthrogram and exam under anesthesia is recommended. If limited abduction is present on exam under anesthesia, then an adductor tenotomy or phenol injection coupled with casting is pursued.

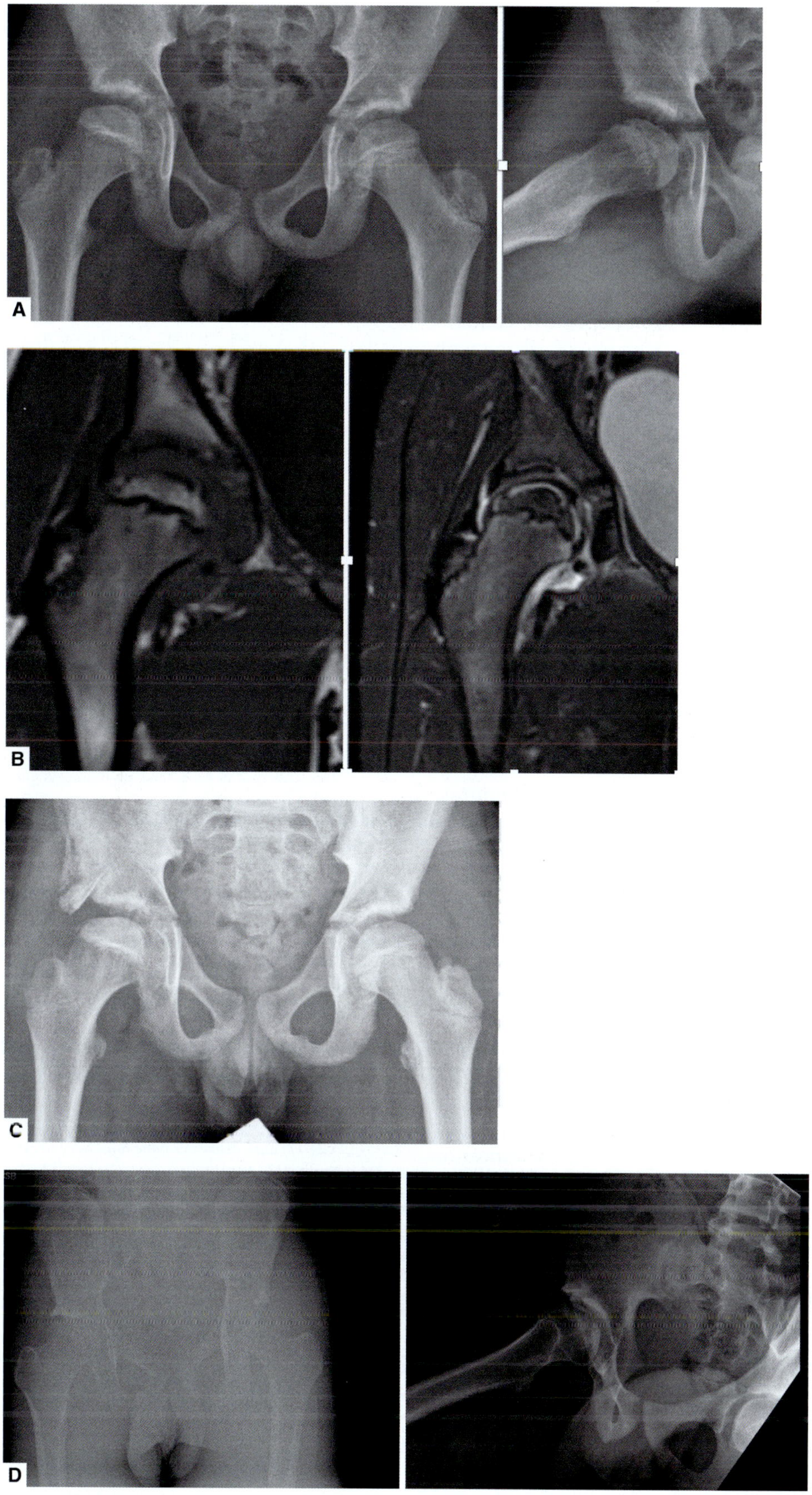

FIGURE 8.5. An example of containment with a shelf osteotomy. This 10-year-old male presented in stage Ia Perthes with sclerosis and minimal collapse (A). Magnetic resonance imaging demonstrated whole head involvement (B). Decision to contain with a shelf pelvic osteotomy was made (C). Five-year follow-up demonstrates Stulberg II hip (D).

The above strategy assumes that the hip is containable. Casting is continued for 6 to 12 weeks, at which point a decision between provider and family is made concerning surgical containment (femoral osteotomy) or nonoperative containment (abduction orthosis). Treatment through fragmentation typically lasts 2 years on average at our institution, and this will vary depending on age of presentation.

Containment remains the primary treatment strategy for children who present between 8 and 11 years of age; however, in this age group surgical containment has been shown to offer superior results to nonoperative containment.[17,46,47] If the hip is irritable, a course of casting with lengthening of the adductor or phenol injection will help gain the hip motion needed to perform the femoral osteotomy. This concept is critical, and if a child does not have enough hip abduction, a varus producing femoral osteotomy should be deferred. In this age group, early surgery can result in improved sphericity; therefore, the use of perfusion MRI is evolving and can potentially be used in the future as a modality to risk-stratify patients in this age group.[48]

In children over 11 years, the reported outcomes have been uniformly poor. Children in this age group demonstrate limited remodeling potential, and the pathophysiology here may parallel adult avascular necrosis rather than typical LCPD.[49] Although a host of variable treatment options have been described, including multiple epiphyseal drilling, core decompression, vascularized fibular grafting, arthrodiastasis, or femoral osteotomy, the functional results are uniformly similar and poor. At our institution, we recommend a period of non–weight-bearing with physical therapy and core decompression supplemented with autologous iliac crest stem cells[50] or shelf arthroplasty as a possible containment method that will not require remodeling with growth.

Perthes is a challenging condition, with an infrequent presentation yet a wide phenotype of disease. The principle of containment is designed to protect the fragile femoral head within the acetabulum as the stages of avascular necrosis and revascularization progress. Stratification according to age at presentation and stage of disease will help guide treatment options. Ongoing multicenter, prospective studies through the *International Perthes Study Group* may help clarify which treatments are indicated, particularly in the 6 to 8 years age group.

REFERENCES

1. Skaggs DL, Tolo VT. Legg-Calve-Perthes disease. *J Am Acad Orthop Surg*. 1996;4(1):9-16.
2. Sundt H. Malum coxae: Calvé-Legg-Perthes. *Zentralk Chir.* 1920;22:538.
3. Molloy MK, MacMahon B. Incidence of Legg-Perthes disease (osteochondritis deformans). *N Engl J Med*. 1966;275(18):988-990.
4. Catterall A. Legg-Calve-Perthes syndrome. *Clin Orthop Relat Res.* 1981(158):41-52.
5. Larson AN, Sucato DJ, Herring JA, et al. A prospective multicenter study of Legg-Calve-Perthes disease: functional and radiographic outcomes of nonoperative treatment at a mean follow-up of twenty years. *J Bone Joint Surg Am*. 2012;999(2):584-592.
6. Stulberg SD, Cooperman DR, Wallensten R. The natural history of Legg-Calve-Perthes disease. *J Bone Joint Surg Am.* 1981;63(7): 1095-1108.
7. Catterall A. Treatment in Legg-Calve-Perthes' disease. *Acta Orthop Belg*. 1980;46(4):431-434.
8. Waldenstrom H. On coxa plana: osteochondritis deformans coxae juveniles: Legg's disease, maladie de Calve, Perthes Krankreit. *Acta Chir Scand*. 1922(55):577-590.
9. Herring JA, Kim HT, Browne R. Legg-Calve-Perthes disease. Part I: Classification of radiographs with use of the modified lateral pillar and Stulberg classifications. *J Bone Joint Surg Am.* 2004;86-A(10):2103-2120.
10. Joseph B, Varghese G, Mulpuri K, Narasimha Rao K, Nair NS. Natural evolution of Perthes disease: a study of 610 children under 12 years of age at disease onset. *J Pediatr Orthop*. 2003;23(5):590-600.
11. Canale ST, D'Anca AF, Cotler JM, Snedden HE. Innominate osteotomy in Legg-Calve-Perthes disease. *J Bone Joint Surg Am*. 1972;54(1):25-40.
12. Harrison MH, Menon MP. Legg-Calve-Perthes disease. the value of roentgenographic measurement in clinical practice with special reference to the broomstick plaster method. *J Bone Joint Surg Am.* 1966;48(7):1301-1318.
13. Salter RB. Experimental and clinical aspects of Perthes' disease. *J Bone Joint Surg Br*. 1966;48(2):393-394.
14. Salter RB, Bell M. The pathogenesis of deformity in Legg-Perthes' disease—an experimental investigation. *J Bone Joint Surg Br.* 1968; 50(2):436.
15. Joseph B, Price CT. Consensus statements on the management of Perthes disease. *Orthop Clin North Am*. 2011;42(3):437-440.
16. Muirhead-Allwood W, Catterall A. The treatment of Perthes' disease. The results of a trial of management. *J Bone Joint Surg Br.* 1982;64(3):282-285.
17. Herring JA, Kim HT, Browne R. Legg-Calve-Perthes disease. Part II: Prospective multicenter study of the effect of treatment on outcome. *J Bone Joint Surg Am*. 2004;86-A(10):2121-2134.
18. Canavese F, Dimeglio A. Perthes' disease: prognosis in children under six years of age. *J Bone Joint Surg Br*. 2008;90(7):940-945.
19. Serlo W, Heikkinen E, Puranen J. Preoperative Russell traction in Legg-Calve-Perthes disease. *J Pediatr Orthop*. 1987;7(3):288-290.
20. Kallio P, Ryoppy S, Kunnamo I. Transient synovitis and Perthes' disease. Is there an aetiological connection? *J Bone Joint Surg Br.* 1986;68(5):808-811.
21. Vegter J. The influence of joint posture on intra-articular pressure. A study of transient synovitis and Perthes' disease. *J Bone Joint Surg Br.* 1987;69(1):71-74.
22. Petrie JG, Bitenc I. The abduction weight-bearing treatment in Legg-Perthes' disease. *J Bone Joint Surg Br*. 1971;53(1):54-62.
23. Purvis JM, Dimon JH 3rd, Meehan PL, Lovell WW. Preliminary experience with the Scottish Rite Hospital abduction orthosis for Legg-Perthes disease. *Clin Orthop Relat Res*. 1980;150:49-53.
24. Rich MM, Schoenecker PL. Management of Legg-Calve-Perthes disease using an A-frame orthosis and hip range of motion: a 25-year experience. *J Pediatr Orthop*. 2013;33(2):112-119.
25. Curtis BH, Gunther SF, Gossling HR, Paul SW. Treatment for Legg-Perthes disease with the Newington ambulation-abduction brace. *J Bone Joint Surg Am*. 1974;56(6):1135-1146.
26. Kamegaya M. Comparative study of Perthes' disease treated by various ambulatory orthoses. *Nihon Seikeigeka Gakkai Zasshi.* 1987;61(7):917-932.
27. Aksoy MC, Caglar O, Yazici M, Alpaslan AM. Comparison between braced and non-braced Legg-Calve-Perthes-disease patients: a radiological outcome study. *J Pediatr Orthop B*. 2004;13(3):153-157.
28. Moya-Angeler J, Abril JC, Rodriguez IV. Legg-Calve-Perthes disease: role of isolated adductor tenotomy? *Eur J Orthop Surg Traumatol.* 2013;23(8):921-925.

29. Axer A. Subtrochanteric osteotomy in the treatment of Perthes' disease: a preliminary report. *J Bone Joint Surg Br*. 1965;47:489-499.
30. Joseph B, Rao N, Mulpuri K, Varghese G, Nair S. How does a femoral varus osteotomy alter the natural evolution of Perthes' disease? *J Pediatr Orthop B*. 2005;14(1):10-15.
31. Leitch JM, Paterson DC, Foster BK. Growth disturbance in Legg-Calve-Perthes disease and the consequences of surgical treatment. *Clin Orthop Relat Res*. 1991(262):178-184.
32. Noonan KJ, Price CT, Kupiszewski SJ, Pyevich M. Results of femoral varus osteotomy in children older than 9 years of age with Perthes disease. *J Pediatr Orthop*. 2001;21(2):198-204.
33. Menelaus MB. Lessons learned in the management of Legg-Calve-Perthes disease. *Clin Orthop Relat Res*. 1986(209):41-48.
34. Kim HK, da Cunha AM, Browne R, Kim HT, Herring JA. How much varus is optimal with proximal femoral osteotomy to preserve the femoral head in Legg-Calve-Perthes disease? *J Bone Joint Surg Am*. 2011;93(4):341-347.
35. Hansson G, Wallin J. External rotational positioning of the leg after intertrochanteric combined varus-derotational osteotomy in Perthes' disease. *Arch Orthop Trauma Surg*. 1997;116(1-2):108-111.
36. Kitakoji T, Hattori T, Iwata H. Femoral varus osteotomy in Legg-Calve-Perthes disease: points at operation to prevent residual problems. *J Pediatr Orthop*. 1999;19(1):76-81.
37. Crutcher JP, Staheli LT. Combined osteotomy as a salvage procedure for severe Legg-Calve-Perthes disease. *J Pediatr Orthop*. 1992;12(2):151-156.
38. Salter RB. Legg-Perthes disease: the scientific basis for the methods of treatment and their indications. *Clin Orthop Relat Res*. 1980; 150:8-11.
39. Vukasinovic Z, Slavkovic S, Milickovic S, Siqeca A. Combined salter innominate osteotomy with femoral shortening versus other methods of treatment for Legg-Calve-Perthes disease. *J Pediatr Orthop B*. 2000;9(1):28-33.
40. Olney BW, Asher MA. Combined innominate and femoral osteotomy for the treatment of severe Legg-Calve-Perthes disease. *J Pediatr Orthop*. 1985;5(6):645-651.
41. Wenger DR, Pring ME, Hosalkar HS, Caltoum CB, Lalonde FD, Bastrom TP. Advanced containment methods for Legg-Calve-Perthes disease: results of triple pelvic osteotomy. *J Pediatr Orthop*. 2010;30(8):749-757.
42. Vukasinovic Z, Spasovski D, Vucetic C, Cobeljic G, Zivkovic Z, Matanovic D. Triple pelvic osteotomy in the treatment of Legg-Calve-Perthes disease. *Int Orthop*. 2009;33(5):1377-1383.
43. Huang MJ, Huang SC. Surgical treatment of severe Perthes disease: comparison of triple osteotomy and shelf augmentation. *J Formos Med Assoc*. 1999;98(3):183-189.
44. Shore BJ, Miller PE, Zaltz I, Schoenecker PL, Sankar WN. Determining Hinge abduction in Legg-Calve-Perthes disease: can we reliably make the diagnosis? *J Pediatr Orthop*. 2019;39(2):e95-e101.
45. Daly K, Bruce C, Catterall A. Lateral shelf acetabuloplasty in Perthes' disease. A review of the end of growth. *J Bone Joint Surg Br*. 1999;81(3):380-384.
46. Wiig O, Terjesen T, Svenningsen S. Prognostic factors and outcome of treatment in Perthes' disease: a prospective study of 368 patients with five-year follow-up. *J Bone Joint Surg Br*. 2008;90(10):1364-1371.
47. Saran N, Varghese R, Mulpuri K. Do femoral or salter innominate osteotomies improve femoral head sphericity in Legg-Calve-Perthes disease? a meta-analysis. *Clin Orthop Relat Res*. 2012;470(9):2383-2393.
48. Kim HK, Burgess J, Thoveson A, Gudmundsson P, Dempsey M, Jo CH. Assessment of femoral head revascularization in Legg-Calve-Perthes disease using serial perfusion MRI. *J Bone Joint Surg Am*. 2016;98(22):1897-1904.
49. Joseph B, Mulpuri K, Varghese G. Perthes' disease in the adolescent. *J Bone Joint Surg Br*. 2001;83(5):715-720.
50. Xu S, Zhang L, Jin H, et al. Autologous stem cells combined core decompression for treatment of avascular necrosis of the femoral head: a systematic meta-analysis. *Biomed Res Int*. 2017;2017:6136205.

CHAPTER 9

Legg-Calve-Perthes Disease: Treatment of Symptomatic Residual Deformity

BACKGROUND

Legg-Calve-Perthes disease (LCPD) is a pediatric disorder characterized by osteonecrosis of the capital femoral epiphysis. The osteonecrosis progresses to fragmentation of the femoral head and eventual revascularization and reossification. Ultimately, LCPD leaves a residual deformity of the proximal femur and acetabulum that can be a cause of progressive hip pain and dysfunction later in life. Previous reports have noted that anywhere between 30% and 50% of individuals affected by LCPD have residual hip symptoms that persist into adulthood.[1-3] The resultant deformities of the hip can lead to pathologic mechanics of femoroacetabular impingement (FAI), hip instability, or a combination of both pathologies.[4] The long-term prognosis of the hip is associated with femoral head sphericity and joint congruence.[5-7] Femoral deformity includes loss of epiphyseal sphericity, coxa magna or breva, a high-riding greater trochanter, and relative retroversion of the femoral head. On the acetabular side, retroversion is commonly encountered, but the acetabular remodeling in response to significant proximal femoral deformity may lead to an adaptive form of acetabular dysplasia.[8] Successful treatment of deformity following LCPD requires an ability to accurately identify and subsequently correct the varied pathomorphology encountered. The goal of treatment is a stable, concentrically reduced joint with an optimized range of motion.

Symptoms caused by the morphologic abnormalities encountered in healed LCPD deformities reflect those encountered in the idiopathic cases of FAI and dysplasia. Classically, FAI is characterized by the abnormal, repetitive contact of the anterior femoral head and neck with the anterior acetabulum. In the healed LCPD hip, this impingement can result from morphologic changes on either the proximal femur or the acetabulum. This abnormal contact leads to progressive damage to the acetabular cartilage, acetabular labrum, or both.[9] Patients with FAI tend to have anterior groin pain and pain in the "c-sign" region of the hip, which is aggravated by physical activity, prolonged sitting, and positions of flexion and internal rotation. Stiffness or loss of motion is also quite common and can at times become symptomatic prior to the onset of pain. Extra-articular FAI, involving contact between the trochanters and the pelvis, can also be seen in the healed LCPD hip. It presents as posterolateral hip pain with extension activities when localized to the greater trochanter and posterior groin pain with extension activities when localized to the lesser trochanter.

Instability symptoms typically manifest during upright activities such as walking or running. Pain may be localized to the anterolateral aspect of the hip and can be associated with pain along the psoas muscle and abductor musculature. Abductor fatigue and a perceived limp can be related to instability but may also be a product of the high-riding greater trochanter and associated inefficiency of the abductor musculature. Symptoms of locking or "catching" of the hip joint with activity may be indicative of articular pathology such as labral tears, cartilage flaps, or loose bodies (**Figure 9.1**).

Initial imaging of patients with healed LCPD deformity should provide a thorough analysis of both proximal femoral and acetabular morphology. Routine radiographs should include a standing anteroposterior (AP) view of the pelvis, lateral view of the proximal femur (45° Dunn or frog-leg lateral), and a false profile view of the acetabulum. Measurements of proximal femoral deformity include assessment of the femoral head-neck sphericity (alpha angle, head-neck offset ratio), the position of the greater trochanter with respect to the femoral head (articulotrochanteric distance), and femoral neck-shaft axis. On the acetabular side, measurements of acetabular coverage (lateral center edge angle, Tönnis roof angle, anterior center edge angle, anterior/posterior wall indices) should be performed. Markers of acetabular retroversion include

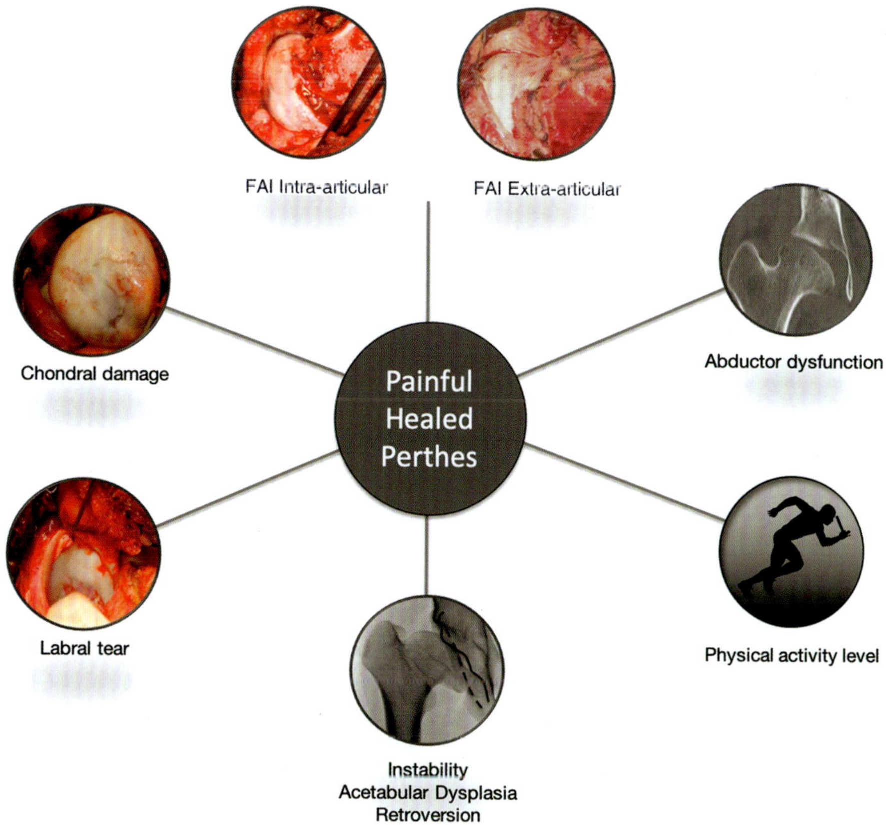

FIGURE 9.1. Diagram showing the etiology of pain in the healed LCPD hip is multifactorial. Pain may be secondary to intra-articular femoroacetabular impingement owing to abnormal femoral head-neck sphericity but also extra-articular owing to a high-riding greater trochanter. Intra-articular biologic damage to the femoral head or acetabular cartilage or to the acetabular labrum can be a cause of pain as well as dysfunction of the abductor musculature, leading to muscle fatigue. Hip instability due to acetabular dysplasia and retroversion may also contribute to symptoms. Finally, patients' level of physical activity may influence the onset and intensity of the symptoms.

assessment of the crossover sign, posterior wall sign, and prominent ischial spine sign. Owing to the often significant deformity associated with LCPD, we recommend routine cross-sectional imaging. Computed tomography of the pelvis, including the distal femur, should be obtained for assessment of the bony morphology, including three-dimensional reconstruction and femoral version. Magnetic resonance imaging is important to determine the extent of articular cartilage and acetabular labral damage.

COMPREHENSIVE STRATEGY FOR DEFORMITY ANALYSIS AND SURGICAL TREATMENT DESIGN

Management of patients with symptomatic healed LCPD requires identification of individual pathomorphologies and associated soft-tissue abnormalities that contribute to the patient's symptoms. It is crucial to distinguish hips with isolated FAI from hips with secondary acetabular dysplasia and instability and from hips with both. Moreover, it is essential to understand the source of the conflict between the proximal femur and the acetabulum rim (femoral vs. acetabular or combined; intra-articular vs. extra-articular) to design the surgical strategy. The most common treatment options on the femoral side of the hip joint include intertrochanteric osteotomy, relative neck lengthening, true femoral neck lengthening, trochanteric advancement, and osteochondroplasty of the head and neck junction. In very severe dysmorphic hips with an incongruent joint, the femoral head reduction osteotomy has recently been described as an option. On the acetabular side, extra-articular procedures include acetabular shelf osteotomy and redirectional osteotomies. In the healed LCPD hip, complex deformities of both femur and acetabulum leading to instability and FAI usually require a combined approach. A comprehensive assessment of the femoral and pelvic pathomorphology

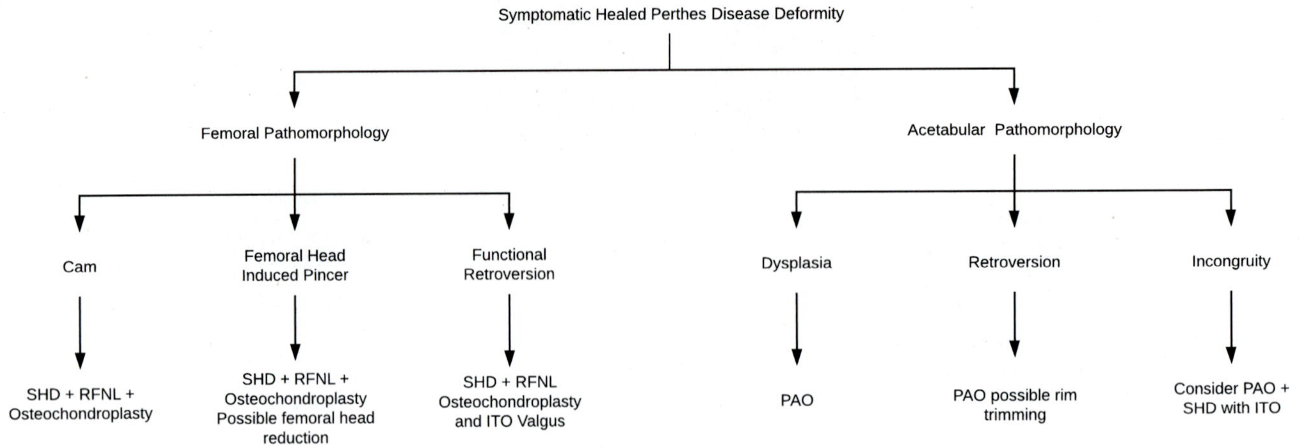

FIGURE 9.2. Diagram showing a comprehensive analysis with planned treatment intervention for each subtype of femoral and acetabular deformity encountered in the healed symptomatic LCPD hip. ITO; PAO, periacetabular osteotomy; RFNL, relative femoral neck lengthening; SHD.

allows for identification of different subtypes and planned treatment according to the altered anatomy. Our strategy for the treatment of symptomatic hip deformity secondary to healed LCPD involves the surgical hip dislocation approach[10] to assess and treat the femoral deformity and intra-articular pathology and the Bernese Periacetabular Osteotomy (PAO)[11] for the treatment of the acetabular deformity (**Figure 9.2**).

A detailed description of the surgical hip dislocation is provided in Chapter 12 and a description of the dissection of the retinacular flap in Chapter 7. Briefly, the surgery is performed with the patient in the lateral decubitus position using a straight lateral incision.[12] The fascia lata is split in line with the femoral shaft, and the interval between the gluteus maximus and medius is dissected. The gluteus medius is retracted, allowing for exposure of the gluteus minimus and the piriformis tendon. The interval between the piriformis tendon and the gluteus minimus is opened by sharp dissection, and the inferior border of the gluteus minimus is dissected from underlying capsule (**Figure 9.3**). Next, a 1 to 1.5-cm thick trochanteric osteotomy is performed with an oscillating saw, leaving the piriformis tendon and short external rotators intact on the base of the stable trochanter (**Figure 9.4**). The trochanteric piece is reflected and flipped anteriorly with the attached vastus lateralis and gluteus medius. The previously exposed capsular

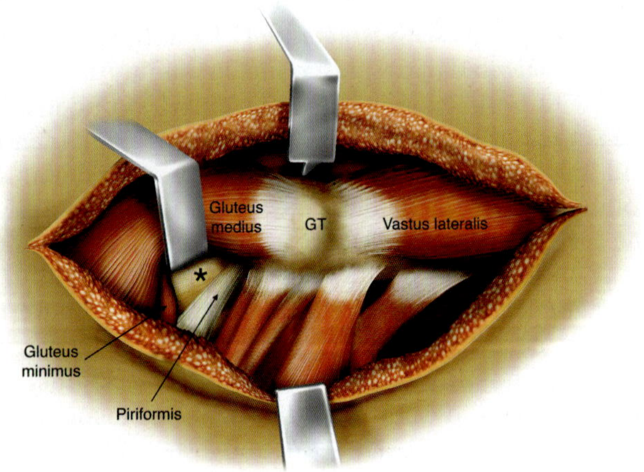

FIGURE 9.3. Illustration showing the gluteus medius insertion is retracted anteriorly, exposing the gluteus minimus and the piriformis tendon. The gluteus minimus fascia is incised on top of the piriformis, and the muscle is retracted anterior-superiorly, exposing the hip capsule (black asterisk). GT, greater trochanter.

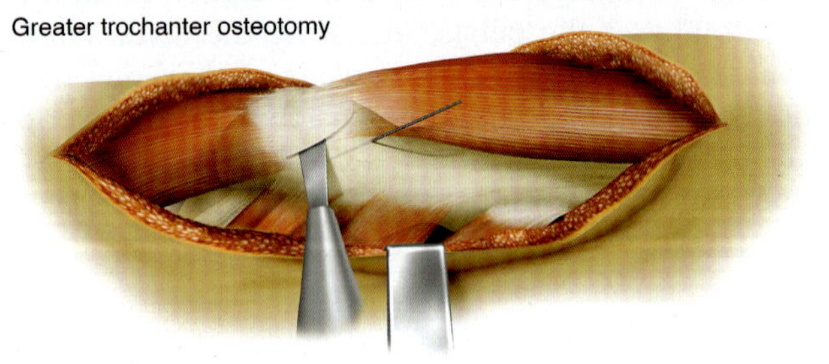

FIGURE 9.4. Illustration showing the trochanteric osteotomy. A Kirschner wire is inserted on the lateral greater trochanter to serve as a guide for the trochanteric osteotomy under fluoroscopy control. Proximally, the osteotomy is usually done 2 to 3 mm anterior to the insertion of the gluteus medius; and distally at the posterior aspect of the origin of the vastus lateralis.

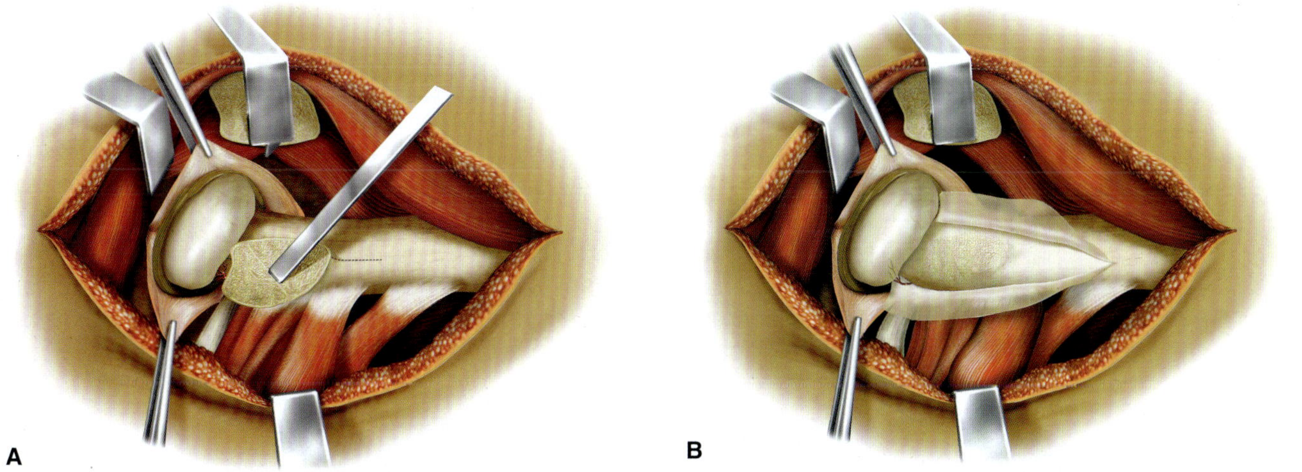

FIGURE 9.5. Dissection of the retinacular flap containing the nutrient vessels to the femoral head. A, Illustration showing the portion of the greater trochanter proximal to the growth plate is mobilized with an osteotome and the cancellous bone carefully removed from the periosteum. The periosteum is incised along the anterior neck, beginning at the anterosuperior corner of the stable greater trochanter (dotted line). The periosteum is incised distally up to the level of the gluteus maximus tendon. B, The periosteum of the neck, including the retinaculum with the blood vessels and the external rotators, is gradually released. The retinacular flap is extended posteriorly along the femoral neck while leaving it secured to the epiphysis, preserving the insertion of the blood vessels.

minimus is further elevated anteriorly off the hip capsule. The anterolateral portion of the vastus lateralis is released from the femur, with the hip in external rotation, until the level of the gluteus maximus insertion. A capsulotomy is performed in a Z-shape fashion (right hip) or reverse Z-shape (left hip), with the longitudinal arm of the Z in line with the anterior femoral neck. With the capsule opened, intra-articular and extra-articular causes of FAI can be dynamically determined. Flexion, adduction, and external rotation allow for the hip to partially dislocate, and the ligamentum teres is divided to allow complete dislocation of the femoral head. The femoral and the acetabular articular cartilage and the labrum are inspected for the presence of labral and chondral lesions.

Most often, LCPD deformity requires a relative lengthening of the femoral neck to improve abductor muscle function and correct extra-articular FAI, which often limits hip abduction and external rotation. An extended retinacular soft-tissue flap should be developed to protect the blood supply to the femoral head[13] (**Figure 9.5**). To develop the retinacular flap, the femoral head is reduced back in the acetabulum. The first step is to trim the posterosuperior portion of the stable greater trochanter down to the level of the femoral neck. The portion of the greater trochanter proximal to the growth plate is mobilized with an osteotome and the cancellous bone carefully removed from the periosteum. The periosteum is incised along the anterior neck beginning at the anterosuperior corner of the greater trochanter growth plate. The periosteum of the neck, including the retinaculum with the blood vessels and the external rotators, is gradually released. The retinacular flap is extended posteriorly along the femoral neck while leaving it secured to the epiphysis. After the retinacular flap is developed, the superior contour of the stable trochanteric segment is further trimmed in line with the femoral neck. The hip is then dislocated, and any nonspherical portion of the femoral head is removed with an osteotome and a high-speed burr. Range of motion after osteochondroplasty should reveal improved hip flexion and internal rotation, external rotation in extension, and abduction without impingement. If an osteochondroplasty and relative femoral neck lengthening (RFNL) is all that is required, then the periosteum is approximated, and the capsule is loosely closed. The trochanteric fragment is fixed distally with three 4.5 mm cortical screws, with its superior border in line with the center of the femoral head to correct the articulotrochanteric distance. When the osteoplasty and neck lengthening is not sufficient to correct the FAI—often when functional retroversion of the proximal femur is present—femoral intertrochanteric osteotomy can be performed.

A full description of the PAO technique is provided in Chapter 5.

Intra-Articular Cam and Extra-Articular Impingement

Clinical Scenario

A 15-year-old female presented with anterolateral and posterior right hip pain aggravated by running and soccer. She was diagnosed and treated nonsurgically for LCPD when she was 8 years old. Her physical examination was consistent with a slight limb length inequality (1 cm) and positive tests for anterior (flexion + adduction + internal rotation) and posterior (extension + abduction + external rotation) impingement. Radiographs of the right hip revealed a slightly nonspherical femoral head, a high-riding greater trochanter with a short femoral neck, and an anterior prominence of the femoral head. She was thought to have intra-articular cam FAI associated with extra-articular impingement, and treatment was performed through a surgical dislocation approach with RFNL and osteochondroplasty of the femoral head and neck junction (**Figure 9.6**).

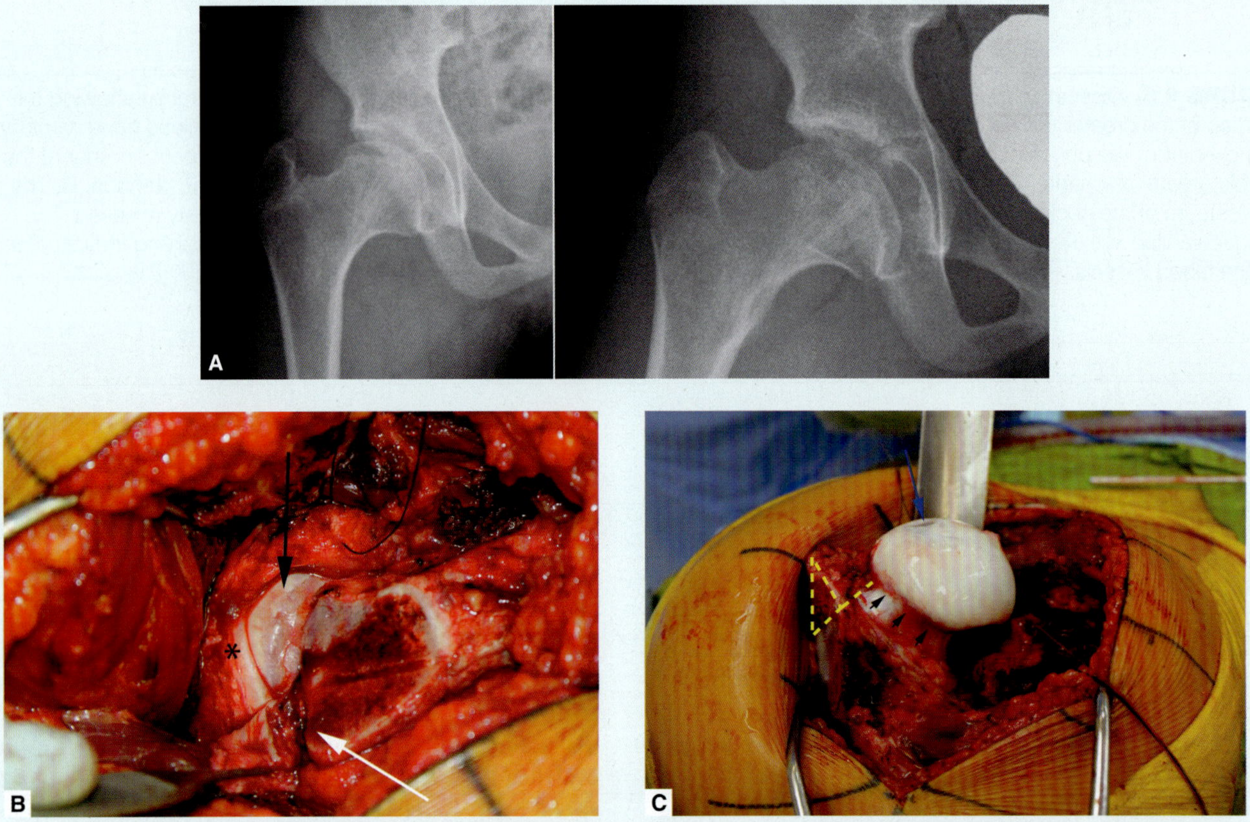

FIGURE 9.6. Residual symptomatic deformity of the hip secondary to LCPD, leading to intra-articular (Cam) and extra-articular impingement. A, Preoperative radiographs showing a nonspherical femoral head, high-riding greater trochanter with a short femoral neck and an anterior prominence of the femoral head. B, Intraoperative picture showing the cam deformity of the femoral head (black arrow) that is prominent and impacts against the acetabular rim and labrum (black asterisk), leading to intra-articular FAI and the high-riding greater trochanter (white arrow) that causes extra-articular impingement against the ilium and posterolateral acetabular rim. C, Intraoperative picture showing the coronal view of the femur. The femoral neck is severely shortened (black arrows), and there is a small area of cartilage loss on the superior aspect of the femoral head (blue arrow). The dashed yellow line marks the superior aspect of the femoral neck, which serves as a reference for the resection of the portion of the stable trochanter proximal to the trochanteric apophysis (yellow dashed triangle).

Clinical Scenario (*continued*)

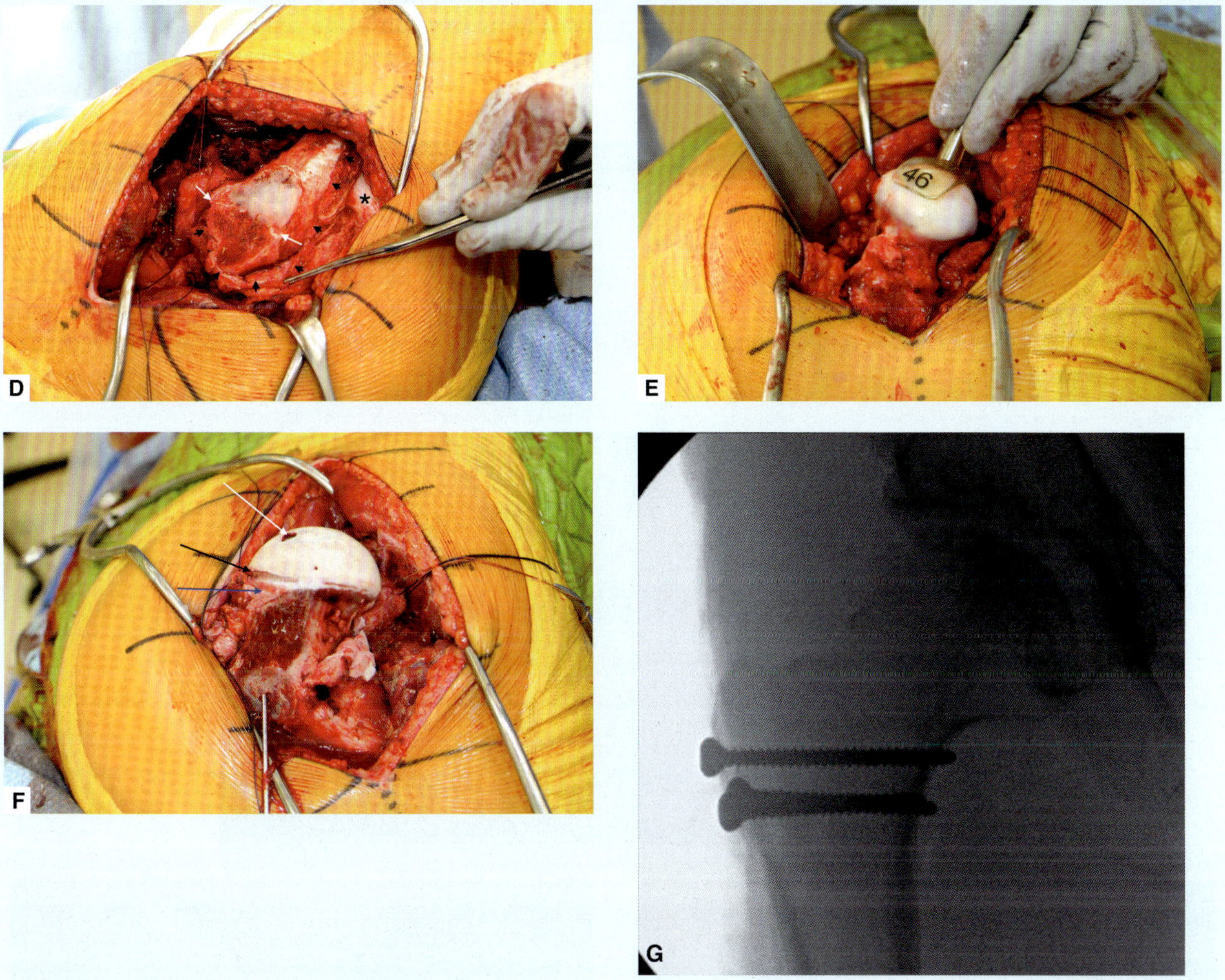

FIGURE 9.6. (*continued*) D, Intraoperative picture showing the lateral aspect of the femur after osteotomy of the greater trochanter and dissection of the periosteum in preparation for the soft retinacular flap dissection. The periosteum (black arrowheads) is dissected from the anterior portion of the femoral neck and trochanter and then posteriorly around the stable trochanteric piece and distally toward the insertion of the gluteal maximus tendon (black asterisk). The portion of the greater trochanter proximal to the apophysis of the greater trochanter (white arrow) should be resected. E, Intraoperative picture showing the application of a spherical template to determine the extent of resection of the femoral head to obtain a spherical morphology. F, Intraoperative picture showing that the osteochondroplasty of the femoral head (black arrow) extends beyond the level of penetration of the nutrient vessels. The femoral epiphysis can be trimmed posteriorly, but the metaphysis should be preserved to avoid damage to the penetrating vessels (blue arrow). Given the very small area of chondral damage to the femoral head, a microfracture with application of juvenile chondrocytes allograft was performed (white arrow). G, Postoperative AP radiograph of the hip showing restoration of the articulotrochanteric distance and improvement of the morphology of the proximal femur.

Intra-Articular Femoral Head–Induced Pincer Impingement

Unlike cam-type deformities, femoral head–induced pincer deformity is associated with severely enlarged and misshapen femoral heads to a degree that prevents the involved portions from entering the acetabulum. One specific pattern of such deformity is hinge abduction defined by limited abduction of the hip and widening of the medial joint space during abduction caused by impaction of the misshapen femoral head on the lateral acetabulum. Functional radiographs of the hip with or without a hip arthrogram are helpful to distinguish hinge abduction preoperatively, but intraoperative inspection of motion restriction is the most reliable means of diagnosis. Treatment of this type of deformity classically involves an intertrochanteric valgus osteotomy that can be performed in combination with an osteochondroplasty of the femoral head and RFNL. However, in hips with asphericity in the coronal plane and associated hinged abduction, a femoral head reduction osteotomy may be the best procedure to improve the morphology of the femur.[14] This procedure involves the development of a retinacular flap to allow a femoral head and neck osteotomy to remove the central necrotic region of the femoral head and reduce its overall volume.

Clinical Scenario

A 10-year-old girl has been followed in clinic since she was 6 years old because of left hip LCPD. She was treated nonsurgically, and gradually over the past few months before her presentation she was found to develop a slight limp and lost range of motion. Under physical examination, her abduction was restricted. Preoperative imaging revealed a severe deformity and enlarged femoral head. She underwent an arthrogram under anesthesia which revealed severe hinge abduction. She subsequently underwent a femoral head reduction osteotomy (**Figure 9.7**).

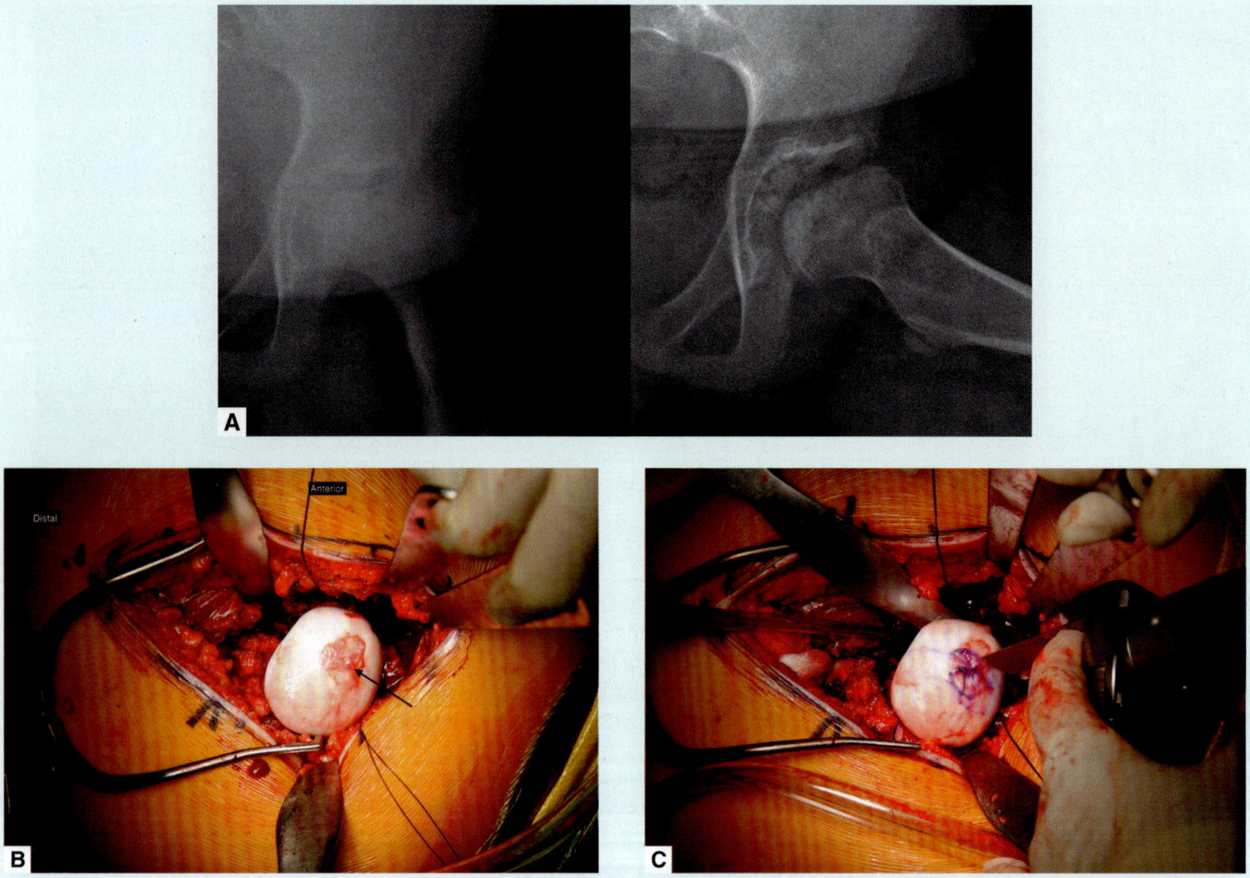

FIGURE 9.7. Residual symptomatic deformity of the hip secondary to LCPD, leading to intra-articular femoral head–induced pincer impingement treated by a femoral head reduction osteotomy in a 10-year-old girl (Courtesy case from Dr. Travis Matheney, MD). A, Preoperative AP and frog-leg lateral radiographs showing severe deformity of the left hip after LCPD with a large portion of the femoral head not well covered by the acetabulum. B, Intraoperative picture showing the dysmorphic femoral head exposed through a surgical hip dislocation approach after development of an extended retinacular soft-tissue flap. The black arrow points to a central area of the femoral head with blistering of the chondral surface. C, Intraoperative picture showing the demarcation for the femoral head osteotomy: the osteotomies are performed in the sagittal plane to protect the blood supply to the femoral head. The medial osteotomy is performed first with an oscillating saw, as shown in the picture.

Clinical Scenario (*continued*)

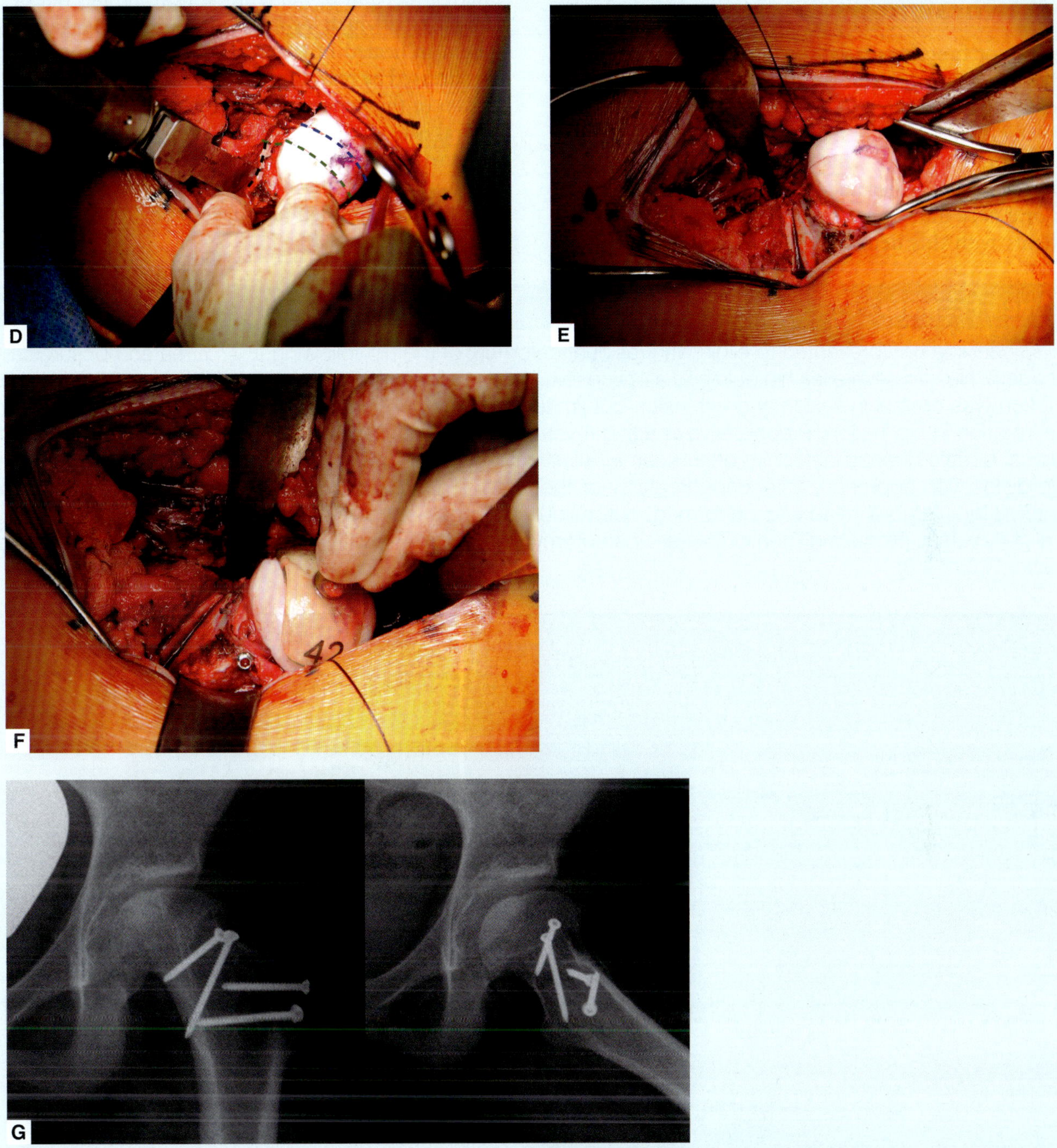

FIGURE 9.7. (*continued*) D, Intraoperative picture showing the lateral osteotomy (dashed green line) has been performed parallel to the medial osteotomy (dashed blue line) to the level of the base of the femoral neck. An osteotomy at the base of the lateral segment is performed (black dashed line) to allow for mobilization of the lateral segment. E, Intraoperative picture showing the femoral head after the central portion had been removed and the lateral segment mobilized medially and held to the medial segment by a pointed clamp. F, After fixation of the head reduction osteotomy, a spherical template is used to confirm the appropriate sphericity of the femoral head. G, Postoperative AP and lateral radiographs at 18-month follow-up showing a well-contained femoral head with improved sphericity index. The patient is asymptomatic with improvement of hip range of motion.

Intra-Articular Impingement: Relative Femoral Head Retroversion

Relative or functional retroversion of the femoral head arises in certain cases of LCPD where there is a significant discrepancy in the positioning between the anterolateral "false" femoral head and the posteromedial "true" femoral head. This discrepant position places the articulating posteromedial head out of line with the femoral neck into a position of relative retroversion.[15-17] Patients with this deformity have notable trouble with hip flexion without significant compensatory external rotation.[18] During hip motion, the anterolateral nonspherical portion of the femoral head rotates out of the acetabulum, which explains the out-toeing gait often present in healed LCPD. Most often, the deformity can be addressed by resection osteoplasty of the anterolateral portion of the femoral head. However, in hips in which femoral osteoplasty does not completely resolve the impingement, an intertrochanteric valgus and slight flexion osteotomy can be performed to improve the alignment of the articulating femoral head with the remainder of the femur (**Figure 9.8**).

Clinical Scenario

A 13-year-old boy presented to clinic with residual deformity of the hip following LCPD treated nonsurgically at age 8. He had severe left hip pain and a noticeable limp, out-toeing, and a marked Trendelenburg sign. Hip motion was normal in flexion and extension but limited in rotation, especially with pronounced loss of internal rotation in hip flexion. Preoperative imaging revealed a severe deformity and enlarged femoral head with typical double-headed deformity often seen in relative retroversion of the femoral head. Through a surgical hip dislocation approach, osteochondroplasty of the femoral head and neck junction with resection of the anterolateral femoral head was performed, but residual impingement persisted. In the same surgical setting, a slightly valgus producing intertrochanteric osteotomy was performed with relative lengthening of the femoral neck. (Figure 9.8)

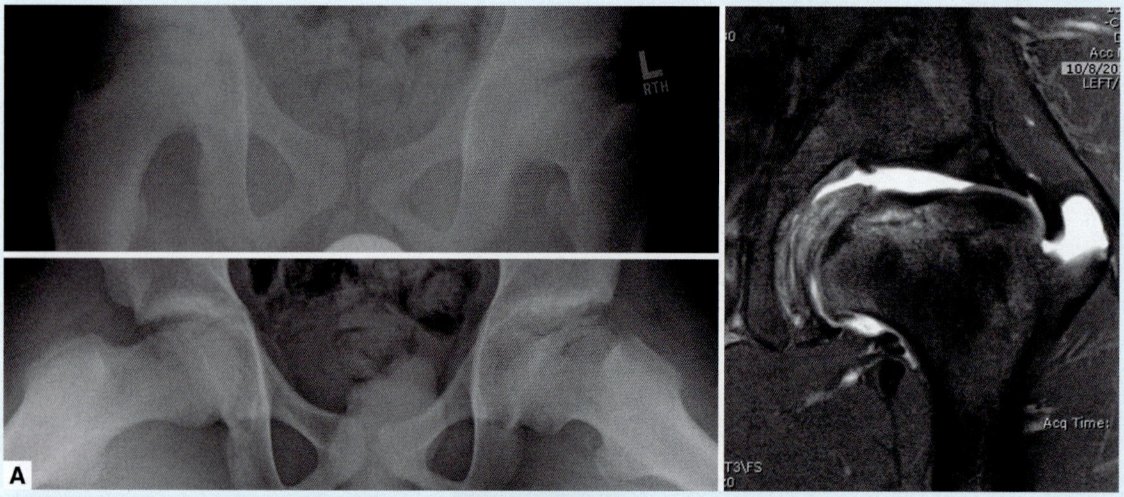

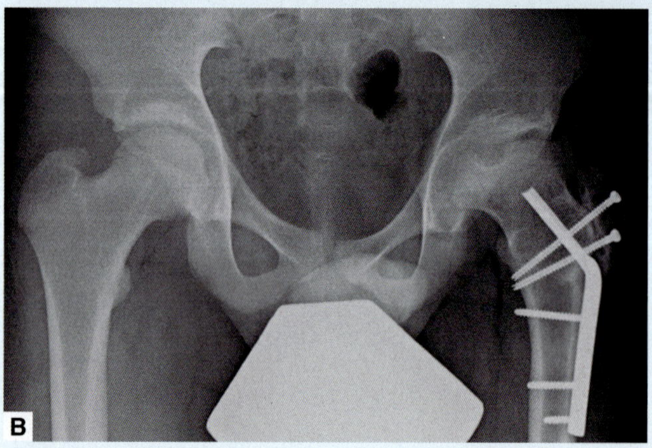

FIGURE 9.8. Residual symptomatic deformity of the hip secondary to LCPD with relative retroversion of the femoral head, leading to pain, limited internal rotation motion, out-toeing gait, and a limp. Surgical treatment consisted of a surgical dislocation approach with osteochondroplasty of the femoral head and neck with excision of the anterolateral portion of the femoral head, RFNL, and a valgus producing osteotomy. A, Preoperative images: AP radiograph (top left panel), frog-leg lateral radiograph (bottom left panel), and coronal MRI (right panel) showing severe deformity of the left hip after LCPD with an enlarged femoral head. B, Postoperative AP pelvis showing improvement of the femoral morphology at 1-year follow-up with corresponding improvement in patient's symptoms and hip range of motion.

Acetabular Dysplasia and Retroversion

The acetabulum morphology is often normal at the time of LCPD onset. Acetabular dysplasia and acetabular retroversion develop as a consequence of the disease process in response to the changes to the femoral head.[8,19] The severity of proximal femoral deformity correlates with the severity of the acetabular deformity.[20] Acetabular dysplasia leads to symptomatic instability, whereas acetabular retroversion leads to anterior FAI and potentially posterolateral instability. The degree of acetabular dysplasia and hip instability must be determined prior to surgery but must also be reassessed after correction of femoral-sided deformity during the surgical hip dislocation approach. Acetabular reorientation with a PAO may be recommended to improve congruency and stability of the hip.[14] In selected hips with acetabular retroversion and relative overcoverage of the femoral head anteriorly, acetabular rim trimming may be performed at the time of the surgical hip dislocation.

Clinical Scenario

A 26-year-old male presented to clinic with residual deformity of the right hip following LCPD treated nonsurgically during childhood. He had right hip pain and slight limp with positive Trendelenburg sign. Hip motion assessment showed limited abduction with preserved flexion. He had a positive anterior impingement test as well as an apprehension test, a positive test for abduction fatigue and pain with abduction of the hip. Preoperative imaging revealed a severe deformity of the proximal femur with an enlarged nonspherical femoral head and a high-riding greater trochanter. Surgical treatment was performed with a surgical hip dislocation approach, osteochondroplasty of the femoral head and neck junction and RFNL, followed by a PAO to correct the dysplastic acetabulum (**Figure 9.9**).

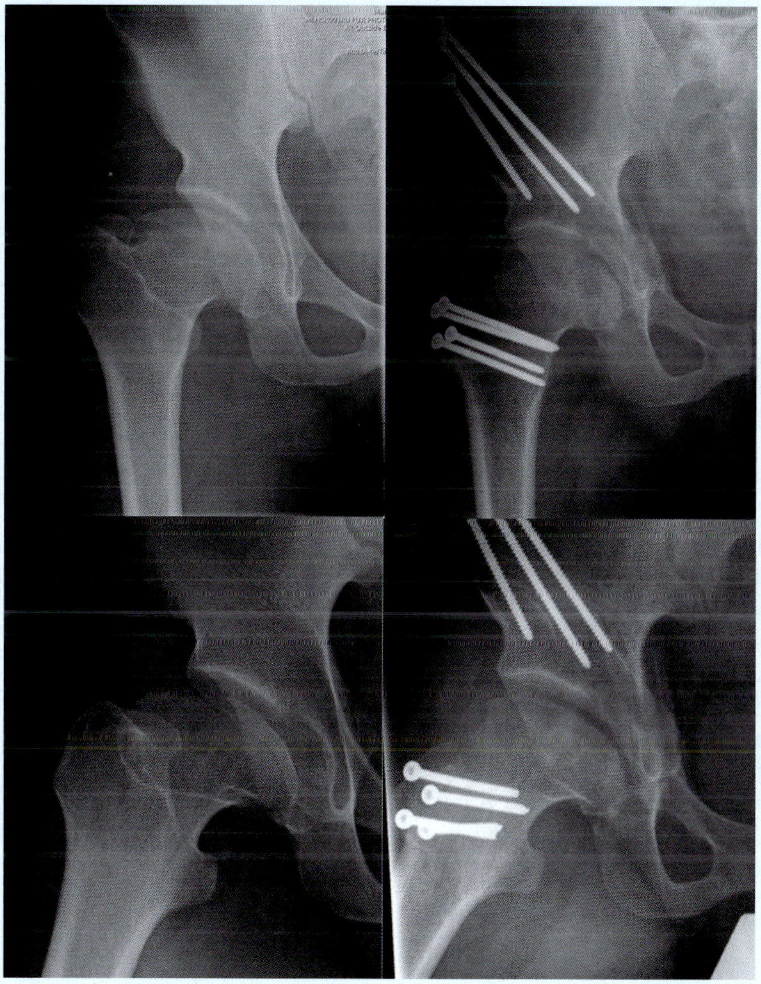

FIGURE 9.9. Residual symptomatic deformity of the hip secondary to LCPD with high riding greater trochanter, short femoral neck, nonspherical femoral head, and acetabular dysplasia in a 26-year old male with pain, limited abduction, positive impingement and apprehension tests, and a slight limp. Preoperative AP (top right) and frog-leg lateral (bottom right) showing the severe deformity. The patient was treated with the surgical dislocation approach with osteochondroplasty of the femoral head and neck, relative femoral neck lengthening, and a periacetabular osteotomy. Postoperative radiographs (left top and bottom) showing improved morphology of the hip.

OUTCOMES

Surgical treatment of residual LCPD using the surgical hip dislocation approach for intraoperative assessment and treatment of femoral deformities with or without a combined PAO for the treatment of acetabular deformities is associated with improved patient reported outcomes in the short- and mid-term with an overall low risk of major complications. A review of the literature[12] found a total of 138 patients with residual LCPD treated with the surgical dislocation approach. The average age at surgery ranged from 14 to 21 years. The majority of hips were classified as Stulberg III (46%) and Stulberg IV (34%). Femoral head-neck osteochondroplasty and RFNL were the most commonly performed procedures (76.8% and 60.9%, respectively). In 22.5% of patients, an intertrochanteric osteotomy was performed, while 9% of the patients underwent a concomitant PAO. Seventy-five percent of patients showed improvement in pain and function, and 40% were reported to be pain free at last follow-up. Six percent of the patients developed a major complication, and 10% of patients had worsening pain and underwent a total hip arthroplasty. The rate of failure (defined as total hip arthroplasty or persistent pain) was about 16%.

In summary, most patients with healed LCPD deformities will present with a wide variety of both proximal femoral and acetabular pathomorphologies. The proximal femoral changes ubiquitously make patients susceptible to FAI and the resultant chondral and labral damage and dysfunction. The proximal femoral deformity should be addressed first with a surgical hip dislocation with extensive femoral osteochondroplasty for intra-articular impingement, followed by an RFNL to correct the reduced articulotrochanteric distance and extra-articular impingement. In cases with significant deformity of the proximal femur that cannot be addressed by osteochondroplasty alone, a femoral head reduction osteotomy or a redirecting intertrochanteric osteotomy to orient the articular femoral head within the acetabulum may be recommended. After complete correction of proximal femoral morphology, the acetabular pathomorphology should be addressed. In cases with residual anterior impingement due to an acetabular retroversion leading to a pincer deformity, acetabular reorientation through a PAO or a focal anterior rim trimming may be performed, and the decision should be based on the global acetabular morphology. In cases with resultant instability of the hip associated with a dysplastic acetabulum, we perform a PAO to reorient the acetabulum into a position to optimize stability while avoiding impingement.

REFERENCES

1. Engelhardt P. Late prognosis of Perthes' disease: which factors determine arthritis risk? *Z Orthop Ihre Grenzgeb.* 1985;123(2):168-181.
2. Lecuire F. The long-term outcome of primary osteochondritis of the hip (Legg-Calve-Perthes' disease). *J Bone Joint Surg Br.* 2002;84(5):636-640.
3. McAndrew MP, Weinstein SL. A long-term follow-up of Legg-Calve-Perthes disease. *J Bone Joint Surg Am.* 1984;66(6):860-869.
4. Novais EN, Clohisy J, Siebenrock K, Podeszwa D, Sucato D, Kim YJ. Treatment of the symptomatic healed Perthes hip. *Orthop Clin North Am.* 2011;42(3):401-417, viii.
5. Mose K, Hjorth L, Ulfeldt M, Christensen ER, Jensen A. Legg Calve Perthes disease. The late of coxarthrosis. *Acta Orthop Scand Suppl.* 1977;169:1-39.
6. Stulberg SD, Cooperman DR, Wallensten R. The natural history of Legg-Calve-Perthes disease. *J Bone Joint Surg Am.* 1981;63(7):1095-1108.
7. Weinstein SL. Legg-Calve-Perthes disease: results of long-term follow-up. *Hip.* 1985;28-37.
8. Ezoe M, Naito M, Inoue T. The prevalence of acetabular retroversion among various disorders of the hip. *J Bone Joint Surg Am.* 2006;88(2):372-379.
9. Ganz R, Parvizi J, Beck M, Leunig M, Notzli H, Siebenrock KA. Femoroacetabular impingement: a cause for osteoarthritis of the hip. *Clin Orthop Relat Res.* 2003;417:112-120.
10. Ganz R, Gill TJ, Gautier E, Ganz K, Krugel N, Berlemann U. Surgical dislocation of the adult hip a technique with full access to the femoral head and acetabulum without the risk of avascular necrosis. *J Bone Joint Surg Br.* 2001;83(8):1119-1124.
11. Ganz R, Klaue K, Vinh TS, Mast JW. A new periacetabular osteotomy for the treatment of hip dysplasias. Technique and preliminary results. *Clin Orthop Relat Res.* 1988(232):26-36.
12. Novais EN. Application of the surgical dislocation approach to residual hip deformity secondary to Legg-Calve-Perthes disease. *J Pediatr Orthop.* 2013;33(1):S62-S69.
13. Ganz R, Huff TW, Leunig M. Extended retinacular soft-tissue flap for intra-articular hip surgery: surgical technique, indications, and results of application. *Instr Course Lect.* 2009;58:241-255.
14. Siebenrock KA, Anwander H, Zurmuhle CA, Tannast M, Slongo T, Steppacher SD. Head reduction osteotomy with additional containment surgery improves sphericity and containment and reduces pain in Legg-Calve-Perthes disease. *Clin Orthop Relat Res.* 2015;473(4):1274-1283.
15. Katz JF. Femoral torsion in Legg-Calve-Perthes disease. *J Bone Joint Surg Am.* 1968;50(3):473-475.
16. Kim HT, Wenger DR. "Functional retroversion" of the femoral head in Legg-Calve-Perthes disease and epiphyseal dysplasia: analysis of head-neck deformity and its effect on limb position using three-dimensional computed tomography. *J Pediatr Orthop.* 1997;17(2):240-246.
17. Upadhyay SS, Burwell RG, Moulton A. Femoral anteversion in Perthes' disease with observations on irritable hips. Application of a new method using ultrasound. *Clin Orthop Relat Res.* 1986;209:70-76.
18. Yoo WJ, Choi IH, Cho TJ, Chung CY, Park MS, Lee DY. Out-toeing and in-toeing in patients with Perthes disease: role of the femoral hump. *J Pediatr Orthop.* 2008;28(7):717-722.
19. Sankar WN, Flynn JM. The development of acetabular retroversion in children with Legg-Calve-Perthes disease. *J Pediatr Orthop.* 2008;28(4):440-443.
20. Madan S, Fernandes J, Taylor JF. Radiological remodelling of the acetabulum in Perthes' disease. *Acta Orthop Belg.* 2003;69(5):412-420.

CHAPTER 10

Congenital Coxa Vara

Coxa vara deformity can be a congenital condition noted at birth, a progressive developmental disorder, or a disorder acquired as a result of trauma, Legg-Calve-Perthes (LCP) disease, slipped capital femoral epiphysis (SCFE), or metabolic or neoplastic conditions.[1-4] The congenital form is believed to result from a limb bud abnormality or another intrauterine process. It is often associated with other limb deficiencies, such as proximal femoral focal deficiency or fibular hemimelia. Congenital coxa vara has an incidence of approximately 1 in 25 000. It affects males and females equally, with no predilection for the right or left side, and occurs bilaterally in 30% to 50% of patients. Most patients first have painless waddling or a Trendelenburg gait between 2 and 6 years of age; a decrease in hip abduction and a limb length discrepancy, if the condition is unilateral, may also be present.[2]

IMAGING

Given the typical age at which coxa vara is diagnosed, plain radiographs are usually sufficient for the initial evaluation. A standing anteroposterior (AP) pelvic radiograph with the hips internally rotated to 15° helps to maximize the ability to obtain an accurate assessment of the neck-shaft angle and the Hilgenreiner epiphyseal angle (**Figure 10.1A**). A frog-lateral view further aids in the assessment of dysmorphic proximal femur changes (**Figure 10.1B**). Owing to the association with other congenital anomalies, additional screening radiographs should be considered to assess for other areas of dysplasia.

INDICATIONS

On plain radiographs, an inverted Y pattern may be seen at the proximal femoral physis, with a resulting fragment at the inferior neck, which is sometimes referred to as the Fairbanks fragment.[1] A neck-shaft angle of less than 90° is considered to be an indication for corrective osteotomy. The Hilgenreiner angle is subtended between the Hilgenreiner line on the AP pelvic radiograph and a line drawn through the proximal femoral physis. A child with a limp and a Hilgenreiner angle (**Figure 10.1A**) greater than 60°, or 45° to 60° with documented progression of varus deformity, should undergo surgical treatment.[2]

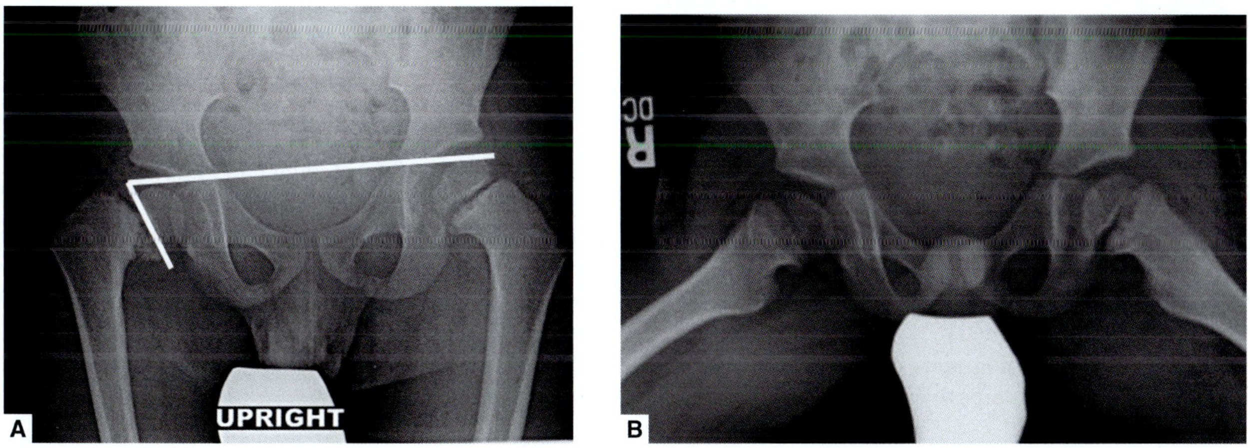

FIGURE 10.1. A-B, Preoperative standing anteroposterior (AP) pelvis with hips internally rotated and frog-lateral view of bilateral hips. Hilgenreiner epiphyseal angle is demonstrated on the AP view. The inferior neck "Fairbanks fragment" is visible on the right hip.

TREATMENT

Nonoperative management for hips with HEA <60° (or <45° to 60° without evidence of progressive deformity) should include routine radiographs as part of a surveillance program. The goal of treatment is to restore a more anatomic alignment and improve the hip range of motion and mechanics. A corrective intertrochanteric or subtrochanteric valgus osteotomy is the preferred treatment to restore the Hilgenreiner angle to approximately 25°, overcorrect the neck-shaft angle to between 150° and 160°, and convert shear forces across the neck into compressive forces across the osteotomy site. A method of performing this osteotomy percutaneously has been described.[4] Additional treatment can include a concomitant adductor tenotomy and proximal femoral shortening to reduce pressure on the femoral head and to reduce the force of correction.

Several complications have been described, including premature physeal closure in as many as 90% of patients, greater trochanter overgrowth, recurrence of the deformity, possibly as a result of undercorrection, osteonecrosis, limb length discrepancy, or degenerative osteoarthritis.[2]

In long-term studies, the predictors of improved clinical and radiographic outcomes include age under 9 years at the time of surgery and overcorrection of the neck-shaft angle to minimize the rate of recurrent deformity.[2] A comparison following operative and nonoperative management has been recorded in small series. Recurrent varus deformity requiring revision osteotomy occurred in as many as nearly 25% of operatively treated cases.[5] Spontaneous correction of coxa vara with an average Hilgenreiner Epiphyseal Angle (HEA) 36° with associated gait abnormalities was not common, warranting surgical correction to the aforementioned angular goal.

Clinical Scenario

The patient is a 4-year-old otherwise healthy male with no other medical issues who presented with painless limp. Overall development was typical for his age, and there was no family history of skeletal dysplasias. There was no history of trauma. Physical exam demonstrated a slight Trendelenburg gait on the right and decreased internal rotation of both hips, more on the right side than on the left.

Initial radiographic evaluation demonstrated coxa vara of both hips with HEA of 70° on the right and 30° on the left. The family wished to try conservative management, but follow-up radiographs demonstrated progression of the HEA on both hips to 75° and 40°, right and left respectively, as well as the appearance of an inferior neck fracture ("Fairbanks") fragment. Given these findings, the family agreed to proceed with treatment of bilateral hips to correct the more affected right side as well as the less affected left owing to concern that it may continue to worsen and out of a desire to avoid the need for subsequent osteotomy.

TECHNIQUE

A direct lateral approach is planned for the proximal femoral intertrochanteric osteotomy. If it is a bilateral case, we prefer to correct both sides under the same anesthetic. In bilateral cases, the patient is positioned supine on multiple folded blankets to elevate the head and torso and allow access to bilateral prepped lower extremities. Based on the preoperative hip abduction, an adductor longus tenotomy may be beneficial.

Plan for a final neck-shaft angle between 140 and 150° because recurrence is possible if there is undercorrection, and your goal will be to end with a Hilgenreiner angle below 25° to maximize compression across the physis. Shortening up to a centimeter and derotating the femur to approximately 15° of anteversion can also be beneficial. To take tension off the repair, the retroversion that is commonly seen must be corrected. Femoral version is marked prior to osteotomy with a thin wire placed percutaneously across the transepicondylar access, which is compared to a similar wire placed in line with the femoral neck based on intraoperative fluoroscopy. Depending on age and patient size, there are several fixed angle options for implants between blade plates and locking proximal femoral plates. In very young patients, multiple prebent smooth wires can be placed into the femoral neck and affixed to the femoral shaft with cerclage wires. Implant should be chosen to lateralize the femoral shaft to restore mechanical axis, as illustrated in **Figure 10.2**. Additional spica casting may be necessary depending on the age of the patient and quality of the bone/fixation.

POSTOPERATIVE CARE

Weight-bearing is restricted for 6 weeks (or until radiographs demonstrate adequate healing). Physical therapy is utilized with the primary goals of improving gait and returning to age-appropriate activities. Implants are typically removed after 6 months depending on patient age and remaining growth. We recommend routine follow-up to at least age 8 to 10 years, given the overall high rate of recurrence and potential need for revision surgery (**Figure 10.2A-B**).

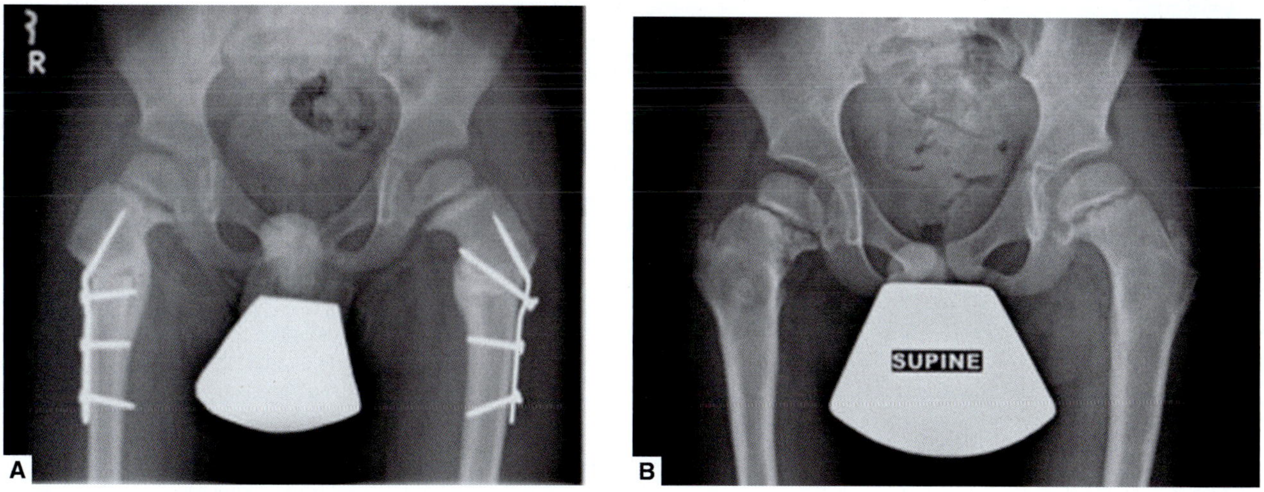

FIGURE 10.2. A-B, Postoperative anteroposterior pelvic radiographs at 1 and 2 years following surgery.

REFERENCES

1. Fairbank HA. Coxa vara due to congenital defect of the neck of the femur. *J Anat*. 1928;62:232-237.
2. Weinstein JN, Kuo KN, Millar EA. Congenital coxa vara: a retrospective review. *J Pediatr Orthop*. 1984;4;70-77.
3. Aarabi M, Rauch F, Hamdy RC, Fassier F. High prevalence of coxa vara in patients with severe osteogenesis imperfecta. *J Pediatr Orthop*. 2006;26:24-28.
4. Sabharwal S, Mittal R, Cox G. Percutaneous triplanar femoral osteotomy correction for developmental coxa vara: a new technique. *J Pediatr Orthop*. 2005;25:28-33.
5. Roberts DW, Saglam Y, De La Rocha A, Frasquillo BN, Tulchin-Francis K, Kim HKW. Long-term outcomes of operative and nonoperative treatment of congenital coxa vara. *J Pediatr Orthop*. 2018;38(4):193-201.

CHAPTER 11

Femoroacetabular Impingement—Cam, Mixed, and Pincer-Type Treatment Decision-Making

INTRODUCTION

Femoroacetabular impingement (FAI) is an abnormal hip kinematics that can lead to joint damage and pain. The modern concept of FAI was proposed by Professor Reinhold Ganz and was based on observations of intra-articular pattern of joint damage and its association with hip morphology, as seen via the surgical hip dislocation approach. Subsequent work demonstrated femoral retroversion, anterior inferior iliac spine (AIIS), prominent anterior trochanter, and other extra-articular morphology as sources of impingement. Surgical management of FAI started via the surgical dislocation approach, but as arthroscopic techniques developed, they gained popularity. At present, there are a range of surgical techniques available to treat the underlying morphologic cause (**Table 11.1**). Optimizing the treatment of patients with FAI-related hip pain requires a thorough thoughtful approach to evaluating the sources of impingement to maximize the outcome of nonoperative measures or surgical correction.

Questions that must be answered during the diagnostic evaluation include:

- What pathomorphology is the source of FAI?
- Can the FAI-related symptoms be managed nonoperatively?
- In cases with multiple sources of pain, how much can reasonably be treated by surgical intervention?
- What is the safest, most reliable means of addressing the sources of FAI?

This chapter will delve into the comprehensive evaluation of FAI symptoms and potential treatment options.

CLINICAL EVALUATION

History

A complete history is essential to the accurate diagnosis of FAI-related hip pain. Important topics to address include location and radiation of pain, activities that alleviate or exacerbate the pain, and the presence of mechanical symptoms such as clicking or locking. Most, but not all, patients with intra-articular pain report the anterior groin or C-sign region as the most common area of pain and describe it as a deep ache or stabbing type of pain. FAI-related pain rarely radiates to the lower leg, unlike pathology commonly encountered in the

TABLE 11.1 Surgical Procedures That Can Be Performed via Surgical Dislocation Vs. Arthroscopic Approaches

Surgical Dislocation	Hip Arthroscopy
Labral debridement, repair, reconstruction	Labral debridement, repair, reconstruction
Cartilage debridement, restoration (microfracture, autologous matrix–induced chondrogenesis, osteoarticular transfers)	Cartilage debridement, restoration (microfracture, autologous matrix–induced chondrogenesis)
Acetabular osteoplasty	Acetabular osteoplasty
Femoral head/neck osteoplasty	Femoral head/neck osteoplasty
Capsular repair/plication	Capsular repair/plication
Femoral neck lengthening	
Trochanteric osteoplasty/transfer	
Intertrochanteric/subtrochanteric osteotomy	

lumbar spine. Positions of flexion and high-impact activities are typically more bothersome for patients with FAI, and complaints of pain or fatigue with prolonged standing or upright activity could suggest the presence of structural instability. Clicking or locking can be from multiple etiologies, including unstable labral tears, iliopsoas snapping, or capsular pathology. It is also important to get a broader perspective on the impact that hip pain has had on the patient's functionality and lifestyle. Often, patients will have been managed by other providers, including physical therapists or primary care physicians, and their previous treatments should be identified. Lastly, it is important to clearly identify the patient's functional goals following treatment, as this may influence the treatment strategy.

Physical Examination

Examination starts with inspection and palpation. Palpation of the greater trochanter can elicit trochanteric bursitis or tendinopathy, which patients often confuse with hip pain. Gait should be evaluated in all patients. A Trendelenburg stance or gait is indicative of gluteal (abductor) dysfunction and may exacerbate the degree of FAI. True abductor tears are rarely encountered in the cohort of young patients undergoing FAI surgery most commonly, but this diagnosis should be considered in older patients with hip pain and evidence of abductor dysfunction.

Supine physical examination should comprehensively evaluate the range of impingement-free motion in all planes of motion. When testing motion, it is essential to quantify the degree of motion specific to the femoroacetabular joint. Compensatory motion through the lumbar spine or rotation through the pelvis can give an inaccurate representation of true femoroacetabular motion. The pelvis should be palpated or observed during motion evaluation, and the limits of femoroacetabular motion should be noted at the onset of pelvic motion. Diminished flexion and flexion/internal rotation (FIR) is commonplace with FAI. When a firm stop is felt during internal rotation testing, femoral retroversion may be present, while offset deformities of the proximal femur typically examine with a softer end point. Diminished hip abduction may indicate lateral sources of impingement either at the proximal femur or at the acetabulum. Prone examination of hip range of motion in extension can provide a good measure of femoral version, with a lack of internal rotation raising suspicion for relative femoral retroversion.

Provocative tests include the following:

- Anterior Impingement Test: Flexion/adduction/internal rotation (FADIR) serves to bring the anterolateral femoral head in contact with the anterior-superior rim. A positive test elicits pain in the anterior groin and may be indicative of cam and/or pincer pathomorphology (**Figure 11.1**).

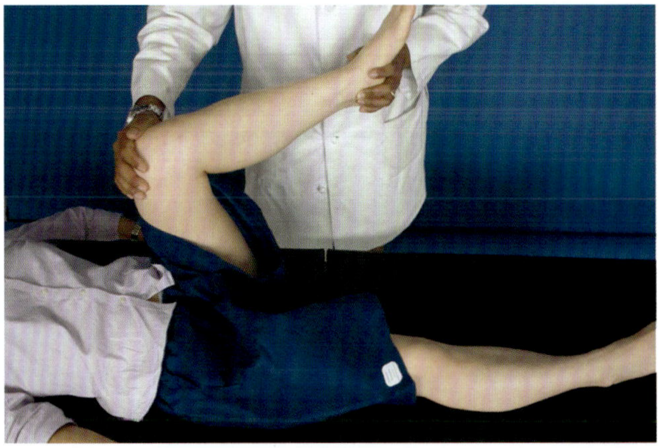

FIGURE 11.1. Impingement test (flexion, adduction, internal rotation [FADIR]) is performed with the hip in FADIR. Anterior groin pain is produced with this maneuver and is a nonspecific test that can indicate anterior labral tear, joint inflammation, and anterior impingement.

- Straight Flexion Test: Anterior groin pain elicited with straight hip flexion may be indicative of AIIS impingement on the anteromedial femoral neck.
- Flexion, abduction, and external rotation (FABER) test could indicate sacroiliac joint pathology, superior/posterior acetabular rim impingement, or psoas irritation depending on the location of pain elicited by this physical examination test (**Figure 11.2**).
- Posterior Impingement Test: Hip extension/external rotation may cause posterior buttock pain (extra-articular impingement) or anterior apprehension/pain (instability).

Chapter 16 outlines the physical examination test and associated anatomic and ultrasound findings in more detail.

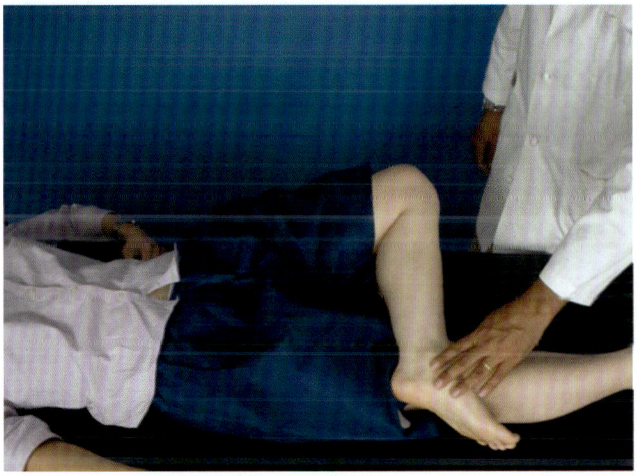

FIGURE 11.2. The FABER (flexion, abduction, external rotation) test can indicate superior rim impingement, anterior instability, or sacroiliac joint irritation depending on the location of the pain with this maneuver.

Imaging

A comprehensive radiographic evaluation of the proximal femur and acetabulum is recommended to fully evaluate hip morphology. The standing anteroposterior (AP) pelvic radiograph evaluates lateral acetabular coverage, anterior and posterior wall coverage, and femoral morphology at the 12 o' clock position (**Figure 11.3**). The false-profile radiograph evaluates anterior acetabular coverage and the femoral morphology at the 3 o' clock position (**Figure 11.4**). The 45° Dunn view evaluates the anterior-superior to superior-anterior (1:30) position on the anterolateral femur, where typical cam deformities are most pronounced (**Figure 11.5**). The combination of these radiographic views provides a comprehensive evaluation of both acetabular and femoral morphology. Important measurements of acetabular coverage include the lateral center-edge angle (AP), Tönnis roof angle (AP), anterior and posterior wall indices (AP), and anterior center-edge angle (FP). Measures of femoral-sided impingement include the alpha angle and femoral head-neck ratio on all three radiographic views. Acetabular retroversion is evaluated on the AP view by the crossover sign, the posterior wall sign, the ischial spine sign, and anterior/posterior wall index (**Figure 11.6**).

Advanced imaging options include magnetic resonance imaging (MRI) and computed tomography (CT) scans. MRI more effectively images the soft tissues, including the labrum and capsule, whereas CT scan more effectively evaluates bony deformity. Three-dimensional reconstruction of CT data can be the most useful in qualitatively evaluating prior cam resection. MRI with cartilage-specific sequences can be helpful in evaluating the quality of the cartilage in the dysplastic or borderline dysplastic hips. Our cartilage imaging of choice is the delayed gadolinium-enhanced MRI of cartilage (dGEMRIC) (**Figure 11.7**). The dGEMRIC index has been shown to determine the early failure of

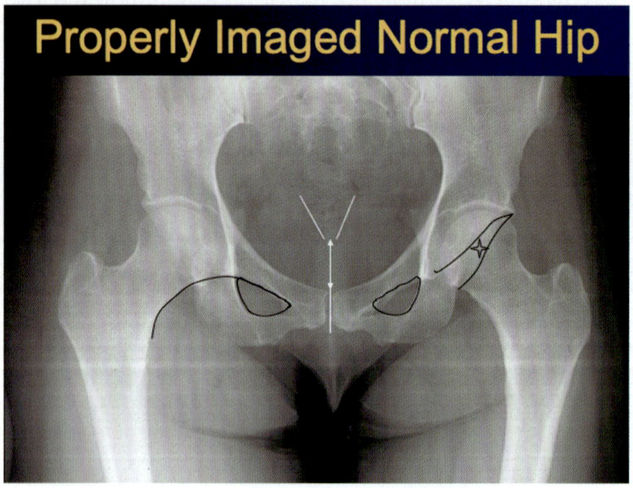

FIGURE 11.3. In a normal hip that is imaged properly with an anteroposterior pelvic x-ray, the symphysis should be right below the coccyx, and the obturator foramina should be symmetric. The Shenton's line should be intact, with the sourcil roughly horizontal and on top of the femoral head. The anterior and posterior walls should meet at the edge of the joint, with the posterior wall just lateral to the femoral head center.

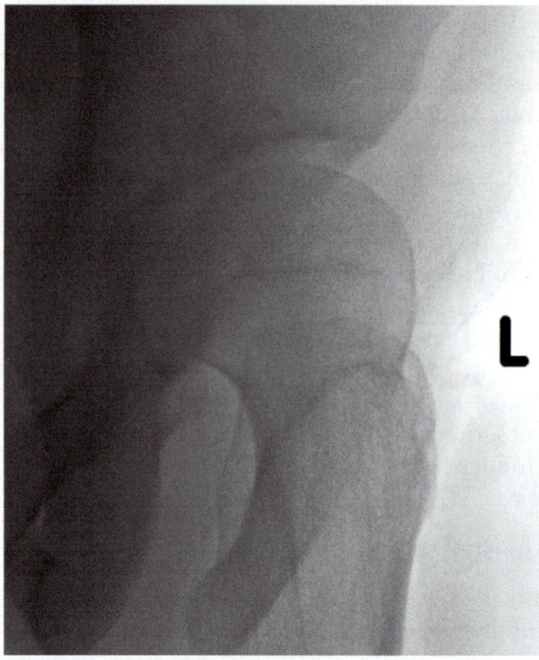

FIGURE 11.4. The false-profile view is obtained in the standing position and is a lateral view of the acetabulum. In a normal hip, the superior joint space is wider than the posterior joint space and is a sensitive view to detect early osteoarthritis as well as anterior hip instability.

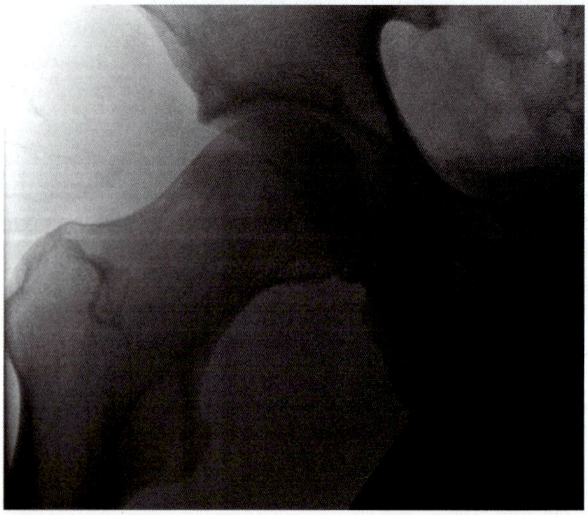

FIGURE 11.5. The modified Dunn lateral view projects the usual location on the head-neck junction where the cam deformity is most prominent.

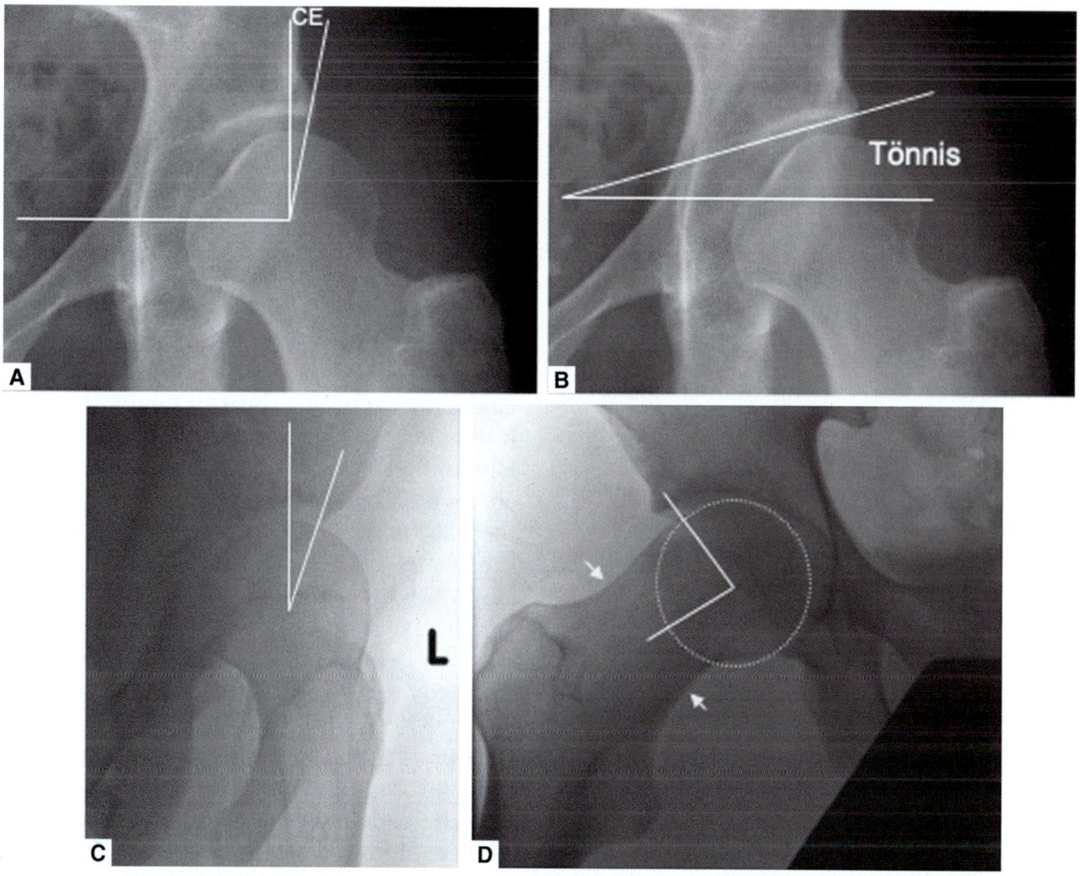

FIGURE 11.6. The center-edge angle of Wiberg (A) measures the femoral head coverage, and less than 16° indicates definite acetabular dysplasia. The horizontal line is found by connecting the centers of both femoral heads, and from this center the edge of the sourcil is connected to define the angle. The Tönnis angle (B) is found by connecting the medial edge of the sourcil in both hips and then the tangent line connecting the medial and lateral-most edge of the sourcil. Normal is between 0° and 10°. The center-edge angle on the false-profile view (C) is found by drawing a vertical line from the center of the femoral head and then another line to the edge of the sourcil. An angle of more than 25° is considered normal. The alpha angle for the cam lesion can be measured on a modified Dunn lateral view (D) by finding the center of the femoral head and the midpoint of the narrowest part of the femoral neck. A second line is then drawn to the edge of the circle where the femoral head starts to become eccentric.

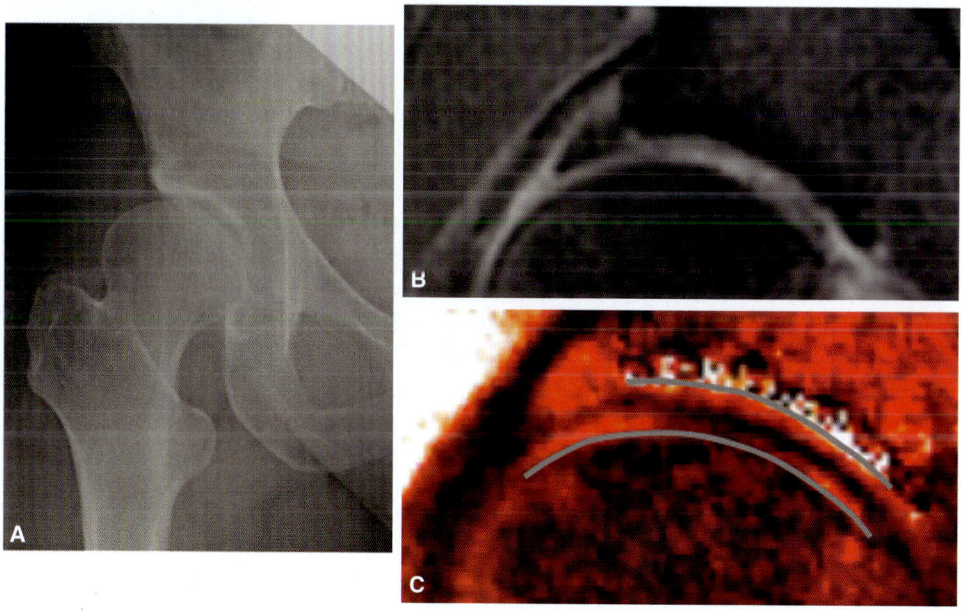

FIGURE 11.7. The delayed gadolinium-enhanced magnetic resonance imaging (MRI) of cartilage (dGEMRIC) is a special MRI technique designed to measure the charge density of articular cartilage. In this dysplastic hip (A), radiographs do not show signs of arthritis. The morphologic MRI (B) shows some signal heterogeneity in the articular surface but is difficult to quantify. The dGEMRIC image (C) shows areas of clear decreased T1 (dark red–black) regions in the articular cartilage, indicating significant loss of tissue integrity.

periacetabular osteotomy for acetabular dysplasia, but its utility in FAI surgery is not well characterized. T2 mapping and T1-rho are other cartilage sequences that are being developed to evaluate cartilage health to help with the identification of early joint degeneration.

Nonoperative Diagnostic and Therapeutic Interventions

Nonoperative interventions should be the first-line treatment in patients with FAI. A structured physical therapy program involving core strengthening, abductor strengthening, lower extremity conditioning, and postural retraining is a good starting point. Activity modification is recommended for patients struggling with inflammatory-type pain. Guided injections of local anesthetic, with or without cortisone, can be a useful adjunct for both diagnostic and treatment purposes. FAI patients commonly present with a variety of complaints that may arise from a number of etiologies. An intra-articular injection is a reliable means of identifying the degree to which intra-articular pathomorphology contributes to the patient's overall symptomatology and their expected symptom improvement following surgery. It is essential to carefully observe the patient's response in the few hours immediately following injection when the local anesthetic is in effect, and repeated examination or patient symptom logs are recommended during this period. The long-term response to intra-articular injections with cortisone, while important, is less predictive of patient improvement following surgical intervention. Diagnostic injections can also target other areas that cause impingement-related pain, including the greater trochanter, the ischiofemoral space, the psoas tendon sheath, and the rectus femoris.

Chapter 15 outlines in detail the use of ultrasound-guided diagnostic injections in the diagnostic and treatment strategies for FAI patients.

FEMOROACETABULAR IMPINGEMENT SUBTYPES

FAI may arise from pathologic morphology occurring in the proximal femur, acetabulum, or both. In the text that follows, we discuss the common pathomorphology subtypes typically encountered in a young patient population. We present each deformity in isolation and discuss relevant parameters toward choosing an arthroscopic versus open (surgical dislocation) approach. Not uncommonly, these deformities will present in clusters, and the sum of the deformities should be taken into consideration when deciding on a surgical approach. In general, the arthroscopic approach to the hip is recommended unless the patient has any of the following pathomorphologic features discussed that could not be addressed via arthroscopy.

Proximal Femoral Deformities

Deformities commonly encountered on the femoral side of FAI hips include cam-type deformities of the femoral head-neck junction and pathologic femoral retroversion. Both of these deformities are discussed here.

Cam-Type Femoral Deformity

Cam-type deformity of the proximal femur has become increasingly recognized since FAI was first noted to be a cause of hip osteoarthritis, and it consists of a loss of convexity of the anterosuperior head-neck junction. Mechanically, it causes a shear strain upon entering the joint, leading to cartilage debonding from the underlying acetabulum and tearing at the chondrolabral junction. The etiology of cam deformity is still uncertain, but several mechanisms have been proposed, including subtle slipped capital femoral epiphysis (SCFE) deformity, epiphyseal overgrowth, and failure of separation of epiphyseal/apophyseal growth centers.

Cam deformities classically arise at the anterosuperior proximal femur, although the position of greatest deformity can vary significantly. AP, modified Dunn, and false-profile lateral views are key in diagnosing cam-type FAI, and cross-sectional imaging can also be of great benefit. The alpha angle was initially described on MR sequences but can easily be calculated on plain radiographs and CT imaging as well. Three-dimensional reconstructions of CT data can provide the clinician with a better overall sense of the proximal femoral anatomy to plan surgical resection (**Figure 11.8**).

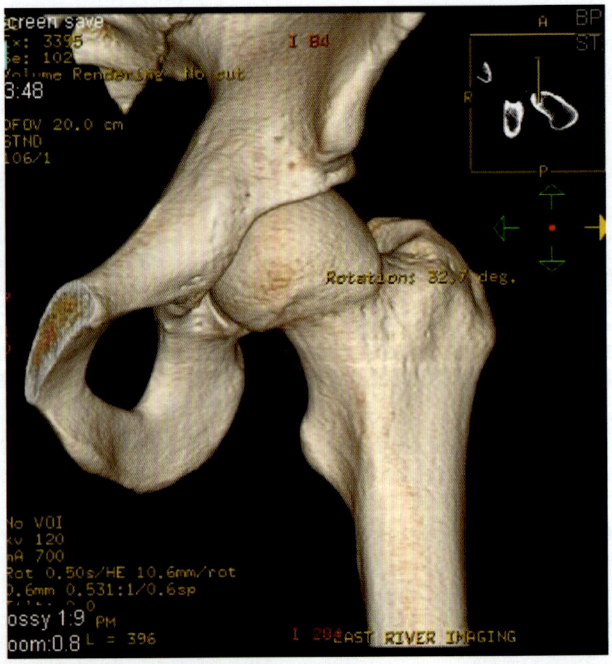

FIGURE 11.8. Three-dimensional rendering of a hip with cam impingement shows clearly the location and size of the cam deformity.

Surgical Decision-Making

Cam-type proximal femoral deformities can be addressed via either open or arthroscopic approaches. Open treatment through a surgical dislocation approach affords complete access to all aspects of the intracapsular femur and acetabulum as well as potential extra-articular sites of impingement. This approach also permits a thorough dynamic examination to directly assess the quality of deformity correction. The downsides of a surgical dislocation include the extent of surgical dissection, including the greater trochanteric osteotomy, and the associated recovery course. Arthroscopic treatment generally affords access to the superior two-thirds of the acetabular rim, the anterolateral half of the femoral head and neck, and pericapsular structures such as the AIIS. The learning curve of hip arthroscopy is steep, and more experienced arthroscopists can access a larger portion of the joint, including the entire acetabulum and posterolateral femoral head-neck region. The benefits of arthroscopy include its limited surgical dissection and more expedient recovery, whereas its limitations involve the inability to access all aspects of the hip and perform a thorough dynamic evaluation of motion.

Ensuring that the proximal femoral deformity can be adequately corrected is the most important goal in choosing a surgical approach. To accurately gauge this decision, it is important to consider both the preoperative physical examination and imaging for each patient. It is important to accurately record the internal rotation of the hip in flexion prior to surgery. Arthroscopic studies document the typical motion improvement following cam resection to be approximately 15°.[1] This level of correction is likely sufficient in most patients but will be insufficient in patients with more limited preoperative motion such as those with obligate external rotation. A surgical dislocation approach in these patients will permit a greater cam decompression, motion analysis, and access for proximal femoral osteotomies if needed.

Location of the cam deformity is important to note as access to the far lateral and posterolateral femur is difficult through an arthroscopic approach. Barriers to complete resection in this region via arthroscopy include both access and concerns for violating the retinacular vessels that pierce the femoral epiphysis around this region. Bedi et al noted that the surgical dislocation approach was a more reliable method to address cam deformities in this region of the femoral head and neck.[2] Patients with a notable cam deformity on AP radiographs likely have a direct lateral or posterolateral component to their deformity. CT scan with 3D reconstructions can confirm this morphologic pattern, and a surgical dislocation approach is recommended.

Femoral Retroversion

Femoral version is an important feature to evaluate prior to FAI surgery. Normal femoral version is typically 15° of anteversion, with an accepted range of normal from 5° to 25°. Excessive anteversion (>25°) is associated with excessive motion and an increased likelihood of instability, whereas excessive retroversion (<5°) is associated with poor motion and increased likelihood of impingement.[3] Retroversion will present clinically with decreased internal rotation on prone examination as well as decreased internal rotation in flexion, often accompanied by a "hard" stop to internal rotation. Femoral retroversion is also hypothesized to increase the severity of cam-type impingement by earlier engagement within the acetabulum. The rotational profile of the femur should be calculated in all patients prior to surgical intervention for FAI with cross-sectional imaging (CT or MRI) through the hip and distal femur.[4,5]

Surgical Decision-Making

In cases of pathologic femoral retroversion, care should be taken to accurately estimate the degree of motion restoration needed by surgical intervention. Again, arthroscopic cam decompression can reliably improve internal rotation by approximately 15°; however, patients with significant retroversion may require further correction to provide normal motion. In these cases, a surgical dislocation approach is advised to address the intra-articular generators of impingement while also allowing access to the proximal femur in case a subtrochanteric, derotational osteotomy is indicated.

Pincer-Type Acetabular Deformity

Pincer-type acetabular deformities are commonly described as a single entity with a predominant feature of "overcoverage" of the femoral head by the acetabulum. This overcoverage impinges on the femoral neck during FIR motions and can lead to compressive damage to the acetabular labrum and cartilaginous rim.[6] Recent work has noted that pincer-type acetabular deformity can result from a variety of pathologic morphologies that should be considered as separate entities when planning surgical interventions. The most common pincer morphologies encountered are: large lunate deep, small lunate deep, and acetabular retroversion.[7,8] These subtypes will be discussed separately in the following sections (**Figure 11.9**).

Large Lunate Deep

A prominent acetabular rim and a normal cotyloid fossa characterize large lunate deep acetabuli. The combination of a prominent rim and normal fossa suggests that these deep hips impinge because of an excessively large lunate cartilage.[7,8] Radiographic features common in this population include excessive wall indices and lateral center-edge angles. On the AP pelvis, the size of the cotyloid fossa should be scrutinized. The Tönnis roof angle should be calculated in all cases for both the current acetabular rim position and the rim position after a rim resection to

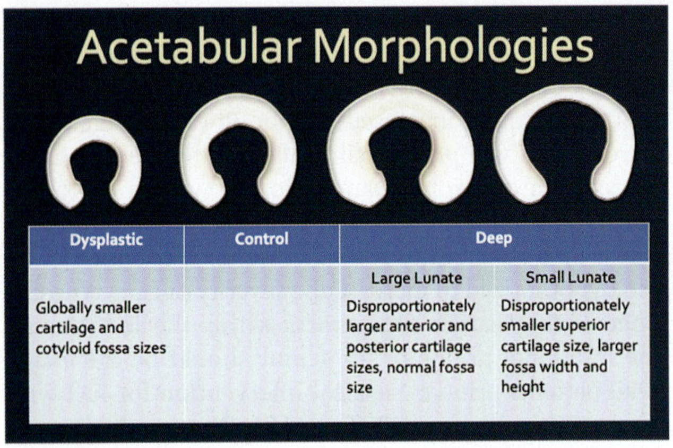

FIGURE 11.9. The lunate surface morphology varies from dysplastic hip with a globally deficient lunate surface. In deep hips, the size of the lunate surface can vary such that even when the hip is overcovered, the lunate surface is not enlarged.

normalize lateral coverage. Often, large lunate deep hips will have a Tönnis roof angle around 0° after template rim resection, indicating a flat sourcil ideal for weight distribution. CT scans with 3D reconstructions are highly beneficial in these patients, and a qualitative evaluation of the cotyloid fossa size (normal vs. large) is often informative (**Figure 11.10**).

Surgical Decision-Making

In hips with pincer-type FAI from large lunate deep acetabular morphology, an osteoplasty-based approach is an option. In mixed impingement cases, involving both cam- and pincer-induced impingement, complete correction of the cam deformity can resolve the FAI symptoms without treatment of the acetabular overcoverage in many cases. In isolated pincer impingement cases, an acetabuloplasty should be performed through either an arthroscopic or an open approach, depending on surgeon comfort and other pathology being addressed at surgery. When planning resection depth, 1 mm of bony resection translates into approximately 1° to 2° of lateral and anterior coverage.[9,10] Care should be taken to avoid overresection because resections of as little as 4 mm have been shown to increase joint contact pressures in cadaveric studies.[11] The acetabular labrum should be repaired to the acetabular rim after the osteoplasty is completed. Techniques for acetabuloplasty by both arthroscopic and open approaches are discussed in subsequent chapters.

Small Lunate Deep

A prominent acetabular rim and a large cotyloid fossa characterize small lunate deep acetabuli. The combination of a prominent rim and enlarged fossa suggests that these deep hips impinge owing to a maloriented acetabulum that has a normal or even hypoplastic lunate cartilage.[7,8] Similar to large lunate deep hips, these hips have

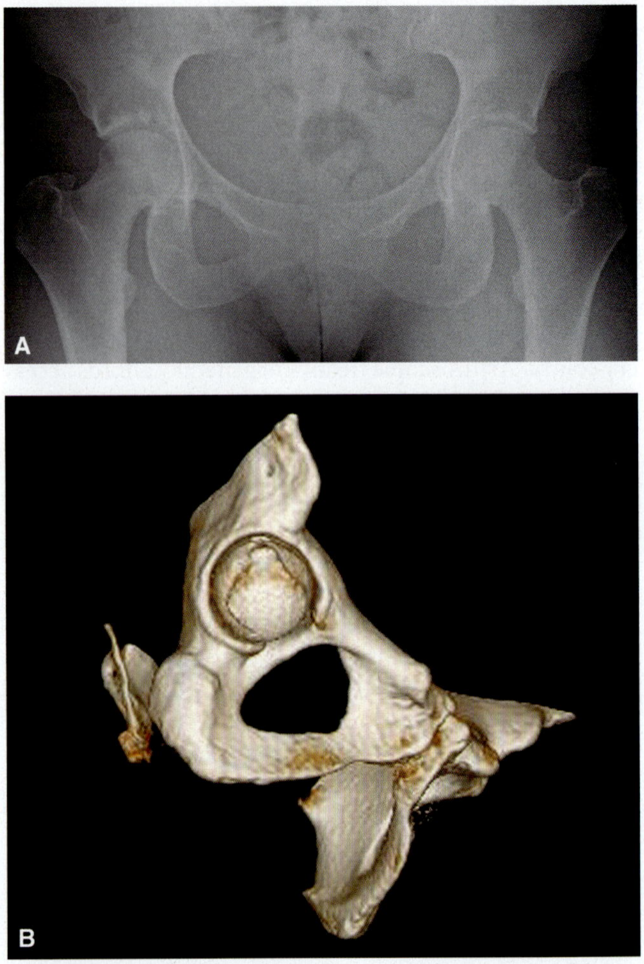

FIGURE 11.10. In this patient, both hips are overcovered (A). On the right the acetabular fossa is high and the Tönnis angle is negative. The CT reconstruction (B) confirms an enlarged acetabular fossa, indicating that an acetabular rim resection would make the lunate surface abnormally small, suggesting a reverse periacetabular osteotomy may be a better solution.

excessive wall indices and lateral center-edge angles. Unlike large lunate deep hips, small lunate deep hips have an enlarged cotyloid fossa. The Tönnis roof angle is often downsloping both at presentation and after templating for an acetabular rim resection. CT scans with 3D reconstructions are especially important in these patients, as an enlarged cotyloid fossa is often easiest to identify by qualitative evaluation of reconstructed pelvis (see Figure 11.10).

Surgical Decision-Making

In hips with pincer-type FAI from small lunate deep acetabular morphology, a reverse periacetabular osteotomy is recommended. In these hips, the acetabulum's orientation results in a medially directed joint reaction force. An acetabular rim trimming will not correct these pathomechanics. Further, as the lunate cartilage in these hips is normal or even low-volume, rim trimming can potentially increase the severity of medial joint loading.

Acetabular Retroversion

Acetabular retroversion is found in hips with normally shaped acetabular rims that are maloriented in a retroverted position. These hips present with concomitant radiographic signs of anterior overcoverage (crossover sign) and posterior undercoverage (posterior wall sign), yet the overall morphology of their acetabular rim is normal and not consistent with focal anterior or posterior pathology.[8] Instead, their normally shaped acetabulum is malrotated into a retroverted orientation, which may occur at the acetabular level or through malrotation of the entire hemipelvis.[12] These hips will often have a positive ischial spine sign, a high retroversion index, and a high PA index on AP pelvic films. Cross-sectional imaging and 3D reconstructions can help better position the acetabular malrotation, with acetabular sector angles providing significant insight into acetabular version.[13]

Surgical Decision-Making

In cases of pincer-type FAI due to isolated acetabular retroversion, an anteverting periacetabular osteotomy is recommended. Rim trimming, via either an arthroscopic or open approach, is not advised because it decreases the volume of a normal lunate surface and may result in increased contact pressure at the hip.

MIXED FEMOROACETABULAR IMPINGEMENT

Earlier, we presented the most common pathomorphologies present in FAI as isolated findings. It is important to note that several pathomorphologies may be encountered in a single hip, and they should all be taken into consideration when determining the optimal surgical treatment approach. A general decision tree for mixed FAI cases is presented in Figure 11.11. Each case should be thoroughly evaluated for potential contributions of FAI in order to identify the best treatment strategy.

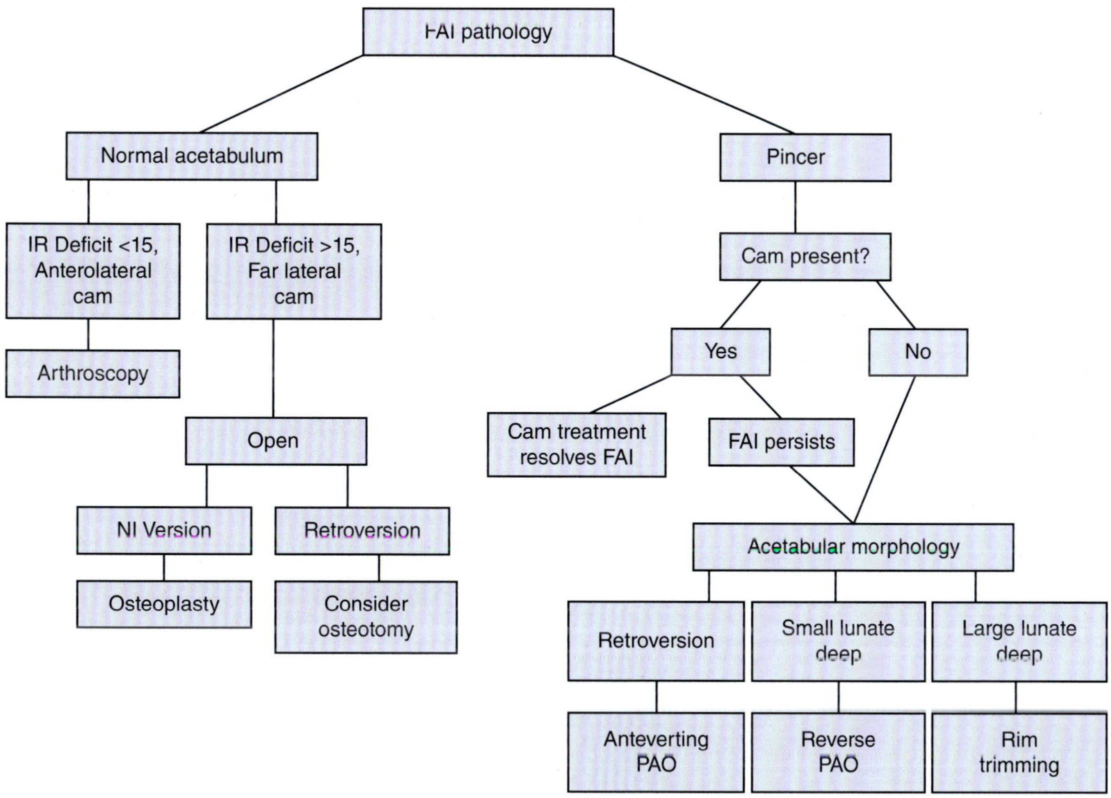

FIGURE 11.11. A proposed decision tree to follow when devising a treatment plan for femoroacetabular impingement.

REFERENCES

1. Kelly BT, Bedi A, Robertson CM, Dela Torre K, Giveans MR, Larson CM. Alterations in internal rotation and alpha angles are associated with arthroscopic cam decompression in the hip. *Am J Sports Med.* 2012;40(5):1107-1112.
2. Bedi A, Zaltz I, De La Torre K, Kelly BT. Radiographic comparison of surgical hip dislocation and hip arthroscopy for treatment of cam deformity in femoroacetabular impingement. *Am J Sports Med.* 2011;39:20S-28S.
3. Fabricant PD, Fields KG, Taylor SA, Magennis E, Bedi A, Kelly BT. The effect of femoral and acetabular version on clinical outcomes after arthroscopic femoroacetabular impingement surgery. *J Bone Joint Surg Am.* 2015;97(7):537-543.
4. Murphy SB, Simon SR, Kijewski PK, Wilkinson RH, Griscom NT. Femoral anteversion. *J Bone Joint Surg Am.* 1987;69(8):1169-1176.
5. Tomczak RJ, Guenther KP, Rieber A, Mergo P, Ros PR, Brambs HJ. MR imaging measurement of the femoral antetorsional angle as a new technique: comparison with CT in children and adults. *AJR Am J Roentgenol.* 1997;168(3):791-794.
6. Ganz R, Parvizi J, Beck M, Leunig M, Notzli H, Siebenrock KA. Femoroacetabular impingement: a cause for osteoarthritis of the hip. *Clin Orthop Relat Res.* 2003(417):112-120.
7. Pun SY, Hingsammer A, Millis MB, Kim YJ. Is increased acetabular cartilage or fossa size associated with pincer femoroacetabular impingement? *Clin Orthop Relat Res.* 2017;475(4):1013-1023.
8. Steppacher SD, Lerch TD, Gharanizadeh K, et al. Size and shape of the lunate surface in different types of pincer impingement: theoretical implications for surgical therapy. *Osteoarthritis Cartilage.* 2014;22(7):951-958.
9. Kling S, Karns MR, Gebhart J, et al. The effect of acetabular rim recession on anterior acetabular coverage: a cadaveric study using the false-profile radiograph. *Am J Sports Med.* 2015;43(4):957-964.
10. Philippon MJ, Wolff AB, Briggs KK, Zehms CT, Kuppersmith DA. Acetabular rim reduction for the treatment of femoroacetabular impingement correlates with preoperative and postoperative center-edge angle. *Arthroscopy.* 2010;26(6):757-761.
11. Bhatia S, Lee S, Shewman E, et al. Effects of acetabular rim trimming on hip joint contact pressures: how much is too much? *Am J Sports Med.* 2015;43(9):2138-2145.
12. Tannast M, Pfannebecker P, Schwab JM, Albers CE, Siebenrock KA, Buchler L. Pelvic morphology differs in rotation and obliquity between developmental dysplasia of the hip and retroversion. *Clin Orthop Relat Res.* 2012;470(12):3297-3305.
13. Anda S, Svenningsen S, Dale LG, Benum P. The acetabular sector angle of the adult hip determined by computed tomography. *Acta Radiol Diagn (Stockh).* 1986;27(4):443-447.

CHAPTER

12

Femoroacetabular Impingement: Surgical Hip Dislocation Approach to the Hip

The surgical hip dislocation (SHD) approach was described by Ganz and colleagues[1] after studying the anatomy of the medial circumflex artery and the blood supply to the femoral head.[2] This approach allows complete access to the femoral head and acetabulum and preserves the blood supply and perfusion to the femoral head without the risk of osteonecrosis.[3] With the development of hip arthroscopy, indications to perform open surgical treatment to femoroacetabular impingement (FAI) deformities are limited. However, some FAI-related deformities may still be better managed by using the SHD approach, given its versatility and wide exposure to the hip. Patients with anterior-superior cam morphology, with cam deformity located between the 1 and 3 o' clock position, are usually treated using an arthroscopic approach (**Figure 12.1**). Our current indications for open treatment of FAI deformity using the SHD approach include the following:

- Patients lacking internal rotation or with negative internal rotation at 90° of hip flexion.
- Patients with cam morphology localized posteriorly to the superior aspect of the femoral head-neck junction.
- Patients with abnormal femoral version, typically femoral retroversion. In addition, those with excessive femoral anteversion may have a specific pattern of acetabular chondral and labral damage and may benefit from open treatment associated with derotational osteotomy.
- Patients with cam-FAI deformity secondary to moderate and severe slipped capital femoral epiphysis (SCFE) and Perthes disease.
- Patients with extra-articular FAI, including those with ischiofemoral and greater trochanter impingement.

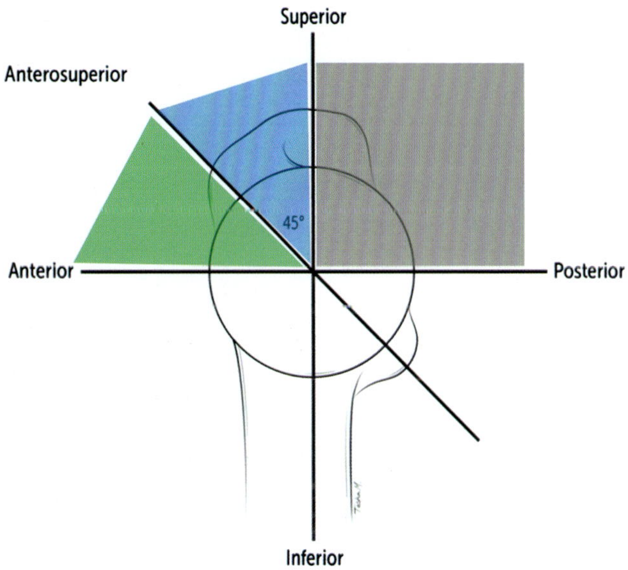

FIGURE 12.1. Illustration representing the femoral head-neck junction regions. Cam deformity localized in the anterior to the anterosuperior region of the femoral head-neck junction can be easily treated by an arthroscopic approach (green area). Cam deformity closer to the superior aspect of the femoral head and neck junction poses more challenge and requires a higher degree of expertise (blue area). When the cam deformity expands posteriorly to the superior aspect of the head-neck junction, arthroscopic resection becomes very difficult (black area). We recommend open treatment using a surgical hip dislocation approach for patients with cam deformity located posterior to the superior aspect of the femoral head-neck junction and for patients with severe restricted motion (those with negative internal rotation with the hip in 90° of flexion).

Clinical Scenario

A 17-year-old male presented with bilateral hip pain aggravated by sitting and sports activities, including being a competitive coxswain. Physical examination revealed that his hip motion was limited to flexion up to 85° to 90°. In 90° of flexion, both hips showed obligatory external rotation with 5° to 10° negative internal rotation. Preoperative radiographs revealed a severe cam deformity of the left hip. Magnetic resonance imaging (MRI) showed chondrolabral damage with potential cartilage delamination. MRI radial reformats around the femoral head-neck junction showed that the cam deformity expanded from the anterior to the posterosuperior head-neck junction (**Figure 12.2**). Given his limited range of motion and extensive cam deformity, surgical treatment was performed using a surgical dislocation approach.

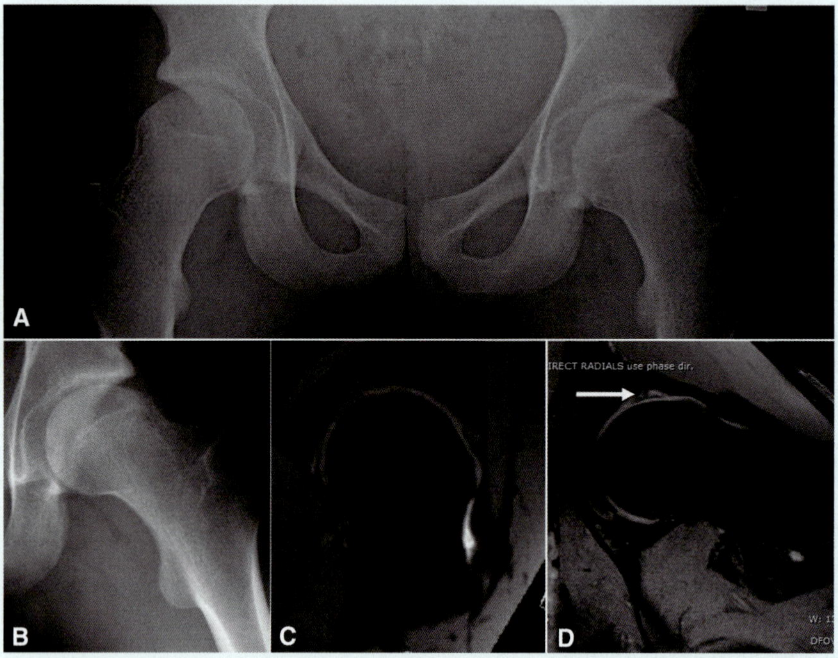

FIGURE 12.2. A 17-year-old male presented with bilateral hip pain aggravated by sitting and sports activities, including being a competitive coxswain. A, Preoperative anteroposterior pelvic radiograph showing bilateral cam-type deformity of the proximal femur. B, Dunn lateral radiograph showing a cam-type femoroacetabular impingement (FAI) deformity with abnormal femoral head-neck offset. C, Magnetic resonance imaging (MRI) of the left hip (double echo steady state [DESS]) confirms a cam deformity extending posteriorly to the superior aspect of the femoral head-neck junction. D, Fat-suppressed proton density MRI showing the acetabular chondrolabral damage with dissociation between the cartilage and the labrum and intrasubstance tear of the labrum in the anterosuperior portion of the rim.

SURGICAL TECHNIQUE

Surgery is performed under general anesthesia with the patient in the lateral decubitus position with the operated leg resting on a U-shaped pillow (**Figure 12.3**). A straight lateral incision approximately 20 cm in length is performed slightly anterior to the top of the greater trochanter (**Figure 12.4**). The subcutaneous tissue is dissected to expose the fascia lata and the gluteal fascia. The anterior border of the gluteus maximus is identified through transparency, and the fascia is divided along the anterior border of the gluteus maximus (**Figure 12.5**). Dissection is carried out to develop the interval between the gluteus maximus that is retracted posteriorly and the gluteus medius according to the Gibson approach[4] (**Figure 12.6**). The Gibson approach is preferred to the classic Kocher-Langenbeck approach because the former does not violate the gluteus musculature and results in an improved cosmetic result. The fascia lata is opened toward the distal end of the incision. The trochanteric bursa is opened from posterior to anterior, exposing the greater trochanter and the insertion of the gluteus medius and origin of the vastus lateralis (**Figure 12.7**).

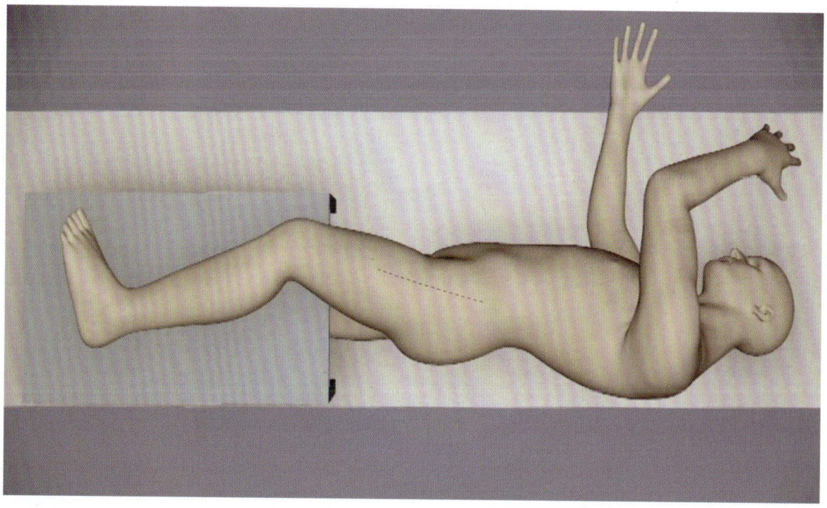

FIGURE 12.3. Illustration showing the patient is in lateral decubitus position with the operated lower extremity placed on top of a U-shaped foam pillow. The entire lower extremity is prepped and draped, allowing visualization of the anterior and the posterior superior iliac spines. A sterile bag drape is placed on the opposite side of the table to receive the leg at the time of the dislocation.

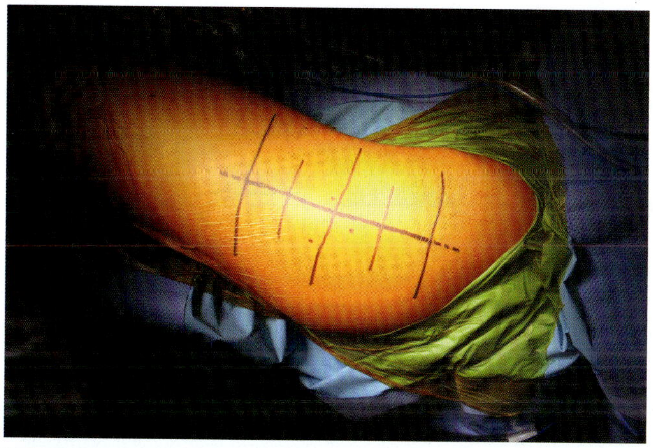

FIGURE 12.4. Intraoperative picture showing a straight incision about 20 cm in length is marked on top of the greater trochanter just anterior to the tip of the trochanter.

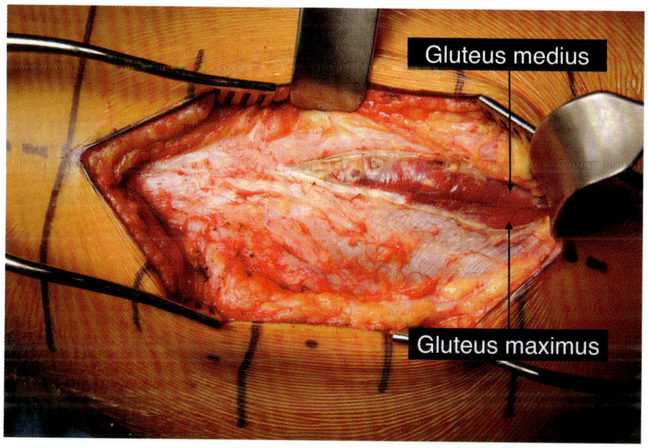

FIGURE 12.6. Intraoperative picture showing the Gibson approach with dissection between the gluteus medius anteriorly and the gluteus maximus posteriorly.

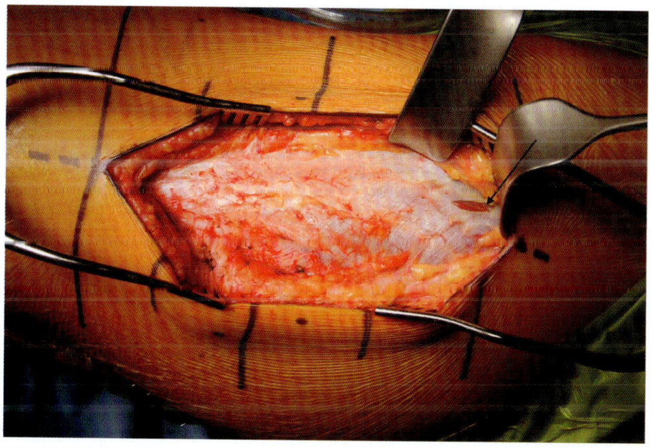

FIGURE 12.5. Intraoperative picture showing the exposure of the fascia lata and gluteal fascia. The fascia is opened proximally just anterior to the gluteus maximus musculature (black arrow).

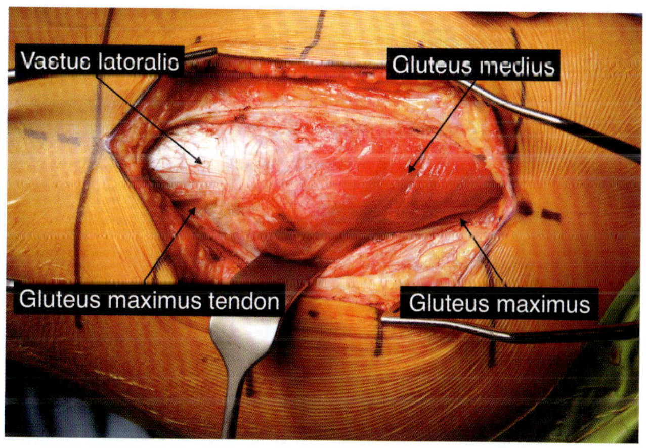

FIGURE 12.7. Intraoperative picture showing the full exposure of the vastus lateralis, greater trochanter, gluteus medius, and gluteus maximus after superficial dissection is undertaken.

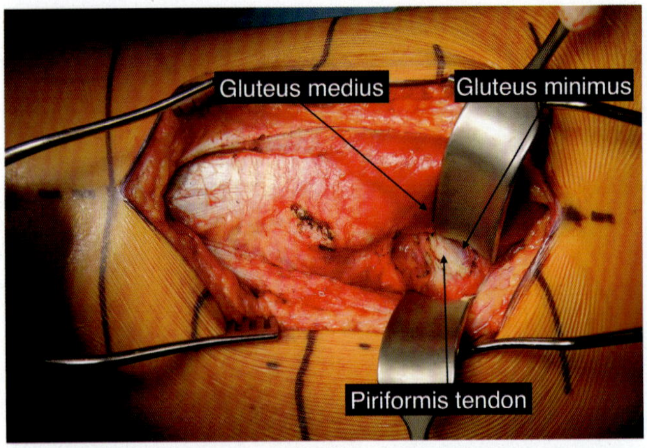

FIGURE 12.8. Intraoperative picture showing the gluteus medius that has been retracted anteriorly, exposing the gluteus minimus and the piriformis tendon underneath.

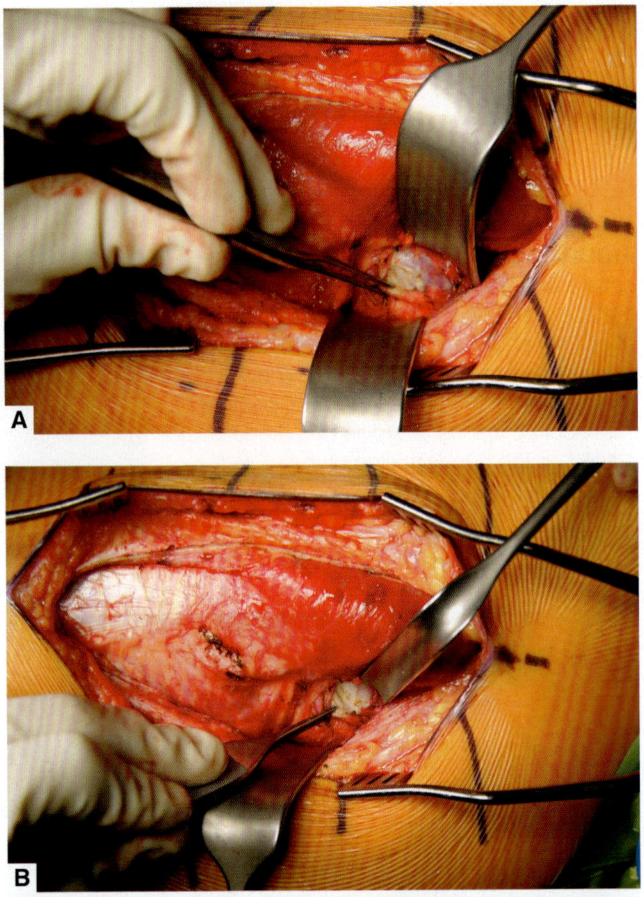

FIGURE 12.9. Intraoperative picture showing the dissection of the interval between the gluteus minimus and the piriformis tendon. A, The piriformis tendon is grasped with forceps and pulled posteriorly, exposing the gluteus minimus insertion in the hip capsule. B, The gluteus minimus fascia is opened, and the muscle is dissected out of the capsule and the posterior ilium to the level of the greater sciatic notch.

Although the original description by Ganz and colleagues[1] recommended that no attempt should be made to mobilize the gluteus medius or to visualize the piriformis tendon, we believe this step is important because it facilitates the correct level of the trochanteric osteotomy and reduces the bleeding at the time of capsular exposure. The gluteus medius insertion on the posterosuperior trochanter is identified and retracted anteriorly to facilitate exposure of the gluteus minimus and the piriformis tendon (**Figure 12.8**). The piriformis tendon is easily palpated and the fascia on top of it incised to expose the tendon. Internal rotation of the hip facilitates exposure of the piriformis. Careful dissection proximal to the piriformis tendon is recommended to avoid damage to the anastomosis between the inferior gluteal artery system and the deep branch of the medial circumflex artery that usually runs distal to the tendon. The fascia on top of the gluteus minimus tendon is incised after the piriformis tendon is pulled posteriorly. The gluteus minimus is then retracted anterior-superiorly exposing the hip capsule (**Figure 12.9**). Distally, the posterior fascia of the vastus lateralis is identified and incised longitudinally, leaving about a 3-mm cuff of fascia for later repair. The vastus lateralis is dissected from the femur anteriorly, and a Hohmann retractor is placed under the muscle, avoiding damage to the periosteum (**Figure 12.10**).

In preparation for the trochanteric osteotomy, an incision is made from the posterosuperior border of the greater trochanter extending distally to the posterior edge of the vastus lateralis (**Figure 12.11**). There are two ways to perform the trochanteric osteotomy:

- Classic osteotomy: The classic osteotomy is a straight and single cut. Proximally, it is usually done 2 to 3 mm anterior to the insertion of the gluteus medius and distally at the posterior aspect of the origin of the vastus lateralis. The oscillating saw is used up to the medial cortex, which should be completely cut with an osteotome. The original technique describes a trochanteric fragment of about 1.5 cm. Having exposed the piriformis tendon previous to the cut allows for the safe performance of a thicker cut without the risk of leaving the piriformis in the mobile trochanter fragment. This technique is preferred when planning for a dissection of the retinacular flap and distal transfer of the greater trochanter (ie, SCFE and Perthes hips).
- Step-cut osteotomy: In this technique, the proximal part of the osteotomy is more superficial, whereas the distal portion of the osteotomy is slightly deeper (more medial). The two cuts are then connected by a third transverse cut done with an osteotome, creating a step in the osteotomy of at least 6 mm. The step-cut osteotomy has the advantage of improving the area of contact of the osteotomy and avoiding rotation or proximal migration of the trochanter fragment (**Figure 12.12**).

The trochanteric piece is flipped and mobilized anteriorly with the attached vastus lateralis and gluteus medius. Posteriorly, the previously exposed gluteus minimus is

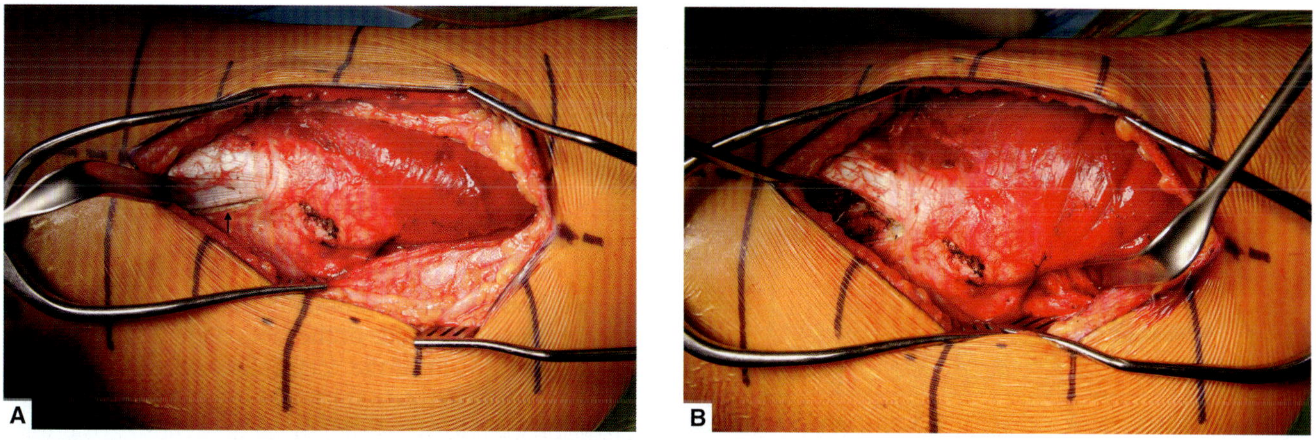

FIGURE 12.10. A, Intraoperative picture showing an incision made in the posterior aspect of the vastus lateralis fascia (black arrow). B, The vastus lateralis is dissected from the femur anteriorly, and a Hohmann retractor is placed underneath it.

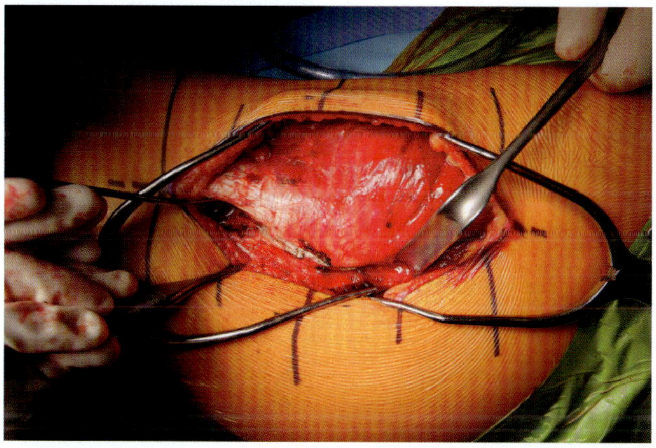

FIGURE 12.11. Intraoperative picture showing the incision made with the cautery connecting the posterosuperior border of the greater trochanter extending distally to the posterior edge of the vastus lateralis. The classic trochanteric osteotomy follows this orientation; however, we prefer to perform the osteotomy using a step-cut technique.

further completely elevated anteriorly off the hip capsule. The gluteus minimus should be released posteriorly as far as the level of the sciatic notch—this will avoid difficulty with acetabular exposure. Distally, the anterolateral portion of the vastus lateralis is released from the femur along with the insertion of the vastus intermedius, which is facilitated by flexion, abduction, and external rotation of the hip. The hip capsule is completely exposed from the anterior to the posterosuperior aspect (**Figure 12.13**). With complete exposure of the capsule, a capsulotomy is performed in a Z shape fashion (right hip) or reverse Z shape (left hip). The capsule is cut initially in line with the longitudinal axis of the anterior neck, starting at the superoanterior corner of the trochanteric osteotomy. The longitudinal flap is only partially opened. The distal capsulotomy extends anterior toward the anteroinferior aspect of the acetabulum. Finishing the distal anteroinferior flap allows for safe completion of the longitudinal flap to the level of the acetabular labrum. At the level of the labrum, the capsular opening is curved posteriorly parallel

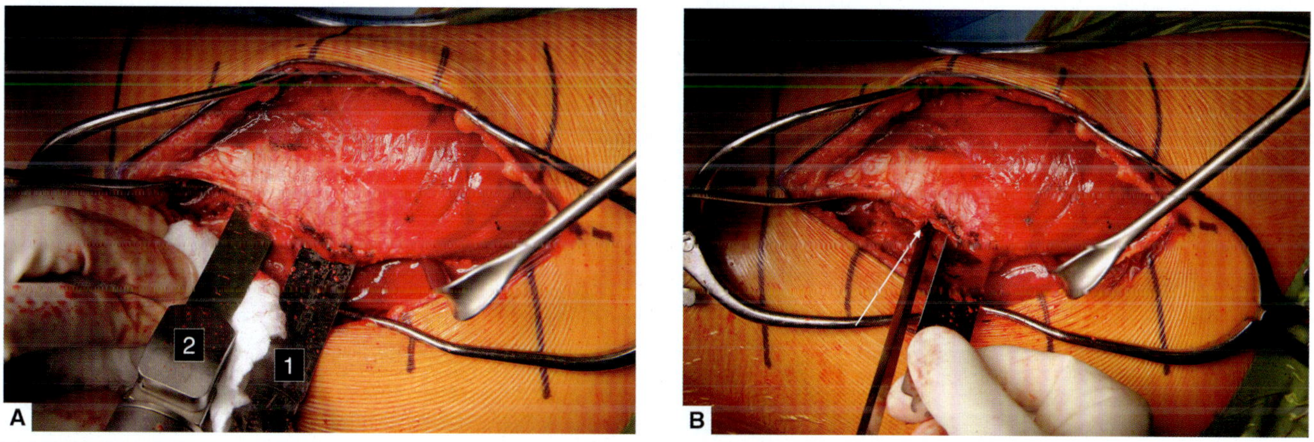

FIGURE 12.12. A, The step-cut technique for the trochanteric osteotomy. The proximal cut (1) is done slightly lateral to the insertion of the gluteus medius. The saw is left in place and the distal cut (2) is performed about 5 mm medial to the first cut. B, Then a small osteotome is placed perpendicularly between the two cuts and is used to complete the osteotomy, creating a step of about 5 mm.

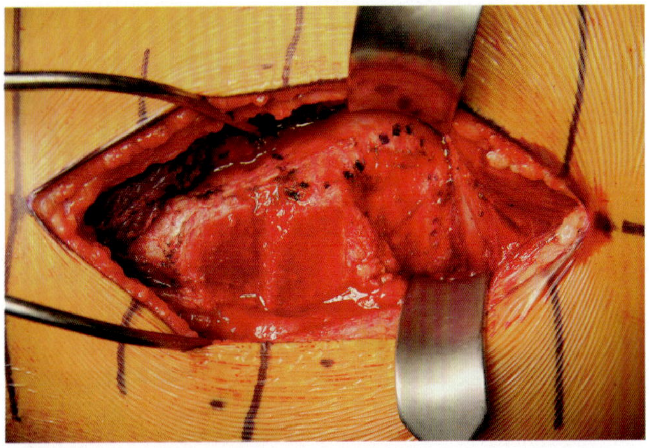

FIGURE 12.13. Intraoperative picture showing the hip capsule has been widely exposed and the capsulotomy (inverted z shaped, left hip) has been marked.

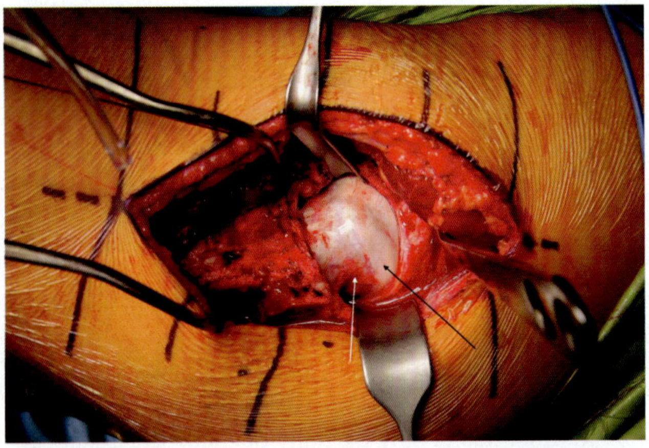

FIGURE 12.14. After the capsulotomy is completed, the hip can be dynamically inspected for femoroacetabular impingement. This intraoperative picture shows how the placement of a Hohmann retractor in the ilium, proximal to the acetabular rim, facilitates the exposure of the joint. An obvious abnormal cam deformity (black arrow) extending posteriorly passed the level of the retinacular vessels (white arrow).

to the acetabular rim and toward the piriformis tendon. With the capsule opened, the joint is inspected for signs of synovitis and for dynamic assessment of range of motion with special attention to flexion and internal rotation. Intra- and extra-articular causes of FAI can be dynamically determined (**Figure 12.14**). Flexion, adduction, and external rotation allow for subluxation of the hip. Further resection of the ligamentum teres allows a complete dislocation of the femoral head. Once the femoral head is dislocated from the acetabulum, the leg is placed in a sterile bag on the opposite side of the table (**Figure 12.15**).

For assessment of the acetabular cavity, the assistant supports the lower extremity, elevating the knee and applying an axial load to bring the femoral head posteriorly to the acetabulum. Two or three Hohmann retractors are placed around the acetabulum (**Figure 12.16**). The

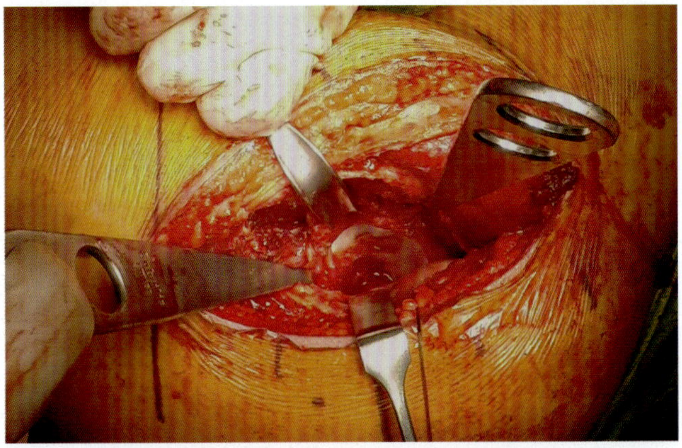

FIGURE 12.16. Intraoperative picture showing exposure of the acetabulum. One Hohmann retractor is placed just distal to the transverse ligament in the inferior aspect of the acetabulum. A second Hohmann retractor is placed in the superior aspect of the acetabulum, proximal to the acetabular rim between the 12 and 1 o'clock positions. In this picture, the anterior (3 o'clock position) is exposed by the assistant holding a Langenbeck retractor, but, if needed, a Hohmann retractor can be placed in the anterior rim.

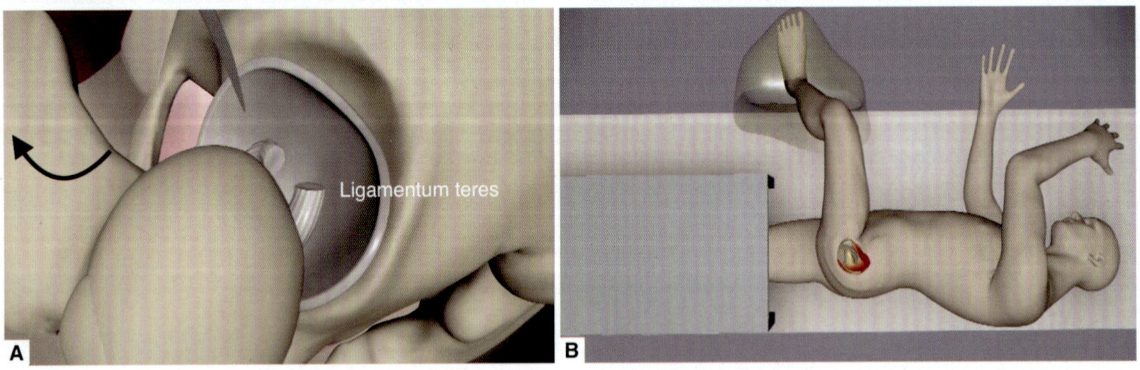

FIGURE 12.15. A, Illustration demonstrating the femur is positioned in flexion and external rotation (black arrow), which breaks the suction seal and subluxates the hip. The ligamentum teres is cut with curved scissors. B, After the ligamentum teres is completely cut, the femoral head should be completely dislocated out of the acetabulum. The hip is positioned in flexion and external rotation, and the leg is placed in a sterile bag on the other side of the surgical table.

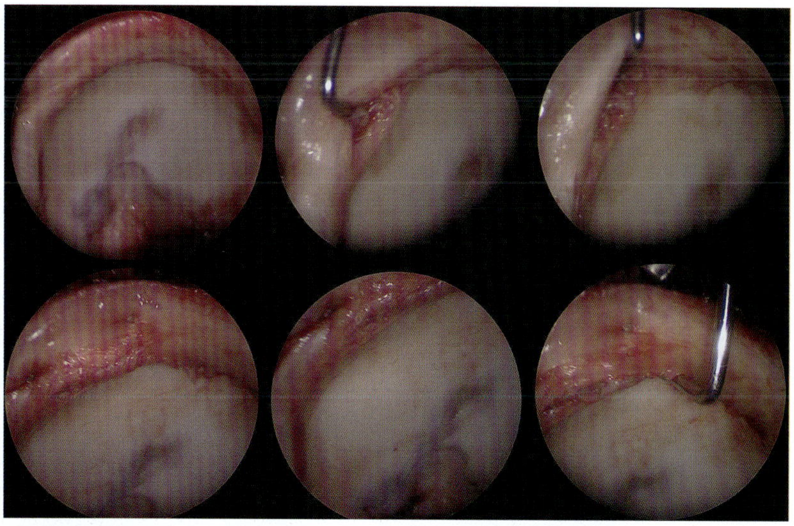

FIGURE 12.17. Treatment of acetabular cartilage and labrum damage can be facilitated by the use of a 70° arthroscopic camera. On top, intraoperative arthroscopic pictures of the acetabular cavity reveal damage to the acetabular cartilage with fraying and delamination. The acetabular labrum is dissociated from the acetabular cartilage and is felt to be unstable. In the bottom half are arthroscopy pictures after repair using two suture anchors with improved stability of the acetabular labrum.

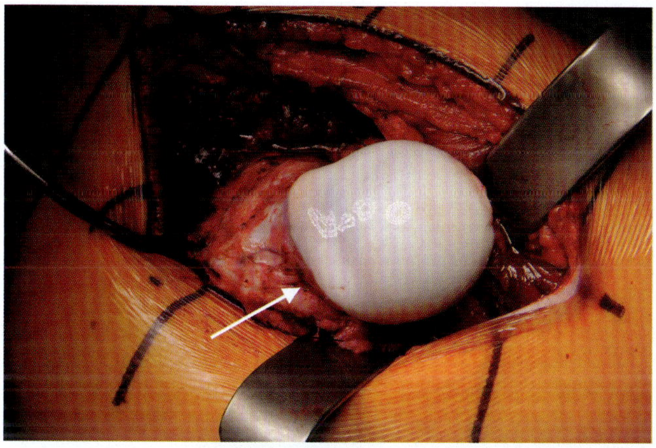

FIGURE 12.18. Intraoperative picture showing the exposure of the femoral head and neck junction after the leg is resting inside the sterile bag on the opposite side of the table and the knee is gently pushing down, allowing the femoral head to stand out of the surgical wound. Note the severe deformity of the femoral head and neck junction with the epiphysis extending distally into the metaphysis and the cam deformity extending posteriorly to the retinacular vessels (white arrow).

acetabular articular cartilage and the labrum are inspected for the presence of labral and chondral lesions, which can be treated with the assistance of a 70° arthroscopic camera (Figure 12.17). A labral tear or chondrolabral dissociation can be treated by complete exposure of the osseous surface just proximal to the labrum without further compromise of the chondral-labral junction and reattachment of the labrum using suture anchors.

Assessment of the femoral head-neck junction is facilitated by lowering the knee, allowing the femoral head to stand out of the wound (Figure 12.18). The sphericity of the femoral head-neck junction is assessed with acrylic spherical templates (Figure 12.19). Resection of the cam deformity is planned and performed in a stepwise fashion, using a scalpel and an osteotome (Figure 12.20). The osteochondroplasty is finished by fine contouring of the epiphysis with the use of a high-speed burr (Figure 12.21). The wound is irrigated, and the femoral head is reduced back in the acetabulum. For reduction of the hip, an assistant applies traction and internal rotation while the surgeon helps the reduction by gently pushing the femoral

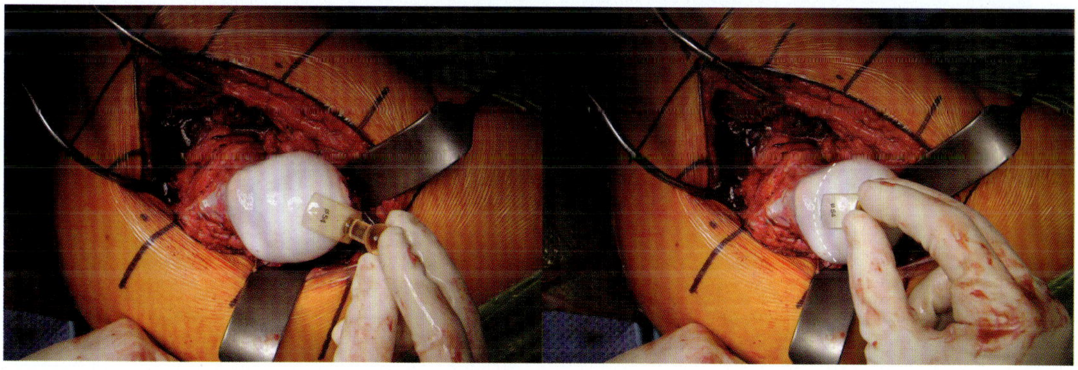

FIGURE 12.19. Intraoperative picture showing the assessment of sphericity of the femoral head and neck junction with the use of acrylic spherical templates. A white dashed line marks the abnormal cam deformity.

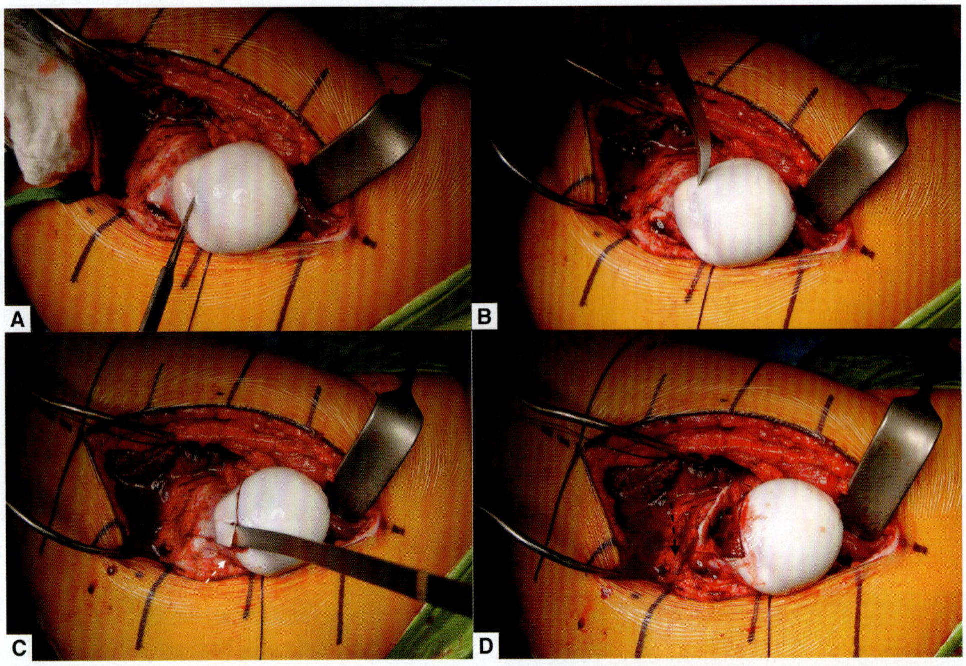

FIGURE 12.20. Intraoperative photographs showing the sequence for osteochondroplasty of the femoral head and neck junction. A, The zone of asphericity identified previously with the spherical templates is delineated using a scalpel. Note that the scalpel marks the head-neck junction to the level of the retinacular vessels. B, The next step is to use a curved sharp Lambotte osteotome in line with the demarcation created by the scalpel. Note the inclination of the osteotome to avoid excessive resection of bone. C, The osteotome is moved progressively in a posterior direction, stopping short at the superior aspect of the head-neck junction to avoid damage to the retinacular vessels (white arrow). D, The osteochondroplasty is completed with the osteotome with removal of the cam deformity to the level of the intertrochanteric line (black dashed arrow). It should be emphasized that the osteotome removes cartilage and bone from the epiphyseal-metaphyseal area up to the superior aspect of the femoral head-neck junction.

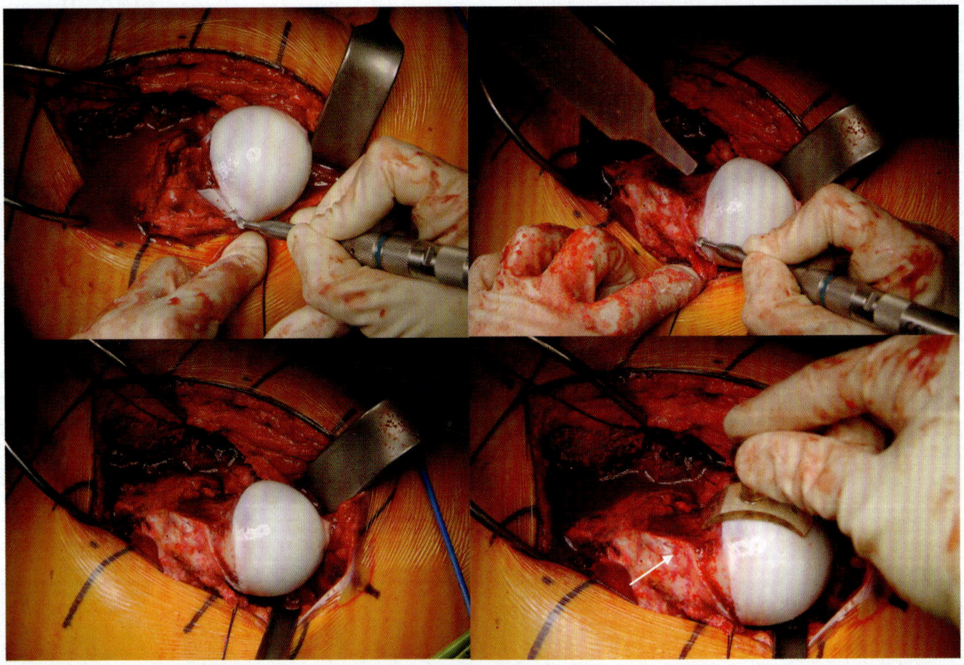

FIGURE 12.21. Intraoperative photographs showing the osteochondroplasty is advanced posteriorly to the retinacular vessels with the use of a high-speed burr. Note that the osteochondroplasty is restricted to the epiphysis and the periosteum remains attached to the metaphyseal-epiphyseal junction at the level of the first retinacular nutrient vessel to the femoral head (white arrow). The femoral head-neck is recontoured with the high-speed burr to the level of the intertrochanteric line, and the osteochondroplasty is complete when sphericity is confirmed by the spherical template.

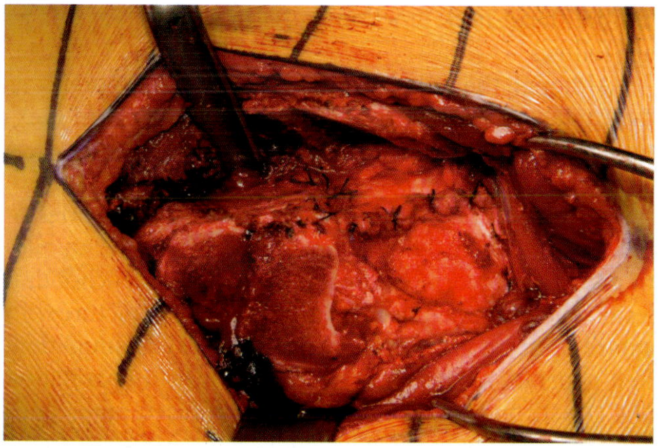

FIGURE 12.22. Intraoperative photograph showing the closure of the hip capsule.

head back in the acetabulum. The hip capsule is closed with separated 0 or 2.0 Vicryl stiches (**Figure 12.22**). The greater trochanter is reattached and fixed with two or three 3.5- or 4.5-mm screws. If a step-cut osteotomy is performed, two bicortical 3.5-mm screws above and below the step are sufficient.

Postoperatively, patients are instructed to limit hip flexion to 90° and avoid active hip abduction for the first 4 to 6 weeks. Naproxen is used as a prophylaxis for heterotopic ossification for 3 weeks. Patients are allowed partial weight-bearing using crutches in the first 4 to 6 weeks after surgery when radiographic healing of the trochanteric osteotomy is confirmed. We have not experienced any complications related to healing of the trochanteric osteotomy because we have adopted the step-cut osteotomy. Physical therapy began at 4 to 6 weeks, and the intensity of the strength and functional training is incrementally increased after week 12. Patients are generally allowed to return to full sports participation after 6 months (**Figure 12.23**).

COMPLEX FEMOROACETABULAR IMPINGEMENT DEFORMITY AND THE APPLICATION OF THE SURGICAL DISLOCATION APPROACH

SHD is a versatile approach to the hip joint. It allows assessment and treatment of acetabular and femoral pathologies beyond the treatment of classic cam and pincer deformities. SHD is our preferred approach for the treatment of complex cases of femoral acetabular impingement, including treatment of residual deformities after SCFE and Perthes disease, which are addressed in other chapters of this book. Additional indications for the SHD approach include focal chondral and osteochondral defects of the femoral head; extra-articular impingement of the greater trochanter against the acetabular rim due to a high-riding greater trochanter or due to abnormal sphericity of the trochanteric neck junction or femoral retroversion; intra-articular hip deformity in association with excessive femoral

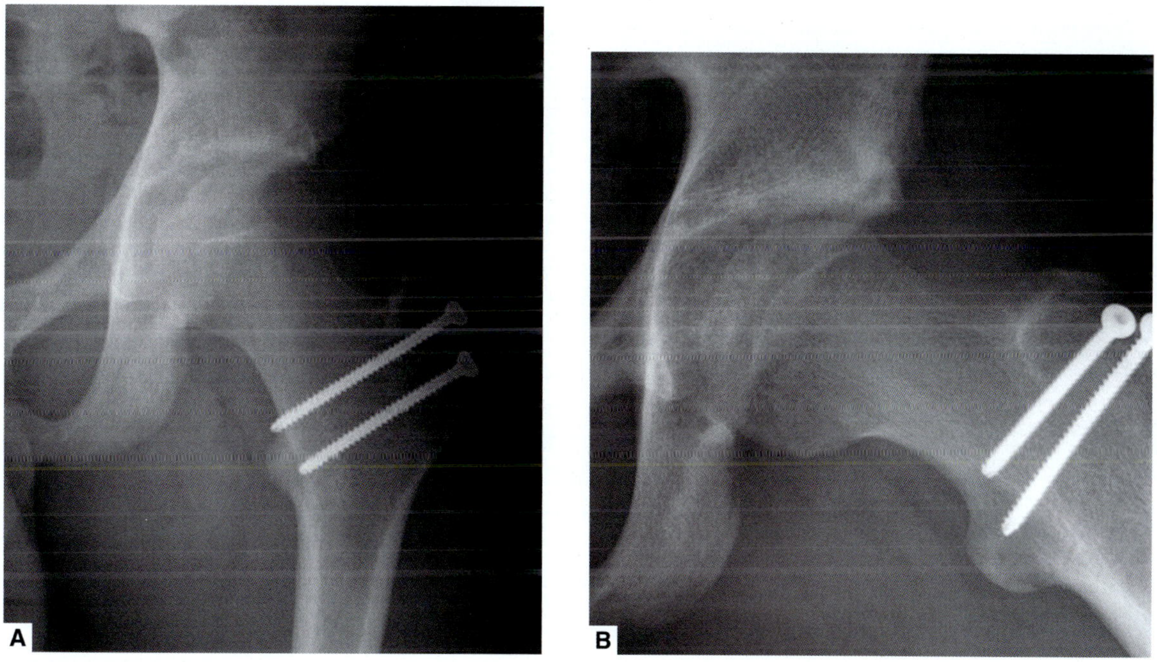

FIGURE 12.23. Postoperative radiograph at 6 months following surgery reveals correction of the femoral head-neck junction concavity in the anteroposterior (AP) and lateral image. The patient resumed his sports activities after 6 months of surgery. A, AP radiograph. B, Dunn lateral radiograph.

anteversion or retroversion and in complex cases with ischiofemoral impingement. The approach can also be applied to the treatment of intra-articular femoral head fractures and to the treatment of posterior acetabular wall fracture in association with posterior dislocation of the hip.

SURGICAL DISLOCATION APPROACH FOR THE TREATMENT OF FOCAL OSTEOCHONDRAL DEFECT OF THE FEMORAL HEAD

Treatment of osteochondral injuries of the femoral head can be relatively easier to perform through the SHD approach in comparison to hip arthroscopy. The surgical approach is standard, as described earlier. After the femoral head is dislocated from the acetabulum, assessment of the femoral head-neck junction and articular cartilage damage follows.

Although the orthopedic literature about femoral condyle, talus, and patellofemoral cartilage restoration is extensive, currently the number of studies reporting cartilage restoration to the femoral head and acetabulum is limited. Moreover, several of the published studies are series of cases lacking high-level comparative studies. Techniques to address and correct a focal chondral or osteochondral lesion of the hip include microfracture; microfracture with suture or fibrin glue repair of the chondral delamination; first-generation autologous chondrocyte implantation (ACI) with periosteal patch; matrix-induced autologous chondrocyte implantation (MACI) with a collagen membrane cultivated with chondrocytes prior to implantation; particulated juvenile cartilage allograft (DeNovo NT), osteochondral autograft transfer (OAT), and osteochondral allograft (OCA).

Clinical Scenario

A 20-year-old basketball player presented with left hip pain aggravated by sports. He has experienced a decrease in his ability to pivot and shift while playing and practicing basketball. Physical examination revealed a rather irritated hip with a positive anterior impingement test and no internal rotation with the hip in 90° of flexion. Preoperative imaging revealed a cam deformity of the left hip and an osteochondral defect of the femoral head (**Figure 12.24**). Surgical treatment was planned through the SHD approach.

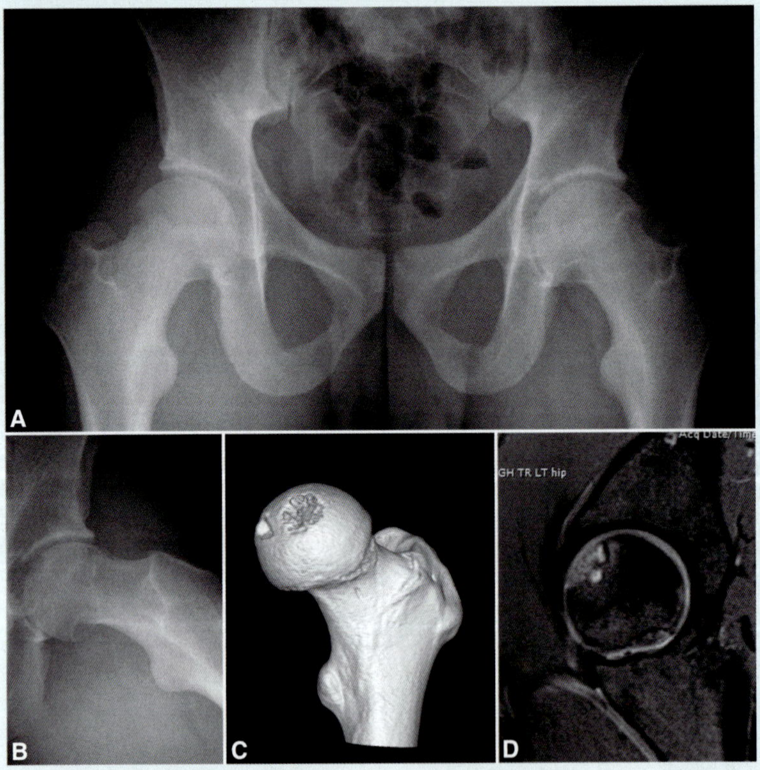

FIGURE 12.24. A 20-year-old male basketball player presented because of hip pain in the left hip. For the past several weeks he has been experiencing difficulty in playing and performing pivoting, shifting at a competitive level with increasing pain and mild stiffness. Surgical treatment was performed through a surgical hip dislocation approach with osteochondroplasty of the head-neck junction and cartilage restoration using implantation of particulated juvenile cartilage allograft (DeNovo NT). A, Preoperative anteroposterior pelvic radiograph showing cystic changes in the medial aspect of the left femoral head. B, Dunn lateral radiograph showing a cam-type femoroacetabular impingement deformity with abnormal femoral head-neck offset. C, Three-dimensional computed tomography scan confirms a cam deformity and shows the parafoveal osteochondral defect in the anteromedial aspect of the femoral head with edema in the subchondral bone. D, Fat-suppressed proton density sagittal magnetic resonance imaging showing the osteochondral defect in the anterior portion of the femoral head.

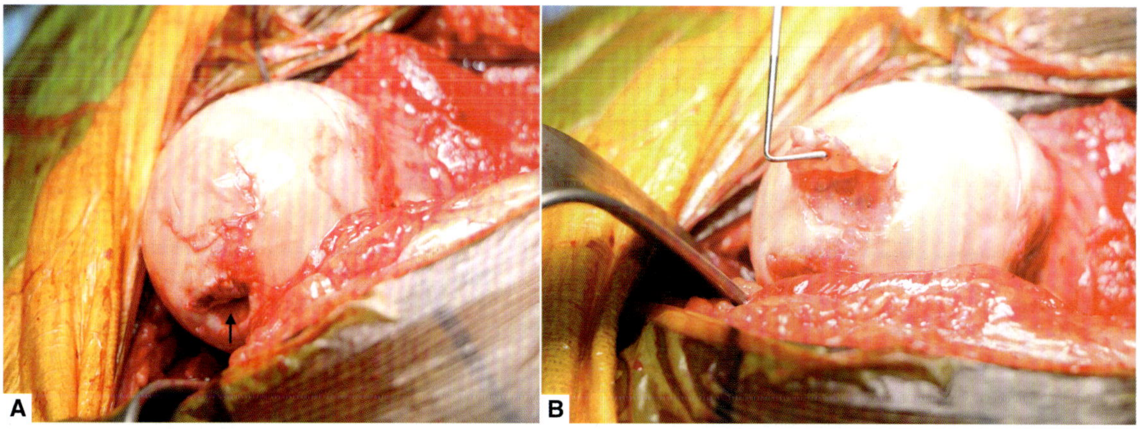

FIGURE 12.25. Assessment of the chondral defect. A, Intraoperative photograph showing a large lesion of the femoral head cartilage adjacent to the fovea (black arrow). B, There is complete cleavage of the cartilage from the bone (Grade IV International Cartilage Repair Society [ICRS]).

Although the etiology of focal chondral defect of the femoral head has not been fully elucidated, an association with cam-FAI has been reported.[5] The advantage of the SHD approach is the extensive exposure of the femoral head, which allows for full assessment, preparation of the defect, and placement of a graft if planned (**Figure 12.25**). In such a situation, the first step is treatment of any acetabular labrum pathology and recontouring of the femoral head-neck junction by osteochondroplasty (**Figure 12.26**). The defect is then carefully prepared to remove all degenerative cartilage and obtain a stable rim with vertical shoulders. Initially, the chondral defect is outlined with a scalpel to the level of the subchondral plate (**Figure 12.27**). Depending on the technique selected for grafting, the level of the defect preparation varies. For instance, if an ACI, MACI, or particulated juvenile cartilage allograft (DeNovo NT) is selected, the defective degenerative cartilage is removed to the level of the subchondral plate. In addition, for those procedures, any bleeding at the depth of the defect should be controlled with fibrin glue. The particulated juvenile cartilage allograft (DeNovo NT) is made of small (1 mm) cartilage cubes from donors younger than 13 years. Because it requires only one surgical procedure, it has been our technique of choice (**Figure 12.28**). The cartilage allograft comes in a packet that is typically enough to cover an area of 2.5 cm^2. After application, the graft should be sealed with fibrin glue and should be stable (**Figure 12.29**). The disadvantage of the particulated juvenile cartilage allograft (DeNovo NT) is the cost associated with the procedure. If there is extensive involvement of the subchondral bone, then OCA using fresh frozen femoral head large plugs or OCA transfers are better options for treatment.

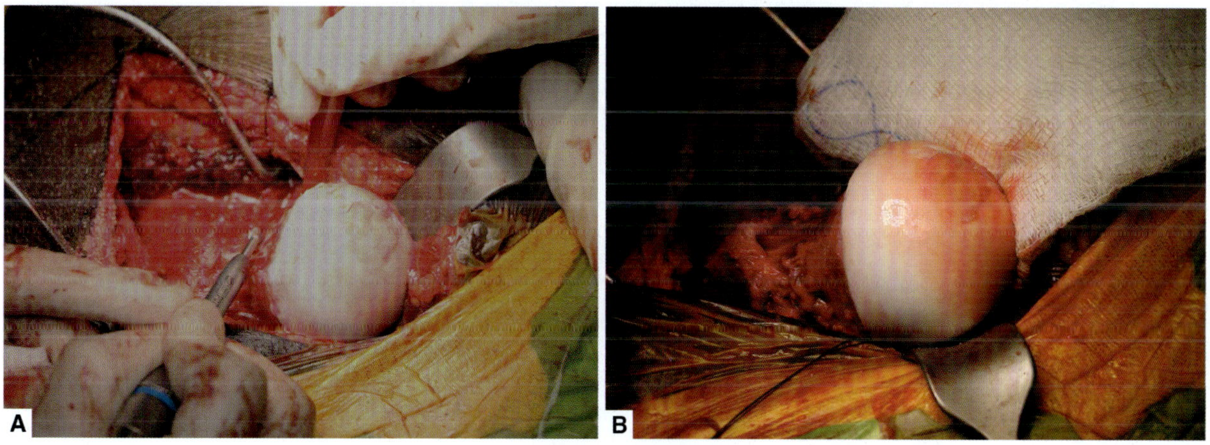

FIGURE 12.26. A, Intraoperative photograph showing the osteochondroplasty of the femoral head-neck junction for treatment of the cam deformity performed with a high-speed burr. B, The osteochondroplasty has been completed to the level of the intertrochanteric line. The chondral lesion is evident on the anterior-medial quadrant of the femoral head.

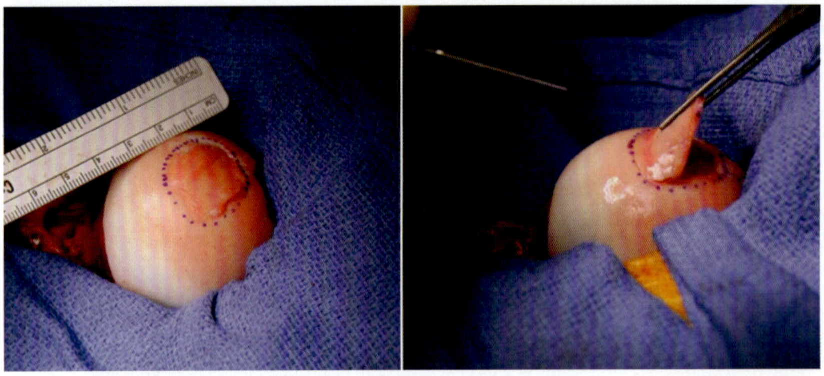

FIGURE 12.27. A, Intraoperative photograph showing measurement and demarcation of the chondral defect. B, The first step in the preparation of the defect is to outline it with a scalpel to the level of the subchondral plate.

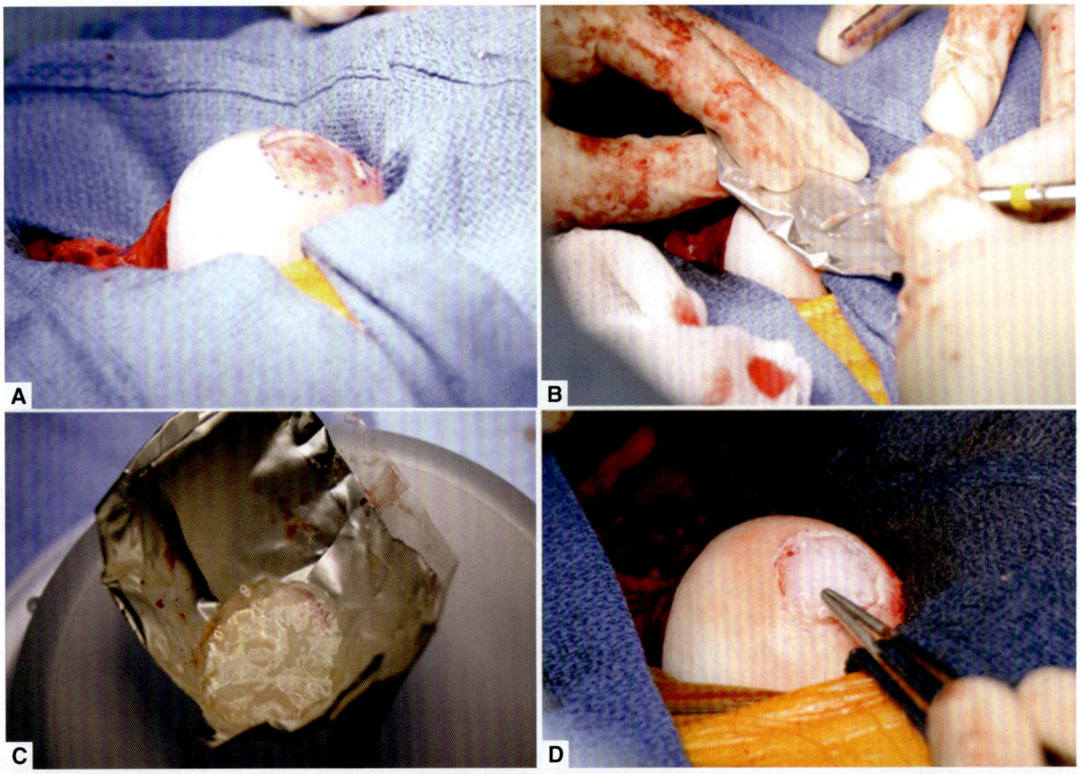

FIGURE 12.28. A, Intraoperative photograph showing the chondral defect has been prepared with removal of the unstable and undermined cartilage back to stable vertical cartilage shoulders without bleeding. B, A piece of sterile aluminum foil is used to mold the chondral defect. C, The particulated juvenile cartilage allograft (Denovo NT) is prepared with fibrin glue on the back table using the aluminum foil as the mold for the graft. D, The graft is placed in the defect, and it should be about 1 mm lower than the edge of the normal surrounding cartilage.

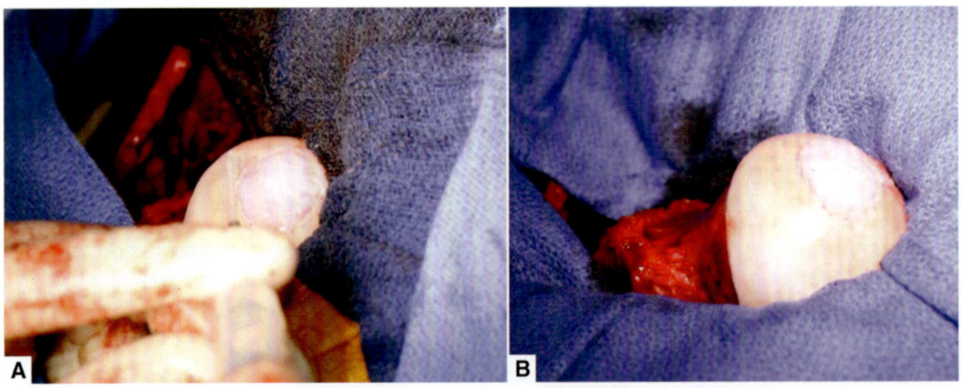

FIGURE 12.29. A, The particulated juvenile cartilage allograft (DeNovo NT) is sealed with fibrin glue. B, Final aspect of the graft sitting nicely in the femoral head chondral defect and sealed by fibrin glue.

SURGICAL DISLOCATION APPROACH FOR THE TREATMENT OF EXTRA-ARTICULAR FEMOROACETABULAR IMPINGEMENT

Extra-articular causes of impingement may be an isolated cause of hip pain in the young athletic population, although they are often associated with hip morphologies leading to intra-articular FAI. Extra-articular FAI include anterior inferior iliac spine (AIIS; subspine impingement), ischiofemoral impingement, and greater trochanteric-pelvic impingement. These conditions are caused by mechanical impact between the proximal femur against the pelvis and the soft tissue between them. Subspine impingement is associated with a prominent AIIS and may be a cause of hip pain typically aggravated by pure hip flexion. Subspine impingement can be addressed during the SHD approach. However, it is not an indication for an open approach because several studies have reported successful outcome of arthroscopic treatment. On the other hand, ischiofemoral and trochanteric-pelvic impingement can be safely corrected using the SHD approach, which is our preferred method of treatment.

Ischiofemoral impingement is described when the space between the lesser trochanter and the ischium is reduced. On examination, pain is elicited by a combination of extension, adduction, and external rotation. Anteroposterior pelvic radiograph may reveal a prominent lesser trochanter often associated with coxa valga. False-profile view of the hip is helpful to confirm decreased space between the ischium and the femur, although the main diagnostic image is MRI. On MRI, the ischiofemoral space is reduced, and an intense signal may be present in the quadratus femoris muscle (**Figure 12.30**). Before surgical treatment is recommended, we favor targeted infiltration of the ischiofemoral space and quadratus muscle, which can be therapeutic but is certainly helpful in confirming that the source of pain is located in the ischiofemoral space. Patients that do not respond well to steroid injection and rehabilitation may be candidates for surgical treatment. Surgical strategies include proximal femoral intertrochanteric varus–producing osteotomy when there is associated anteversion and persistent anteversion. Osteoplasty and resection of the lesser trochanter may be performed arthroscopically, but this requires extensive experience and is quite laborious. We prefer to perform resection of the lesser trochanter through the SHD approach after dissection of the soft tissue flap containing the retinacular vessels (**Figure 12.31**).

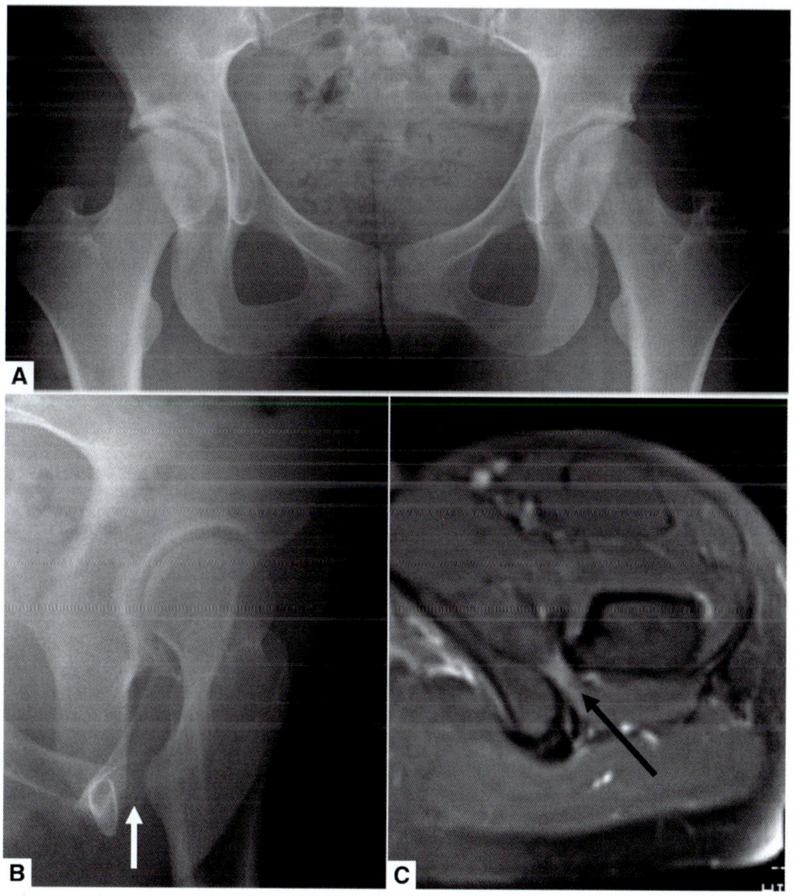

FIGURE 12.30. A 19-year-old female presented to clinic with left gluteal pain aggravated by sitting for long periods of time and walking. A, Anteroposterior pelvic radiograph reveals mild coxa valga bilaterally but otherwise normal bony structure. B, False-profile radiograph showing narrowing between the lesser trochanter and the ischium (white arrow). C, T2 fat-suppressed axial magnetic resonance imaging of the hip shows a very narrow ischiofemoral space with edema present in the quadratus muscle (black arrow).

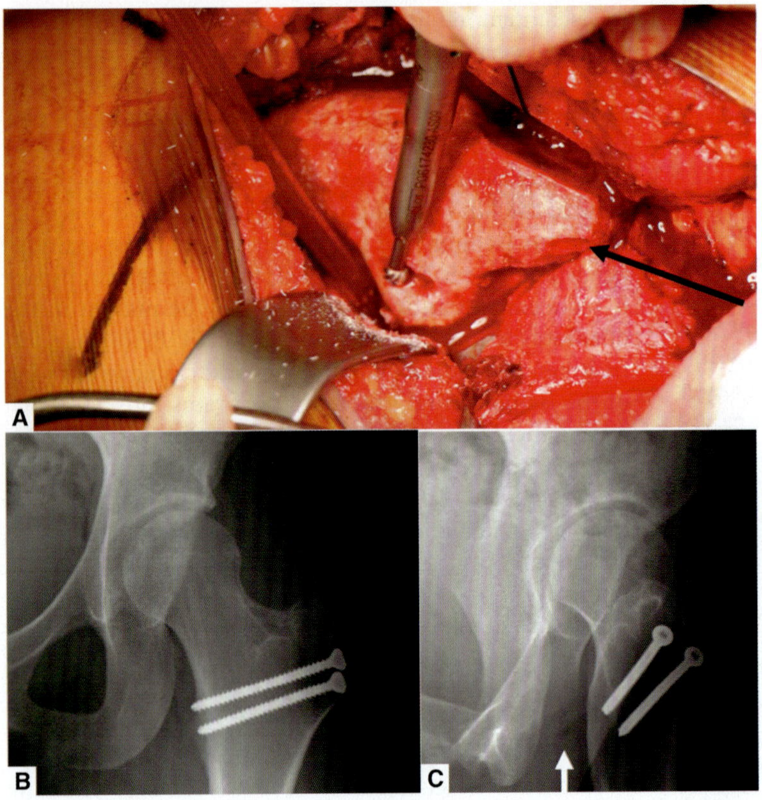

FIGURE 12.31. A, Intraoperative photograph during surgical hip dislocation showing resection of the posterior and superior aspects of the greater trochanter to allow for dissection of the soft tissue containing the retinacular vessels all the way around the lesser trochanter. The lesser trochanter is resected using a high-speed burr. If needed, the psoas tendon can be reattached by suture anchors. B, Postoperative anteroposterior radiograph at 18 months from surgery shows healing of the osteotomy and improved morphology of the lesser trochanter. C, Postoperative false-profile radiograph at 18 months shows correction of the ischiofemoral space (white arrow).

Trochanteric-pelvic impingement typically presents with posterior or posterolateral hip pain that is aggravated on physical examination by hip extension, abduction, and external rotation (the so-called posterior impingement test). The classic example of trochanteric-pelvic impingement is the residual deformity following Perthes disease during infancy with a high-hiding greater trochanter. However, we have observed that several patients with cam-type FAI have an abnormal transition between the femoral neck and the greater trochanter in association with cam deformity. These patients have a rather large anterior facet of the greater trochanter and an abnormal waist/contour and excessive bone at the transition with the femoral neck. During an SHD approach, impingement can be noted between the anterior facet of the trochanter and the lateral aspect of the ilium and acetabular rim, which can be treated by resection of the anterior facet of the trochanter (**Figure 12.32**).

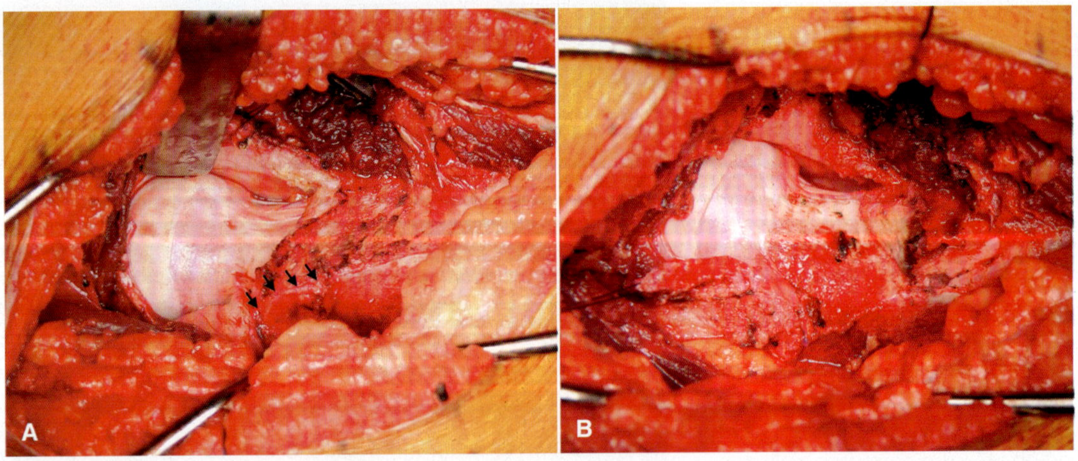

FIGURE 12.32. A 24-year-old female presented with residual hip pain aggravated by sitting following surgical treatment by a hip arthroscopy with cam decompression and acetabular labral repair. A, Intraoperative photograph during surgical hip dislocation showing a relatively short femoral neck with a large anterior facet of the greater trochanter (black arrows), leading to impingement against the acetabular rim with flexion and internal rotation. B, Intraoperative photograph after resection of the anterior facet of the greater trochanter and the osteochondroplasty extended to the level of the intertrochanteric line with improvement of the head-neck trochanter morphology and hip motion.

Finally, abnormal femoral version can be a source of intra- and extra-articular impingement. Excessive femoral anteversion, especially when associated with valgus deformity, may lead to posterior impingement and has been associated with a more anterior pattern of chondral and labral pathology in the acetabular side. Excessive femoral retroversion may lead to impingement between the distal aspect of the neck against the acetabular rim, aggravating the mechanism of pincer FAI. Surgical treatment of such complex deformities through the SHD approach allows for correct identification and treatment of the sources of impingement along with a subtrochanteric derotational osteotomy to normalize femoral version.

SUMMARY

In summary, the SHD approach is a versatile surgical approach to the hip that grants complete access to the femur and the acetabulum. Intra- and extra-articular pathologies leading to hip pain and dysfunction may be treated using the approach. Although the vast majority of patients with FAI are currently managed through an arthroscopic approach, we continue to use the SHD to treat residual deformities of the hip after pediatric disorders such as SCFE and Perthes and for complex deformities leading to FAI. Those include cam morphology involving the posterosuperior aspect of the head-neck junction, extra-articular impingement, including ischiofemoral and pelvic-trochanteric impingement, FAI associated with femoral version abnormality, and complex pincer impingement requiring extensive acetabular rim trimming. Our experience with the SHD approach has been very satisfactory overall. We have reported improvement in patients' reported outcomes and physical activity level and a high proportion of return to athletic activities following open treatment of FAI using this approach.[6-9]

REFERENCES

1. Ganz R, Gill TJ, Gautier E, Ganz K, Krugel N, Berlemann U. Surgical dislocation of the adult hip a technique with full access to the femoral head and acetabulum without the risk of avascular necrosis. *J Bone Joint Surg Br*. 2001;83(8):1119-1124.
2. Gautier E, Ganz K, Krugel N, Gill T, Ganz R. Anatomy of the medial femoral circumflex artery and its surgical implications. *J Bone Joint Surg Br*. 2000;82(5):679-683.
3. Notzli HP, Siebenrock KA, Hempfing A, Ramseier LE, Ganz R. Perfusion of the femoral head during surgical dislocation of the hip. Monitoring by laser Doppler flowmetry. *J Bone Joint Surg Br*. 2002;84(2):300-304.
4. Gibson A. Posterior exposure of the hip joint. *J Bone Joint Surg Br*. 1950;32-B(2):183-186.
5. Zaltz I, Leunig M. Parafoveal chondral defects associated with femoroacetabular impingement. *Clin Orthop Relat Res*. 2012;470(12):3383-3389.
6. Novais EN, Mayo M, Kestel LA, Carry PM, Mayer SW. Return to play following open treatment of femoroacetabular impingement in adolescent athletes. *J Am Acad Orthop Surg*. 2016;24(12):872-879.
7. Novais EN, Heyworth BE, Stamoulis C, Sullivan K, Millis MB, Kim YJ. Open surgical treatment of femoroacetabular impingement in adolescent athletes: preliminary report on improvement of physical activity level. *J Pediatr Orthop*. 2014;34(3):287-294.
8. Rebello G, Spencer S, Millis MB, Kim YJ. Surgical dislocation in the management of pediatric and adolescent hip deformity. *Clin Orthop Relat Res*. 2009;467(3):724-731.
9. Spencer S, Millis MB, Kim YJ. Early results of treatment of hip impingement syndrome in slipped capital femoral epiphysis and pistol grip deformity of the femoral head-neck junction using the surgical dislocation technique. *J Pediatr Orthop*. 2006;26(3):281-285.

CHAPTER 13

Hip Arthroscopic Approach for Femoroacetabular Impingement Treatment

BACKGROUND

Hip arthroscopy is being increasingly utilized to manage femoroacetabular impingement.[1] It provides excellent access to the central compartment as well as the ability to resect bone from the peripheral compartment. As discussed previously, the benefits of hip arthroscopy compared to more traditional open approaches include a more limited surgical dissection with resultant decreased perioperative discomfort and a more rapid recovery. The potential benefits of hip arthroscopy also serve as its limitations. With a more limited approach, obtaining safe, reliable access to the deformities associated with femoroacetabular impingement is dependent on surgical technique and experience.[2] In this chapter, we will discuss the indications and limitations of the arthroscopic approach, surgical technique, postoperative management, complications, and reported results.

Clinical Scenario

SL is a 22-year-old male with persistent left hip pain for more than 6 months. He did finish a course of physical therapy to alter his posture and body mechanics to relieve his hip pain but without much relief. On physical exam, his left hip flexes from 0° to 90° with flexion/internal rotation (IR) of 15° and flexion/external rotation (ER) of 45° with a positive impingement sign. In full extension, his abduction is 35° and adduction is 15°. His radiographs (**Figure 13.1A**) show a cam deformity

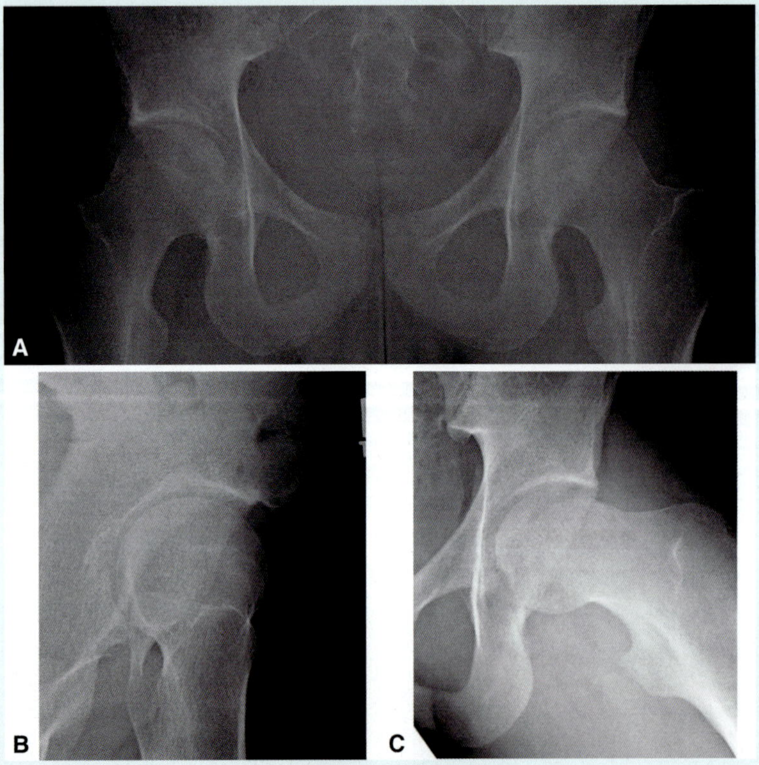

FIGURE 13.1. 22-year-old male with symptomatic left hip impingement. The anteroposterior pelvic radiograph (A) shows normal acetabular coverage and normal acetabular version. The decreased head-neck offset is visible. The false-profile view (B) shows normal anterior coverage but a prominent anterior inferior iliac spine, which may cause subspine impingement. The modified Dunn lateral view (C) is the best view to show the cam deformity.

visible on the anteroposterior (AP) pelvis view with normal acetabular coverage and acetabular version. On the false-profile view (**Figure 13.1B**), there is normal coverage but a prominent inferior iliac spine, and on the modified Dunn lateral view (**Figure 13.1C**), the cam deformity is clearly visible. The magnetic resonance imaging (MRI) (not shown) did not show significant chondral damage and femoral anteversion of 19°, and the patient underwent an arthroscopic cam decompression (**Figure 13.2**) with excellent pain relief and returned to all activities in 4 months.

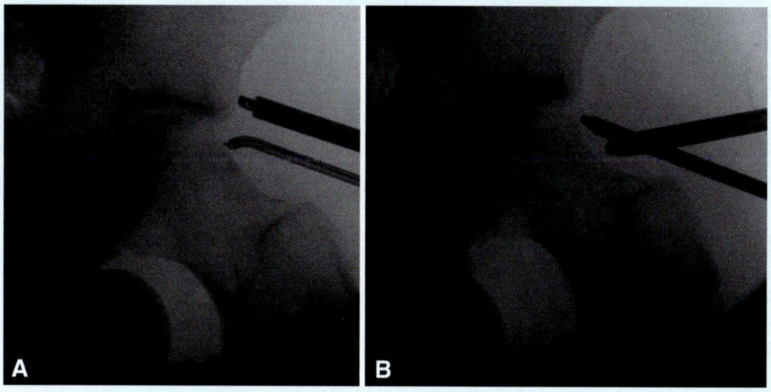

FIGURE 13.2. Intraoperative Dunn lateral view of the proximal head-neck junction before (A) and after (B) after arthroscopic cam decompression in a 22-year-old male.

This case represents a good candidate for arthroscopic cam decompression that has normal acetabulum, minimal joint damage, no proximal femoral retroversion, and limited motion and pain likely on account of the cam deformity.

INDICATIONS

- What deformity does well with arthroscopic approach?
  - Anterior-superior cam deformity with normal acetabular coverage
  - Peripheral rim osteophytes limiting hip flexion/IR and flexion/ER
- How much deformity is too much?
  - Hip flexion/IR <0°[3]
  - Acetabular dysplasia (LCE <15°)[4]
  - Excessive femoral retroversion[5]
  - Circumferential femoral osteophytes[3]

TECHNIQUE

Patient Positioning and Prep (Figure 13.3; Table 13.1)

Traction

Limiting the duration of operative traction is important and can be influenced by numerous factors prior to starting the surgical procedure. The following is a list of steps recommended prior to applying traction (**Table 13.2**).

Traction Process

Gentle traction is placed on the contralateral hip as a means of stabilizing the pelvis.

Operative hip is moved to a position of flexion (20°), abduction (20°), and maximal internal rotation. (The greater trochanter should be maximally prominent.) This position serves to relax the iliofemoral ligament and facilitates traction application.[6] Approximately 30 to 50 lbs of gross traction is applied in this position and held in place. The leg is then brought to a position of neutral flexion/extension and abduction/adduction. Fluoroscopy can confirm the degree of distraction (**Figure 13.4**).

Draping

Drapes

Sticky towels × 4 in a block-drape configuration (**Figure 13.5**). Hip arthroscopy drape placed such as to ensure adequate access to all relevant portal sites. A sterile mayo stand should be placed cranial to hold commonly used instruments (**Table 13.3**).

Hip Access

Skin Marking

Prior to starting the procedure, the anterior-superior iliac spine (ASIS) and greater trochanter should be marked to assist portal placement. In our technique, we prefer to use the anterolateral (AL) and midanterior (MA) portals

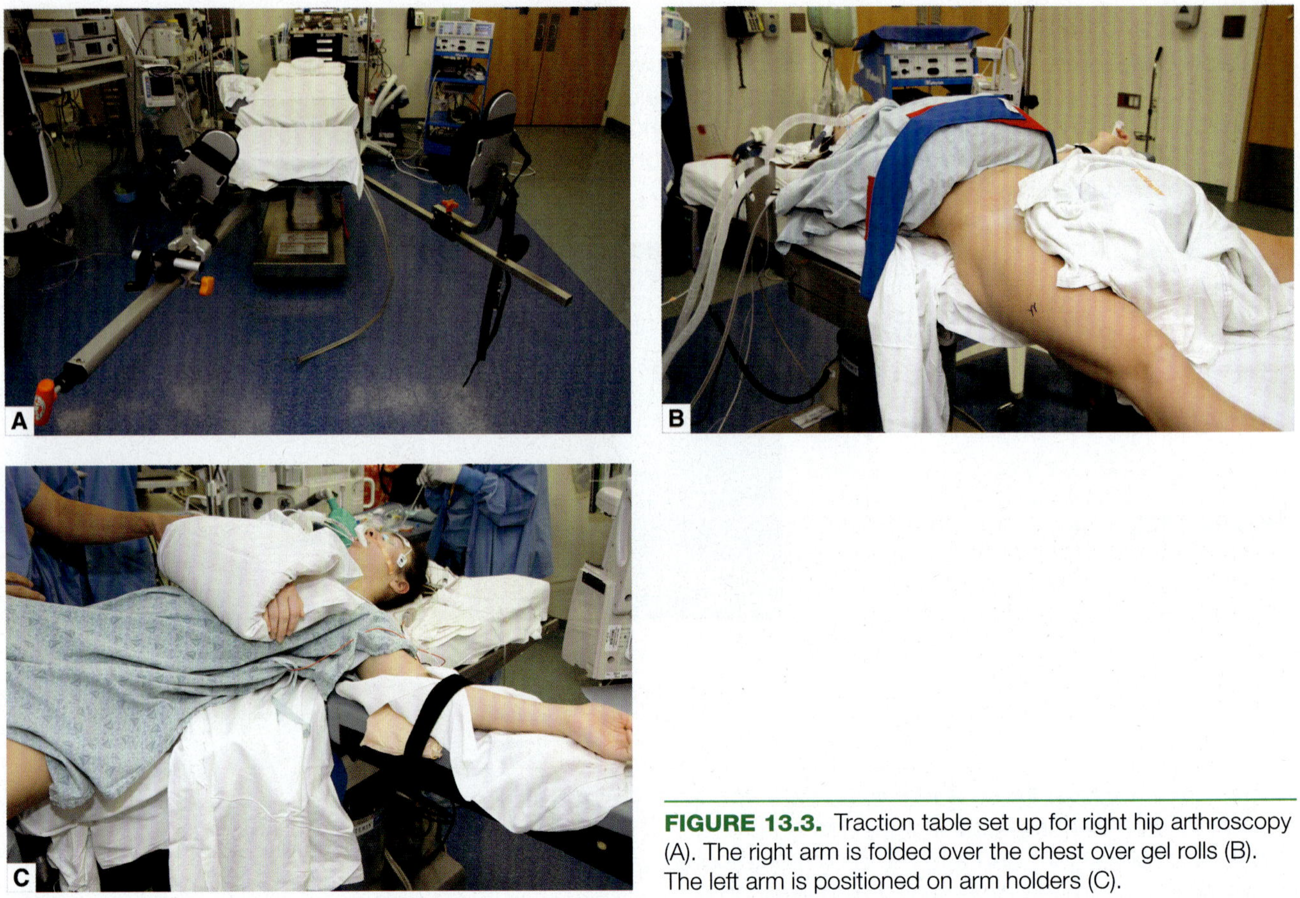

FIGURE 13.3. Traction table set up for right hip arthroscopy (A). The right arm is folded over the chest over gel rolls (B). The left arm is positioned on arm holders (C).

TABLE 13.1 Equipment Needed for Patient Positioning

Site	Needs
FEET	ABD × 4 (2 per side) Webril × 2 (1 per side)
HIP	POST and PAD Plastic U-Drape × 1 Plastic Strips × 2
ARMS	Contralateral—Armboard @ 90° Ipsilateral—Foam/Gel Pad × 2 Belt/Tape

TABLE 13.2 Surgical Checklist Prior to Traction

- Anesthesia team completed with airway management/sedation
- Patient translated onto hip post and plastic drapes applied
- Arms secured onto arm-board/across chest
- Feet well padded and secured within traction apparatus
- C-Arm is in the room and turned on (ready for imaging)
- Fine traction mechanism is set at zero (ie fully shortened)
- Skin is ready for prep application

as our working portals. The posterolateral (PL) and distal anterolateral accessory (DALA) portals are used on a much less frequent basis (**Figure 13.6**).

AL Portal Access

Steps for AL access to hip joint:

1. Switching stick at proposed AL portal site is used to identify the ideal starting point. (**Figure 13.7**) The following should be considered:
   a. Cranial/caudal location should start at the level of or just proximal to the greater trochanter on fluoroscopic imaging.
   b. Antero/posterior location depends on the femoral version. A normal version femoral starting point should be midway between the tip and the anterior border by skin marking/palpation. In anteverted femurs, this position will move further anterior, whereas in retroverted femurs this will move posterior.

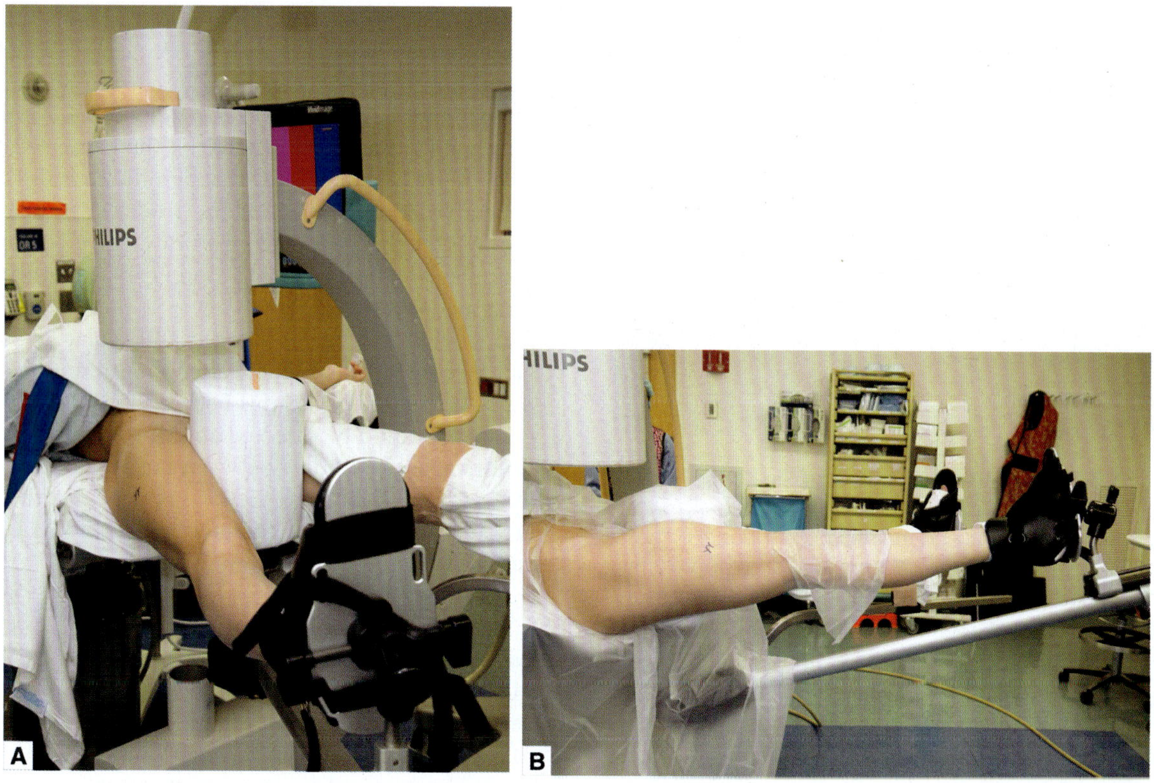

FIGURE 13.4. The leg is initially placed into some abduction and neutral rotation (A) to place the plastic drapes. For traction, the leg is maximally internally rotated (B) to place the femoral head deep in the acetabulum and to place the trochanter laterally.

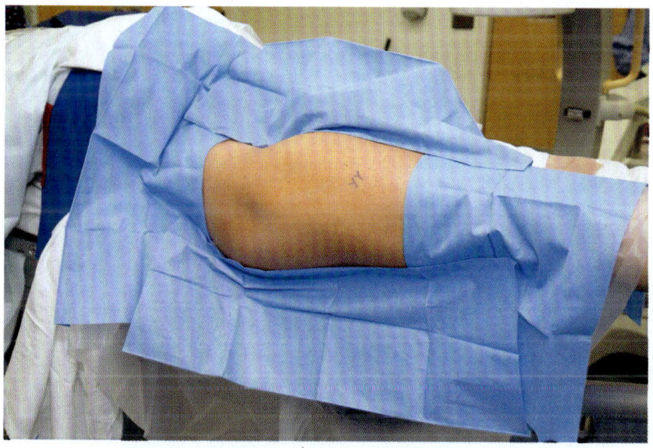

FIGURE 13.5. Sterile blue paper drapes are placed around the hip before the clear plastic drape is applied.

TABLE 13.3 Items for Mayo Stand
Arthroscope (70°), light source, camera, trocar connector
Arthroscopic shaver
Radiofrequency Ablation wand (RFA)
2 Hip Access Needles
1 Nitinol Wire
11 Blade Scalpel
4.5-mm cannula with blunt trocar
5-mm cannula with blunt trocar
5.5-mm cannula
Switching stick/Wissinger rod
Switching slot

2. 18 gauge needle is inserted to the level of the capsule under fluoroscopy. Typically, the trajectory is 10° to 15° cranial and posterior from the starting point in order to pierce the capsule at the 12 o' clock position. The targeted space lies between the femoral head and the acetabular labrum. The needle tip should face away from the labrum during capsular penetration, then reversed (away from the femoral head) if inserted further (**Figure 13.8A, B**).
3. Needle trochar is removed, and air (~15 cc) is injected into the joint. The air arthrogram will break the fluid seal of the hip and permit fine-tuned traction if needed at this stage. Fluoroscopic imaging of this air arthrogram should show the inferior border of the labrum "float" away from the needle. In cases where this is not observed, repositioning the needle should be considered. **Figure 13.8C** shows the labrum and femoral head moving out of the way after injection of air into the joint.

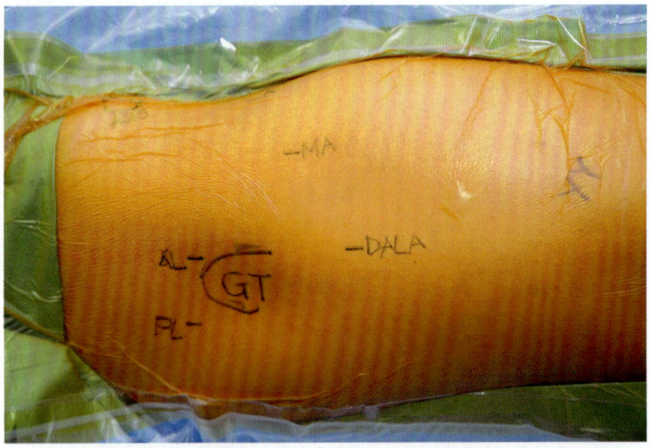

FIGURE 13.6. The greater trochanter and the portals are marked after traction application. The two main working portals are the anterolateral and the midanterior portals. The posterolateral portal is useful to vent the joint or to approach the posterior acetabular rim. The distal anterolateral accessory portal is useful for acetabular rim anchor placement and for head-neck junction resection.

4. Nitinol wire is inserted. When judging portal placement, the nitinol wire should cross the entire sourcil to the cotyloid fossa. If the wire stops short of the fossa, the portal is likely malpositioned in the anteroposterior plane (typically aimed too posterior). The needle should be repositioned. **Figure 13.8D** shows correctly placed nitinol wire.
5. Once the nitinol is well positioned, the needle is removed and a skin incision is made. The 4.5-mm cannula with blunt entry trochar is then inserted to the level of the capsule. Entry through the capsule is made with a twisting motion of the trochar/cannula along the axis of the nitinol wire until a "give" is felt. The cannula's position within the joint can be confirmed by imaging (**Figure 13.8E**).
6. The trochar can be disengaged and replaced with the arthroscope at this point. Water should not be started until the second portal has been established. The camera's lens should be directed anteriorly to bring the anterior capsular window between the acetabular labrum and femoral head into view. This provides the intra-articular view needed to safely place the MA portal cannula (**Figure 13.9A**).

MA Portal Access

Steps for MA access to the hip joint:

1. The MA portal starting point was marked out prior to surgical start; however, the final AL portal position may change from its initial marking. The MA portal should be adjusted for these changes.
2. 18 Gauge needle is inserted through the MA portal site and triangulated into position with the known AL portal. This step is best performed initially by looking

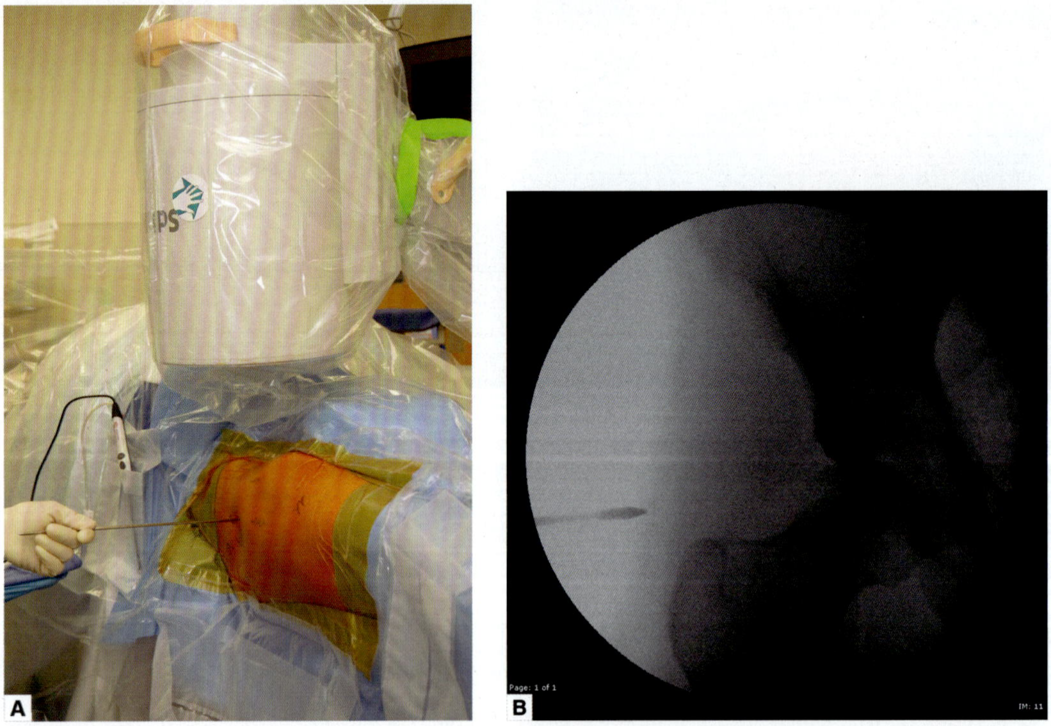

FIGURE 13.7. The anterolateral portal is placed by inserting a needle just above the femoral head on the anteroposterior view (A). The trajectory is typically about 10° to 15° cranial (B) and slightly posterior in angle.

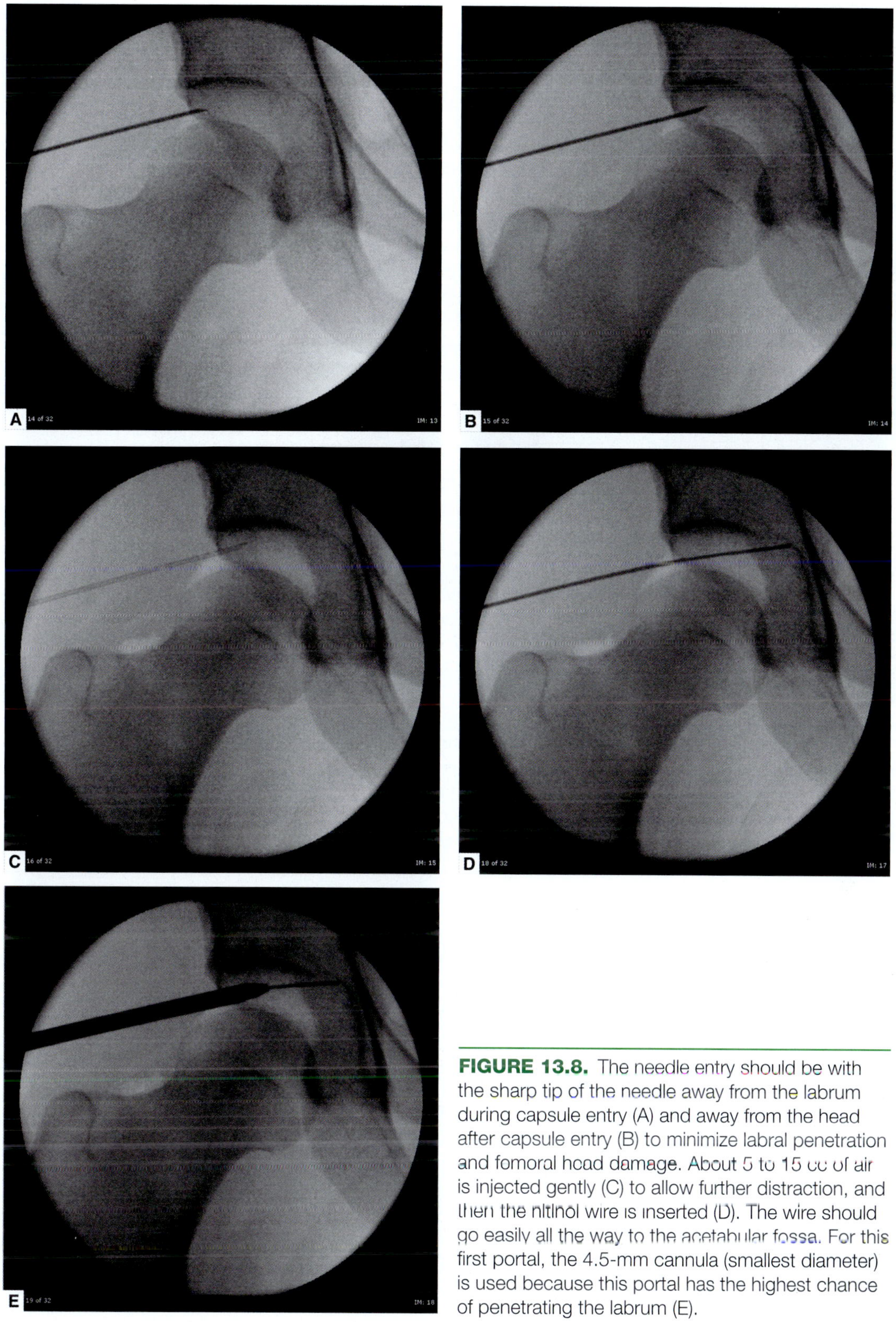

FIGURE 13.8. The needle entry should be with the sharp tip of the needle away from the labrum during capsule entry (A) and away from the head after capsule entry (B) to minimize labral penetration and femoral head damage. About 5 to 15 cc of air is injected gently (C) to allow further distraction, and then the nitinol wire is inserted (D). The wire should go easily all the way to the acetabular fossa. For this first portal, the 4.5-mm cannula (smallest diameter) is used because this portal has the highest chance of penetrating the labrum (E).

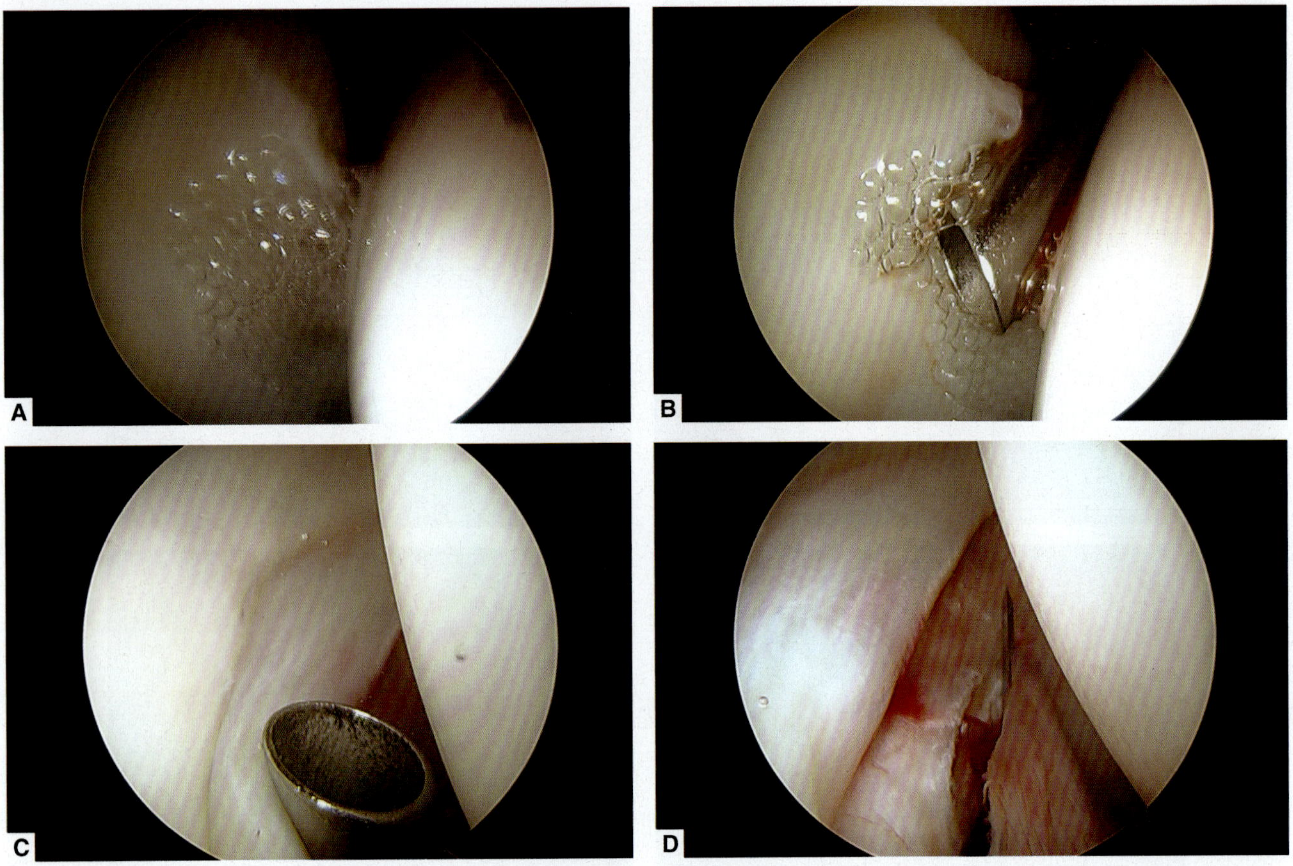

FIGURE 13.9. The anterolateral portal is entered and the anterior labrum visualized without fluid (A) because there is no vent. The triangular space between the femoral head and the labrum is the target for the midanterior portal (B). The camera is then switched to the midanterior portal, and the fluid is turned on and the anterolateral portal inspected to make sure it did not penetrate the joint (C). The interconnecting capsulotomy is started through the anterolateral portal (D).

at the external hip to establish an accurate trajectory. Typically, the needle needs to be pointed more medial and distal than is expected. Fluoroscopy can be used to guide this trajectory, looking at the needle tip's relationship to the anterior wall. Once a reasonable trajectory is obtained, the view should be transitioned to the arthroscope as you prepare to pierce the capsule. The needle should be positioned as close as possible to the femoral head to ease peripheral compartment access and facilitate capsular closure.

3. Nitinol wire is placed through the needle and a skin incision is made.
4. 5-mm cannula with blunt trochar is inserted to the level of the capsule. Again, twisting motion is used to insert the trochar/cannula under direct visualization (**Figure 13.9B**).

- Capsulotomy
  1. After establishing the MA portal, the arthroscope is moved to this portal. The AL cannula should be maintained. The camera is directed posteriorly to allow visualization of the AL portal position (**Figure 13.9C**). Arthroscopic fluid can be started to flush the joint after this transition. The AL portal can be readjusted if needed.
  2. A capsular blade (banana blade or other) is then inserted through the AL cannula, and the cannula is removed. The capsulotomy is started posterior and parallel to the labrum until the blade-capsule relationship is no longer visible (**Figure 13.9D**). The piriformis tendon is the absolute limit for posterior extension of the capsulotomy. The blade is then directed anteriorly toward the MA portal, again paralleling the labrum as far as possible.
  3. The blade is returned to the original AL portal position, and the switching slot is placed over it. The blade can then be removed from the joint. A switching stick is then inserted along the slot, and the slot can be removed once the stick is within the joint. The 5.5-mm cannula is then placed into the joint over the switching stick. The arthroscope can now be moved to the AL cannula, and the camera is aimed anteriorly to localize the MA cannula.
  4. The capsule blade is inserted through the anteromedial (AM) cannula, which is then removed. The

blade is directed anteriorly first along the labrum. The psoas tendon is the absolute limit to this limb of the capsulotomy. The blade is then directed posteriorly along the labrum toward the AL cannula, completing the capsulotomy. A switching slot can then be inserted over the blade to enable its removal.

Central Compartment Work

After gaining adequate access to the central compartment, work can begin on the acetabular rim, anterior inferior iliac spine, acetabular cartilage, and labrum. All central compartment work will be performed under traction, so efficiency is important. The goal for total traction time should be less than 2 hours to minimize the risk of traction-related complications.[7]

- Photo documentation of injuries
  A standard approach to imaging the hip joint should be followed. Our sequence is as follows: (1) anterior wall (**Figure 13.10A**), (2) weight-bearing dome, (3) posterior wall (**Figure 13.10B**), (4) cotyloid fossa and ligamentum (**Figure 13.10C**), (5) femoral head (**Figure 13.10D**), (6) anterosuperior acetabular rim and labrum. In cases with identifiable pathology, an arthroscopic probe can be inserted to manipulate the affected regions of acetabular labrum and/or cartilage.
- Acetabular rim osteoplasty
  The indications for acetabular rim osteoplasty were discussed in Chapter 11. In short, large lunate deep hips with symptomatic overcoverage can undergo acetabular rim osteoplasty through either an open or an arthroscopic approach. Our technique for acetabular rim osteoplasty is as follows:

1. With the arthroscope in the AL portal, instrumentation is performed via the MA portal. The RFA wand is inserted, and the interval between the acetabular labrum and hip capsule is defined. It is important to clearly demarcate the acetabular rim to enable visualization during the acetabular osteoplasty.
2. The acetabular labrum must be elevated on its capsular insertion to give access to the true acetabular rim. This is performed with the RFA wand with care to avoid injuring the labrum during the elevation process. The chondrolabral junction should

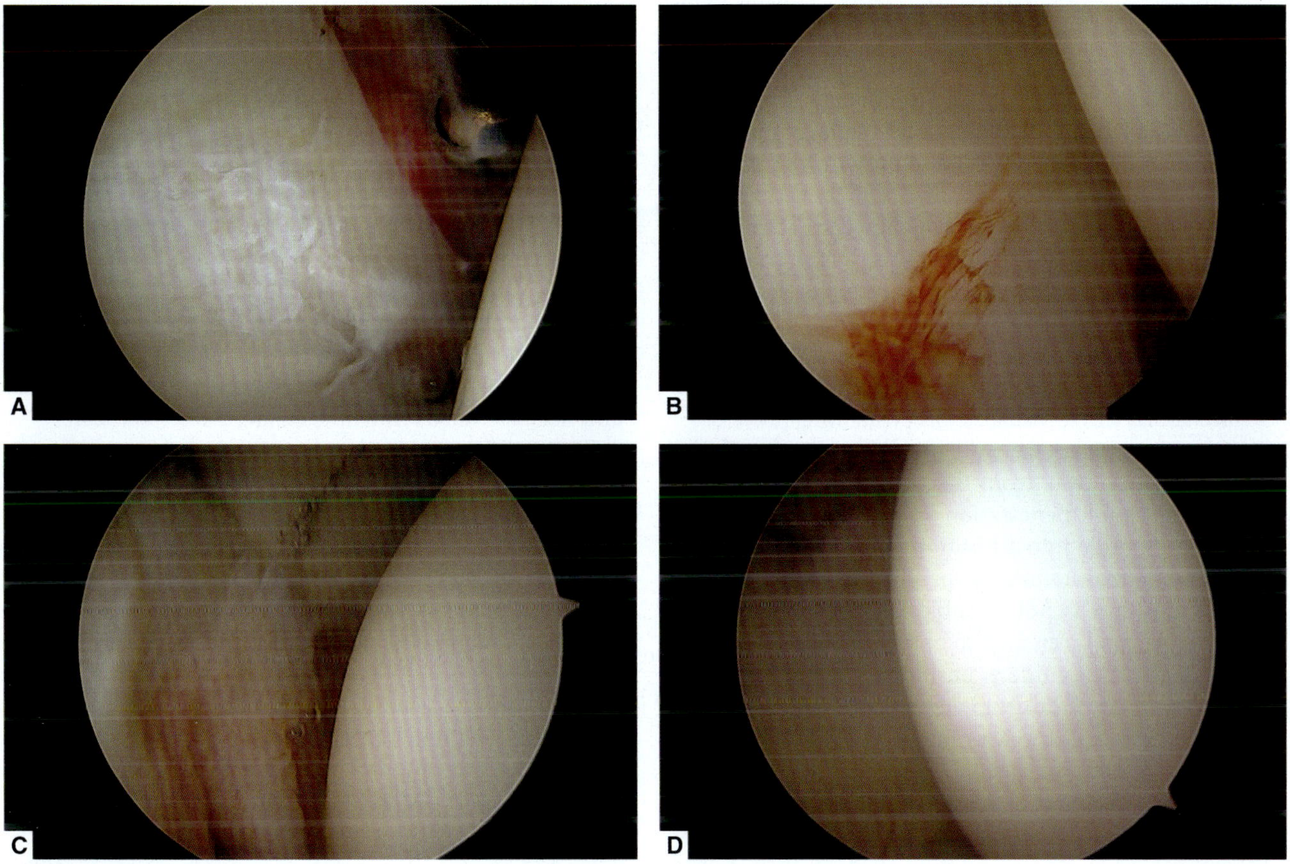

FIGURE 13.10. Standard inspection of the joint should be performed. First the anterior wall of the acetabulum is visualized (A), and the scope is turned to look at the superior weight-bearing dome and then the posterior wall (B). The acetabular (cotyloid) fossa and the round ligament is visualized (C) and the femoral head (D) inspected.

be maintained, if at all possible, to improve chondrolabral stability and to maintain the suction seal of the labrum following the acetabular osteoplasty. Once the labrum is elevated to the point that the undersurface of the acetabular cartilage is barely visible at the acetabular rim, the rim is ready for recession.

3. The RFA wand is removed, and an arthroscopic burr (5.5 mm) is inserted through the MA portal via a slotted cannula. AP fluoroscopic views can help in localizing the anterior-most extent of the acetabular osteoplasty. We typically begin anteromedially and work posterolaterally. The burr size (5.5 mm) is used as a template for the planned resection.
4. After adequate bony resection, repeat AP fluoroscopic views should be obtained to assess the completeness of osteoplasty. The acetabular labrum should then be repaired to the new acetabular rim. This technique is discussed later in this chapter.

- Acetabular Labrum
  In general, the labrum should be preserved whenever possible. Its benefits include improved mechanical load transmission and stability through its suction seal.[8]
- Acetabular Labral Repair Technique:
  1. Labral repairs typically begin anteromedially and proceed posterolaterally. The arthroscope is typically used in the AL portal, and the MA portal is used for instrumentation. Insertion of a cannula through the MA portal is often beneficial while repairing a labrum to assist suture management.
  2. Suture anchors are deployed to perform the labral repair, either knotted or knotless. Our preference is to use a knotless construct to avoid knot irritation within the capsulolabral fold. The first anchor is inserted at the anterior margin of the unstable portion of the labrum. The drill guide is inserted through the MA cannula and positioned approximately 1 to 2 mm away from the acetabular rim. The arthroscope is positioned above the acetabular rim to visualize this positioning process.
  3. Once positioned, the drill guide must be placed into a trajectory away from the acetabular concavity to prevent joint penetration. This involves levering the drill guide into a position closer to the patient's leg while maintaining its previous starting point. If this position is not possible, an alternative portal (DALA) can be created to obtain this trajectory.
  4. Once the drill guide is positioned, the arthroscope is moved into a position viewing the acetabular cartilage. The drill can then be used to create the anchor's path on full speed. Drilling should be stopped if there is evidence of pending joint penetration. The drill guide can be repositioned as above and the process repeated. If using knotted anchors, they should be inserted immediately after drilling through their respective guides. If using knotless anchors, a nitinol wire can be inserted into the anchor base to use as a placeholder for later anchor placement.
  5. The repair sutures should now be passed through the acetabular labrum in either a looped or labra-based mattress fashion using a bird-beak or similar passer (**Figure 13.11**). See technical note for recommended suture conformations.[9]
  6. The anchor can be definitively fixed by sliding arthroscopic knots (we recommend Weston knot, followed by three half-hitches) or impaction of the knotless anchor. When tensioning the labral repair, the sutures should be snug to ensure stability, but care must be taken to avoid "overreduction" of the labrum onto the rim. If the labrum is overreduced, the efficacy of its suction seal function may be reduced (**Figure 13.11C**).
- Acetabular cartilage
  - Fraying—Gentle abrasion arthroplasty is our treatment of choice for frayed acetabular cartilage with a goal of achieving a stable cartilaginous base with minimal resection
  - Delamination—Delamination-type injuries characteristic of cam-type impingement are frequently left alone or stabilized through the labral repair procedure. We do not advocate resection of delaminated cartilage flaps except for cases with significant instability and risk for loose body formation
  - Defect—Acetabular microfracture is a reasonable alternative for full thickness (Outerbridge 4) cartilage defects of the acetabulum and/or femoral head. Addition of a microfracture prolongs crutch use and partial weight-bearing restrictions for 6 weeks following surgery.

Peripheral Compartment Work

After completing all work in the central compartment, traction can be released. The femoral head should be observed because it reduces within the acetabulum. Focus can now be directed toward the peripheral compartment, which provides access to the intracapsular femoral head and neck as well as the hip capsule.

- Femoral Osteochondroplasty
  The femoral osteochondroplasty is arguably the most important portion of the majority of hip arthroscopies for femoroacetabular impingement. The cam-type lesion of the proximal femur is typically the greatest mechanical stress to the hip and is associated with a heightened risk for the future development of osteoarthritis.
- Femoral Osteochondroplasty Technique:
  1. After traction release, the hip can be brought into a position of 20° of flexion with neutral abduction/adduction. With the arthroscope in the AL portal, the RFA wand can be introduced through the MA portal. The region of the cam lesion should be delineated at this point, with any region of sclerosis, erythema, or other signs of abrasion being included within the identified cam-deformity region. The templated resection region should be clearly

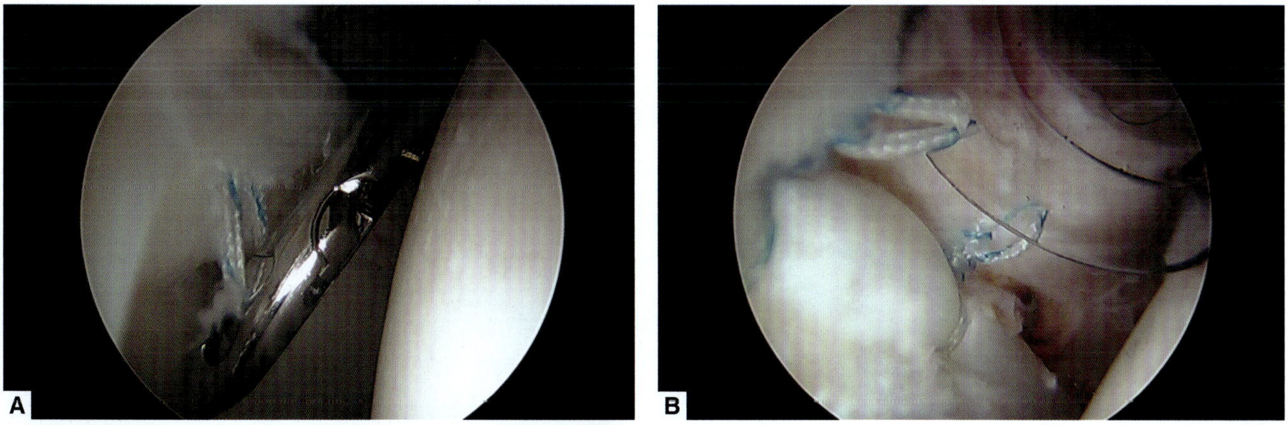
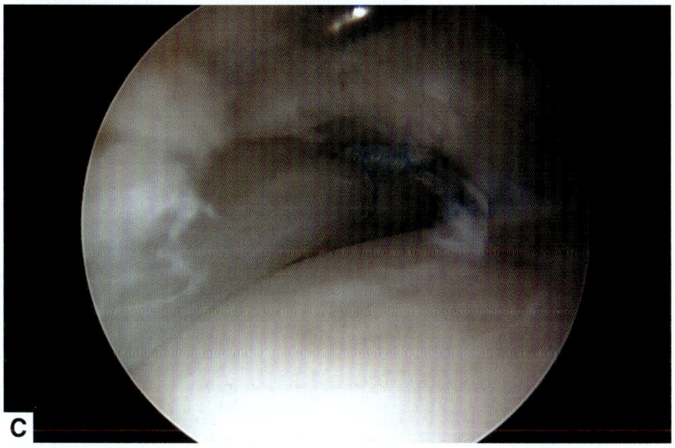

FIGURE 13.11. Labral repair can be performed using knotless versus a knot-tying suture anchor. Various suture passers are available (A), and the suture can be placed either in a loop configuration (B) or in a mattress configuration. Care should be taken not to overreduce the labrum (C) and thereby compromise its sealing function.

marked, especially at the proximal extent, and should parallel the contour of the acetabular labrum with 2 to 3 mm of femoral head cartilage left intact distal to the labrum.

2. After the cam resection region has been identified, the arthroscope is transitioned to the MA portal, and the arthroscopic shaver is introduced through the AL portal. The arthroscope should be positioned along the axis of the femoral neck with the lens directed laterally, visualizing the more lateral portion of the femoral head/neck junction. Pericapsular soft tissue can be shaved at this time to improve visualization, exercising care to avoid a capsulectomy.
3. After adequate visualization is obtained, the shaver can be replaced with the arthroscopic burr. The burr should be positioned at the most lateral portion of the accessible femoral head, which should still lie anterior to the retinacular vessels. The vessels can and should be visualized at this time to avoid iatrogenic injury.
4. Once position is confirmed, the arthroscopic burr is used to template the depth and extent of the superolateral proximal femur osteochondroplasty, with the goal of creating adequate offset and roundness of the proximal femur. As a rule of thumb, decortication of the sclerotic bony regions is a good starting point for resection.[10] The C-arm can be used at this time with a 10° oblique image of the proximal femur to localize the site of osteoplasty and judge the depth and extent of resection. Focusing on the distal aspect of resection depth is key to restoring adequate head/neck offset.
5. Once the template depth and extent are confirmed visually and fluoroscopically, this template is then used for the remainder of the osteochondroplasty, which proceeds anteromedially. As the burr is brought further anterior, the camera lens is gradually adjusted to give a bird's eye view down the neck of the femur. As the burr moves into the anterior portion of the neck, care should be taken to avoid overresection. Again, decortication is a reasonable goal for the first pass of bony resection (**Figure 13.12**).
6. Fluoroscopy can be used after the initial osteoplasty to confirm adequate resection. AP and oblique laterals at 10° to 15° intervals can provide a fluoroscopic evaluation of femoral osteochondroplasty. Typically, residual deformities identified by fluoroscopy will be distal on the femoral neck. To access these lesions, the hip can be abducted (for lateral lesions) and further flexed (for anterior lesions) in an effort to improve capsular mobility. The arthroscopic burr's shield can be used as a retractor on the capsule to

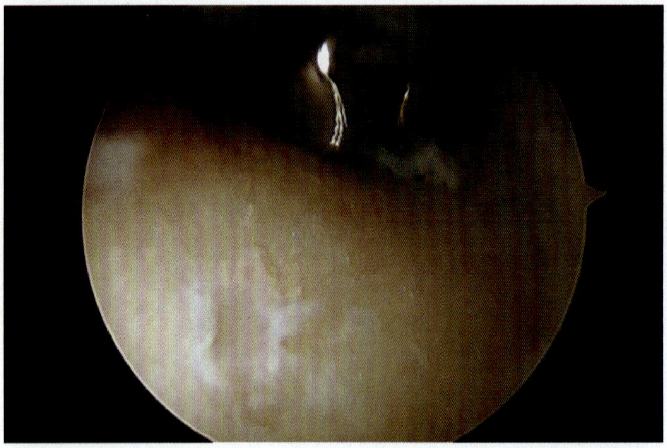

FIGURE 13.12. Femoral head-neck junction is performed using a burr, and we usually perform the resection until the cortical bone is removed, and then fluoroscopic images are obtained to check the depth of resection.

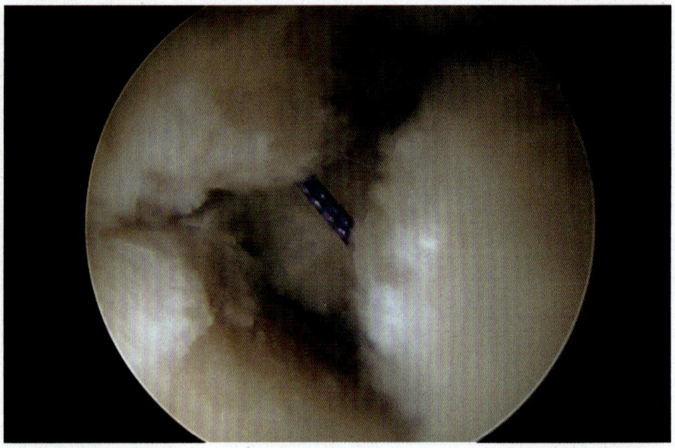

FIGURE 13.13. Increasingly, the importance of capsule management is becoming evident. Various suture passers are available that will enable routine closure of the capsule.

permit more distal access. Osteoplasties should be carried distally to a level near the intertrochanteric line, if possible.

7. Final fluoroscopic views should confirm a restored femoral head-neck offset carried through the length of the neck on all radiographic views.
    - Capsular preparation and closure
      Capsular management has gained increased attention in the field of hip arthroscopy. Several studies have documented risks of iatrogenic instability or instability-related pain following hip arthroscopy in which the capsulotomy was not closed.[11] Our indications for capsulotomy include:
        - All female patients
        - Male patients with concomitant:
            - Soft tissue laxity (ie Beighton score ≥5), collagen disorder (ie Ehlers-Danlos, Marfans, etc)
            - Acetabular dysplasia—usually patients with a symptomatic cam deformity with mildly reduced acetabular coverage

Technique for Capsular Repair/ Plication

1. Capsular repair starts with the preparation of both the femoral and acetabular capsular leaflets. The RFA wand is used to define the superficial aspects of each leaflet and sweep away soft tissue, which will hinder visualization and suture placement.
2. For capsular repairs, the camera is placed in the MA portal, and a disposable cannula is inserted over a switching stick through the AL portal.
3. A Slingshot device is used to shuttle sutures across the capsular defect in a simple suture fashion. The initial pass is made on the acetabular (less mobile) side. The capsular penetrator is then passed through the femoral side, and the width of this pass determines the final capsular tension (**Figure 13.13**).
4. After a suture has been passed through both leaflets, it is tied over the capsule under direct visualization using an arthroscopic knot pusher and simple square knots.
5. Sutures are passed every 7 to 10 mm, typically requiring three to four stitches for an average-sized capsulotomy. The switching stick can be used between suture passages to reposition the cannula for optimal access to the capsule as the repair moves anteromedially.

Wound Closure

- After capsular closure, all instruments are withdrawn from the hip. A 16G spinal needle is then reinserted through the MA site onto the capsular repair/femoral neck.
- Both AL and MA portals are provisionally closed with 2-0 Vicryl. Next, 20 cc of 0.2% ropivacaine is injected into the periarticular space, and the spinal needle is removed. The arthroscopy portals are then closed with 3-0 Monocryl.

POSTOPERATIVE MANAGEMENT/ COMPLICATIONS

- Crutch use is employed postoperatively with partial weight-bearing restrictions (approximately 25% of body weight).
    - Arthroscopy alone: 2 weeks
    - Arthroscopy with microfracture: 6 weeks

- Heterotopic ossification (HO) prophylaxis is used in all patients for 4 weeks following surgery involving bony intra-articular resections (cam and/or pincer). We typically prescribe naproxen 500 mg BID for routine HO prophylaxis. Patients with gastrointestinal (GI) diagnoses or intolerance to naproxen are prescribed celecoxib 100 mg BID.
- Deep vein thrombosis (DVT) prophylaxis is used in all patients for 4 weeks following surgery. Typically, patients are prescribed aspirin 81 mg daily for routine prophylaxis, but patients with known clotting disorders (Factor V Leiden, Lupus anticoagulant, etc) or with a history of DVT/pulmonary embolism (PE) are typically managed with subcutaneous enoxaparin.
- Physical therapy (PT) and return to sports:
  - Referral to PT typically occurs after the first postoperative visit (2 weeks). Early PT efforts focus on maintenance of motion and muscular activation (quads, glutes, core). Care is taken to avoid extension and external rotation positioning so as to minimize the risk of dislocation through the anterior capsulotomy.
  - Between 4 and 12 weeks, range of motion (ROM) restrictions are typically lifted, and patients begin progressive strengthening protocols, moving from double limb to single limb exercises for both closed and open chain movements. Exercise bike (4 weeks) and elliptical (8 weeks) are commonly employed at this time for motion and light endurance activities.
  - Return to running typically occurs at 3 months following surgery, and a graduated program of increased distance and intensity is followed. Patients are progressed to jumping/plyometrics at 4 months, followed by a graduated return to sports-specific activity. Generally speaking, full return to play can be expected to be achieved between 4.5 and 6 months following surgery.

Outcomes

- Hip arthroscopy has been shown to be safe and highly effective in the treatment of femoroacetabular impingement in multiple case series. Nearly 80% of patients note significant functional improvements on patient reported outcomes using modern surgical techniques such as labral repair and capsular closure.[12] Postoperative return to sports is achieved in 87.5% of patients, similar to other sports-related surgical procedures.[13]
- Failed hip arthroscopy has been linked to errors in both technical performance and patient selection. From a technical standpoint, inadequate bony resection has been shown to be a common cause for continued impingement symptoms.[14,15] From an indication standpoint, the presence of acetabular dysplasia or osteoarthritis should be considered relative contraindications for an isolated hip arthroscopy owing to their known risk for early failure.[4,16]

Complications

Complications following hip arthroscopy for femoroacetabular impingement are typically low and are shown to occur in 1% to 8% of cases in large-scale reviews.[13,17] Traction-related neurologic injuries are the most common intraoperative complications, involving the sciatic, femoral, or pudendal nerves. These injuries are frequently avoided by limiting traction time (<2 hours) and force (<50 lbs). Postoperatively, DVT (3% to 5%) and HO (2% to 4%) are the most common complications, which we have mitigated with the use of a baby aspirin and naproxen, respectively.[17] Rare complications such as iatrogenic instability (excessive acetabular rim resection) and iatrogenic femoral neck fracture (excessive proximal femoral resection) are avoided with appropriate preoperative and intraoperative precautions. Avascular necrosis, although a theoretical concern, has not been reported in a case of hip arthroscopy for femoroacetabular impingement.[17]

REFERENCES

1. Colvin AC, Harrast J, Harner C. Trends in hip arthroscopy. *JBJS.* 2012;94(4):e23. doi:10.2106/JBJS.J.01886.
2. Hoppe DJ, de SA D, Simunovic N, et al. The learning curve for hip arthroscopy: a systematic review. *Arthroscopy.* 2014;30(3):389-397. doi:10.1016/j.arthro.2013.11.012.
3. Bedi A, Zaltz I, De La Torre K, Kelly BT. Radiographic comparison of surgical hip dislocation and hip arthroscopy for treatment of cam deformity in femoroacetabular impingement. *Am J Sports Med.* 2011;39:20S-28S. doi:10.1177/0363546511412734.
4. Yeung M, Kowalczuk M, Simunovic N, Ayeni OR. Hip arthroscopy in the setting of hip dysplasia: a systematic review. *Bone Joint Res.* 2016;5(6):225-231. doi:10.1302/2046-3758.56.2000533.
5. Fabricant PD, Fields KG, Taylor SA, Magennis E, Bedi A, Kelly BT. The effect of femoral and acetabular version on clinical outcomes after arthroscopic femoroacetabular impingement surgery. *J Bone Joint Surg Am.* 2015;97(7):537-543. doi:10.2106/JBJS.N.00266.
6. Hewitt JD, Glisson RR, Guilak F, Vail TP. The mechanical properties of the human hip capsule ligaments. *J Arthroplasty.* 2002;17(1):82-89. doi:10.1054/arth.2002.27674.
7. Frandsen L, Lund B, Grønbech Nielsen T, Lind M. Traction-related problems after hip arthroscopy. *J Hip Preserv Surg.* 2017;4(1):54-59. doi:10.1093/jhps/hnw044.
8. Cadet ER, Chan AK, Vorys GC, Gardner T, Yin B. Investigation of the preservation of the fluid seal effect in the repaired, partially resected, and reconstructed acetabular labrum in a cadaveric hip model. *Am J Sports Med.* 2012;40(10):2218-2223. doi:10.1177/0363546512457645.
9. Fry R, Domb B. Labral base refixation in the hip: rationale and technique for an anatomic approach to labral repair. *Arthroscopy.* 2010;26(9):S81-S89. doi:10.1016/j.arthro.2010.01.021.
10. Atkins PR, Aoki SK, Whitaker RT, Weiss JA, Peters CL, Anderson AE. Does removal of subchondral cortical bone provide sufficient resection depth for treatment of cam femoroacetabular impingement? *Clin Orthop Relat Res.* 2017;475(8):1977-1986. doi:10.1007/s11999-017-5326-5.

11. Domb BG, Stake CE, Finley ZJ, Chen T, Giordano BD. Influence of capsular repair versus unrepaired capsulotomy on 2-year clinical outcomes after arthroscopic hip preservation surgery. *Arthroscopy.* 2015;31(4):643-650. doi:10.1016/j.arthro.2014.10.014.
12. Cvetanovich GL, Weber AE, Kuhns BD, et al. Clinically meaningful improvements after hip arthroscopy for femoroacetabular impingement in adolescent and young adult patients regardless of gender. *J Pediatr Orthop.* 2016;38(9):465-470. doi:10.1097/BPO.0000000000000852.
13. Minkara AA, Westermann RW, Rosneck J, Lynch TS. Systematic review and meta-analysis of outcomes after hip arthroscopy in femoroacetabular impingement. *Am J Sports Med.* 2019;47(2):488-500. doi:10.1177/0363546517749475.
14. Bogunovic L, Gottlieb M, Pashos G, Baca G, Clohisy JC. Why do hip arthroscopy procedures fail? *Clin Orthop.* 2013;471(8):2523-2529. doi:10.1007/s11999-013-3015-6.
15. Burrus MT, Cowan JB, Bedi A. Avoiding failure in hip arthroscopy: complications, pearls, and pitfalls. *Clin Sports Med.* 2016;35(3):487-501. doi:10.1016/j.csm.2016.02.011.
16. Menge TJ, Briggs KK, Dornan GJ, McNamara SC, Philippon MJ. Survivorship and outcomes 10 years following hip arthroscopy for femoroacetabular impingement: labral debridement compared with labral repair. *J Bone Joint Surg Am.* 2017;99(12):997-1004. doi:10.2106/JBJS.16.01060.
17. Nakano N, Khanduja V. Complications in hip arthroscopy. *Muscles Ligaments Tendons J.* 2016;6(3):402-409. doi:10.11138/mltj/2016.6.3.402.

CHAPTER 14

Pelvic Osteotomy Technique for Pincer Impingement

INTRODUCTION

Although the proximal femur is the most common source of femoroacetabular impingement, acetabular morphology can also serve as a source of impingement pathomorphology. Acetabular sources of femoroacetabular impingement usually result from a state of either acetabular retroversion or global acetabular overcoverage (ie, acetabular protrusio). In cases of pathologic version or overcoverage (retroverted or small lunate deep hips), where the lunate cartilage is not amenable to rim reduction, a reorienting periacetabular osteotomy (PAO) is advised to optimize the spatial orientation of the acetabulum.

INDICATIONS FOR SURGERY

The following are the relevant examination and imaging findings of patients with femoroacetabular impingement symptoms who may be considered for a PAO, either anteverting or reverse in nature, to address their abnormal hip mechanics.

Anteverting Periacetabular Osteotomy

Acetabular retroversion is a diagnosis made by clinical examination and imaging analysis. Patients frequently complain of impingement-related difficulties, including pain with sitting and impact activities. There are frequent findings of anterior impingement on examination with pain during flexion and internal rotation of the hip. In severe cases, patients can present with significant limitations to internal rotation and may have findings of obligate external rotation in flexion. Occasionally, patients may also have the sensation of instability during impingement testing, which is the result of the femoral head levering on the anterior acetabular wall, causing subluxation of the femoral head on an insufficient posterior wall.[1]

Radiographic findings in these patients include a crossover sign, posterior wall sign, and ischial spine sign on anteroposterior (AP) pelvis radiographs. Frequently, the entire hemipelvis is externally rotated in acetabular retroversion, which explains why a focal acetabular prominence or insufficiency is seldom encountered.[2] It is imperative that the AP pelvis radiograph be taken with the coccyx overlying the pubic symphysis, as any rotation of the pelvis on this projection will alter the appearance of acetabular version. The AP pelvis should also be scrutinized for the anterior and posterior wall indices, the lateral acetabular coverage (lateral center-edge angle [LCEA], Tönnis angle), and deformity of the proximal femur. Dunn lateral and false profile views should also be obtained to look for femoral cam deformity and anterior acetabular coverage, respectively. Cross-sectional imaging, including both computed tomography (CT) and magnetic resonance imaging (MRI), are essential to accurately quantify the version angle of both the acetabulum and femur and evaluate the articular cartilage and acetabular labrum, respectively.[3,4]

Reverse Periacetabular Osteotomy

Acetabular overcoverage is a diagnosis made by clinical examination and imaging analysis. Patients frequently complain of impingement-related difficulties, including pain with sitting and impact activities. There are frequent findings of anterior impingement on examination with pain during flexion and internal rotation of the hip. In severe cases, patients can present with significant limitations to hip motions including flexion, abduction, and internal rotation.

Radiographic findings in these patients indicate global acetabular overcoverage. AP pelvis radiographs will show elevated lateral acetabular coverage (LCEA >35, Tönnis <0), high anterior and posterior wall indices, and coxa profunda or protrusion. False profile radiographs will similarly show anterior overcoverage. The proximal femur morphology on both AP pelvis and Dunn lateral radiographs should be noted, but cam-type deformity is infrequently encountered in the presence of a truly overcovered acetabulum.[5] Cross-sectional studies, specifically CT scans, are beneficial in these patients to accurately identify the bony pathomorphology. CT is particularly helpful by its 3-D reconstructions that help define the size of the lunate cartilage in deep hips. Large lunate hips may be managed with acetabular rim trimming, but small lunate hips are better suited with a reorientation acetabular osteotomy.[6,7]

SURGICAL TECHNIQUE

The positioning, approach, and osteotomy technique for both the anteverting and reverse PAO procedures mirror those of the standard PAO for acetabular dysplasia.[8] An in-depth description of this surgical technique is presented in Chapter 5, but a brief description of this procedure will be. After completion of all osteotomies, the reorientation of the acetabulum for both anteverting and reverse PAOs differ from the traditional PAO and are discussed in greater depth in this chapter.

Positioning and Preparation

Patients undergoing PAO should be placed supine on a radiolucent (ie Jackson) table. Typically, a combination of general anesthesia without motor paralysis and a lumbar plexus block catheter are used. A urinary catheter is placed prior to prep and drape. We typically use a blood collection suction device allowing us an autologous transfusion at the end of surgery.

Approach

A modified Smith-Peterson approach is utilized through a bikini incision to access the hip and pelvis for the periacetabular osteotomies. Briefly, the aponeurosis of the abdominal musculature is elevated from the iliac wing, and the iliac periosteum is sharply divided and elevated medially, giving access to the lateral window of the ilioinguinal approach. Next, the interval between the tensor fascia lata and the sartorius is developed with care to avoid violation of the sartorial compartment in an effort to preserve the lateral femoral cutaneous nerve. This interval is developed proximally to the pelvis, where the sartorius insertion is osteotomized at the anterior superior iliac spine, allowing it to be elevated medially. The distal extent of this interval is typically the ascending branch of the lateral femoral circumflex artery, which should be preserved.

The rectus femoris tendon and iliocapsularis muscle is found at the base of the tensor/sartorius interval. The iliocapsularis is elevated off the rectus tendon and the underlying joint capsule in a lateral to medial direction, with its proximal fibers being released from the anterior inferior iliac spine. As the iliocapsularis is elevated medially, flexion of the hip will facilitate mobilization of both the iliocapsularis muscle and psoas musculotendinous unit. Ultimately, these must be medialized beyond the level of the pubic eminence. The periosteum of the iliac and pubic bones is divided and elevated to the level of the ischial spine medially. Distally, the interval between the hip capsule and the psoas is developed by blunt dissection, allowing access for the first osteotomy cut of the ischium.

Osteotomies

A total of four periacetabular osteotomies are made in order to completely mobilize the acetabular fragment. The typical sequence of osteotomy is the ischial, pubic, iliac, and posterior column. The ischial osteotomy is done under fluoroscopic guidance, using a 30° angled chisel (Ganz osteotome). The goal of this step is an incomplete osteotomy of the ischium (leaving a segment of posterior column bone intact) immediately distal to the hip capsule insertion. This osteotomy will eventually be joined by the posterior column osteotomy.

The pubic osteotomy is made just medial to the pubic eminence and can be made with a variety of tools (Gigli saw, osteotome, burr), but our preference is the Gigli saw. The periosteum of the pubic ramus is elevated both anteriorly and posteriorly around the superior ramus, and retractors are placed to avoid injury to the nearby obturator nerve and vessels. The Gigli saw is passed from anterior to posterior around the ramus using a silk passing suture. Unlike the traditional PAO technique, the pubic osteotomy should have a slight reverse obliquity, allowing the fragment to rotate without impingement of the pubic segments.

The iliac osteotomy is performed with an oscillating saw. First, the ideal starting point for the posterior column cut is identified via fluoroscopy. Next, a small (1-cm) incision is made along the abductor insertion on the lateral ilium in line with the posterior column starting point, and a narrow Hohmann retractor is inserted along the lateral ilium to protect the gluteal muscles. The osteotomy is started at the lateral ilium and is directed toward the pelvic brim in a line perpendicular to the body's longitudinal axis, aiming for the posterior column starting point. For anteverting PAOs, a standard iliac cut suffices. For true reverse PAOs, rounding of the junction of the iliac and posterior column osteotomies is beneficial for later fragment reorientation and can be facilitated with a curved osteotome.

Last, the posterior column osteotomy is created using a variety of osteotomes to connect the iliac and ischial osteotomies. First, a narrow straight osteotome is used to start the medial cut of the posterior column, using manual palpation and fluoroscopy to guide the cut. The medial cut is finished with the 30° Ganz osteotome to the level of the ischial osteotomy. Next, the iliac/posterior column corner is completely osteotomized with the Ganz osteotome. After freeing this corner, a laminar spreader is inserted to put tension across the iliac osteotomy. The lateral aspect of the posterior column cut is then made with the 30° Ganz osteotome, connecting distally to the ischial

Clinical Scenario

A 24-year-old female presented for evaluation of bilateral hip pain, left more symptomatic than the right, which had become significantly worse over a 2-year period. She had tried and failed multiple rounds of physical therapy to improve gluteal strength and pelvic positioning. She had impingement symptoms with pain on flexion (90°) and internal rotation (10°). She was evaluated with radiographs (**Figure 14.1A, B**) and an MRI. Her radiographs demonstrated acetabular retroversion with a large crossover sign, posterior wall sign, and ischial spine sign. All of these were most notable on her supine AP pelvis radiograph but also present on standing films. Her acetabuli had borderline lateral (23° LCEA, 8° Tönnis) and anterior coverage (20° ACEA). She had a spherical femoral head on AP imaging as well as a lateral image (not shown). MRI indicated acetabular retroversion and mild degenerative changes within the acetabular labrum, but the femoral and acetabular cartilage appeared normal. Taken together, her morphology was considered consistent with a retroverted acetabulum causing femoroacetabular impingement. She was considered a candidate for an anteverting PAO for acetabular redirection.

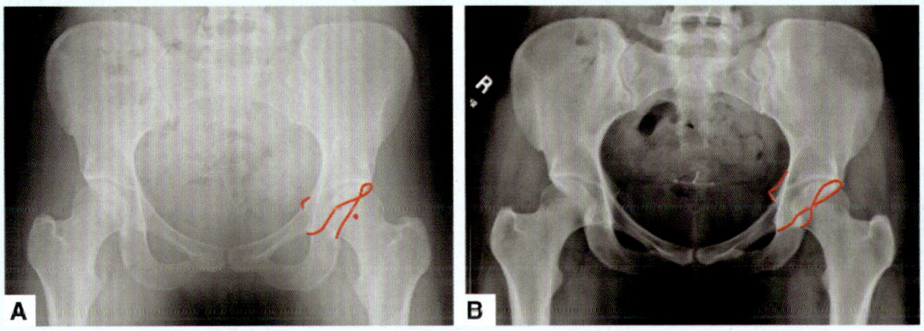

FIGURE 14.1. Supine (A) and standing (B) anteroposterior pelvis radiographs showing the presence of a crossover sign, posterior wall sign, and ischial spine sign on both views.

osteotomy. At this point, the acetabular fragment should be completely freed from the remainder of the pelvis with an intact portion of the posterior column remaining.

Reorientation and Fixation

Anteverting Periacetabular Osteotomy

The goal of an anteverting PAO is to only change the acetabular version with minimal effect on the anterior and lateral coverage of the femoral head. In order to effectively antevert the acetabulum, it is absolutely essential that the acetabular fragment be completely free from the pelvis. Inserting a Schanz screw helps to mobilize the fragment and ensure its free rotation. **Figure 14.2** shows the positioning of the acetabular fragment before and after the anteversion displacement was performed. To achieve this, the first step involves displacing the acetabular fragment's superomedial corner (at the junction of the iliac and posterior column cuts) posterior to the inner table of the iliac osteotomy cut on the stable pelvis (**Figure 14.3**).

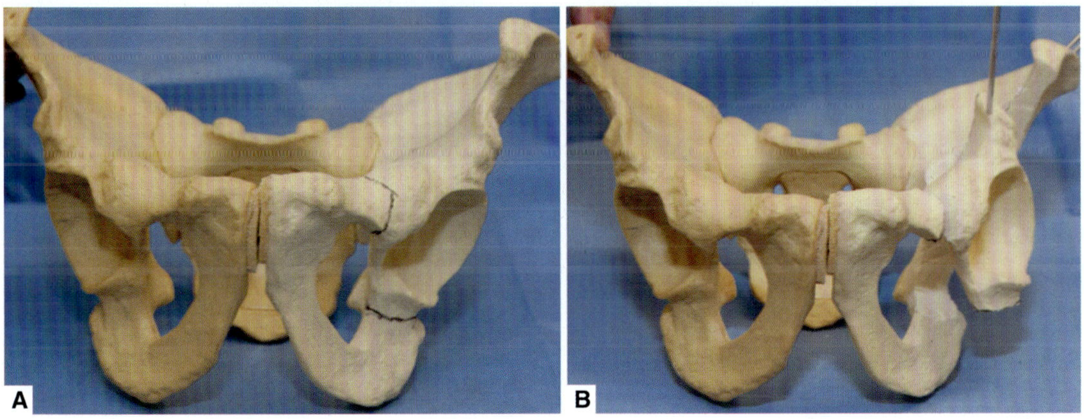

FIGURE 14.2. Diagram of the acetabular position pre- (A) and post reduction (B) during an anteverting PAO.

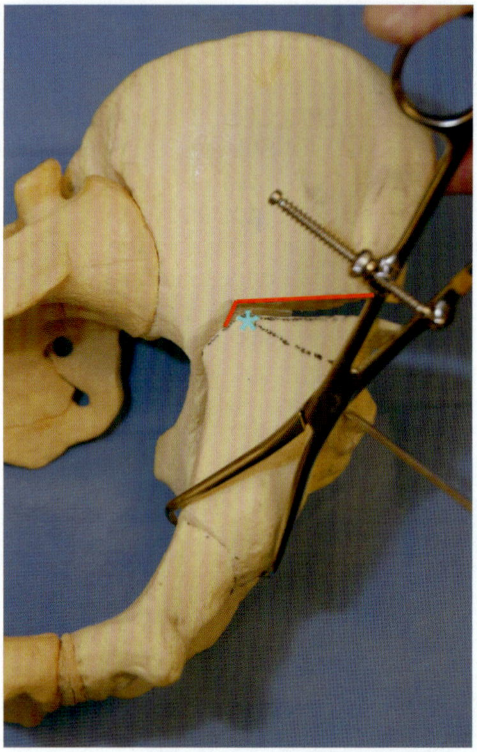

FIGURE 14.3. Diagram of the first step in anteverting PAO reorientation. The superomedial corner (blue star) of the acetabular fragment must be mobilized and displaced medial to the inner table of the iliac osteotomy to allow acetabular anteversion.

The lamina spreader is inserted into the superomedial corner and is gradually rotated as tension is applied. Once this is accomplished, it is possible to apply medial rotation of the acetabular fragment (ie anteversion) through the Schanz screw without resulting in displacement of the hip joint's center of rotation (**Figure 14.4**). The fragment can be provisionally fixed with two 3/32″ k-wires, and fluoroscopic images can be obtained.

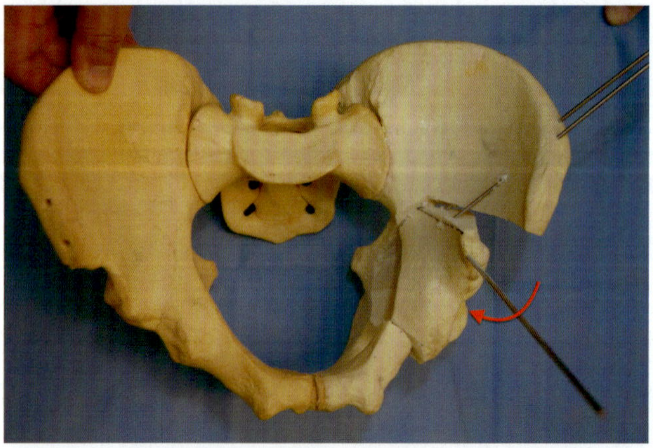

FIGURE 14.4. The acetabulum is anteverted by pure medial rotation of the Schanz pin (red arrow) to perform a purely anteverting reorientation of the acetabulum.

Fluoroscopic technique is essential in assessing the fragment position. The C-arm should be brought into an AP view of the operative hip with the "boom" of the C-arm in a fully extended position. The "boom" is then pulled back toward the midline for an AP pelvis view while the C-arm's base is kept in a fixed position. Care must be taken to ensure that the tip of the coccyx is in perfect alignment with the pubic symphysis so that no artificial rotation is being projected, and subtle rotational adjustments of the imaging arm can be done to accomplish this. Once the perfect rotational view is obtained, the C-arm base is again left in position while the "boom" is again fully extended to center on the operative hip.

With this radiographic view, the position of the anteverted acetabulum can be assessed.

The goals of reduction are as follows:

- No crossover sign
- No posterior wall sign
- AWI 30% to 40%, PWI 90%
- LCEA 28° to 33°, Tönnis 3° to 10°
- Note: Ischial spine sign will not change

Once the appropriate acetabular correction is achieved, a third 3/32″ k-wire is inserted. These wires will all be sequentially exchanged for 3.5-mm or 4.5-mm cortical screws. When performing an anteverting PAO, it is important to exchange the middle k-wire for a cortical screw first in order to maximize the rotational control while placing this initial screw. After the acetabular fragment is fixed with cortical screws, hip range of motion should be assessed. Internal rotation at 90° of flexion should specifically be observed, and lack of motion (<30°) is likely indicative of a cam-type proximal femoral deformity.[9] The cam lesion can be addressed by an anterior capsulotomy through the PAO approach.

Case Resolution

Bilateral anteverting periacetabular osteotomies were performed for the diagnosis of femoroacetabular impingement due to acetabular retroversion. Most recent radiographs (**Figure 14.5**) at 1 year show healed left periacetabular

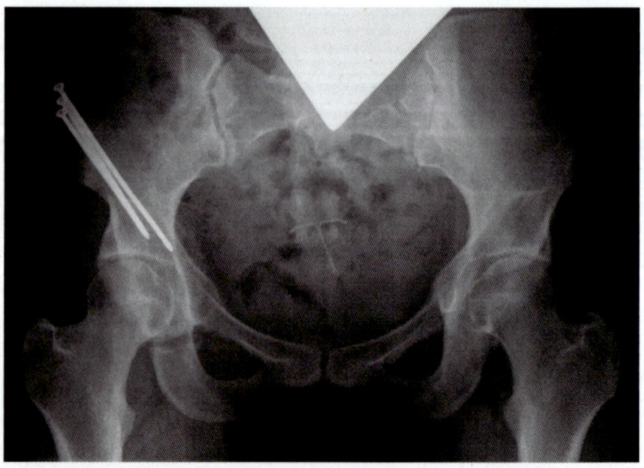

FIGURE 14.5. Postoperative radiographs at 1 year (left hip) and 4 months (right hip) following anteverting periacetabular osteotomies.

osteotomy site and progressive healing of the right osteotomy (4 months out) with improved acetabular version and coverage. Her motion is significantly improved with flexion to 100° and easy internal rotation to 30° in flexion.

Reverse Periacetabular Osteotomy

The goal of a reverse PAO is to reduce both anterior and lateral acetabular coverage in a globally overcovered hip. Again, the acetabular fragment must be completely free to rotate prior to attempted reorientation. A Schanz screw is inserted, as for a traditional PAO; however, in reverse PAOs it is placed with a trajectory parallel to the acetabular sourcil, as seen on the false profile view. This will place the Schanz screw at an oblique angle to the iliac osteotomy (**Figure 14.8**). After the fragment is fully mobilized and the Schanz screw is in place, the reduction maneuver can be started.

The order of correction in these hips is (1) anteversion, (2) uncover laterally, and (3) uncover anteriorly. Lateral and anterior coverage are linked, so changing lateral coverage may effectively reduce anterior coverage. To achieve anteversion and reduce lateral coverage, the superomedial corner of the acetabular fragment must be rotated into a position posterior to the iliac wing's inner table and is impacted medially into this corner. "Rounding" of the junction between the iliac and the posterior column osteotomies facilitates this maneuver, which can be accomplished during the osteotomy or afterward by the use of a rongeur to contour this junction (**Figure 14.9**). The Schanz pin, which is a surrogate of anterior coverage, should reorient into a more perpendicular relationship with the body following this maneuver (**Figure 14.10A, B**). The acetabular fragment can be pinned in this position with 3/32″ k-wires. AP and false profile radiographs can be obtained to check correction.

Clinical Scenario

A 38-year-old female presented for evaluation of bilateral hip pain, left more symptomatic than the right, which was significantly exacerbated by an increase in running mileage while training for a marathon. She had impingement symptoms with pain on flexion (90°) and internal rotation (0°). She was evaluated with radiographs (**Figure 14.6A, B**), MRI, and a CT scan (**Figure 14.7**). Her radiographs demonstrated protrusio with acetabular overcoverage (LCEA: 46°), a down-sloping acetabular sourcil (Tönnis angle −10°), and a spherical femoral head. MRI indicated degenerative changes within the acetabular labrum, but the femoral and acetabular cartilage appeared normal. CT scan was noteworthy for a large cotyloid fossa, best appreciated on 3-dimensional reconstructions. Taken together, her morphology was considered consistent with a deep, small lunate hip. She was considered a candidate for a reverse PAO for acetabular redirection.

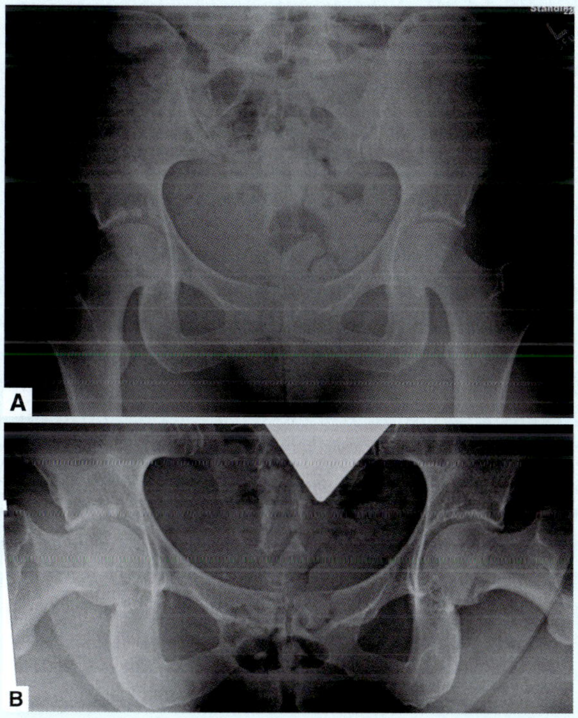

FIGURE 14.6. A and B: Standing anteroposterior and 45 Dunn lateral views showing acetabular protrusion and overcoverage with spherical femoral heads.

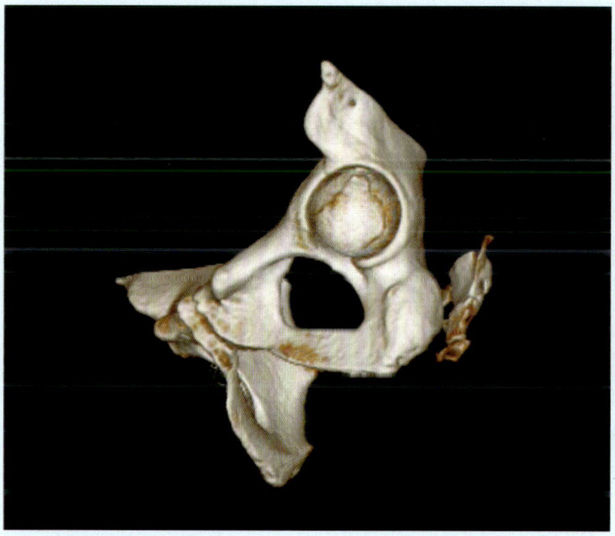

FIGURE 14.7. 3-Dimensional CT reconstruction showing a large acetabular cotyloid fossa in the setting of a deep hip.

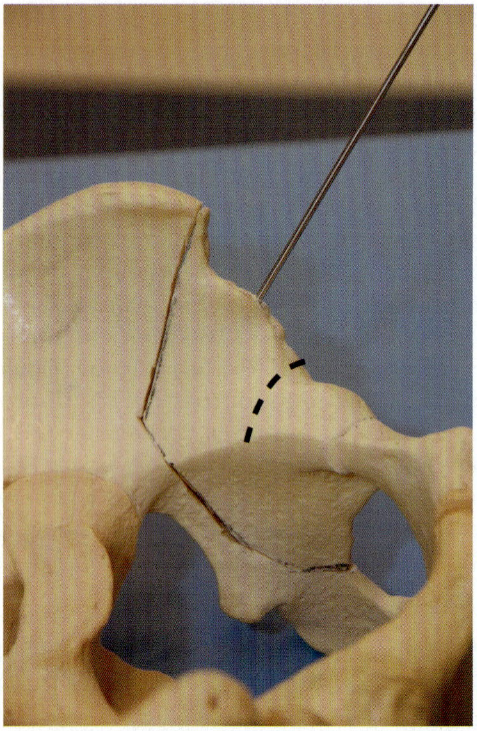

FIGURE 14.8. Pelvic model shown from a false profile view. The Schanz pin is inserted parallel to the acetabular sourcil (dashed line) in this view during the reverse PAO.

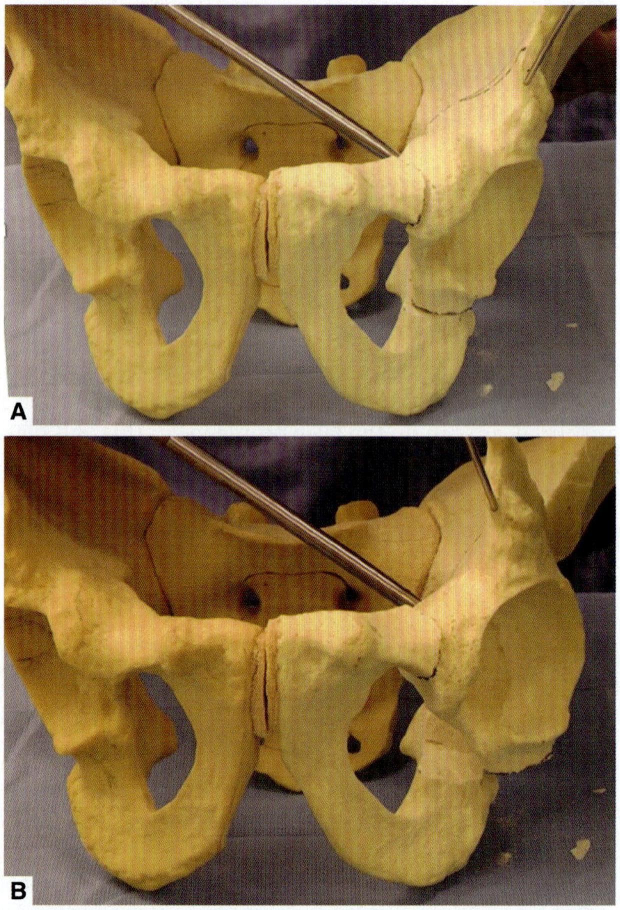

FIGURE 14.10. A, Anteroposterior view of the pelvic model after all osteotomies have been completed and a Schanz pin inserted. B, The acetabular fragment is reoriented with increased anteversion and decreased lateral coverage. The Schanz pin is rotated medially and more perpendicular to the axial skeleton during this maneuver.

If lateral coverage has been effectively reduced but anterior coverage remains excessive, a wedge of iliac bone should be resected from the acetabular fragment parallel to the Schanz pin (**Figure 14.11**). After resection and closure of this osteotomy, the Schanz pin should be fully perpendicular to the body, indicating adequate improvement of the anterior coverage (**Figure 14.12A, B**). This should not overly influence the lateral coverage. The acetabular fragment can again be fixed in this position, and repeat AP and false profile images can be obtained. In cases where an iliac wedge is resected, after fragment reduction there is typically a gap in the osteotomy sites at the posterior column. This area is at risk for settling with weight-bearing activity. To prevent this occurrence, we recommend bone grafting of this defect (the iliac wedge segment can be morselized and used) and strategically placing acetabular fragment fixation in an oblique orientation (**Figure 14.13**) as well as the use of larger 4.5-mm screws for fixation.

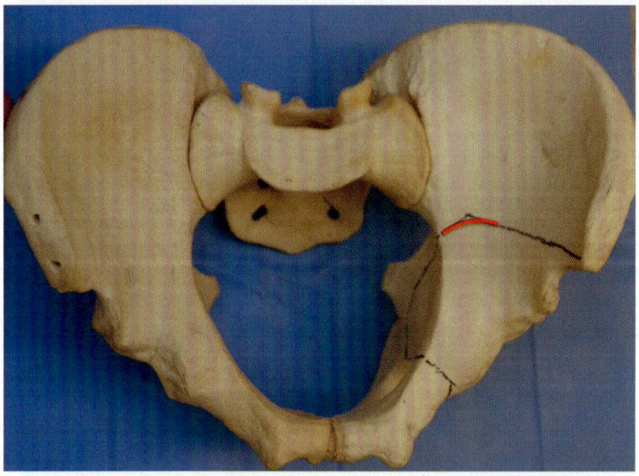

FIGURE 14.9. The red line indicates the ideal "rounded" connection between the iliac and posterior column cuts to facilitate reorientation. This can be performed with a curved chisel at the time of creating the iliac cut or by use of a rongeur after completion of all four osteotomies.

After fragment fixation, range of motion should again be assessed, specifically flexion-internal rotation (FIR) and extension-external rotation (EER). Diminished FIR is unlikely following the acetabular reorientation procedure because cam-type deformities are fairly uncommon in overcovered hips.[5] Diminished EER can be encountered in certain cases where acetabular reorientation results in

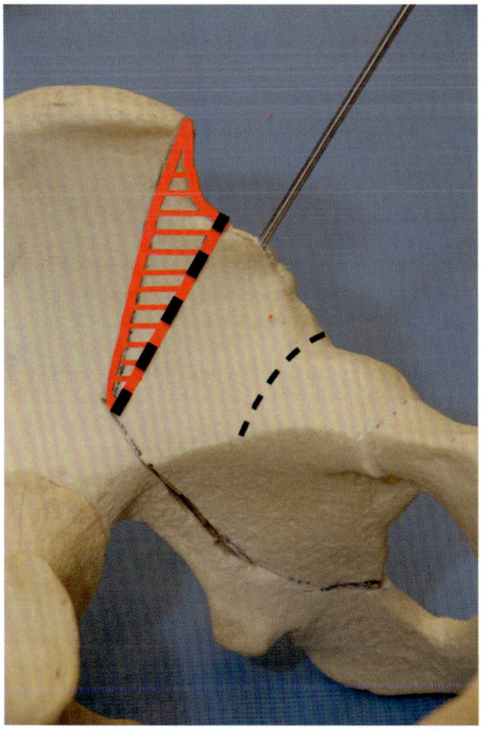

FIGURE 14.11. In cases with persistently increased anterior coverage on the false profile radiograph following initial acetabular reorientation, an iliac wedge (red hashmarks) can be resected to facilitate a decrease in anterior coverage on the fase profile radiograph.

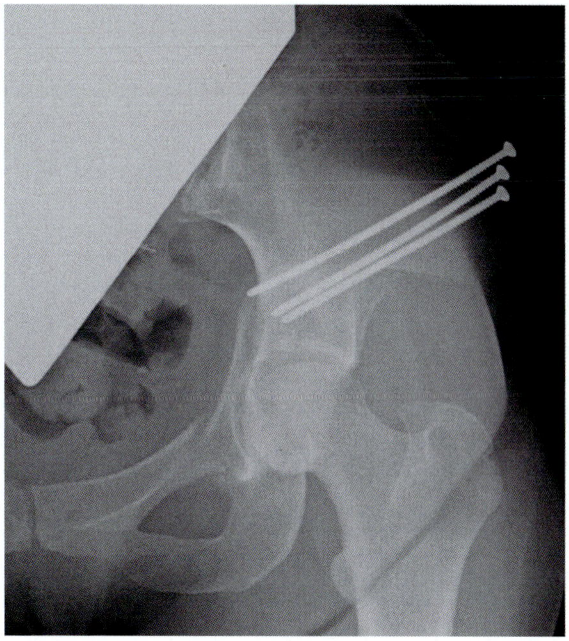

FIGURE 14.13. Acetabular fragment fixated by three cortical screws with an oblique trajectory to stabilize the fragment and prevent settling at the iliac osteotomy site.

overcoverage of the acetabulum's posterior wall, which can result in posterior impingement. In these cases, an additional surgical dislocation with posterior-inferior rim resection may be considered on a case-by-case basis.

Case Resolution

Bilateral reverse periacetabular osteotomies were performed for the diagnosis of femoroacetabular impingement due to deep, small lunate hips. Most recent radiographs (Figure 14.14) at 6 years show healed osteotomy sites with diminished anterior and lateral coverage. She is now 7 years out from the reverse PAOs and has returned to running at a high level. She continues to train for and participate in marathons on an annual basis.

OUTCOMES

Anteverting Periacetabular Osteotomy

Siebenrock et al have the largest series of anteverting periacetabular osteotomies for symptomatic acetabular retroversion.[9,10] They showed significant improvement

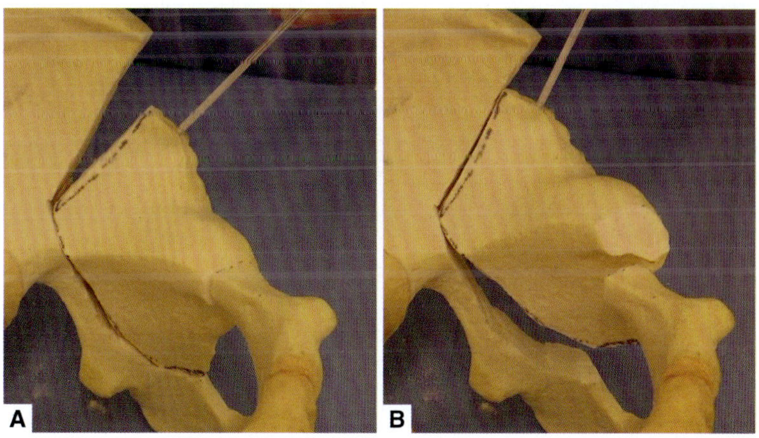

FIGURE 14.12. Correction of excessive anterior coverage in a pelvic model. A, False profile view of the hemipelvis after iliac wedge resection. B, The Schanz pin is brought into a position perpendicular to the axial skeleton, closing the gap after wedge resection to decrease anterior coverage.

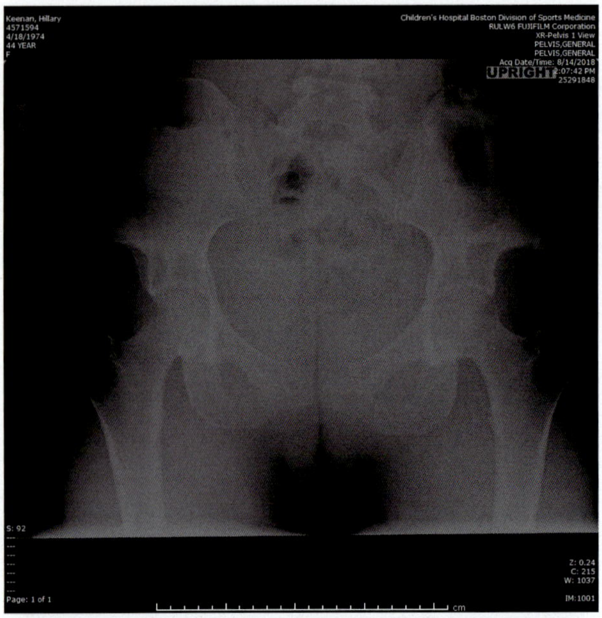

FIGURE 14.14. 6-year postoperative anteroposterior pelvis radiograph after bilateral reverse periacetabular osteotomies showing united osteotomies, maintenance of diminished lateral acetabular coverage, and preserved joint space.

in subjective scores and range of motion following surgery. At a mean 10-year follow-up, no hips had undergone conversion to a total hip arthroplasty, although 29% were experiencing pain and/or dysfunction or had required a secondary hip procedure. The majority of these patients were also treated with a proximal femoral osteoplasty at the time of PAO.

Reverse Periacetabular Osteotomy

True reverse PAOs for global acetabular overcoverage are infrequently reported in the literature. Pun et al have the largest case series of 31 hips in 26 patients with short-term outcomes data.[11] Reverse PAO showed improvements in subjective scores, range of motion, and radiographic appearance of coverage at an average of 30 months postoperatively.

REFERENCES

1. Steppacher SD, Albers CE, Siebenrock KA, Tannast M, Ganz R. Femoroacetabular impingement predisposes to traumatic posterior hip dislocation. *Clin Orthop Relat Res.* 2013;471(6):1937-1943.
2. Tannast M, Pfannebecker P, Schwab JM, Albers CE, Siebenrock KA, Buchler L. Pelvic morphology differs in rotation and obliquity between developmental dysplasia of the hip and retroversion. *Clin Orthop Relat Res.* 2012;470(12):3297-3305.
3. Murphy SB, Simon SR, Kijewski PK, Wilkinson RH, Griscom NT. Femoral anteversion. *J Bone Joint Surg Am.* 1987;69(8):1169-1176.
4. Anda S, Svenningsen S, Dale LG, Benum P. The acetabular sector angle of the adult hip determined by computed tomography. *Acta Radiol Diagn (Stockh).* 1986;27(4):443-447.
5. Steppacher SD, Tannast M, Werlen S, Siebenrock KA. Femoral morphology differs between deficient and excessive acetabular coverage. *Clin Orthop Relat Res.* 2008;466(4):782-790.
6. Pun SY, Hingsammer A, Millis MB, Kim YJ. Is Increased acetabular cartilage or fossa size associated with pincer femoroacetabular impingement? *Clin Orthop Relat Res.* 2017;475(4):1013-1023.
7. Steppacher SD, Lerch TD, Gharanizadeh K, et al. Size and shape of the lunate surface in different types of pincer impingement: theoretical implications for surgical therapy. *Osteoarth Cartilage.* 2014;22(7):951-958.
8. Matheney T, Kim YJ, Zurakowski D, Matero C, Millis M. Intermediate to long-term results following the bernese periacetabular osteotomy and predictors of clinical outcome: surgical technique. *J Bone Joint Surg Am.* 2010;92(1):115-129.
9. Siebenrock KA, Schaller C, Tannast M, Keel M, Buchler L. Anteverting periacetabular osteotomy for symptomatic acetabular retroversion: results at ten years. *J Bone Joint Surg Am.* 2014;96(21):1785-1792.
10. Siebenrock KA, Schoeniger R, Ganz R. Anterior femoro-acetabular impingement due to acetabular retroversion. Treatment with periacetabular osteotomy. *J Bone Joint Surg Am.* 2003;85(2):278-286.
11. Pun SY, Merz M, Bowen G, et al. Periacetabular osteotomy to uncover the hip: uncommon variations on a common procedure. *J Hip Preserv Surg.* 2016;3(1).

CHAPTER 15

Nonarticular Hip Pain With a Special Focus on Hip Ultrasonography

INTRODUCTION

Pediatric patients with complex hip pain can be challenging to care for in many ways, as the exact source of pain is often difficult to discern. Extra-articular hip pain in young active children is common, with many possible etiologies. Teasing out pain generators clinically is often one of the most difficult jobs of the clinician caring for young patients with hip pain. Understanding the interplay between the biomechanics of the hip in young children and injury patterns, especially during periods of growth and development, is critical for making an accurate diagnosis and treatment plan of care. Pediatric athletes, in this light, place high physical demands on the hip joint routinely, including increased mechanical load to the physis, as in the ice hockey athlete and gymnast, and supraphysiologic ranges of motion, as in the dancer. Furthermore, rapid periods of growth and development result in peripelvic strength and flexibility imbalances. A comprehensive physical examination of the hip and peripelvic structures is a critical requirement in the care of patients with hip pain and extra-articular pathology. Overreliability on diagnostic studies is problematic because the prevalence of an asymptomatic bony deformity may be as high as 37% and up to 55% in athletes versus 23% in the general population.[1]

Nonoperative care of the patient includes a thorough history, comprehensive knowledge of physical examination technique, and proper diagnostic testing. Dynamic hip ultrasonography and selective diagnostic and therapeutic ultrasound (US)-guided injections now play an important role in the assessment and treatment of young patients with hip pain and injury. The aim of this chapter is to review the evaluation and treatment of pediatric patients with extra-articular hip pain, including the role of diagnostic and dynamic ultrasonography and selective injections.

ILIOPSOAS AND RECTUS FEMORIS TENDINITIS

Injury to the hip flexor tendons in young active children is a common cause of extra-articular hip pain. In athletes that rely heavily on the hip joint for speed and skill, injuries to the hip flexor tendons can be even more prevalent. For example, in soccer, groin injuries account for 8% to 18% of all injuries, with an incidence of 0.4 to 1.3 groin injuries per 1000 hours of exposure.[2-7] The iliopsoas musculotendinous unit is located directly anterior to the hip joint and is composed of the iliacus, psoas major, and psoas minor.[8,9] The most common cause of groin injury stems from the adductor, followed by the iliopsoas.[7,10-12] The iliopsoas has recently been implicated in 25% of acute groin injuries.[2] Other studies have, similarly, indicated that iliopsoas disorders were found in 25% to 30% of athletes with acute groin injury and 12% to 36% of athletes with chronic groin pain.[2,8,13,14] Common injury mechanisms for injury to the iliopsoas involve kicking, sprinting, and change of direction in sports such as soccer, basketball, and handball.[2,13] In artistic performing athletes, repetitive and extreme range of hip flexion is often inherent to the discipline. Injury and pain related to a snapping iliopsoas, also known as the "dancer's tendon" was found in 58% of dancers.[15] If not diagnosed and treated appropriately, iliopsoas injuries can become chronic and greatly impair sport performance.[7,10,14]

The anatomy of the iliopsoas complex includes the confluence of three main structures, namely, the iliacus, psoas major, and psoas minor.[8] The main origin of the psoas major includes the vertebral bodies, intervertebral discs, and transverse processes of T12-L5.[0] The psoas minor originates from the vertebral bodies of T12 to L1 and is present in roughly 60 to 65% of individuals.[16] Recent cadaveric studies have identified five individual muscle bundles comprising the iliopsoas muscle complex,[17] and

US studies have documented four of the five bundles reported in cadaveric studies.[18] Cadaveric studies have reported a bifid tendon in up to 4 out of 24 cases,[17] and magnetic resonance (MR) studies of children revealed bifid tendon anatomy in 26% of cases imaged and bilateral bifid tendon anatomy in 14% of cases.[19]

The anatomy of the rectus femoris involves a confluence of two main tendon insertions, designated as the direct head and indirect head. A third head is described arising from the inferior edge of the indirect tendon, merging superficially with the gluteus minimus muscle and deeply with the lateral iliofemoral ligament.[20]

The comprehensive examination of the iliopsoas/rectus femoris complex is performed in both a static and a dynamic manner. Notably, significant variations exist concerning physical examination tests performed by hip specialists and interpretation of the findings. Careful palpation of the anterior soft tissue structures is an important component of the hip examination. Hammoud et al.[21] bring to light the layered complex structures of the hip and the importance of recognizing compensatory injury patterns associated with hip joint pathology. In this light, pain with palpation of the iliopsoas tendon complex may be indicative of iliopsoas tendinitis, iliopsoas bursitis/impingement, and or injury and inflammation of the underlying joint structures. Taken together with dynamic provocative physical examination tests and US static and dynamic imaging, clinicians can improve the accuracy of diagnosis in patients with complex hip pain.

The hip tests most commonly performed consistently include flexion external and internal range of motion (ROM); log roll; flexion, adduction, internal rotation (FADIR); straight leg raise against resistance (Stinchfield test); flexion, abduction, external rotation (FABER), femoral anteversion analysis, and standing gait analysis.[22] Of these maneuvers, the Stinchfield test is a test of iliopsoas strength, as well as a sign of inter-articular pathology, as the psoas places pressure on the underlying structures, including the acetabular labrum.[22] Other helpful tests for iliopsoas pathology include hip extension internal rotation (iliopsoas stretch test), FABER against resistance, and seated resisted straight leg raise (Ludloff test).

Injury to the rectus femoris may present as pain anteriorly, in the case of injury to the direct head and conjoined tendon, and laterally, in the case of injury to the indirect head. Palpation of the direct head along with selective provocation tests for pain, including seated hip flexion against resistance, and Ludloff test, can help support or negate injury to the rectus tendon. Clinically, injury to the rectus femoris complex may present with insidious onset of anterior pain with chronic injury, inflammation, and tear versus acute traumatic rupture of the direct head, with swelling, deformity, and pain anteriorly.

Clinical management of iliopsoas/rectus femoris pathology consists of rest, activity modification, nonsteroidal anti-inflammatories, physical therapy, and corticosteroid injections.[8] In cases where there is notable tendinopathy, emphasis on eccentric strengthening is important. When nonoperative treatment is unsuccessful, iliopsoas tendon release, along with correction of existing underlying Intra-articular (IA) abnormality can be performed.[8,23-27]

ILIOPSOAS IMPINGEMENT AND SNAPPING

Iliopsoas impingement commonly occurs in active young females, and is provoked by activities involving hip flexor tendon use, including walking distances, stair climbing and prolonged sitting ordriving.[8] Iliopsoas snapping is more common in females[24] and has been reported to occur in up to approximately 60% of elite-level dancers[15] and 5 to 10% in the general population.[28] Physical examination reveals a pain with hip excursion, positive impingement test, positive scour test, iliopsoas provocative tests, including Stinchfield and Ludloff testing. Commonly, there is tenderness to palpation directly over the anterior hip and iliopsoas complex.

Dynamic US evaluation can be very helpful in making the diagnosis. Dynamic hip excursion may reveal iliopsoas tendon snapping over the iliopectineal eminence when the patient flexes, abducts, externally rotates, and extends the hip.[28] Deslandes et al. describes movement of the iliopsoas tendon abruptly into the iliopsoas muscle complex during active hip motion.[29] Iliopsoas impingement refers to anterior labral injury seen during arthroscopy, as a result of impingement and trauma to the labrum by the iliopsoas tendon.[30] Iliopsoas impingement may be demonstrated using dynamic ultrasonography of the hip joint during hip flexion and may show compression of the acetabular labrum by the muscle tendon unit of the iliopsoas and/or rectus femoris. Domb et al. identified 25 patients with direct anterior labral tears at the 3 o'clock position (right hip) in the absence of bony abnormalities.[31] Similarly, Blankenbaker et al. reported MR findings of iliopsoas impingement in patients diagnosed during hip arthroscopy and found that the labral injury typically occurs at the 3 o'clock position.[30] Labral tears occurring at the 3 o'clock position should therefore suggest iliopsoas impingement, especially in the setting of female athletes with normal bony anatomy.

The iliopsoas bursa is a potential space that lies just deep to the iliopsoas muscle tendon complex and superficial to the joint. The iliopsoas bursa is often compressed with repetitive hip motion, resulting in thickening and irritation to the underlying structure. The iliopsoas bursa has been reported to communicate with the underlying joint in 15% of people.[8] US imaging of the hip is very useful for imaging of the iliopsoas bursa in both the transverse and sagittal planes. Iliopsoas bursitis appears as thickening of the bursa with or without the presence of a hypoechoic center, signifying the presence of fluid.

The normal US anatomy has been documented with four bundles of the iliopsoas muscle (inferior, medial, lateral, ilioinfratrochanteric muscle) seen in all study subjects, with the psoas major tendon depicted as a thick hyperechoic ovoid structure, when imaged in the transverse plane, resting against the anterior aspect of the superior pubic ramus, acetabular rim, or the upper coxofemoral joint capsule.[18]

Iliopsoas peritendinous injection with US guidance for diagnostic and therapeutic reasons is useful and safe when performed by an experienced sonographer. Iliopsoas peritendinous injections have been shown to provide both short-term (6 weeks)[32] and sustained (2 to 10 months) pain relief.[33]

US of the rectus femoris complex begins with the anterior hip and direct tendon in the neutral position. The axial plane depicts the direct head nicely, beginning at the anterior superior iliac spine (ASIS) and progressing to the anterior inferior iliac spine (AIIS). Imaging the tendon in the longitudinal plane is important and can be done by rotating the transducer 90° in the sagittal plane. This view allows for US examination of the insertion of the tendon as well as morphologic characteristics of the AIIS (see subspine impingement section).[20] US of the indirect head can be achieved by scanning at the level of the conjoined tendon in the sagittal plane and applying a curvilinear ascending motion following the path of the indirect head from distal to the origin of the supraacetabular ridge at the lateral hip.[20] A lateral approach to imaging the indirect head has been described scanning the lateral hip in the axial plane, just lateral to the AIIS, and localizing the indirect head deep in the gluteus minimus and medius muscles and overlying the supraacetabular ridge and lateral iliofemoral ligament.[20,34] Bianchi et al. utilized cadaveric anatomic dissection of the rectus femoris to confirm the presence of the central aponeurosis as a sagittally oriented fibrous band located within the proximal two-thirds of the muscle belly. This same study has been described in vitro US showing the central aponeurosis as a curvilinear hyperechoic structure.[35]

Bianchi et al. further describe the US findings of injury to the rectus femoris tendon in three ways; a hyperechoic band surrounding an intact central aponeurosis; mixed hypo- and hyperechoic bands surrounding an intact central aponeurosis but associated with globular enlargement of the rectus femoris; and complete discontinuity of the rectus femoris, reflecting small partial tears, larger partial tears, and complete musculotendinous junction tears respectively.[35]

EXTRA-ARTICULAR HIP IMPINGEMENT

Ischiofemoral Impingement

Ischiofemoral impingement (IFI) is characterized by compression of the quadratus femoris muscle between two bony prominences, the femoral lesser trochanter, and the lateral aspect of the ischial tuberosity. The clinical evaluation and assessment of patients with IFI can be complex and challenging because the clinical presentation is nonspecific and pain location can vary with posterior buttock pain to groin or medial thigh pain. Patients with IFI commonly present with deep gluteal pain that may be mild or moderate in severity and that often has a gradual onset.[36] Often, there is no precipitating event, and limitation by patients of sitting time and physical activities, including long-stride walking, are reported.[36] Physical examination tests, as described by Hernando et al.[36] include positive IFI test if pain is provoked when the affected hip is extended and adducted with the patient in the contralateral decubitus position; the long-stride walking test is positive when posterior pain is produced during the terminal phase of gait and relieved by walking with short strides and hip abduction.[36] Concordant pathology that may result is narrowing of the IF space, including hamstring tendinosis with tendon thickening and edema, bone tumors, including osteochondromas, history of fracture, and hip dysplasia, pelvic and spinal instability.[36] Chronic inflammatory changes and adhesions of the quadratus femoris muscle (QFM) area may cause sciatic nerve symptoms and contribute to chronic pain and deep gluteal syndrome.[37]

Diagnostic MR may reveal quadratus muscle atrophy, narrowing of the ischiofemoral (IF) and quadratus femoris space (QFS) as well as quadratus muscle edema.[38,39] Meta-analysis of data by Singer et al. showed that IFI can be diagnosed with 77% accuracy with a combination of clinical symptomatology and MR findings of ischiofemoral space (IFS) measurement of <15 mm.[40] Ultrasound has been shown to accurately assess the IFS when compared to MR imaging in healthy study subjects.[41] US may show hyperemia of the QF space but does not always correlate with MR findings showing IFI.[36,42]

Treatment of IFI should start with, and consistently include, activity modification and peripelvic, spine, and lower extremity stretching and strengthening of the deep hip stabilizers with special attention to the hip abductors and internal rotators, spine and lower abdominals. Nonsteroidal anti-inflammatory medications and corticosteroid injections may have a role in the treatment of IFI. CT-guided anesthetic and corticosteroid injections that provide temporary symptom relief are described in the literature[36,42] Specifically, Backer et al. investigated the effectiveness of US-guided quadratus femoris (QF) injections to treat IFI and found that injection groups had significantly better short-term pain reduction versus controls who did not receive injections for MR-documented IFI.[42]

Anterior Inferior Subspine Impingement

Prominence of the AIIS has been described as a cause of extra-articular hip impingement. Subspine impingement (SSI) causes hip/groin pain and limitation in ROM during hip flexion as the femoral neck impinges on the most caudal aspect of the AIIS.[43] Clinical examination reveals limitation of hip internal rotation, adduction with hip flexion to 90°.[44] Early case reports of subspine impingement in the literature describe athletes (two soccer players and one hockey athlete) with groin pain, sitting intolerance, and limitation in ROM.[45]

Patients with SSI often have a history of prior hip flexor injury during their adolescent years.[44] AIIS bony morphology may be the result of chronic traction injury, acute avulsion fractures, or congenital deformity.[44] Three anatomic types of AIIS morphology have been described on the basis of 3D CT reconstruction data analysis. In Type I, there is a smooth ilium bony wall between the caudal AIIS and the acetabular rim; in Type II the AIIS sits at the level of the acetabular rim with a "rooflike" bony prominence; and in Type III the AIIS extends distally to the anterior superior acetabular rim with a downward bony "spur" appearance.[43] Awareness of SSI, and close attention to AIIS anatomy and the physical examination findings, along with the proper diagnostics including radiographs and US, can help make an accurate diagnosis.

ULTRASOUND UTILIZATION IN THE EVALUATION OF HIP PAIN IN THE YOUNG ATHLETE

US is a useful imaging modality for hip assessment in three respects. The first two comprise static and dynamic imaging. Combining the two methods enhances the understanding of anatomic abnormalities and their potential relationship to pain. Often, it is not until the dynamic exam is performed that a potential abnormality such as a painful snapping psoas tendon is detected. Furthermore, the US exam should be considered complementary to the other images such as plain radiographs, computed tomography, and magnetic resonance imaging (MRI). The third component of the US exam may include the response to diagnostic anesthetic injections into the joint or periarticular tissues. The US hip exam is anatomically divided into the anterior, medial, lateral, and posterior exam. The examination may require changing between the high-frequency linear probes (12 to 5 MHz) and the curvilinear probes (5 to 1 MHz) to accommodate different depths of interest. The combination of all these methods is often useful in detecting the etiology of the painful hip both preoperatively and with the postoperative painful hip.

Anterior Exam

The exam should be done in a routine manner and may progress from the most lateral portion of the anterior exam, the AIIS, across the hip medially. Images are obtained with multiple orthogonal views. The probe may start in the sagittal plane (**Figure 15.1**) with a view of the rectus tendon and the direct head attachment to the AIIS. This view will demonstrate the position of the AIIS in relation to the acetabulum for potential subspine impingement. The classification of AIIS morphology is similar to the CT categories noted previously: Type I with a smooth flat AIIS, Type II with the AIIS to the level of the acetabulum, and Type III below the acetabulum. In this position, one also notes the integrity of the direct head of the rectus attachment for signs of tendinopathy as well as ossification in the tendon. Sono-palpation at this site may elicit pain of the proximal rectus attachment. Once the direct head is visualized, the probe is moved laterally and obliquely to see the indirect head move in a more posterolateral direction to the acetabulum. There is usually much anisotropy of the indirect head as it curves to its deeper position (**Figure 15.2**). If the rectus is in question, the probe is turned 90° to visualize the direct anterior attachment in a short-axis view and rotated laterally to visualize the indirect head.

Next, the probe is moved to a sagittal oblique position in the plane of the femoral neck. In this position, the femoral head, neck, and acetabulum are well visualized (**Figure 15.3**). The anterior synovial recess is also well seen for signs of collection of fluid, which is compressible. Alternatively, it may show synovial thickening, which is noncompressible and may show uptake on color flow doppler. This is best determined by comparing side to side. The labrum is a hyperechoic triangular structure that is well seen.

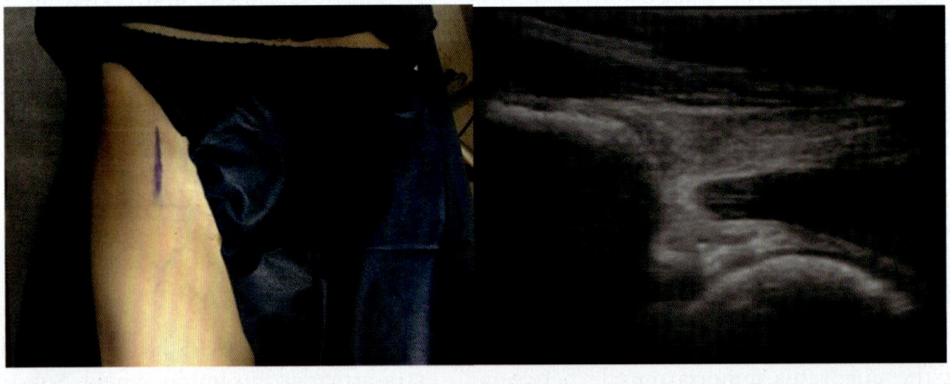

FIGURE 15.1. Sagittal view of the anterior inferior iliac spine with attachment of rectus femoris.

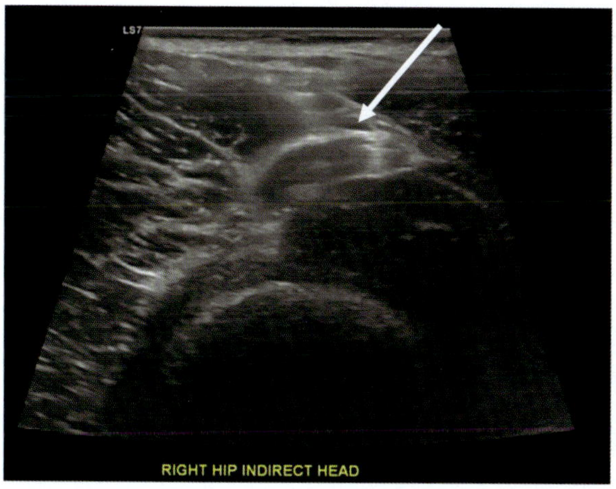

FIGURE 15.2. Reflected head rectus femoris.

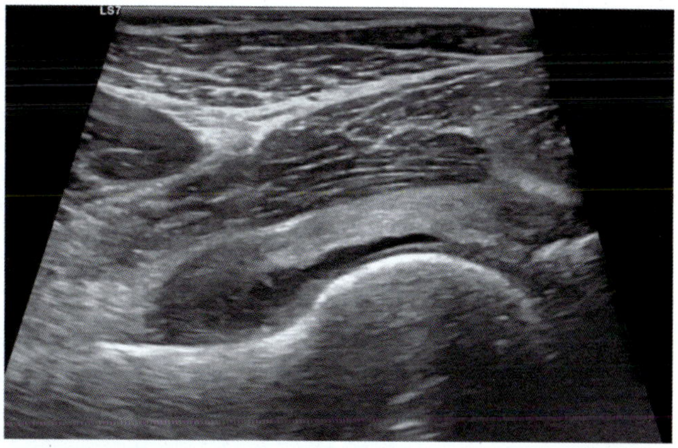

FIGURE 15.3. Sagittal oblique view.

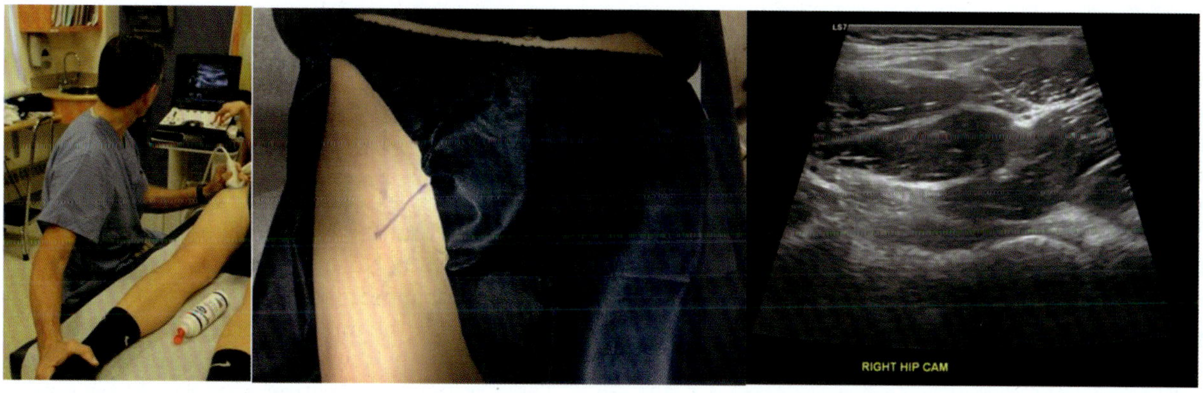

FIGURE 15.4. Sagittal oblique CAM view.

The capsule is superimposed on this. Next, with the probe in this orientation, the labrum is scanned from the area of the rectus medially to the psoas tendon. This is a common area of labral pathology such as degenerative labrum, paralabral cyst and frank labral tears. It must be done with care to avoid anisotropic error in reading. This sagittal oblique position also allows evaluation of a camshaft (CAM) or decreased femoral head-neck offset (**Figure 15.4**). This is enhanced by holding the leg in internal rotation, which brings the superolateral prominence into view.

A transverse axial view is best obtained by turning the probe 90° essentially parallel to the inguinal ligament. In this view, one can appreciate the AIIS and the iliopectineal line. Overlying this is the medial psoas tendon and muscle (**Figure 15.5**). Hypoechoic fluid from an iliopsoas bursitis may be detected under and around the tendon. Moving the probe more distally allows a view of the femoral head and acetabulum. In this position, dynamic examinations are performed.

Anterior Dynamic Examinations

The anterior dynamic examinations include assessment of the snapping hip, impingement, and instability. In the transverse axial view, two dynamic examinations are achieved depending on the clinical scenario. First, a snapping psoas is often seen by holding the probe steadily in this position while asking the supine patient to flex, abduct, and externally rotate the hip. The psoas tendon is seen to move up laterally into the iliopsoas muscle. Next, the patient actively straightens the hip. The psoas tendon is seen to snap out of the muscle onto the iliopectineal line. This may also be noted to reproduce the patient's symptoms.

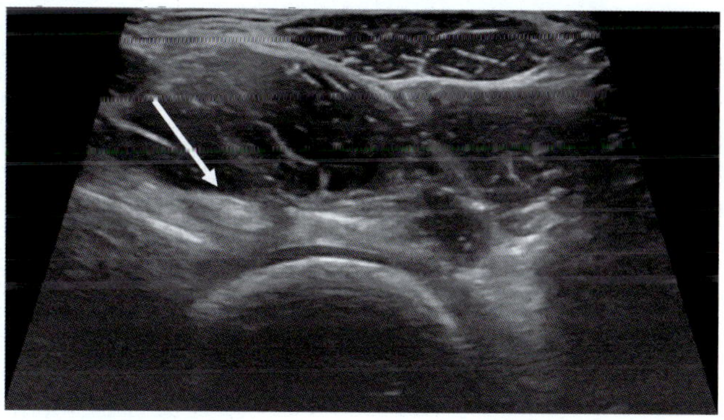

FIGURE 15.5. Hyperechoic psoas tendon on axial view.

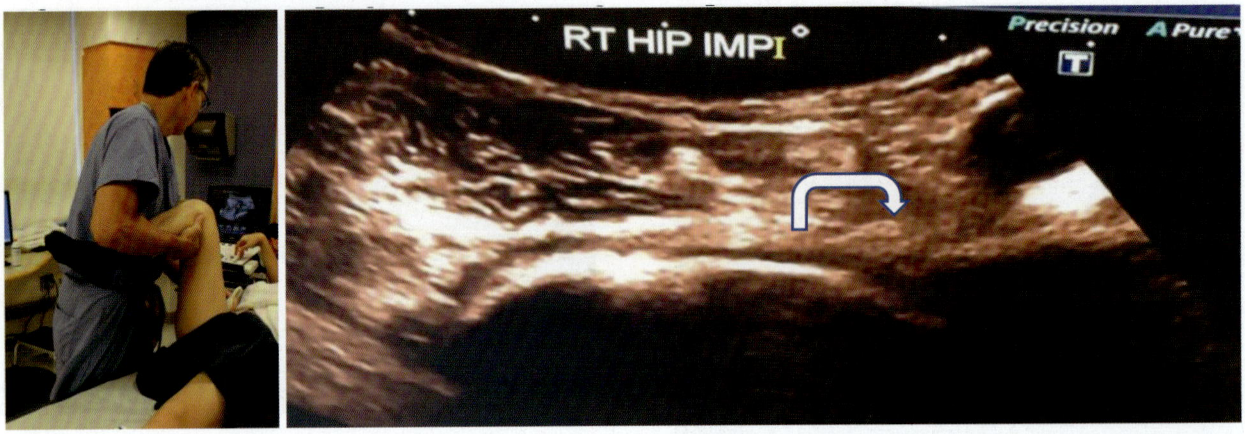

FIGURE 15.6. Anterior impingement at 90° hip flexion with internal rotation.

With this same transverse axial position, hip impingement may be tested. The hip is flexed up close to 90° while maintaining the view of the femoral head and the medial acetabulum. This must be done slowly in order to avoid losing visualization. At about 90° of hip flexion, the hip is internally rotated, and any impingement of the femoral neck pushing up on the labrum is noted (**Figure 15.6**). This impingement may at times also be noted from a lateral view by placing the probe coronal to the femur proximal to the trochanter with an approximately 20° anterior tilt (**Figure 15.7**). Internal rotation in this position may also demonstrate labral impingement from a CAM impingement as well as trochanteric impingement.

Anterior hip instability may also be assessed. Particularly in the borderline dysplastic patient, excessive translation due to capsular insufficiency may be another clinical factor in determining operative interventions. In the apprehension position, the leg is held in extension and external rotation (EER) on the side of the examination table. This translates the femoral head anteriorly with respect to the acetabulum. The US can reliably measure this translation from neutral to the EER position.[46] With the probe held in a sagittal oblique plane, the patient will first flex the contralateral hip to get a baseline neutral position of the ipsilateral femoral head in relation to the acetabulum. Next, the patient is placed in the apprehension position, and the level of anterior translation is assessed (**Figure 15.8**). Normative values have not been fully established but appear to be about 3 to 4 mm.

Finally, the more superficial lateral cutaneous nerve of the thigh is visualized. The probe is held in a direct transverse position over the ASIS. As the probe is moved distally, the medial sartorius muscle is seen, and laterally the tensor fascia latae muscle is seen. The lateral femoral cutaneous nerve is seen between these two. As the probe continues distally, the rectus femoris will appear from the AIIS, and the nerve will travel superficial to the rectus. The probe may also be translated more proximally to the inguinal ligament where the nerve has a variable emergence.

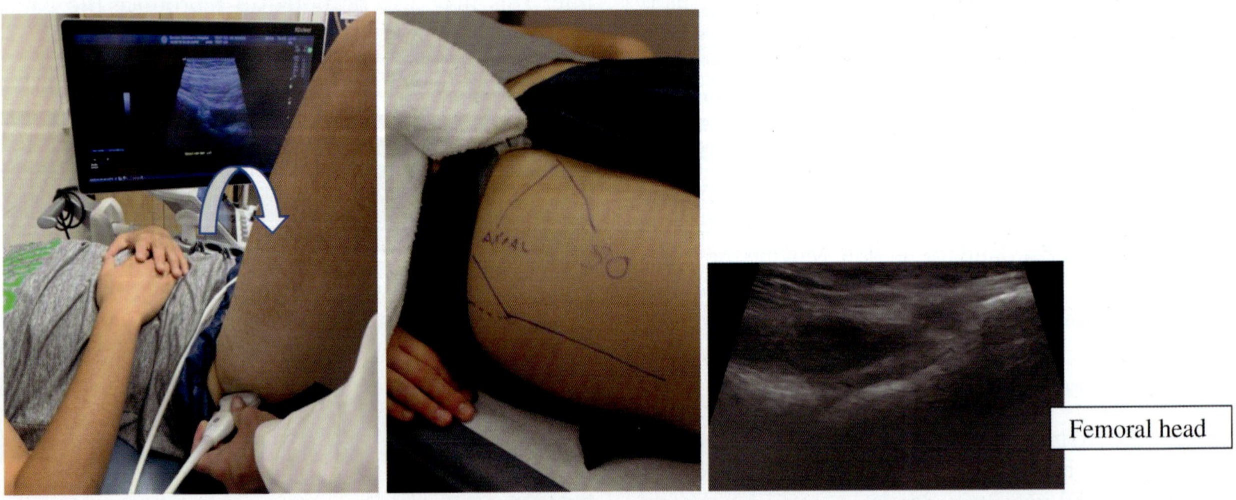

FIGURE 15.7. Lateral hip impingement with probe about 25° from the femur coronal view with internal rotation.

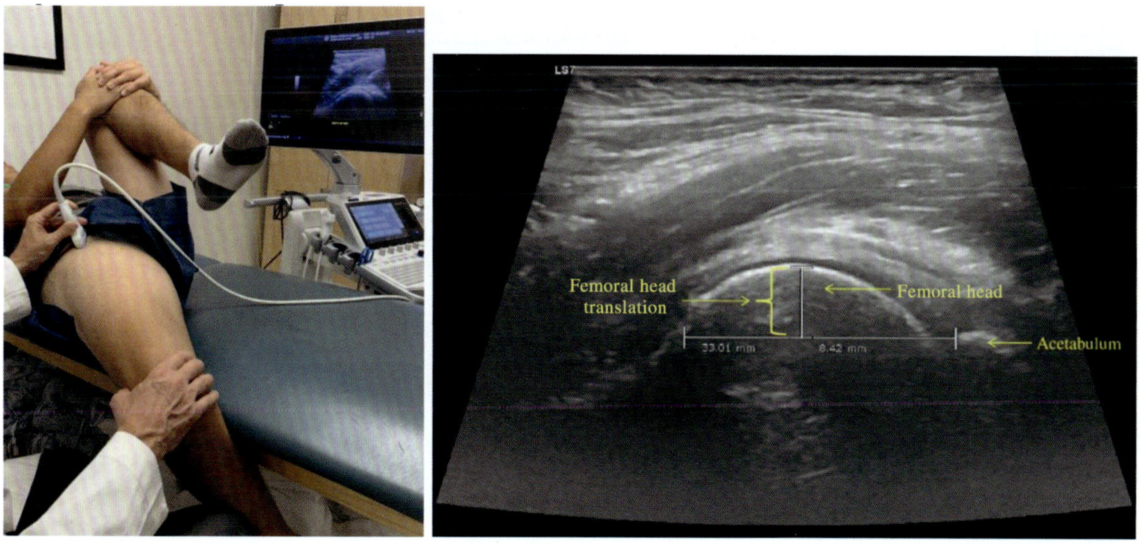

FIGURE 15.8. Anterior hip translation in the apprehension position. Used with permission from d'Hemecourt P, Sugimoto D, McKee-Proctor M, et al. Can dynamic ultrasonography of the hip reliably assess anterior femoral head translation? *Clin Orthop Relat Res*. 2019;477(5):1086-1098.

Ultrasound Examination of the Postoperative Painful Hip

Postoperative hip arthroscopy pain can be challenging, and many causes must be explored, including incomplete rehabilitation, persistent femoroacetabular impingement (FAI), labral re-tear, instability, adhesions, heterotopic ossification, tendinopathies, and psoas bursitis. The US exam is an effective complementary imaging study to evaluate these issues, and many of these diagnoses may be made using multiple orthogonal views. In the sagittal oblique view, the persistence of a cam may be seen as well as an anterior labral tear. Scanning the anterior hip in the sagittal view from lateral to medial may demonstrate heterotopic ossification, rectus tendinopathies, capsular defects from the arthrotomy, and joint effusions or synovitis. The transverse axial view may reveal the presence of excess extra-articular scar, often seen under the rectus. Psoas bursa enlargement may also be appreciated in this view.

Dynamic examination here may demonstrate hip instability with excessive anterior translation in the apprehension position. This may be correlated with any capsular defect seen on the sagittal views. In the transverse axial view, any scar tissue that is appreciated may be further demonstrated by logrolling the extremity; this shows the scar tissue stuck to the capsule and limiting full rotation.

ANTERIOR HIP ULTRASOUND-GUIDED INTERVENTION

The response to intra-articular hip injections has demonstrated utility both therapeutically and diagnostically to predict successful surgical interventions. The immediate anesthetic response is often very helpful in predicting intra-articular pathology. The addition of corticosteroid may also help therapeutically but should be limited in the amount of repeated cartilage exposure. The addition of hyaluronic acid, while still needing investigation, may maximize the anti-inflammatory effect as well as diminish the intra-articular adhesions.

The hip intra-articular injection is best approached in the sagittal oblique view. The subcutaneous tissue is anaesthetized down to the level of the psoas but not into the psoas if it is being performed for diagnostic purposes. Care is taken to visualize the surrounding circumflex arteries. Once the spinal needle is at the femoral head-neck juncture, the probe is turned 90° to get a short-axis view of the needle tip to confirm location (**Figure 15.9**). The needle is then entered through the capsule and confirmed with a single cc of anesthetic to confirm position.

Psoas bursa injections have a number of approaches. A common one is the axial view demonstrating the psoas in short axis overlying the femoral head and acetabulum. Placing a towel under the foot with hip flexion and a little external rotation will diminish the pressure on the bursa and facilitate the injection. The needle is approached from lateral into the bursa. Conversely, another approach is to view the psoas long axis as one would do an intra-articular injection but position the probe more medially, visualizing the psoas tendon and bursa. An in-plane approach to the bursa is then used.

Extra-articular scar tissue hydrodissection may be attempted when a postoperative patient demonstrates adhesions with restricted ROM. These adhesions are often noted along the path of the arthroscope subjacent to the rectus tendon. In this case, a transverse view is obtained just below the AIIS. Logrolling the extremity in this view will help clarify the scar tissue. An in-plane lateral

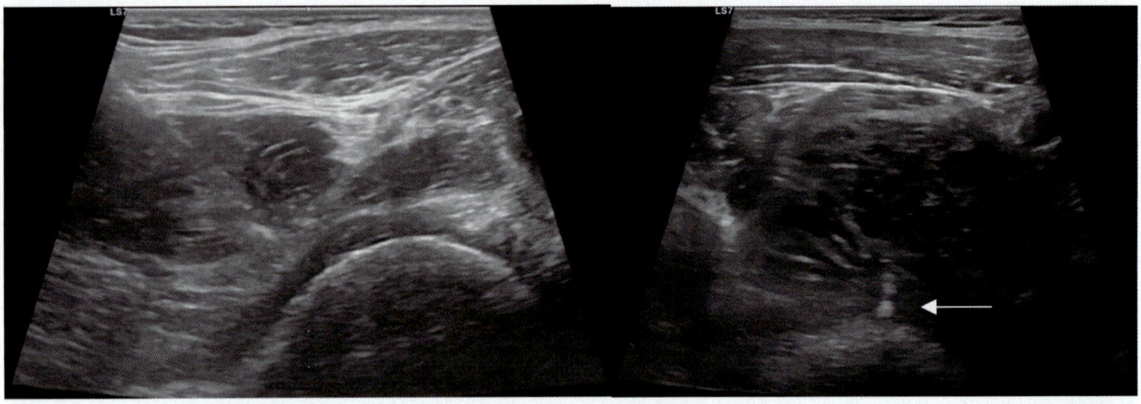

FIGURE 15.9. Intra-articular injection in long axis (left) and short axis (right) showing the single dot above the femoral neck confirmation.

approach with a spinal needle will help break up this tissue next to the capsule using a combination of long-acting ropivacaine, saline, and a small dose of corticosteroid.

Regenerative medicine techniques are still in need of rigorous investigation. Platelet-rich plasma (PRP) may be used in a few pathologies around the hip. If there is a demonstrated capsular defect postoperatively, PRP may assist in the capsule closing. PRP may also be utilized for rectus tendinopathies along with other regenerative intervention. Extracorporeal shock wave therapy (ECSWT) may also be useful for these tendinopathies.

In the setting of gonarthrosis, leukocyte-poor PRP in small studies has shown prolonged efficacy. Combining with hyaluronic acid may also have a positive effect in symptom scores. Finally, intra-articular adipose stem cells have had some positive symptom effect.

Medial Hip Examination

The medial hip is usually visualized with the leg abducted and externally rotated. The probe is then placed in an axial plane to visualize the three muscles overlying each other from the superficial adductor longus over the adductor brevis followed by the adductor magnus. The pectineus muscle is medial to these. The probe can be taken proximally to the insertion on the pubic tubercle to look for any tendinopathy or tears. The probe is then turned 90° to visualize the attachments in the long-axis view. The probe is next turned transversely over the symphysis pubis to visualize this joint and the overlying fibrocartilaginous plate that connects the rectus abdominis and adductor muscles.

Lateral Hip Examination

The lateral hip examination is approached with the patient in the lateral decubitus position with a towel between the knees and the hip flexed about 25°. The axial view starts on the lateral aspect of the femur below the greater trochanter. From this orientation, the probe is moved proximally until it overlies the facets of the greater trochanter. Here, there is usually a well-demarcated hyperechoic anterior and lateral facet (**Figure 15.10**). The posterior facet is more posterior with a less dramatic transition. The probe is then moved anteriorly over the anterior facet. However,

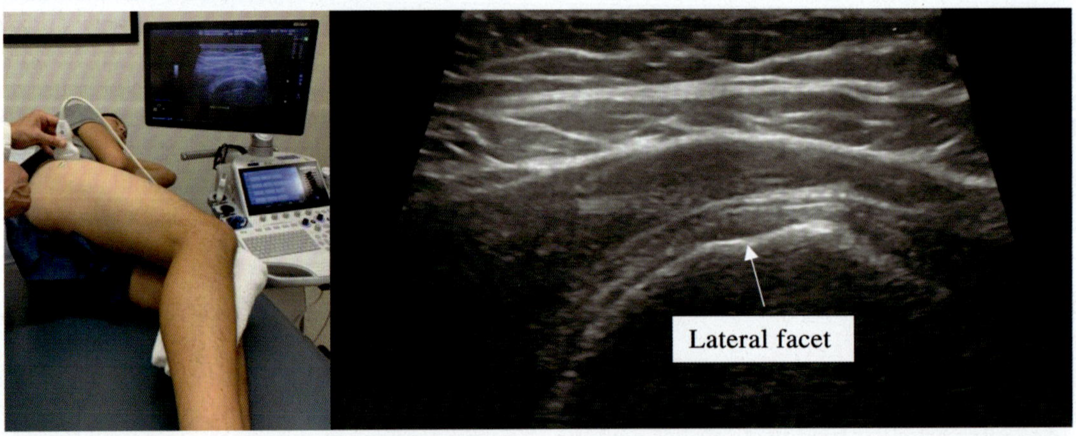

FIGURE 15.10. Lateral hip demonstrating the anterior and lateral facets in the short-axis view.

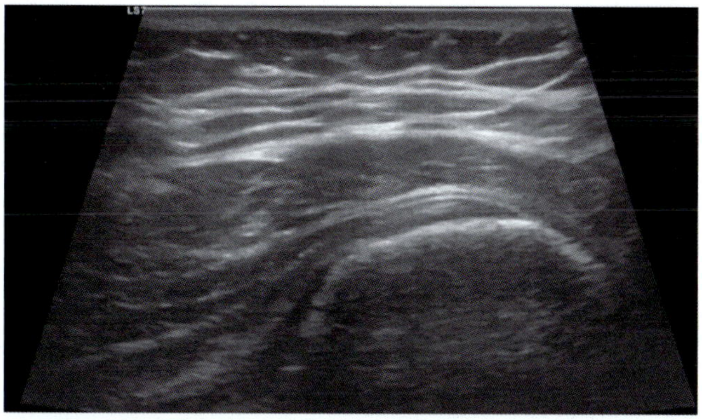

FIGURE 15.11. Long-axis view of gluteus medius.

to be in true short axis to the attaching gluteus minimus, the probe's lateral side is pointed toward the ASIS. In order to visualize the gluteus minimus long axis, the probe is turned 90°, to reveal the subjacent bursa and attachment site of the tendon.

The probe is then moved posteriorly in an axial plane over the lateral facet for a short-axis view of the gluteus medius attachment. The probe is again directed toward the ASIS to obtain a true short-axis view. The probe is moved more superiorly, which should also demonstrate the thicker attachment of the posterior band of the gluteus medius onto the superoposterior facet. The long-axis view is obtained by turning the probe orthogonally again to the AIIS and scanned from anterior to posterior over the lateral facet. The anterior band is thinner and goes over the trochanteric ridge (**Figure 15.11**). The posterior band is a thicker, more direct attachment (**Figure 15.12**). One may see a subjacent bursa or tendinopathy, especially over the greater trochanteric ridge. This will be manifested with a spectrum of tendon thickening, hypoechoic changes, frank tears, and cortical irregularities.

The posterior facet has no attachments. The gluteus maximus (GM) is overlying this, as it traverses anteriorly for a partial attachment to the iliotibial band (ITB). The greater trochanteric bursa lies between the GM and the posterior facet. This large bursa traverses forward between the ITB and the gluteus medius.

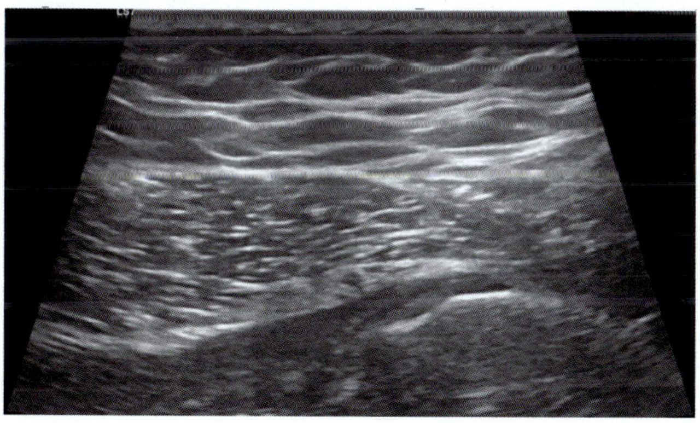

FIGURE 15.12. Gluteus medius posterior band long-axis view.

Snapping Lateral Hip

The snapping lateral hip is called external coxa saltans. It involves some portion of the proximal ITB snapping over the greater trochanter. The ITB has an origin on the iliac crest. The two muscles that attach into it are the anterior fibers of the GM and the tensor fascia latae muscle. It is possible for the snapping to occur from either of these insertions. It is best viewed from an axial US view starting at the greater trochanter and scanning proximally as well as anteriorly and posteriorly to see the two muscle attachments. The patient is then asked to reproduce the snapping. This may be achieved in the lateral decubitus position while the patient is asked to perform a bicycle motion. Alternately, the patient may be standing to reproduce the snapping.

LATERAL HIP INTERVENTIONS

In youth, lateral hip pain may simply be a bursitis, but as one approaches the age of 40, there is usually a coexisting tendinopathy of the gluteal tendons. This must be considered in the choice of interventions as overuse of corticosteroids may be detrimental to tendinopathy. Although small doses into bursopathy may enhance the physical therapy strengthening. Furthermore, one needs to understand that spinal pathology may radiate to the lateral hip. Finally, intra-articular hip pathology may radiate to the lateral hip.

The most common lateral bursa injection is the greater trochanteric bursa. It is best approached in the axial view of the posterior facet and gluteus medius over the lateral facet. A posterior approach is used placing the needle into the bursa, distending it under the ITB. The subgluteus medius and minimus bursa may be approached in the long-axis view of either tendon. Either an in-plane or an out-of-plane approach may be used.

Regenerative techniques are often employed for gluteal tendinopathy. Certainly, appropriate strengthening is the first step. Needling with the addition of PRP or autologous whole blood may be utilized. This has been successfully used in moderate to severe gluteus medius tendinopathy. Recently, there has been strong interest in a less invasive regenerative technique, ECSWT. This therapy may be either a focused shock wave with electromagnetic pulses directed specifically and deeply at a defined area of tendinopathy. Alternately, radial shock wave is a pneumatic source of energy aimed more superficially at the myotendinous junctures. The focus is often enhanced by delineating the area with US guidance. ECSWT has shown some efficacy with gluteal tendinopathies.

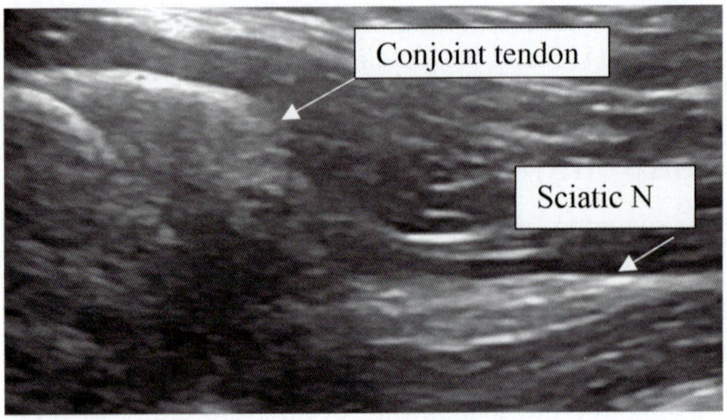

FIGURE 15.13. The sciatic nerve is next to the conjoint tendon over the quadratus femoris muscle.

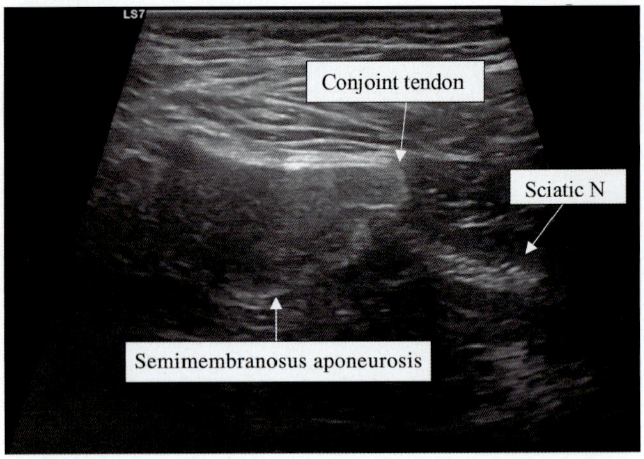

FIGURE 15.14. Hyperechoic triangle. Biceps femoris muscle above sciatic nerve, and semitendinosus muscle above the semimembranosus aponeurosis.

Posterior Hip Examination

The posterior hip examination is started at the distal level of the ischial tuberosity. In the axial view, one can visualize the superficial attachment of the conjoint tendon with the semimembranosus tendon deeper on the tuberosity. The sciatic nerve is lateral and adjacent to the conjoint tendon over the quadratus femoris muscle (**Figure 15.13**). One can then scan caudally. One will see the hyperechoic triangle. This is represented by superficial conjoint tendon, with the lower medial semimembranosus tendon and the lateral sciatic nerve (**Figure 15.14**). Each of the hamstrings can be followed down, with the first muscle developing as the semitendinosus and then, laterally, the biceps femoris. Finally, the semimembranosus muscle develops medially. It should also be noted that the adductor magnus on the medial side of the ischium may involve some tendinopathy and mask as a hamstring injury (**Figure 15.15**).

As one moves back cranially to the ischial tuberosity, the probe is moved laterally to see the lesser trochanter. This is an area of concern for IFI (**Figure 15.16**). As one moves more cranially, one visualizes the sciatic nerve over the obturator internus (OI) and then up to the posterior hip joint (**Figure 15.17**). Here, the probe is moved more medially and pointed toward the sciatic notch to visualize the piriformis muscle inserting on the greater trochanter. Lower extremity rotation will help delineate the piriformis from the overlying GM.

Posterior Hip Interventions

Posterior hip injections include the piriformis injection, OI bursa injection, IFS injections, and ischiogluteal bursa injections.

All of these require identification of the sciatic nerve and careful observation of the needle tip all through the injection.

The piriformis is usually performed in the axial oblique view of the piriformis from the sciatic notch to the greater trochanter. It is important to confirm that the sciatic nerve is not traversing through the piriformis muscle as an anatomic variant. The injection may be typically performed medial to lateral.

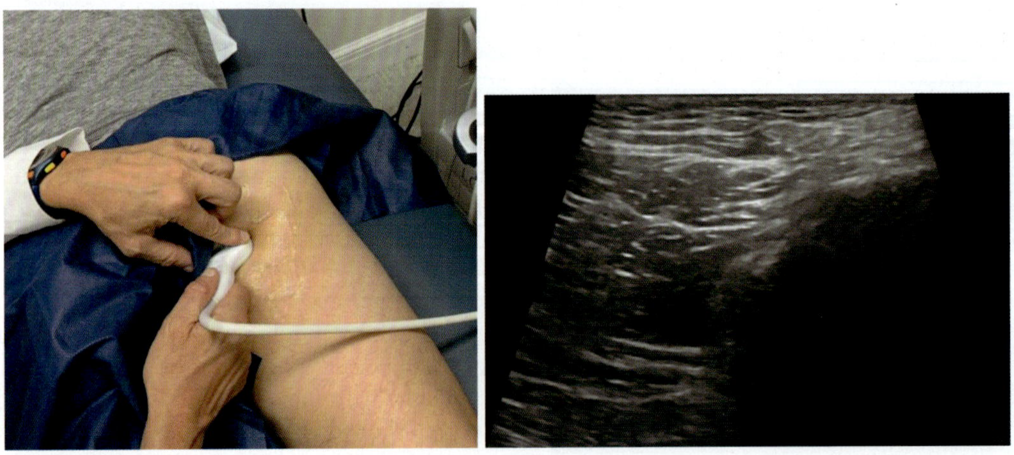

FIGURE 15.15. Adductor magnus.

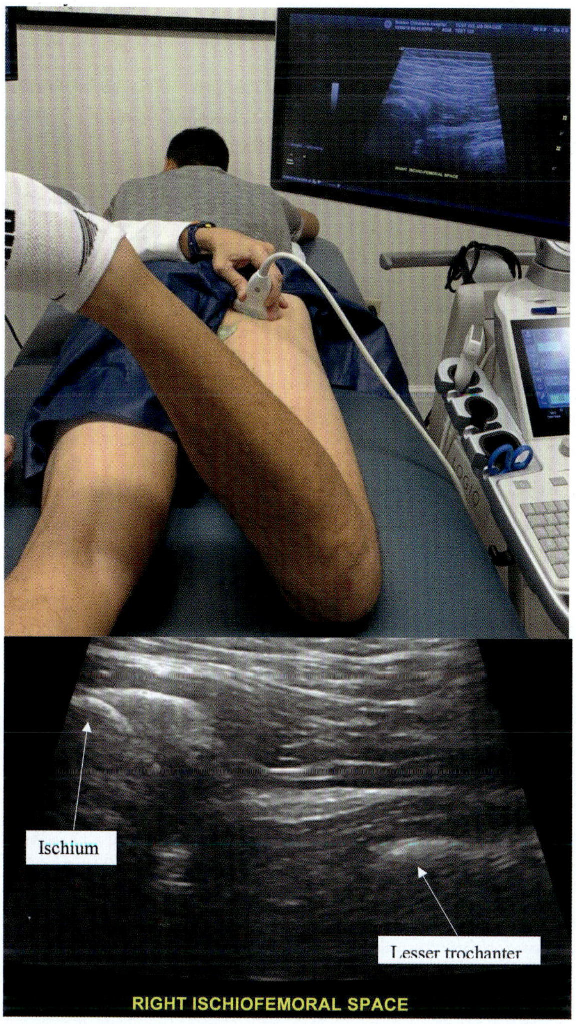

FIGURE 15.16. Ischiofemoral space with hip externally rotated and probe slightly oblique downward laterally.

The OI injection is identified caudad to the piriformis. Using the doppler at the level of the piriformis, the inferior gluteal artery is identified. The probe is moved more medially to see the slight prominence of the medial ischium, which is the ischial spine. The OI is just below these two structures. The bursa sits between the ischium and the OI. To inject this bursa, the needle usually approaches lateral to medial but can be done conversely. This same approach may be done to perform a sheath injection of the OI. Careful visualization of the sciatic nerve is important.

The IFS is a common area of impingement and responds well to corticosteroid injections here. The quadratus femoris is identified at the lower ischium along with the lesser trochanter. If the hip is extended, adducted, and externally rotated, the space may significantly narrow, and the sciatic nerve may be forced superficially. These injections are performed from a lateral to a medial approach typically. The needle tip is seen entering the quadratus femoris below the sciatic nerve.

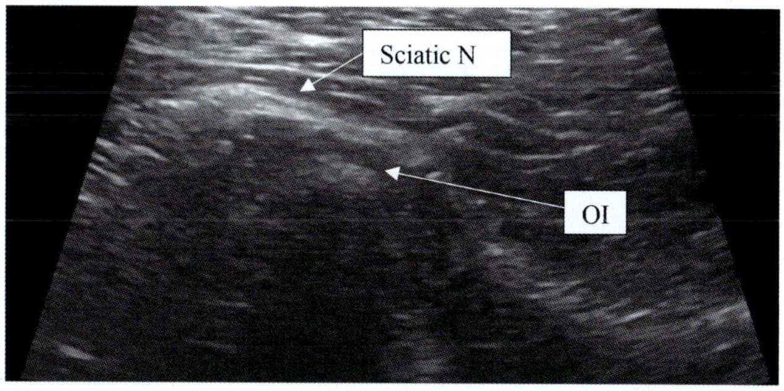

FIGURE 15.17. Obdurator internus over the ischium with sciatic nerve.

The ischiogluteal bursa may also be injected. This is simply the space between the ischium and the GM. It is approached with an axial view from the lateral side.

Regenerative techniques may also be performed on the proximal hamstrings for tendinopathy. One should always look to see if the adductor magnus medially is involved as well. Regenerative techniques include needle fenestration with an axial view from a lateral approach. This allows constant visualization of the sciatic nerve. Autologous blood products may be added along with the needle fenestration such as PRP. This has shown some efficacy.

REFERENCES

1. Frank JM, Harris JD, Erickson BJ, et al. Prevalence of femoroacetabular impingement imaging findings in asymptomatic volunteers: a systematic review. *Arthroscopy*. 2015;31(6):1199-1204.
2. Serner A, Tol JL, Jomaah N, et al. Diagnosis of acute groin injuries: a prospective study of 110 athletes. *Am J Sports Med*. 2015;43(8):1857-1864.
3. Arnason A, Sigurdsson SB, Gudmundsson A, Holme I, Engebretsen L, Bahr R. Risk factors for injuries in football. *Am J Sports Med*. 2004;32(1):5s-16s.
4. Ekstrand J, Hilding J. The incidence and differential diagnosis of acute groin injuries in male soccer players. *Scand J Med Sci Sports*. 1999;9(2):98-103.
5. Hagglund M, Walden M, Ekstrand J. Injuries among male and female elite football players. *Scand J Med Sci Sports*. 2009;19(6):819-827.
6. Renström P, Peterson L. Groin injuries in athletes. *Br J Sports Med*. 1980;14(1):30-36.
7. Werner J, Hagglund M, Walden M, Ekstrand J. UEFA injury study: a prospective study of hip and groin injuries in professional football over seven consecutive seasons. *Br J Sports Med*. 2009;43(13):1036-1040.
8. Anderson CN. Iliopsoas: pathology, diagnosis, and treatment. *Clin Sports Med*. 2016;35(3):419-433.
9. Jacobson JA, Bedi A, Sekiya JK, Blankenbaker DG. Evaluation of the painful athletic hip: imaging options and imaging-guided injections. *Am J Roentgenol*. 2012;199(3):516-524.
10. Hölmich P, Thorborg K. Epidemiology of groin injuries in athletes. In: Diduch D, Brunt LM, eds. *Sports Hernia and Athletic Pubalgia*. New York, NY: Springer; 2014:13-21.
11. Hölmich P, Thorborg K, Dehlendorff C, Krogsgaard K, Gluud C. Incidence and clinical presentation of groin injuries in sub-elite male soccer. *Br J Sports Med*. 2014;48(16):1245-1250.
12. Brophy RH, Wright RW, Powell JW, Matava MJ. Injuries to kickers in American football: the National Football League experience. *Am J Sports Med*. 2010;38(6):1166-1173.

13. Serner A, Weir A, Tol JL, et al. Characteristics of acute groin injuries in the hip flexor muscles—a detailed MRI study in athletes. *Scand J Med Sci Sports*. 2018;28(2):677-685.
14. Hölmich P. Long-standing groin pain in sportspeople falls into three primary patterns, a "clinical entity" approach: a prospective study of 207 patients. *Br J Sports Med*. 2007;41(4):247-252.
15. Winston P, Awan R, Cassidy JD, Bleakney RK. Clinical examination and ultrasound of self-reported snapping hip syndrome in elite ballet dancers. *Am J Sports Med*. 2007;35(1):118-126.
16. Neumann DA, Garceau LR. A proposed novel function of the psoas minor revealed through cadaver dissection. *Clin Anat*. 2015;28(2):243-252.
17. Tatu L, Parratte B, Vuillier F, Diop M, Monnier G. Descriptive anatomy of the femoral portion of the iliopsoas muscle. Anatomical basis of anterior snapping of the hip. *Surg Radiol Anat*. 2001;23(6):371-374.
18. Guillin R, Cardinal E, Bureau NJ. Sonographic anatomy and dynamic study of the normal iliopsoas musculotendinous junction. *Eur Radiol*. 2009;19(4):995-1001.
19. Crompton T, Lloyd C, Kokkinakis M, Norman-Taylor F. The prevalence of bifid iliopsoas tendon on MRI in children. *J Child Orthop*. 2014;8(4):333-336.
20. Moraux A, Balbi V, Cockenpot E, et al. Sonographic overview of usual and unusual disorders of the rectus femoris tendon origins. *J Ultrasound Med*. 2018;37(6):1543-1553.
21. Hammoud S, Bedi A, Voos JE, Mauro CS, Kelly BT. The recognition and evaluation of patterns of compensatory injury in patients with mechanical hip pain. *Sports Health*. 2014;6(2):108-118.
22. Martin HD, Kelly BT, Leunig M, et al. The pattern and technique in the clinical evaluation of the adult hip: the common physical examination tests of hip specialists. *Arthroscopy*. 2010;26(2):161-172.
23. Agten CA, Rosskopf AB, Zingg PO, Peterson CK, Pfirrmann CW. Outcomes after fluoroscopy-guided iliopsoas bursa injection for suspected iliopsoas tendinopathy. *Eur Radiol*. 2015;25(3):865-871.
24. Kroger EW, Griesser MJ, Kolovich GP, Ellis TJ. Efficacy of surgery for internal snapping hip. *Int J Sports Med*. 2013;34(10):851-855.
25. Anderson SA, Keene JS. Results of arthroscopic iliopsoas tendon release in competitive and recreational athletes. *Am J Sports Med*. 2008;36(12):2363-2371.
26. Contreras ME, Dani WS, Endges WK, De Araujo LC, Berral FJ. Arthroscopic treatment of the snapping iliopsoas tendon through the central compartment of the hip: a pilot study. *J Bone Joint Surg Br*. 2010;92(6):777-780.
27. Flanum ME, Keene JS, Blankenbaker DG, Desmet AA. Arthroscopic treatment of the painful "internal" snapping hip: results of a new endoscopic technique and imaging protocol. *Am J Sports Med*. 2007;35(5):770-779.
28. Piechota M, Maczuch J, Skupinski J, Kukawska-Sysio K, Wawrzynek W. Internal snapping hip syndrome in dynamic ultrasonography. *J Ultrason*. 2016;16(66):296-303.
29. Deslandes M, Guillin R, Cardinal E, Hobden R, Bureau NJ. The snapping iliopsoas tendon: new mechanisms using dynamic sonography. *Am J Roentgenol*. 2008;190(3):576-581.
30. Blankenbaker DG, Tuite MJ, Keene JS, del Rio AM. Labral injuries due to iliopsoas impingement: can they be diagnosed on MR arthrography? *Am J Roentgenol*. 2012;199(4):894-900.
31. Domb BG, Shindle MK, McArthur B, Voos JE, Magennis EM, Kelly BT. Iliopsoas impingement: a newly identified cause of labral pathology in the hip. *HSS J*. 2011;7(2):145-150.
32. Han JS, SD, McKee-Proctor *MH*, Stracciolini A, d'Hemecourt PA. Short-term effect of ultrasound-guided iliopsoas peritendinous injection in athletes with iliopsoas tendonitis. *J Ultrasound Med*. 2019; 38(6): 1527-1536.
33. Blankenbaker DG, De Smet AA, Keene JS. Sonography of the iliopsoas tendon and injection of the iliopsoas bursa for diagnosis and management of the painful snapping hip. *Skeletal Radiol*. 2006;35(8):565-571.
34. Moraux A, Wawer R, Lefevbre G, Cotten H, Demondion X, Cotten A. An anatomical study of the indirect tendon of the rectus femoris using ultrasonography. *Eur Radiol*. 2015;25(12):3614-3619.
35. Bianchi S, Martinoli C, Waser NP, Bianchi-Zamorani MP, Federici E, Fasel J. Central aponeurosis tears of the rectus femoris: sonographic findings. *Skeletal Radiol*. 2002;31(10):581-586.
36. Hernando MF, Cerezal L, Perez-Carro L, Canga A, Gonzalez RP. Evaluation and management of ischiofemoral impingement: a pathophysiologic, radiologic, and therapeutic approach to a complex diagnosis. *Skeletal Radiol*. 2016;45(6):771-787.
37. Hernando MF, Cerezal L, Perez-Carro L, Abascal F, Canga A. Deep gluteal syndrome: anatomy, imaging, and management of sciatic nerve entrapments in the subgluteal space. *Skeletal Radiol*. 2015;44(7):919-934.
38. Tosun O, Algin O, Yalcin N, Cay N, Ocakoglu G, Karaoglanoglu M. Ischiofemoral impingement: evaluation with new MRI parameters and assessment of their reliability. *Skeletal Radiol*. 2012;41(5):575-587.
39. Taneja AK, Bredella MA, Torriani M. Ischiofemoral impingement. *Magn Reson Imaging Clin N Am*. 2013;21(1):65-73.
40. Singer AD, Subhawong TK, Jose J, Tresley J, Clifford PD. Ischiofemoral impingement syndrome: a meta-analysis. *Skeletal Radiol*. 2015;44(6):831-837.
41. Finnoff JT, Johnson AC, Hollman JH. Can ultrasound accurately assess ischiofemoral space dimensions? a validation study. *PM R*. 2017;9(4):392-397.
42. Backer MW, Lee KS, Blankenbaker DG, Kijowski R, Keene JS. Correlation of ultrasound-guided corticosteroid injection of the quadratus femoris with MRI findings of ischiofemoral impingement. *Am J Roentgenol*. 2014;203(3):589-593.
43. Hetsroni I, Poultsides L, Bedi A, Larson CM, Kelly BT. Anterior inferior iliac spine morphology correlates with hip range of motion: a classification system and dynamic model. *Clin Orthop Relat Res*. 2013;471(8):2497-2503.
44. Carton P, Filan D. Anterior inferior iliac spine (AIIS) and subspine hip impingement. *Muscles Ligaments Tendons J*. 2016;6(3):324-336.
45. Larson CM, Kelly BT, Stone RM. Making a case for anterior inferior iliac spine/subspine hip impingement: three representative case reports and proposed concept. *Arthroscopy*. 2011;27(12):1732-1737.
46. d'Hemecourt P, Sugimoto D, McKee-Proctor M, et al. Can dynamic ultrasonography of the hip reliably assess anterior femoral head translation? *Clin Orthop Relat Res*. 2019;477(5):1086-1098.

CHAPTER 16

Evaluating the Failed Hip Arthroscopy

INTRODUCTION

The incidence of hip arthroscopy has been increasing over the last two decades.[1] Alongside, there is also an increase in the number of patients where hip arthroscopy fails to improve their pain and/or function. Certain populations have been identified that have less improvement after primary hip arthroscopy. These include patients over 40 years of age, females, those with acetabular dysplasia, and patients with relative femoral retroversion.[2-4] As with most procedures, revision hip arthroscopy has less improvement in patient-reported outcomes than has primary hip arthroscopy.[5]

Evaluating the failed hip arthroscopy requires a thoughtful evaluation of why the primary procedure failed. Sometimes, the patient should not have been treated with hip arthroscopy in the first place, as in the setting of acetabular dysplasia, where a pelvic osteotomy would have likely been a more appropriate primary surgery. Alternatively, hip arthroscopy may have been appropriate but underresection of the cam deformity led to a poor outcome, requiring revision for complete resection of the pathoanatomy. These patients require a thorough and thoughtful approach to an evaluation of why their hip arthroscopy failed to maximize the outcome of nonoperative measures or revision surgery.

Clinical Scenario

A 25-year-old male comes in with recurrent left hip pain for the last 12 months. He has had two prior left hip arthroscopies. He had some improvement of his pain for approximately 1 year after the first surgery, which included a femoroplasty and labral repair, but his deep aching groin pain returned after a year. He then had a second surgery for debridement of adhesions and revision femoroplasty. He got no relief from the second surgery. Both surgeries were performed through an interportal capsulotomy without repair, and his presenting anteroposterior (AP) and lateral radiographs are presented in **Figure 16.1**.

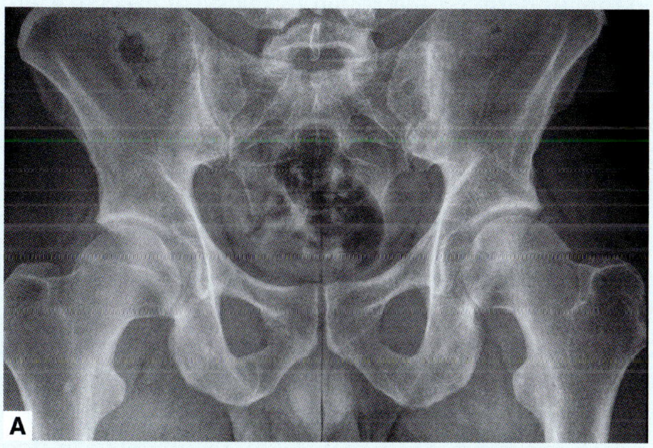

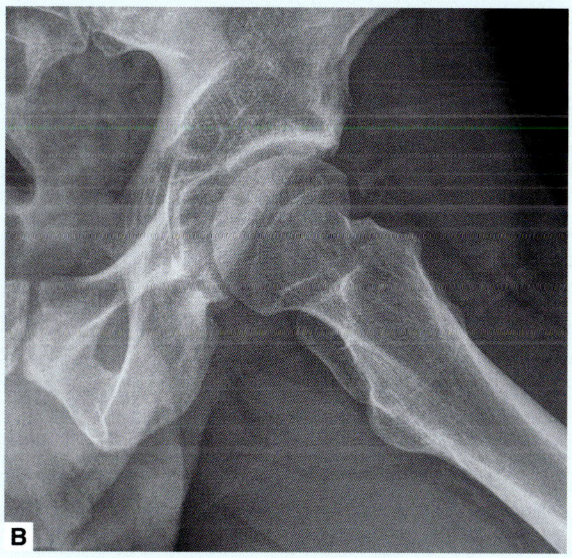

FIGURE 16.1. A, Anteroposterior pelvis radiograph of a male who has had two prior hip arthroscopies. He has borderline acetabular dysplasia (lateral center edge [LCEA] 20°) and unresected lateral cam lesion (alpha angle of 82°). B, Lateral radiograph shows overresection in the anterior aspect of the femoral head-neck junction.

APPROACH

A series of questions must be answered in evaluating the failure of a prior hip arthroscopy. This approach is similar to that which can be used for a failed surgery of any kind. These questions are:

- What was the original diagnosis and was it correct?
- Had the patient failed appropriate nonoperative therapy before undergoing surgery?
- What procedure was performed, and was it appropriate for the diagnosis?
- Was the procedure technically well done?
- Was the rehabilitation done appropriately, or are they underrehabilitated?
- Are there other patient factors that may be clouding the patient's outcome?
- Has the patient developed degenerative disease that precludes revision preservation surgery?
- How do you best address the failure with nonoperative or surgical interventions?

A systematic way of answering these questions should be developed to understand the reason for failure of the index surgery. There are many techniques that can be used to help answer these questions. As with the evaluation of any patient, the first step is history and physical examination. This is then augmented by a comprehensive radiographic evaluation of the hip, including all aspects of femoral and acetabular anatomy. Advanced imaging techniques, including computed tomography (CT) scanning and magnetic resonance imaging (MRI), are useful adjuncts to the radiographic evaluation. This chapter will go into comprehensive evaluation of the failed hip arthroscopy along with potential treatment options with case-based examples to illustrate the principles of evaluation and management of this difficult problem.

CLINICAL EVALUATION

History

In the setting of a failed surgery, the history has two important aspects to it. The first of these is the traditional patient-reported history of their symptoms and prior treatments, including their postoperative course after their first surgery. The second involves gathering all patient records available in regard to the prior surgery. This includes prior clinic notes, imaging tests, operative reports, and arthroscopic pictures from the previous surgery, when available.

The patient-reported history is important to obtain in relation to the current patient symptoms as well as the symptoms prior to the original surgery. Although patients suffer from some degree of recall bias, asking a complete history of their symptoms prior to the first surgery can be enlightening. This allows the surgeon to get an idea of how they would have approached the patient's original problem. Important questions to ask in both settings are similar to evaluating any patient with hip pain. This starts with the locations of the patient's pain and whether it radiates or whether there are other associated pains in the lower back or more distally in the extremity. Most, but not all, patients with intra-articular pain report the anterior groin as the most common area of pain. An important exacerbating factor is sitting or standing for long periods. Patients with structural instability from acetabular dysplasia commonly report increased pain while standing or walking for long periods, whereas patients with impingement have more pain with activities in positions of deep hip flexion including sitting for long periods of time or taking long car rides. Clicking or catching can be from multiple etiologies, including unstable labral tears, iliopsoas (or internal hip) snapping, iliotibial band (or external) snapping, or capsular insufficiency. Arthrofibrosis or intra-articular adhesions, commonly capsule-labral, can lead to patient-reported painful stiffness of the hip joint or pain with motion. Deep pain in the posterior aspect of the hip and/or radiation of pain down the leg could be indicative of missed lumbar spine pathology or ischiofemoral impingement, which may have been the etiology of the patient's pain at initial presentation. However, ischiofemoral impingement is uncommon in the young patient population commonly treated with arthroscopy for femoroacetabular impingement (FAI).

In collecting the interval history after their index surgery, it is important to understand the degree of improvement the patient had after surgery. Some patients report an interval of improved symptoms, only to have the pain return after seemingly successful return to sport. This is common in the patients with undercorrection of impingement that have a soft tissue repair that is injured by continued bony deformity. In patients with structural instability from underlying acetabular dysplasia or excessive femoral anteversion, there is commonly lack of any improvement from surgery because hip arthroscopy can further destabilize an already unstable hip. Patients with impingement treated with cam decompression in the setting of femoral retroversion report improvement in symptoms but to less of an extent than those with normal femoral version. The amount of physical therapy and the type of exercises performed can evaluate the appropriateness of the rehabilitation. Exercises should focus on core strengthening and stabilization and hip abductor strengthening focusing on closed kinetic chain exercises, along with a comprehensive and progressive lower extremity–conditioning program.

It is important to acquire all documentation possible from the patient's prior evaluation and treatment. This can include talking to the prior surgeon about the patient's preoperative evaluation and postoperative course. Preoperative imaging and clinical notes can be used to evaluate the indications for the prior surgery, and operative notes and arthroscopic images can, in some cases, be used to evaluate the quality and completeness of the procedure. The operative report and pictures are important for the technical aspects of the case that may or may not have been performed. For example, was the labrum torn, and was it repaired or was it torn and debrided? Is there a lack of labral tissue remaining? Was the labrum torn, and was it just left in this condition? In addition, it is important to determine how the capsule was managed. If there was an unrepaired capsulotomy or capsulectomy, then the patient may be suffering from hip instability without dislocation, referred to by some as hip microinstability.

Physical Examination

Examination starts with inspection and identification of prior operative scars. Palpation can sometimes elicit pain at portal sites or dysesthesias in the lateral femoral cutaneous nerve distribution. Palpation of the greater trochanter can elicit trochanteric bursitis or tendinopathy. Gait should be evaluated in all patients. In patients with a Trendelenburg stance or gait, one should worry about abductor tears or significant underrehabilitation after surgery. True abductor tears are much more common in the older patient population and are not commonly associated with younger patients undergoing surgery for FAI.

Supine physical examination should comprehensively test range of motion in hip flexion and internal rotation and external rotation at 90° of flexion. In underresected impingement, there is commonly decreased internal rotation in flexion. In the setting of adhesions or arthrofibrosis, there is generally a lack of internal and external rotation in flexion. Provocative tests include the impingement examination in flexion-adduction-internal rotation, which can be positive in unresected cam or unaddressed labral tear. Hip flexion with internal and external rotation in abduction can be painful with an underresected lateral cam lesion. Posterior impingement and/or anterior apprehension can be elicited in hip extension and external rotation with the contralateral knee held to the chest. Posterior buttock pain is indicative of posterior impingement and anterior apprehension or anterior-based pain is indicative of anterior instabilities or loading of an injured anterior chondrolabral junction. An axial traction test or dial test can be performed to further evaluate anterior capsular integrity after a failed hip arthroscopy. A toggling of the hip joint on axial traction or lack of an end point on dial testing can be signs of lack of iliofemoral ligament integrity after prior arthroscopy. Range of motion of the hip in extension in the prone position can be a good measure of femoral version where lack of internal rotation should raise suspicion for relative or absolute femoral retroversion. It is also important to note the symmetry of the exam, as commonly the symptomatic side has more femoral retroversion or lack of internal rotation. Excessive femoral anteversion can be seen with excessive internal rotation in both the prone and the supine positions. In patients with excessive internal rotation in flexion (>40°) after a hip arthroscopy for cam impingement, you should question whether cam impingent was the correct diagnosis, to begin with.

Strength testing can be helpful to understand functional deficits. In patients with prior psoas release, seated hip flexion is commonly weaker compared to the nonoperative side. Side-lying abduction strength testing should be performed in hip flexion, neural and extension. Patients who are still unable to engage their gluteus maximus and co-contract the maximus and medius commonly have weakness with resisted hip abduction in the extended position. This may be a sign of underrehabilitation or poor rehabilitation after prior surgery.

Imaging

A comprehensive radiographic evaluation of the proximal femur and acetabulum is needed to fully evaluate the prior operative interventions.[6] The standing anteroposterior pelvis radiograph evaluates the lateral acetabular coverage and the femoral morphology at the superior position. In addition, the anterior and posterior wall indices can give you an idea of the anterior and posterior coverage of the acetabulum. The false profile radiograph evaluates anterior acetabular coverage and the anterior position on the femoral head-neck junction. We combine these two views with the 45° Dunn view, which evaluates approximately the anterior-superior to superior-anterior position on the anterolateral femur, which is the most common site of the cam morphology. We find that the lateral or superior position on the femur is the most common area of the cam deformity that is underresected in the revision setting. Important measurements to perform on these images include the lateral center edge angle (LCEA), Tönnis angle, anterior center edge angle, and the alpha angle on the femoral side. Acetabular retroversion can also be evaluated with the crossover sign, the posterior wall sign, the ischial spine sign, and the anterior and posterior wall indices, as well as the ratio between these indices. A summary of important radiographs to obtain and measurements to perform are presented in **Table 16.1**.[6]

Advanced imaging options include MRI and CT scans. MRI more effectively images the soft tissues including the labrum and capsule, while CT scan more effectively evaluates prior bony resection. MRI-arthrograms can be used to evaluate for capsular defects/instability after prior hip arthroscopy. Generally, in evaluating the failed hip arthroscopy, an arthrogram is preferred over a noncontrast hip MRI. Three-dimensional reconstruction of CT data can be the most useful in qualitatively evaluating prior cam resection. Obtaining imaging through the distal femur is important to evaluate femoral version because versional abnormalities can lead to residual impingement (femoral retroversion) or residual instability (femoral anteversion). MRI with cartilage-specific sequences can

TABLE 16.1 Radiographs and Important Measures

Radiographic View	Important Measurements
Standing anteroposterior pelvis	Lateral center edge angle Tönnis angle Anterior wall index Posterior wall index Femoro-epiphyseal acetabular roof index Femoral neck shaft angle Femoral alpha angle Crossover sign Posterior wall sign Ischial spine sign
False profile	Anterior center edge angle
Laterals: 45° Dunn lateral Frog lateral	Femoral alpha angle

be helpful to evaluate the quality of the cartilage in the dysplastic or borderline dysplastic acetabulum. Our cartilage imaging of choice is the delayed gadolinium-enhanced MRI of cartilage (dGEMRIC). The dGEMRIC index can be used to predict the early failure of periacetabular osteotomy (PAO) as a treatment for dysplasia.[7] T2 mapping and T1-rho are other cartilage sequences that are being developed to evaluate cartilage health to help with identification of early joint degeneration. Working with a trusted radiologist or team of radiologists can be helpful to completely evaluate these advanced imaging tests in the patients with prior hip arthroscopy. Dynamic hip ultrasound has recently been described to evaluate functional hip motion and instability and impingement. As we move forward, ultrasound of the hip will likely be utilized more in evaluating the painful hip after failed arthroscopy.

Nonoperative Diagnostic and Therapeutic Interventions

Nonoperative measures are the first-line treatment in the failed hip arthroscopy patient. In patients without obvious operative needs, we generally start with a structured physical therapy program involving core strengthening, abductor strengthening, and lower extremity conditioning. This should focus on closed kinetic chain functional exercises. Guided injections of local anesthetic with or without cortisone can be a useful adjunct for diagnostic purposes. When patients have a confusing picture and multiple areas of pain, starting with an intra-articular injection and determining how much relief in pain this provides helps determine whether the pain is intra-articular. Other areas that can cause pain include the greater trochanter/abductor tendons, the ischiofemoral space, the psoas tendon sheath, and the prior portal site or the lateral femoral cutaneous nerve (LFCN). If intra-articular injection does not provide pain relief, but injection into these other sites relieves the patient's pain, then this could help direct further intervention or treatment.

CASE EXAMPLES AND TREATMENT OPTIONS

Return to Physical Therapy With Improvement in Symptoms

Not all failed hip arthroscopies require surgery. Some patients do well for a while after surgery but return to busy day-to-day lives and stop all stretching and strengthening exercises for their hip. Occasionally, we see these patients come back with a return of deep aching groin pain 1 to 2 years after surgery. If imaging shows good radiographic correction, then physical therapy can improve symptoms in some of these patients with return to a core and closed kinetic chain focused physical therapy program improving hip and pelvic strength and mechanics. This is why appropriate physical therapy with a trusted therapist is our first mainstay of treatment in these patients. In addition, this gives you the time to get to know the patients, send them to therapy for a few months, and ask them to come back to their follow-up appointment with any missing information and records from their prior treatment. This can commonly be combined with an intra-articular cortisone injection to give the patients pain relief if indicated and allow them to engage better in the physical therapy program.

Revision Hip Arthroscopy for Residual Cam With Capsular Repair

Returning to our case example of the 25-year-old male with continued pain after two prior left hip arthroscopies, he had some relief with his original surgery but had

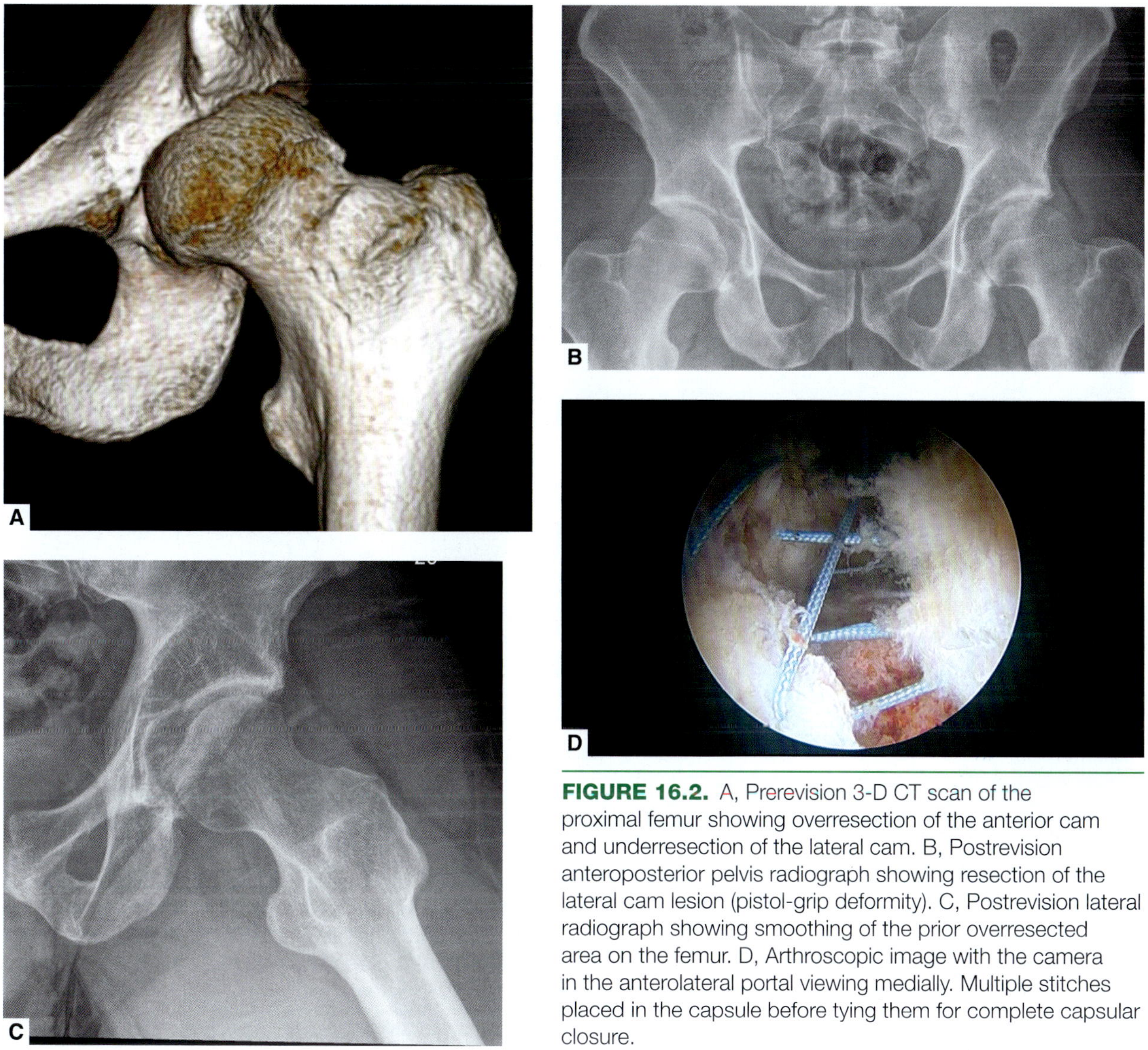

FIGURE 16.2. A, Prerevision 3-D CT scan of the proximal femur showing overresection of the anterior cam and underresection of the lateral cam. B, Postrevision anteroposterior pelvis radiograph showing resection of the lateral cam lesion (pistol-grip deformity). C, Postrevision lateral radiograph showing smoothing of the prior overresected area on the femur. D, Arthroscopic image with the camera in the anterolateral portal viewing medially. Multiple stitches placed in the capsule before tying them for complete capsular closure.

recurrence of pain a year later with revision surgery for debridement and revision osteoplasty. His radiographs are presented in Figure 16.1, and his CT scan 3-D reconstruction is presented in **Figure 16.2A**. He has obvious overresection in the anterior aspect of the femur and underresection of the lateral or pistol-grip region of the cam deformity. From review of his prior operative reports, there had been no attempt at capsular repair at either of his prior hip arthroscopies. The labrum had been repaired at the first surgery. After failure of a repeat course of physical therapy, revision arthroscopy was performed with revision osteoplasty with removal of the unresected lateral cam lesion (**Figure 16.2B**), smoothing of the overresected area (**Figure 16.2C**), and capsular repair with multiple high-tensile strength sutures (**Figure 16.2D**). In these patients with revision including capsular plication or repair of a prior unrepaired capsulotomy, it is important to slow their rehabilitation down for the first 6 weeks and avoid hip extension beyond neutral and external rotation to avoid stressing the capsular repair.

Revision Arthroscopy With Heterotopic Ossification Resection

An important aspect of postoperative care is the use of anti inflammatorics to decrease the risk of developing heterotopic ossification (HO). When this develops in the anterior aspect of the hip, this can lead to continued deep groin pain. Patients generally develop pain at about 3 months after surgery after an initial pain-free interval. They can then have symptoms similar to those of their FAI with pain sitting for long periods of time, with deep hip flexion activities and with flexion and internal rotation.

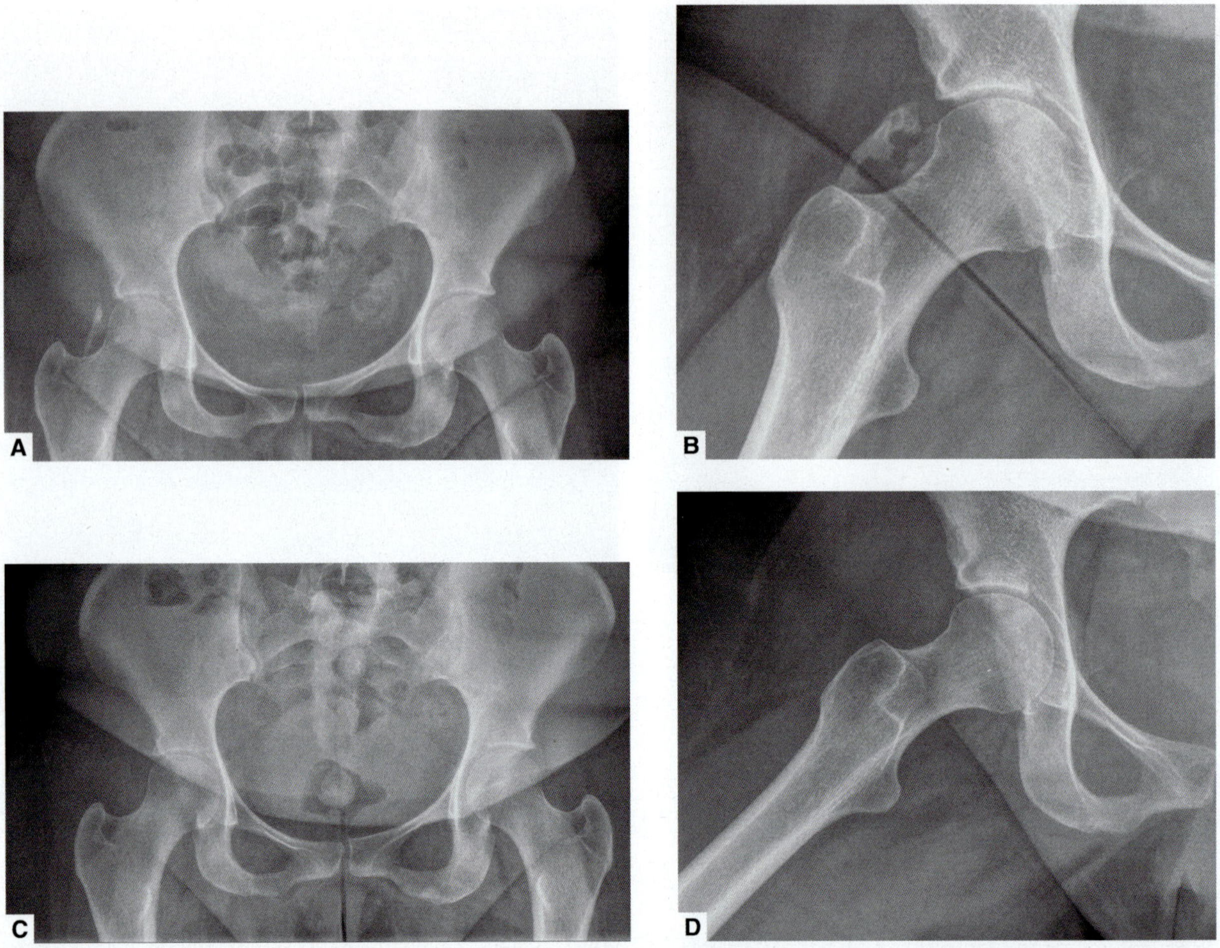

FIGURE 16.3. A, Prerevision anteroposterior (AP) radiograph shows significant anterior heterotopic ossification of the anterior capsule but with good prior cam resection. B, Prerevision lateral radiograph shows significant anterior heterotopic ossification of the anterior capsule but with good prior cam resection. C, Postoperative AP radiograph showing resection of the heterotopic ossification. D, Postoperative lateral radiograph showing resection of the heterotopic ossification.

Figure 16.3 shows radiographs of a 30-year-old female who is 1-year out from hip arthroscopy for FAI with a good cam resection, but who was not treated with nonsteroidal anti-inflammatory drugs (NSAIDs) for HO prophylaxis. She developed significant HO on the anterior capsule and had return of her pain (Figure 16.3A, B). She was treated with an endoscopic extracapsular approach to remove the HO, but this could also be done open. Postoperative radiographs showed complete resection of the HO (Figure 16.3C, D). The patient had significant improvement in her pain after surgery and was prophylaxed with Naprosyn 500 mg twice daily for 4 weeks after surgery.

Revision of Hip Arthroscopy With Periacetabular Osteotomy

Despite preliminary studies that suggested arthroscopy had favorable outcomes in dysplasia, our experience has been that patients may do well for a short period after hip arthroscopy, and then their symptoms commonly return within a few years. Others have no relief of pain from their arthroscopy or have progressive worsening of their symptoms. The surgical treatment of these patients is normally straightforward with periacetabular dysplasia to address their bony instability. Labral pathology and femoral-sided asphericity/cam lesion have commonly been appropriately addressed during the prior arthroscopy. This leaves the open hip preservation surgeon to address the underlying dysplasia. Important radiographic and advanced imaging measurements in evaluating the patient with mild or borderline dysplasia are the LCEA and anterior center edge angle (ACEA) (measured to the sourcil edge, not the bone edge).

A case example of this is illustrated here. This is a 20-year-old female collegiate high jumper. She had a hip arthroscopy with labral repair and femoral osteoplasty done 9 months prior to presentation. She went through an appropriate progressive postoperative physical therapy program and attempted return to high jumping around 4.5 months postoperatively. After her first track meet with high intensity high jumping requiring forceful hip extension, she had a return of her anterior groin pain. Activities were decreased, and the patient returned to physical therapy. She was unable to improve and progressed to daily pain with normal activities. Postoperative radiographs showed mild dysplasia with appropriately addressed femoral cam deformity (**Figures 16.4A, B**). On examination, the patient had 40° of internal rotation inflexion and significant pain and apprehension with extension, slight abduction, and external rotation. MR-arthrogram showed a small capsular defect at area of prior repair (of a longitudinal capsulotomy) with repaired labrum and normal appearing articular cartilage (**Figure 16.4C**). Preoperative CT scan showed femoral anteversion of 4°. Discussion with the patient revolved around revision to repair/tighten the capsule versus addressing the bony deficiency. Recommendation was for PAO to address the bony instability of the hip. Postoperative radiographs show improved acetabular coverage (**Figure 16.4D, E**). At 3 months after surgery, the patient had radiographic healing and significant improvement in symptoms. They were back training with a goal of returning to sport by 6 months post surgery.

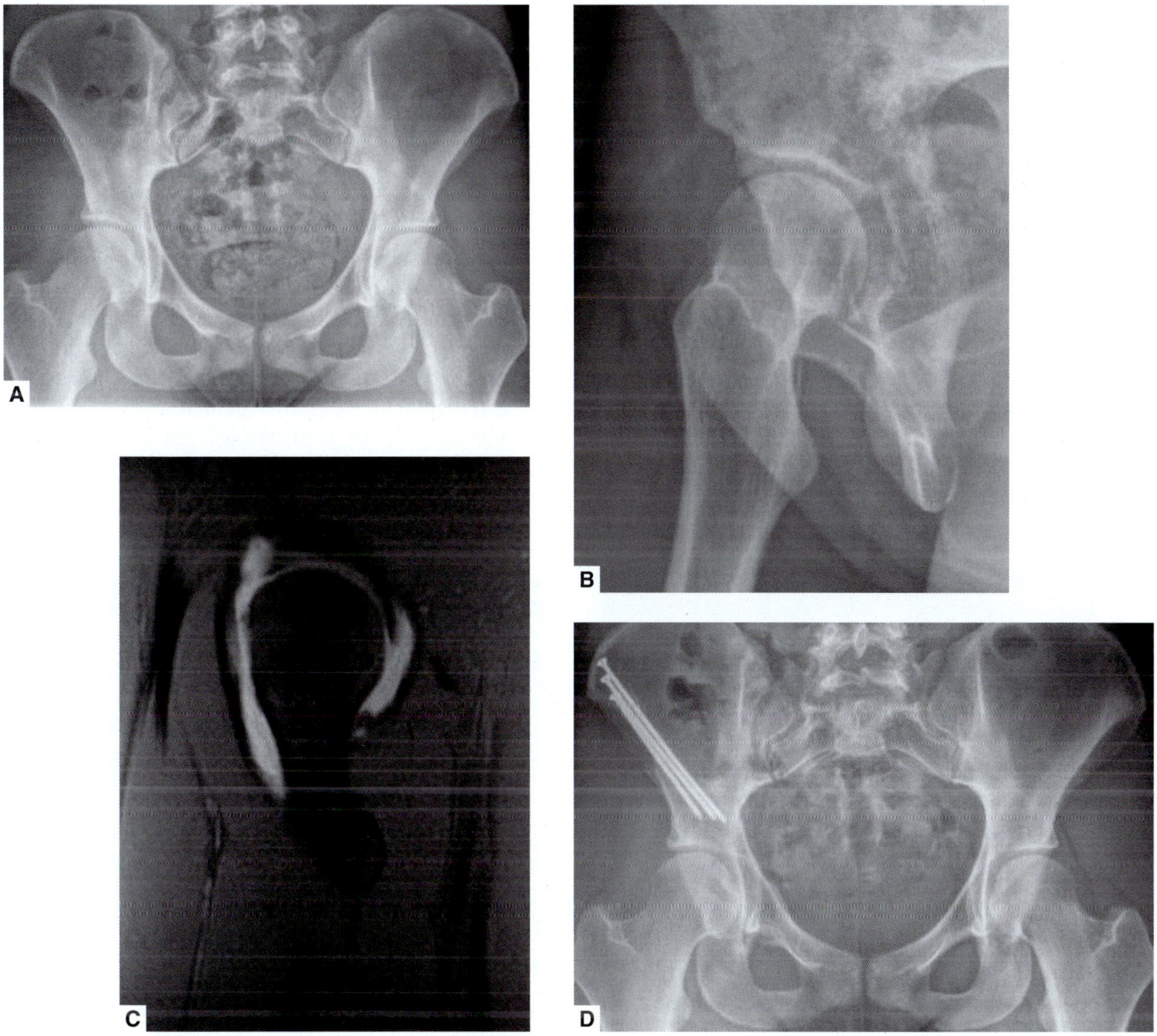

FIGURE 16.4. A, Anteroposterior (AP) pelvic radiograph showing mild dysplasia with a lateral center edge angle (LCEA) of 17°. B, False profile radiograph showing mild dysplasia with an anterior center edge angle of 19°. C, MR-arthrogram showing contrast leak through prior longitudinal capsulotomy. D, AP pelvic radiograph showing correction of dysplasia with an LCEA of 27°.

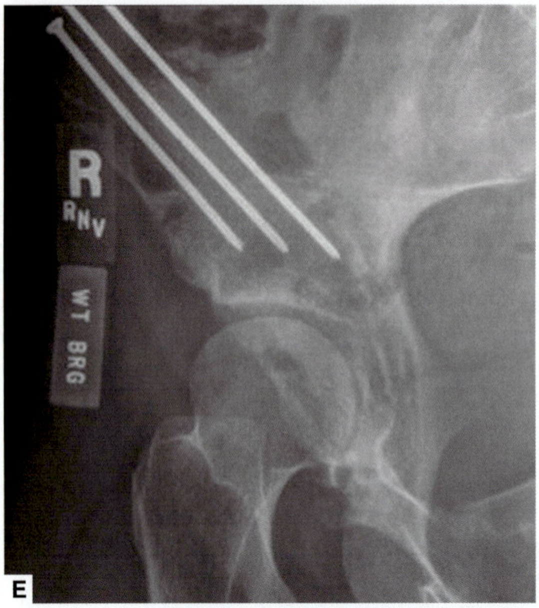

FIGURE 16.4. (*continued*) E, False profile radiograph showing correction of dysplasia with an anterior center edge angle of 30°.

Revision Hip Arthroscopy With Labral Reconstruction

In the setting of continued hip pain with a prior labral debridement or resection, revision hip arthroscopy with labral reconstruction may be needed for labral deficiency. In small defects, a segmental reconstruction may be needed, whereas larger defects may require a circumferential reconstruction. Other aspects of the prior surgery can be addressed as well, including revision osteoplasty for unresected cam deformity and capsular repair or plication for capsular deficiency. **Figure 16.5A** shows an MRI of a 39-year-old female who had prior hip arthroscopy with femoroplasty and labral debridement. **Figure 16.5B** shows the deficient anterosuperior labrum with scarring and erythema. **Figure 16.5C** and **D** show the labral deficiency addressed with debridement and a segmental labral reconstruction.

Revision of Hip Arthroscopy With Open Surgical Dislocation ± Femoral Rotational Osteotomy or Anterior Trochanteric Osteoplasty

Patients with relative or absolute femoral retroversion have worse outcomes after hip arthroscopy for FAI. In these patients that are doing poorly, there can be continued impingement despite a well-done femoral osteoplasty. This can result from contact between the anterior facet of the greater trochanter and the anterior inferior iliac spine. This can be revised through a surgical dislocation approach, with or without femoral rotational osteotomy. **Figure 16.6A** shows 3D-CT reconstruction of the hip of a 34-year-old patient with hip pain for many years. He had not had prior arthroscopy but had significant pain with flexion, adduction, and internal rotation (FADIR), and 0° of internal rotation in both supine with the hip flexed and prone physical examination. The images from his CT scan show 20° of true femoral retroversion (**Figure 16.6B**). The impingement from this deformity was thought to be untreatable with arthroscopy. He was treated with surgical dislocation with femoral rotational osteotomy (**Figure 16.6C**).

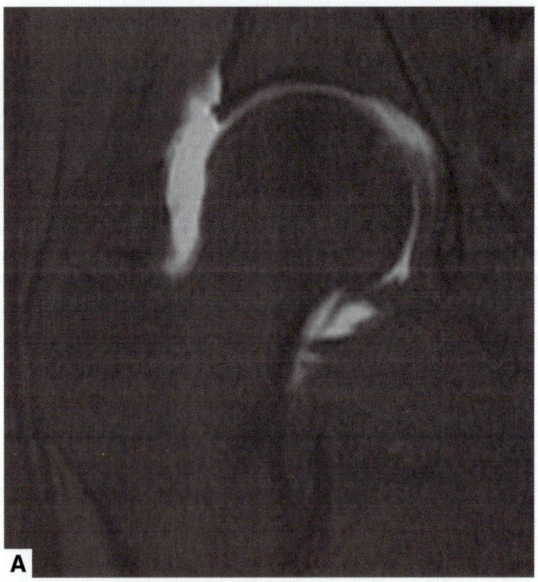

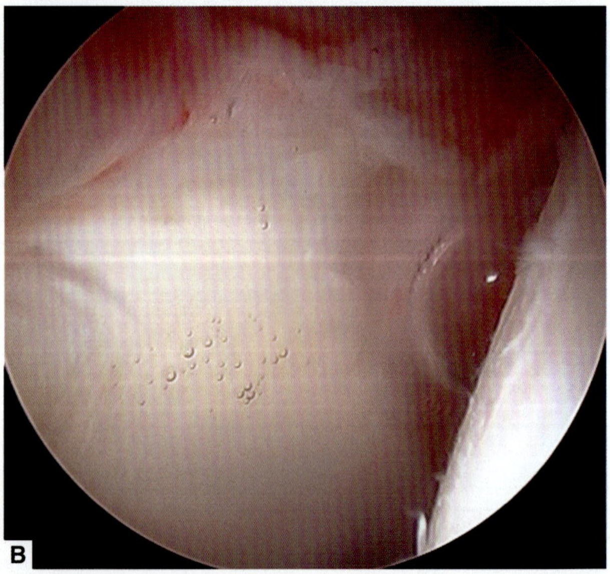

FIGURE 16.5. A, Coronal T1 Fat-Sat MRI image in area of prior labral debridement with diminutive appearing labrum. B, Intraoperative arthroscopic image showing area of prior labral debridement with erythema and scar formation.

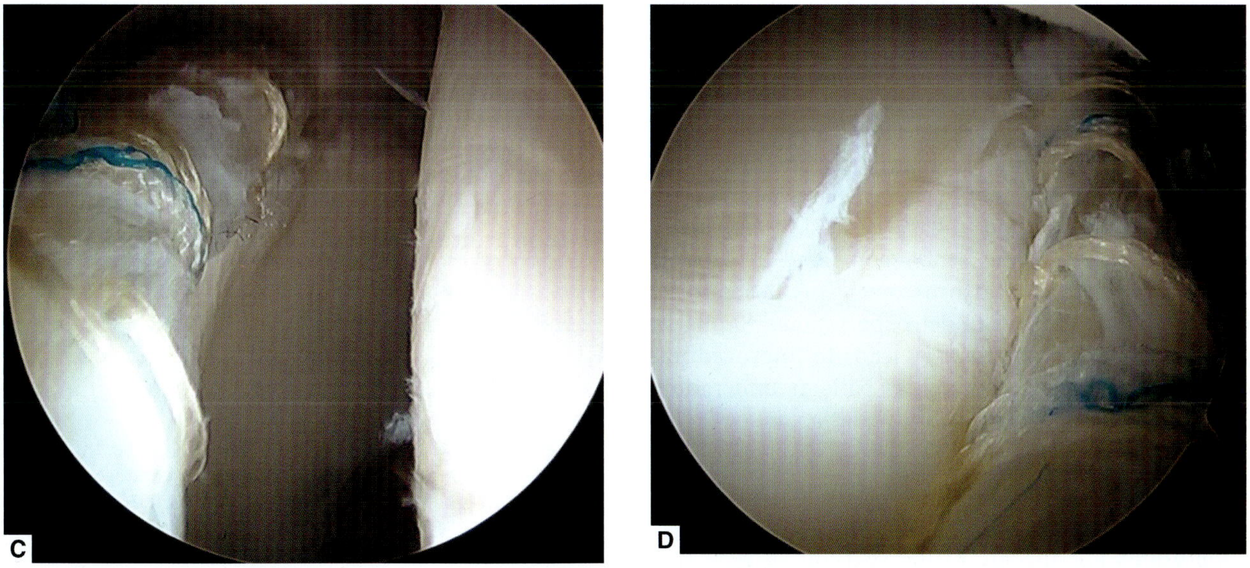

FIGURE 16.5. (*continued*) C and D, Arthroscopic images after segmental labral reconstruction.

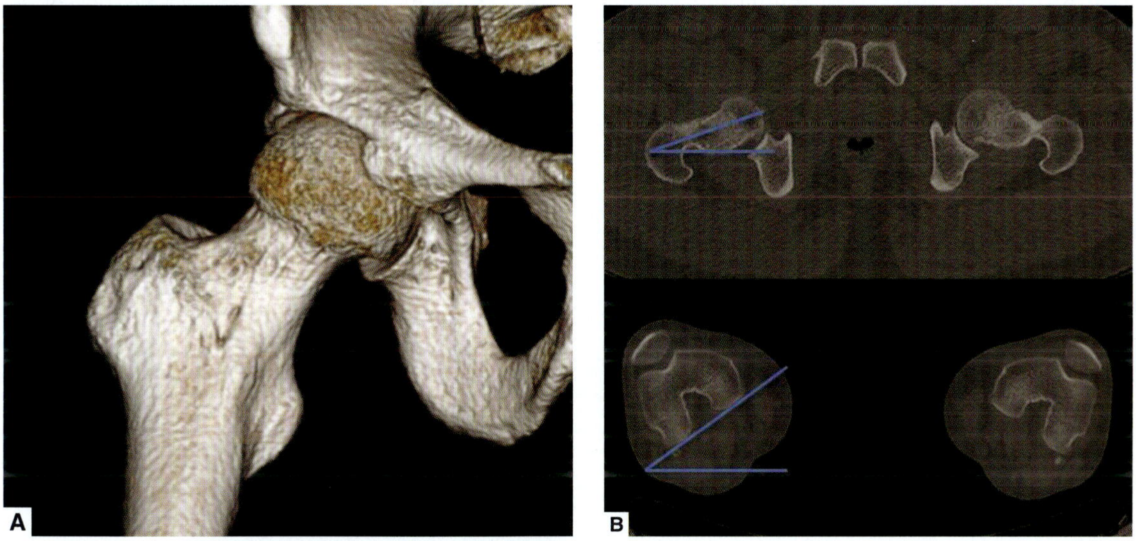

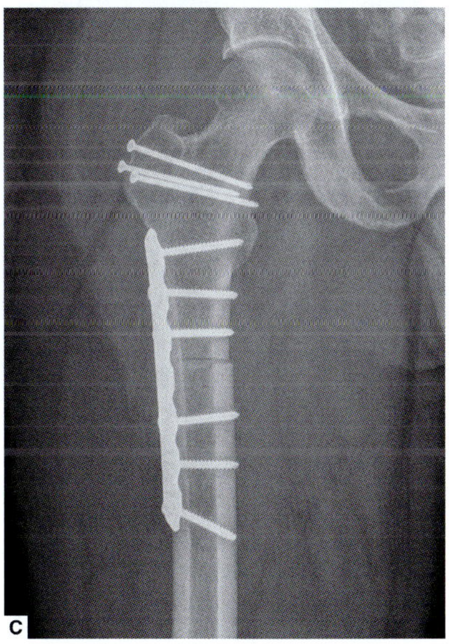

FIGURE 16.6. A, 3D CT reconstruction of the proximal femur showing a pincer trough in the proximal femur from femoral retroversion. There was no elevated alpha angle on any radiographic view. B, Axial images from the distal femur and the proximal femur showing 20° of absolute femoral retroversion. C, Anteroposterior femur radiograph after surgical dislocation with femoral derotational osteotomy.

EXPECTED OUTCOMES

Outcomes studies of revision surgery after failed hip arthroscopy report that most patients have significant improvement after revision surgery. However, the degree of improvement is generally less than is obtained from the same primary hip surgery.[7] On average, a revision hip arthroscopy can be expected to have 10 to 20 points lower patient-reported outcomes scores compared to patients undergoing primary hip arthroscopy.[7] This needs to be discussed before surgery to set expectations. Similarly, PAO after failed hip arthroscopy leads to improved patient outcomes but not as much as patients undergoing PAO as their index procedure for dysplasia.

COMPLICATIONS

Complications are specific to the revision surgery that is chosen to address the etiology of the patient's failure. Please see other chapters that go into depth on the techniques used for revision surgery, including hip arthroscopy, PAO, and surgical dislocation with or without femoral osteotomy for a complete discussion of complications of these techniques.

SUMMARY

Hip arthroscopy can fail for many reasons, and it takes a thoughtful approach to evaluate the patient with continued pain after hip arthroscopy. There can be multiple reasons for continued pain. A thoughtful approach generally starts with a structured physical therapy program with or without an intra-articular injection. This allows time to obtain outside records and images. Answering the series of questions posed earlier, a structured physical examination and radiographic and advanced imaging can help determine the appropriate treatment through nonoperative, revision arthroscopy or open treatment methods.

REFERENCES

1. Bozic KJ, Chan V, Valone FH, Feeley BT, Vail TP. Trends in hip arthroscopy utilization in the United States. *J Arthroplasty.* 2013;28(8):140-143.
2. Frank RM, Lee S, Bush-Joseph CA, Salata MJ, Mather RC 3rd, Nho SJ. Outcomes for hip arthroscopy according to sex and age: a comparative matched-group analysis. *J Bone Joint Surg Am.* 2016;9(10):797-804.
3. Fabricant PD, Fields KG, Taylor SA, Magennis E, Bedi A, Kelly BT. The effect of femoral and acetabular version on clinical outcomes after arthroscopic femoroacetabular impingement surgery. *J Bone Joint Surg Am.* 2015;97(7):537-543.
4. Haynes JA, Pascual-Garrido C, An TW, Nepple JJ, ANCHOR Group, Clohisy JC. Trends of hip arthroscopy in the setting of acetabular dysplasia. *J Hip Preserv Surg.* 2018;5(3):267-273.
5. O'Connor M, Steinl GK, Padaki AS, Duchman KR, Westermann RW, Lynch TS. Outcomes of revision hip arthroscopic surgery: a systematic review and meta-analysis. *Am J Sports Med.* 2020;48(5):1254-1262.
6. McClincy MP, Wylie JD, Yen YM, Novais EN. Mild or borderline hip dysplasia: are we characterizing hips with a lateral center-edge angle between 18° and 25° appropriately? *Am J Sports Med.* 2019;47(1):112-122.
7. Kim SD, Jessel R, Zurakowski D, Millis MB, Kim YJ. Anterior delayed gadolinium-enhanced MRI of cartilage values predict joint failure after periacetabular osteotomy. *Clin Orthop Relat Res.* 2012;470(12):3332-3341.

CHAPTER 17

Hip Instability in Down Syndrome

Down syndrome or trisomy 21 is one of the most common chromosomal abnormalities. Patellofemoral dislocation, foot deformities, atlantoaxial instability, scoliosis, and hip instability are the most common musculoskeletal manifestations that may negatively impact the quality of life in patients with Down syndrome.[1,2] Instability of the hip has been reported to affect between 1% and 7% of children with Down syndrome.[1,3] However, as much as 28% of adults with Down syndrome have been reported to have abnormalities of the joint.[4]

The etiology of hip instability in Down syndrome is multifactorial, including ligamentous laxity, hip capsule insufficiency, and muscular hypotonia, and, most importantly, osseous abnormalities of the femur and acetabulum are accepted as the mainstay of hip instability in Down syndrome. We investigated 42 patients with Down syndrome and found that the acetabulum is retroverted, shallow, and globally insufficient.[5] Moreover, hip instability was associated with more severe global acetabular insufficiency and increased femoral anteversion, but not with more severe acetabular retroversion. In line with a previous study, we found no difference in the mean femoral neck-shaft angle between the stable and unstable hips.

Hip instability presents differently based on patients' age.[6] The initial stage is characterized by a stable but hypermobile hip. Then, hypermobility may progress into habitual dislocation. Hypotonia and delayed walking are common, and children with hyperlaxity may present with a nonpainful *popping* of the hip when the child is carried by the caregivers. Radiographs at this stage may be normal, although physical examination may reveal the instability. With growth, progressive subluxation progresses, leading to loss of concentric reduction and acetabular dysplasia that is easily recognized on radiographs. With progression to subluxation and acetabular dysplasia, the child may present with a limp, fatigue, and decrease in ability to walk. The final stage is typically seen in early adulthood and corresponds to a fixed dislocation of the hip. Pain is not typically present until later in life when patients may lose the ability to walk independently.

Anteroposterior (AP) radiograph of the pelvis and frog-leg lateral radiograph of the femur are the mainstay of imaging of the hip in patients with Down syndrome. However, three-dimensional imaging including magnetic resonance imaging (MRI) and computed tomography (CT) or MRI including the femoral condyles give additional information about the morphology of the acetabulum and femur and are helpful when planning for surgical intervention.

Preserving hip joint concentric reduction is important given the poor natural history.[4,7] The goals of treatment depend on the patient's age and the phase of the disease. Nonsurgical treatment including bracing and casting have not been reported to achieve and maintain hip stability in patients with Down syndrome. With habitual dislocation, the goal is to stabilize the hip and to prevent secondary acetabular dysplasia. One previous study reported that all 14 hips remained stable at an average of 5 years after isolated femoral varus intertrochanteric osteotomy.[8] During subluxation phase, the goal is to obtain a concentric reduction of the hip and correct the dysplastic acetabulum. Historically, the Salter, Chiari, and Pemberton pelvic osteotomies have been used in combination with capsular plication and/or femoral procedures. However, we have consistently reported that the acetabulum is retroverted in patients with Down syndrome.[5,9] Because those osteotomies may further compromise the posterior acetabular coverage, their role may be limited in patients with Down syndrome. Our preference has been to perform a triple osteotomy of the pelvis in patients with open triradiate cartilage and a Bernese periacetabular osteotomy (PAO) in patients close to skeletal maturity age.[10-13] For a fixed dislocated hip, the goal is to preserve walking ability, which may require a hip salvage procedure or total hip replacement.[14-16]

Clinical Scenario

A 6-year-old female patient with Down syndrome presented to clinic with her parents who reported that she had a constant pop in both hips. During evaluation in clinic, she was noted to have frank posterior dislocation of both hips when the hips were positioned in adduction, internal rotation with an axial force applied to the knees. Imaging revealed a relative concentric hip bilaterally. CT imaging revealed the severe acetabular retroversion and insufficient coverage of the femoral head posteriorly (**Figure 17.1**).

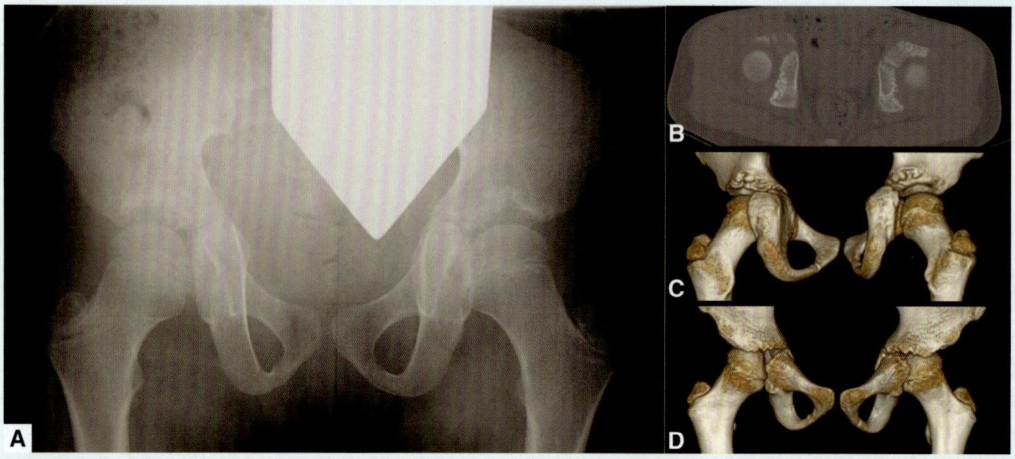

FIGURE 17.1. A 6-year-old female with Down syndrome presented with bilateral habitual dislocation of the hips. A, Anteroposterior pelvic radiograph shows a concentric relationship between the femoral heads and the acetabulum without clear subluxation or severe dysplasia. B, Axial computed tomography (CT) image showing severe acetabular retroversion bilaterally. C, Three-dimensional reconstructed CT image view from posterior showing decreased femoral head coverage because of acetabular retroversion. D, Three-dimensional reconstructed CT image view from anterior shows relatively excessive coverage of the femoral head anteriorly because of acetabular retroversion.

THE BOSTON TECHNIQUE FOR TRIPLE PELVIC OSTEOTOMY

Surgery was performed under general anesthesia with a lumbar plexus catheter for pain management. The patient was positioned supine on a radiolucent table with the entire hemipelvis and lower extremity draped free. Although a single incision is possible, our preference is to perform our modified version of a triple osteotomy using two incisions: a longitudinal medial incision in the groin and an oblique bikini-like iliofemoral incision in the pelvis (**Figure 17.2**).

The medial approach is performed with a longitudinal incision over the posterior border of the adductor longus. The adductor fascia is incised in line with the skin incision and the adductor longus muscle is dissected (**Figure 17.3**). The plane between the adductor longus and the adductor brevis is dissected, and the anterior division of the obturator nerve is identified overlying the adductor brevis (**Figure 17.4**). The anterior branch of the obturator nerve is protected, and the nerve is traced to the obturator foramen. The pectineus muscle is retracted proximally, and a finger is placed laterally in the foramen to identify the ischium (**Figure 17.5**). The ischium should be cleared of soft tissue with blunt dissection and a Lane retractor is placed through the obturator foramen toward the ischial spine

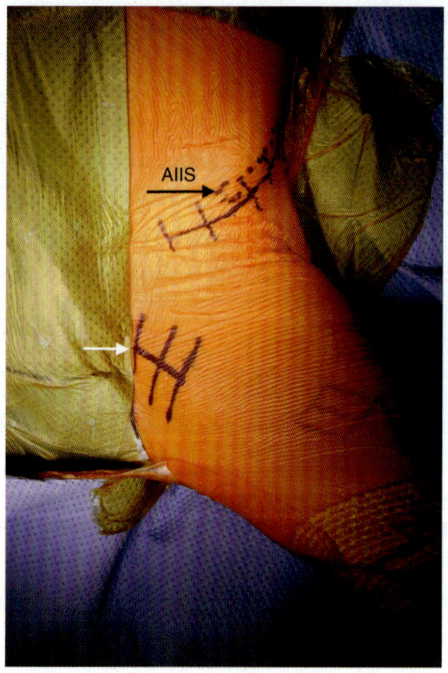

FIGURE 17.2. Two incisions are marked in the skin for the triple pelvic osteotomy. The medial incision extends about 8 cm longitudinally along the posterior aspect of the adductor longus muscle (white arrow). A bikini iliofemoral incision is made, beginning medial and distal to the anterior superior iliac spine (black arrow) and continuing laterally to a point just beyond the summit of the iliac crest (marked with dotted line). AIIS, anterior inferior iliac spine.

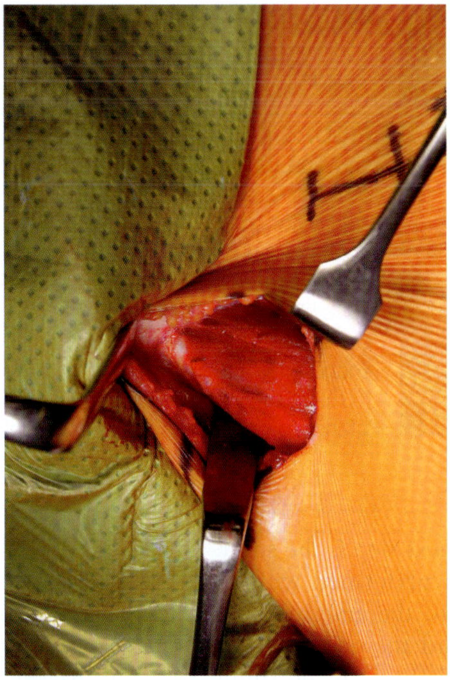

FIGURE 17.3. The adductor longus muscle is exposed after the fascia has been split in line with the incision. A retractor is placed distally to the adductor longus, facilitating the dissection of the plane between the adductor longus and the adductor brevis.

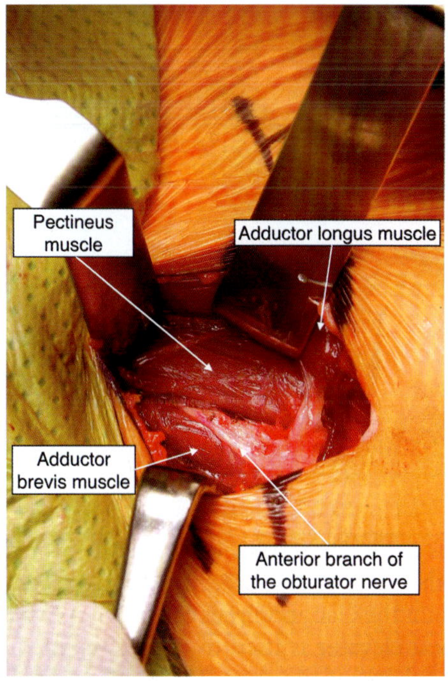

FIGURE 17.4. The adductor longus muscle is retracted anteriorly and the plane between the adductor longus and the brevis is bluntly dissected. The anterior branch of the obturator nerve is identified overlying the adductor brevis.

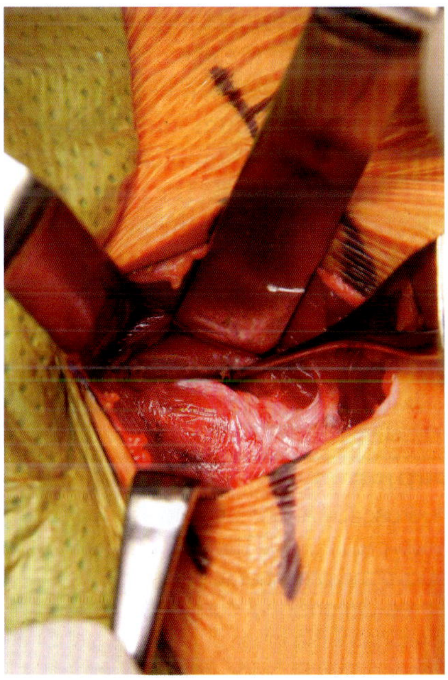

FIGURE 17.5. The pectineus muscle is retracted proximally to protect the femoral neurovascular bundle. The anterior branch of the obturator nerve is traced proximally to the point at which it exits the obturator foramen. In this photograph, a forceps is placed laterally in the foramen to identify the ischium. Avoid cutting into a leash of vessels that are usually encountered in this area.

using fluoroscopic guidance. A Ganz-type chisel is placed just lateral to the Lane retractor (**Figure 17.6**). It is important to use fluoroscopy to be certain that the Lane retractor and the chisel are in the correct location. The Ganz chisel is advanced aiming proximal to the ischial spine. A lateral window is created with the blunt elevator to protect the sciatic nerve. The Lane retractor is removed from the medial aspect of the ischium and redirected toward the lateral. The retractor is introduced laterally, again extraperiosteally but hugging the lateral cortex of the ischium. The Ganz chisel is repositioned laterally, and the oblique osteotomy of the ischium is completely above the ischial spine and sacrospinous ligament (**Figure 17.7**). A few additional passes with the Ganz chisel may be needed to ensure that the ischial cut is complete. It is important to note that the ischial osteotomy is slightly oblique, angling from proximal and medial to distal and lateral when visualized on the AP projection. The medial wound is packed with a sponge. The superior pubic ramus can be cut through the medial incision. However, it is our preference to perform the pubic osteotomy through the anterior approach.

The oblique bikini skin incision is made and the external oblique muscle is elevated from its insertion on the iliac crest (**Figure 17.8**). The iliac apophysis is completely exposed. Distally in the wound, the interval between the tensor fascia lata laterally and the sartorius medially is dissected. The muscular fascia of the tensor fascia lata is opened parallel to the interval between the sartorius and tensor, avoiding the exposure of the lateral femoral

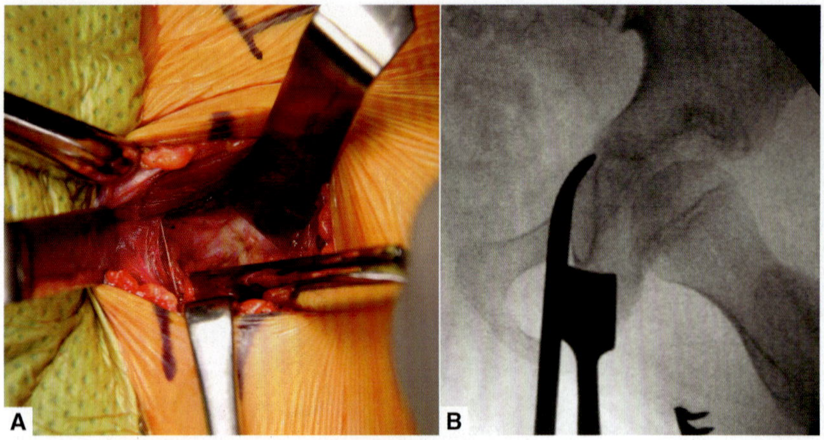

FIGURE 17.6. A, Intraoperative photograph showing the pectineus muscle retracted proximally, and the ischium has been cleared of soft tissue. A Lane retractor has been placed through the obturator foramen hugging the periosteum of the quadrilateral plate all the way to the ischial spine. B, The correspondent intraoperative fluoroscopy image after a long Ganz-type chisel is placed to make the ischial cut from a point just inferior to the margin of the acetabulum.

cutaneous nerve. Dissection is carried out through this interval to the origin of the direct head of the rectus femoris. At this point the iliac apophysis can be sharply incised and a periosteal elevator is used to elevate the medial aspect of the apophysis of the crest. The iliopsoas muscle is retracted medially, and the superior pubic ramus is exposed while leaving the periosteum intact. Positioning the hip in flexion and adduction helps the exposure of the superior pubic ramus.

After the superior pubic ramus is exposed extraperiosteally, a long curved large clamp is passed into the obturator foramen from distal to proximal extraperiosteally. Careful passage of the clamp is crucial to avoid entrapment of the obturator nerve and vessels. A #0 silk tie is attached to the tip of the clamp under direct visualization and the silk tie is pulled distally. The distal end of the silk tie is attached to a Gigli saw and the saw is passed extraperiosteally under the superior pubic ramus from distal to proximal and the pubic ramus is cut with the saw (**Figure 17.9**). The thick periosteum of the ramus may need to be incised to improve the acetabular fragment positioning.

The next step is the supra-acetabular iliac osteotomy, which is performed with an oscillating saw from just inferior to the anterior inferior iliac spine (AIIS) aiming toward the proximal aspect of the sciatic notch but ending about 1 cm off the pelvic brim. An angle chisel completes the iliac osteotomy similar to that used for a Bernese PAO. However, instead of cutting through the posterior column, it is angled down into the sciatic notch. In preparation from the iliac osteotomy, a reverse Hohmann retractor is placed into the sciatic notch to protect the sciatic nerve and the remaining contents of the notch (**Figure 17.10**). The lateral aspect of the iliac apophysis is partially detached from the ilium to create a window where a small thin long Hohmann retractor is placed (**Figure 17.11**). Although the osteotomy can be fully done with an oscillating saw, we often use a bone scalpel to cut the medial cortex of the ilium and mark the osteotomy line. The iliac osteotomy is completed with an oscillating saw and a Ganz angled chisel. The oscillating saw should stop short at about 1 cm from the pelvic brim before the osteotomy is curved into the sciatic notch using the chisel

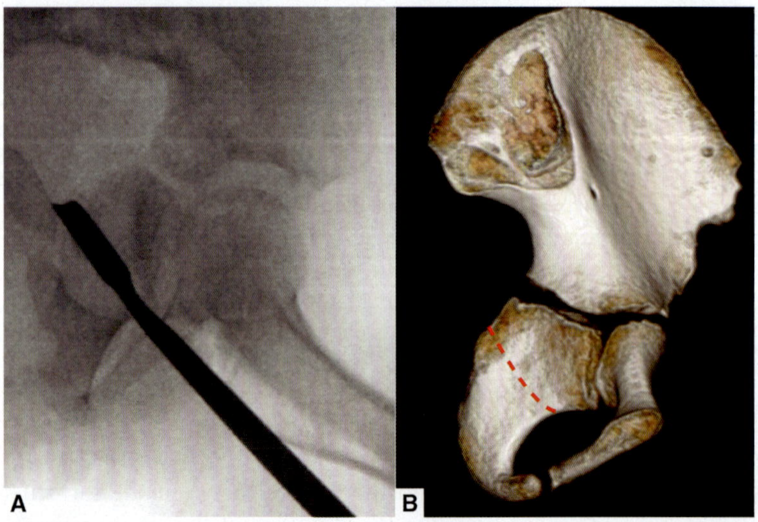

FIGURE 17.7. A, Intraoperative oblique fluoroscopy at 50° of obliquity corresponding to a false-profile view. The Ganz chisel is placed aiming above the proximal aspect of the ischial spine. B, Three-dimensional computed tomography (CT) imaging of the inner pelvis. The ischial cut (red dashed line) is made from a point just inferior to the margin of the acetabulum to a point above the proximal aspect of the ischial spine staying away from the greater sciatic notch. Making the osteotomy cut at this level ensures that the sacrospinous ligament that is attached to the ischial spine will not affect the mobility of the acetabular fragment.

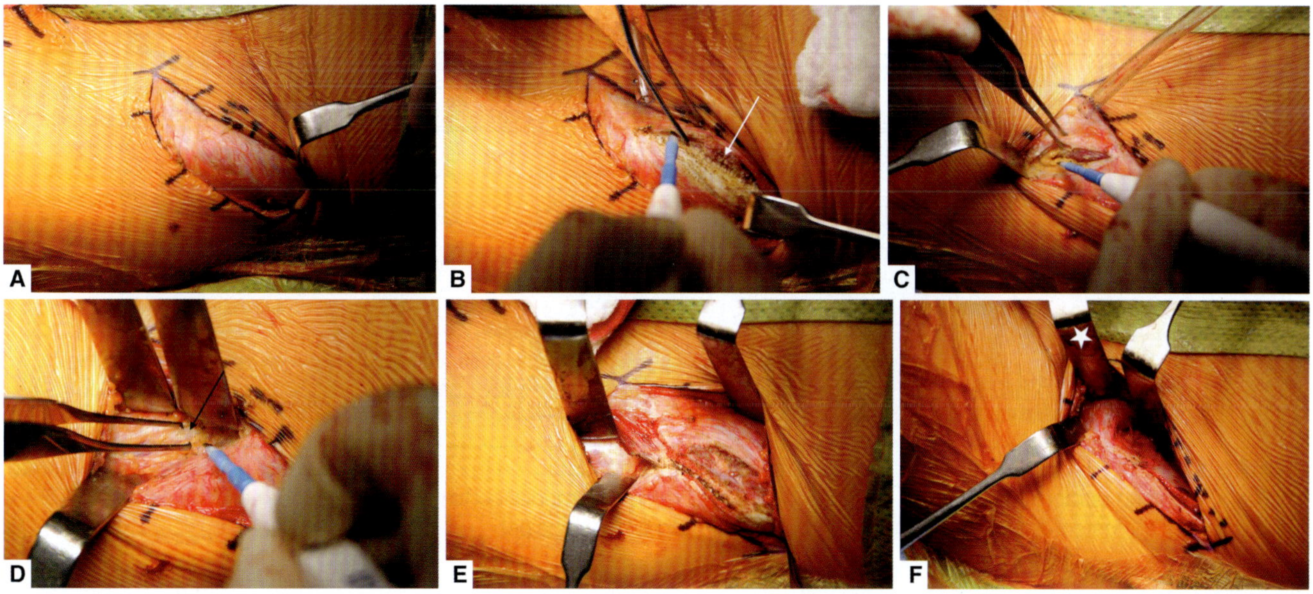

FIGURE 17.8. Anterior bikini approach for the superior pubic and iliac osteotomies. A, The skin incision is performed, and the subcutaneous tissue is dissected exposing the external oblique muscle inserting into the iliac crest. B, The external oblique muscle (white arrow) is elevated from the iliac crest preserving the periosteum up to the level of the anterior superior iliac spine (ASIS). C, Distally in the wound the fascia on top of the tensor fascia lata muscle is opened and the muscle is exposed. Opening the tensor fascia decreases the risk of lateral femoral cutaneous nerve injury as the nerve runs in the sartorius fascia. D, The tensor fascia lata muscle is retracted laterally and the sartorius is retracted medially, which grants exposure of the direct head of the rectus femoris muscle (black arrow) inserting into the anterior inferior iliac spine (AIIS). E, Two retractors are placed distally in the wound as described earlier and another retractor is placed proximally exposing the entire iliac apophysis. The apophysis is split with a scalpel from proximal to distal. By exposing the tensor fascia lata-sartorius interval the surgeon can split the apophysis to the level of the AIIS without risking damage of the ASIS cartilage. F, The iliac apophysis has been split sharply incised and a periosteal elevator elevated the medial aspect of the apophysis of the crest. The lateral aspect of the apophysis is maintained intact. A retractor (white star) is placed under the iliopsoas muscle to retract the muscle medially, granting exposure to the superior pubic ramus.

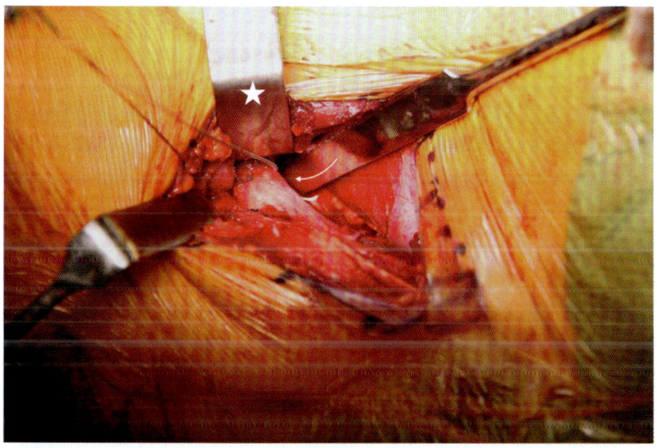

FIGURE 17.9. Intraoperative picture shows a Hibbs retractor (white star) is placed on top of the superior pubic ramus to retract the iliopsoas muscle medially. A Lane retractor has been placed extraperiosteally from proximal to distal in the obturator foramen to protect the contents of the foramen while a Gigli saw is used to perform the superior pubic ramus osteotomy.

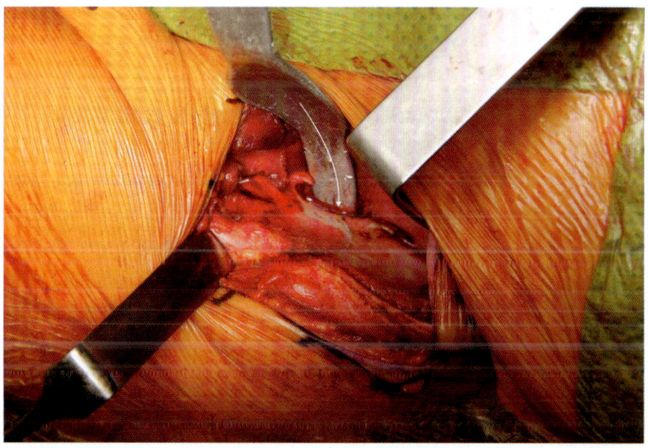

FIGURE 17.10. Intraoperative picture shows a radiolucent reverse curved Hohmann placed in the sciatic notch (white arrow) to protect the contents of the notch.

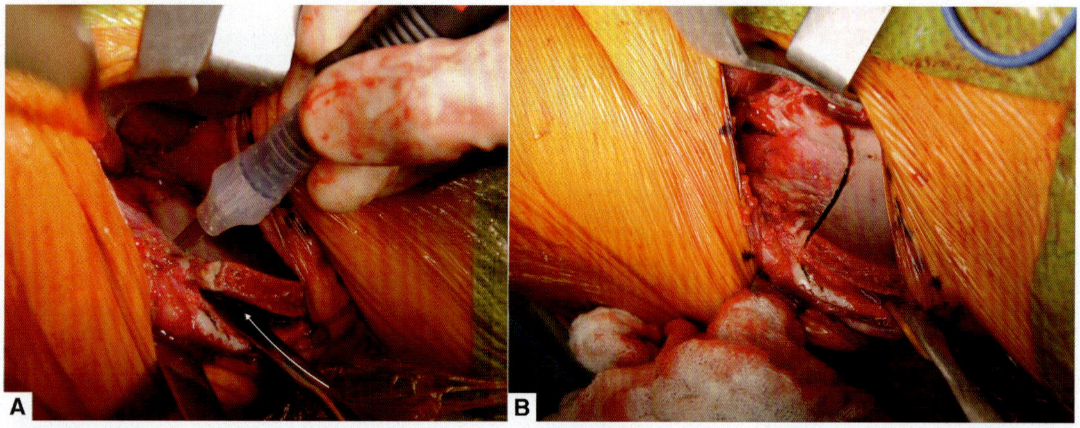

FIGURE 17.11 A, The lateral portion of the iliac apophysis is partially detached from the ilium to create a window where a small thin long Hohmann retractor is placed. A bone scalpel is used to cut the medial cortex of the ilium and mark the osteotomy. B, Final aspect of the osteotomy after the medial cortex is cut using a bone scalpel.

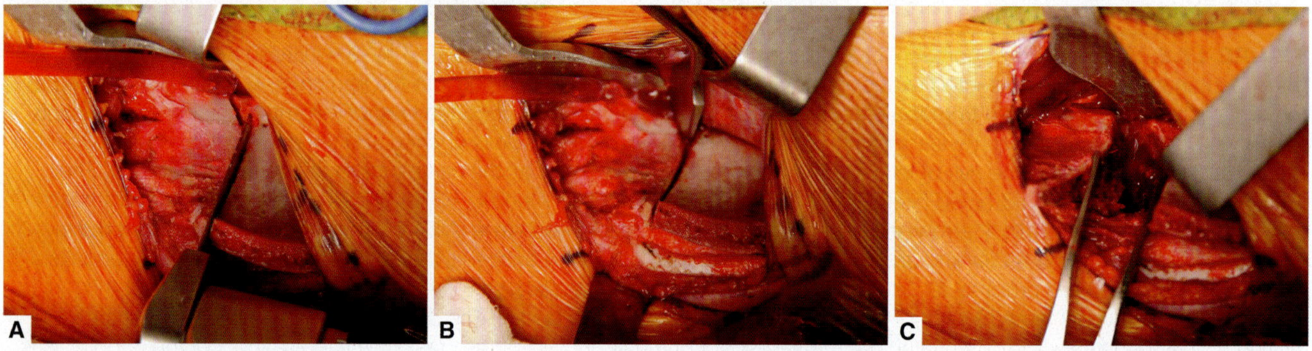

FIGURE 17.12. A, An oscillating saw is used to complete the supra-acetabular iliac osteotomy to about 1 cm from the pelvic brim. B, The osteotomy is completed by placing an angled Ganz chisel in the corner aiming toward the sciatic notch that is protected by a radiolucent reverse curved Hohmann retractor. C, A laminal spreader is inserted in the osteotomy to spread it open and reassure its completeness.

(**Figure 17.12**). A laminal spreader is inserted into the osteotomy and spread open to help with completion of the cut.

After the three osteotomies are completed, the acetabular fragment should be mobilized and a 3.5 mm Schanz pin is introduced in the supra-acetabular region above the AIIS. The acetabulum is manipulated to correct the posterior and lateral acetabular deficiency by anteversion and adduction of the fragment with respect to iliac osteotomy. The fragment is held in place with two or three 3/32 K-wires drilled through the ilium (**Figure 17.13**). Clinically, the proximal aspect of the fragment should be medial in relation to the AIIS. AP and false-profile imaging are obtained with fluoroscopy to ensure adequate correction of acetabular coverage and the position of the K-wires. The continuity in Shenton line, the degree of acetabular coverage, the femoral head migration index, the position of the teardrop, and the acetabular sourcil are the radiographic parameters to be checked. Hip stability is tested in flexion and internal rotation. If the hip persists with instability, further anteversion of the fragment is recommended. Rarely a concomitant intertrochanteric femoral varus derotational osteotomy is needed to improve the stability of the hip. Fixation is performed by replacing the K-wires with three to four 3.5-mm cortical screws. The iliac crest apophysis is reapproximated and the wounds are closed in layers.

In some cases, a concomitant femoral derotation osteotomy may need to be performed in the event that the hip becomes unstable anteriorly. The pelvic osteotomy will stabilize the posterior instability; however, because of extreme femoral anteversion, in extension and external rotation, the hip is seen to be unstable anteriorly on the false-profile view. In this case, a femoral derotation osteotomy should be performed to correct the anterior instability.

A spica cast is applied and kept for about 6 weeks when an abduction brace is applied in clinic at nighttime for 3 to 6 months after surgery. Patients are seen at 3, 6, and 12 months postoperatively and monitored until skeletal maturity (**Figure 17.14**).

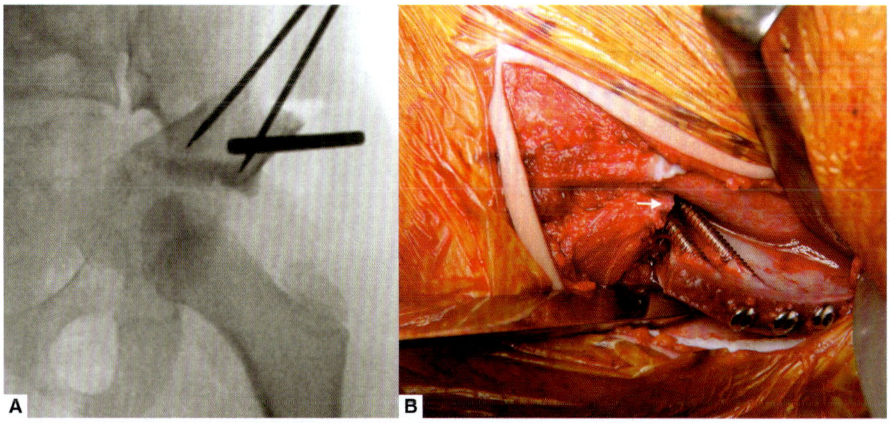

FIGURE 17.13. A, Intraoperative fluoroscopy showing the acetabular fragment has been mobilized with the aid of a Schanz pin in abduction and internal rotation to increase the lateral coverage and acetabular anteversion, respectively. Two K-wires hold the fragment provisionally. B, Intraoperative picture after the acetabular fragment has been fixed with 3.5 mm cortical screws showing the proximal aspect of the acetabular fragment is medial to the anterior superior iliac spine (ASIS) corresponding to achieve anteversion of the fragment.

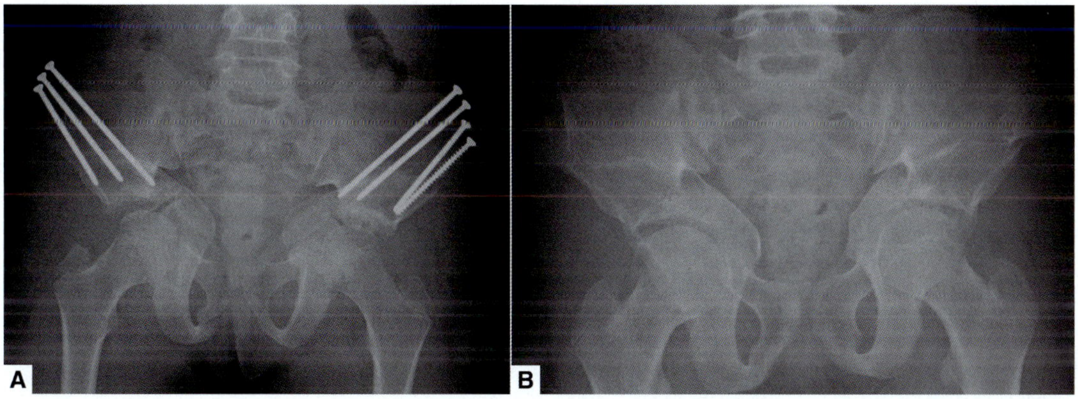

FIGURE 17.14. A, Postoperative anteroposterior (AP) pelvic radiograph at the 2-year follow-up visit following bilateral triple pelvic osteotomy. B, Postoperative AP pelvic radiograph at skeletal maturity after all implants have been removed showed adequate healing and corrected acetabular retroversion bilaterally.

OUTCOMES AND SPECIAL CONSIDERATIONS

We have reported the results of this modified anteverting triple pelvic osteotomy in 16 patients (21 hips) who were followed for a mean of 4 years (±2.6 years).[11] There were nine females and seven males and the mean age at surgery was 7.4 years (±2 years). After an average of 4 years, 20/21 hips (95%) remained clinically stable. However, we found a relatively high proportion of asymptomatic ischial and/or pubic nonunions (24%) and stress fracture of the pubis or ischium (14%). Only one patient developed an infection. Since recently reviewing this series of patients, we have started to use bone grafting to the ischium and pubis.

Surgical management of hip instability in Down syndrome is difficult and challenging. We believe that reorientation of the acetabulum through our modified anteverting triple osteotomy as described herein is the best pelvic osteotomy to achieve hip instability. Two previous studies reported that bilateral varus intertrochanteric osteotomy performed early (before age 7 years) may grant stability of the hip in select patients.[8,17] The recommended technique of varus osteotomy aims to decrease the neck-shaft angle to 105° and restore Shenton line. Correction of anteversion should be planned based on preoperative axial image. Typically, a minimum of 20° of femoral anteversion should remain. Patients who present with subluxation and acetabular dysplasia typically after 8 years of age require a pelvic reorientation procedure. Those authors agree with our philosophy that a triple pelvic osteotomy is the best technique for acetabular reorientation in patients with Down syndrome.

The Adolescent and Young Adult Down Syndrome Patient with Acetabular Dysplasia and Hip Subluxation

Hip instability may not present during childhood in patients with Down syndrome because they typically do not complain of pain. During adolescence or early years of adulthood, Down syndrome patients with hip subluxation and acetabular dysplasia may present because of decrease in the endurance and ability to walk. A full workup is necessary to reassure that there is no compromise of the spinal cord because of atlantoaxial instability. Once the hip is identified as the source of decreased function and eventually pain, a CT scan is recommended to evaluate the morphology of the pelvic and proximal femur. In general, we have found that acetabular dysplasia and subluxation in Down syndrome are associated with global acetabular insufficiency and acetabular retroversion.[5,9] MRI of the hip may also be helpful to assess the acetabular morphology, but its main indication is to investigate the health of the articular cartilage. Dynamic radiographs including an abduction and internal rotation AP pelvic view and a flexion false-profile view should be obtained preoperatively to confirm a concentric reduction of the femoral head in the native acetabulum. The presence of a pseudo-acetabular cavity with excessive proximal and lateral migration of the femoral head that does not reduce concentrically to the native hip socket is a potential contraindication for a reorientation osteotomy.

The surgical treatment of the young adult with hip dysplasia secondary to Down syndrome is challenging. We have reported our preliminary[9,18] and mid-term[19] experience with an anteverting Bernese PAO. We evaluated 19 patients with Down syndrome (26 hips) who underwent PAO at a mean age of 16 years (±5 years). At an average follow-up of 13 years (±5 years; range, 5 to 24 years), 13 (62%) of 21 hips demonstrated good or excellent Harris hip scores. Ninety-five percent of the patients were independent in ambulation. Nearly 70% of the hips were preserved; however, one in three hips met the criteria for failure, which was associated with older age at the time of the procedure and a moderate osteoarthritis grade (Tönnis grade 2) at the time of the procedure. The technique of acetabular reorientation using the Bernese PAO is described in detail in Chapter 5. PAO for the Down syndrome patient aims to correct the insufficient coverage of the femoral head and acetabular retroversion. Therefore, during mobilization of the fragment, the surgeon should internally rotate the acetabulum to increase the posterior coverage of the femoral head while rotating the fragment to also increase lateral coverage.

Older adult patients with advanced osteoarthritis (Tönnis grade 3) may benefit from a total hip arthroplasty (THA) to improve symptoms and function. The expected hip survivorship at 10 years is around 85%.[15] However, a higher risk of THA complications, including loosening, infection, and short-term surgical-related complications such as hemorrhage, pneumonia, and urinary tract infections, has been reported in patients with Down syndrome after THA.[14,16]

REFERENCES

1. Caird MS, Wills BP, Dormans JP. Down syndrome in children: the role of the orthopaedic surgeon. *J Am Acad Orthop Surg.* 2006; 14(11):610-619.
2. Diamond LS, Lynne D, Sigman B. Orthopedic disorders in patients with Down's syndrome. *Orthop Clin North Am.* 1981;12(1):57-71.
3. Shaw ED, Beals RK. The hip joint in Down's syndrome. A study of its structure and associated disease. *Clin Orthop Relat Res.* 1992(278):101-107.
4. Hresko MT, McCarthy JC, Goldberg MJ. Hip disease in adults with Down syndrome. *J Bone Joint Surg Br.* 1993;75(4):604-607.
5. Bulat E, Maranho DA, Kalish LA, Millis MB, Kim YJ, Novais EN. Acetabular global insufficiency in patients with down syndrome and hip-related symptoms: a matched-cohort study. *J Bone Joint Surg Am.* 2017;99(20):1760-1768.
6. Bennet GC, Rang M, Roye DP, Aprin H. Dislocation of the hip in trisomy 21. *J Bone Joint Surg Br.* 1982;64(3):289-294.
7. Roberts GM, Starey N, Harper P, Nuki G. Radiology of the pelvis and hips in adults with Down's syndrome. *Clin Radiol.* 1980;31(4):475-478.
8. Knight DM, Alves C, Wedge JH. Femoral varus derotation osteotomy for the treatment of habitual subluxation and dislocation of the pediatric hip in trisomy 21: a 10-year experience. *J Pediatr Orthop.* 2011;31(6):638-643.
9. Sankar WN, Schoenecker JG, Mayfield ME, Kim YJ, Millis MB. Acetabular retroversion in Down syndrome. *J Pediatr Orthop.* 2012; 32(3):277-281.
10. Maranho DA, Fuchs K, Kim YJ, Novais EN. Hip instability in patients with Down syndrome. *J Am Acad Orthop Surg.* 2018;26(13):455-462.
11. Maranho DA, Kim YJ, Williams KA, Novais EN. Preliminary results of an anteverting triple periacetabular osteotomy for the treatment of hip instability in Down syndrome. *J Child Orthop.* 2018;12(1):55-62.
12. Sankar WN. Complete redirectional acetabular osteotomies for neurogenic and syndromic hip dysplasia. *J Pediatr Orthop.* 2013;33 Suppl 1: S39-S44.
13. Sankar WN, Millis MB, Kim YJ. Instability of the hip in patients with Down Syndrome: improved results with complete redirectional acetabular osteotomy. *J Bone Joint Surg Am.* 2011;93(20):1924-1933.
14. Boylan MR, Kapadia BH, Issa K, Perfetti DC, Maheshwari AV, Mont MA. Down syndrome increases the risk of short-term complications after total hip arthroplasty. *J Arthroplasty.* 2016;31(2): 368-372.
15. Gross AE, Callaghan JJ, Zywiel MG, et al. Total hip arthroplasty in Down syndrome patients: an improvement in quality of life: replacement arthroplasty in Down syndrome (RADS) study group. *J Arthroplasty.* 2013;28(4):701-706.
16. Zywiel MG, Mont MA, Callaghan JJ, et al. Surgical challenges and clinical outcomes of total hip replacement in patients with Down's syndrome. *Bone Joint J.* 2013;95-B(11 Suppl A):41-45.
17. Kelley SP, Wedge JH. Management of hip instability in trisomy 21. *J Pediatr Orthop.* 2013;33 Suppl 1:S33-S38.
18. Katz DA, Kim YJ, Millis MB. Periacetabular osteotomy in patients with Down's syndrome. *J Bone Joint Surg Br.* 2005;87(4):544-547.
19. Maranho DA, Williams KA, Millis MB, Kim YJ, Novais EN. Mid-term results of periacetabular osteotomy for the treatment of hip dysplasia associated with Down syndrome: minimum follow-up of five years. *J Bone Joint Surg Am.* 2018;100(5):428-434.

CHAPTER 18

Osteonecrosis of the Femoral Head in Sickle Cell Disease

FUNDAMENTALS AND BACKGROUND

Sickle cell disease (SCD) is an inherited disorder of the red blood cells that leads to chronic hemolytic anemia and microvascular occlusion. One of the most common musculoskeletal complications associated with SCD is osteonecrosis of the femoral head. The incidence of osteonecrosis of the femoral head in patients with SCD is 2 to 4.5 cases per 100 patient-years with an overall prevalence of 10%.[1] Typically, children with SCD who developed osteonecrosis of the femoral head present with new onset of hip pain and a limp. A high suspicion for osteonecrosis of the femoral head in patients with SCD encourages early advanced imaging. Often, in the initial phase of necrosis, plain films, including an anteroposterior (AP) and frog-lateral radiographs, may not suffice for the diagnosis, and a magnetic resonance imaging (MRI) should be obtained. Femoral head involvement can be assessed by measuring the arc of the necrotic segment (the necrotic arc angle).[2] The size of the lesion is defined by the sum of the necrotic arc angles measured on the AP and frog-lateral radiographs. Collapse of the femoral head is measured as the distance from a perfect concentric circle around the femoral head to the area of collapse.[3] Multiple classifications exist for quantifying the extent of osteonecrosis of the femoral head. We use the University of Pennsylvania system (Steinberg staging).[4] According to the staging system, stage 0 is preclinical with normal radiographs and MRI; stage I has normal radiographs with abnormal MRI; stage II reveals diffuse or localized areas of cystic and sclerotic changes in the femoral head; in stage III, there is subchondral collapse without flattening of the femoral head (crescent sign); stage IV is identified by flattening of the femoral head but no acetabular involvement; stage V is characterized by the development of acetabular changes in addition to the collapse of the femoral head with joint space narrowing; stage VI is defined by advanced degenerative changes of the hip joint.[4] Grades I to IV are subdivided into A (<15% femoral head is affected), B (15% to 30% of the femoral head is affected) and C (>30% of the femoral head is affected).

Osteonecrosis of the femoral head can have a deleterious impact on patient's function and quality of life. Osteonecrosis can not only have a major impact on patient's function and quality of life, but can also affect the long-term survival of the native hip. Osteonecrosis may ultimately lead to deformity of the femoral head and osteoarthritis of the hip. The natural history of patients with SCD and osteonecrosis during childhood or adolescence is unsatisfactory, with 80% of hips developing pain, restricted motion, limb-length inequality, and limp.[5] Most asymptomatic patients develop symptoms later in life and may have radiographic progression to femoral head collapse.[6] A recent prospective study of children with SCD followed by MRI for an average of 2 years reported that 65% of the patients developed progression of their necrotic lesions.[7]

Treatment of osteonecrosis of the femoral head in patients with SCD includes nonsurgical strategies and surgical treatment. There is no medical treatment to prevent femoral head collapse. Physical therapy is typically recommended along with provisional limitation of weight-bearing. A randomized prospective study compared 21 adult patients with SCD treated with physical therapy alone versus 17 patients treated with core decompression and physical therapy. After a mean follow-up of 3 years, there was no difference in patient-reported outcomes and hip survival between the two groups.[8] Isolated core decompression was performed in the past for SCD osteonecrosis. However, contemporary techniques, including injection with osteoinductive cells, have improved the outcome of core decompression alone. Gangji et al[9,10] reported better symptom resolution and lower risk of femoral head collapse in patients undergoing core decompression with implantation of autologous bone marrow cells compared to core decompression alone. Hernigou et al[11] investigated 38 skeletally mature patients with SCD followed from 10 to 17 years and showed that core decompression with autologous bone marrow implantation brought about pain improvement and delayed progression to collapse of the femoral head in 87% of the hips. Although adults with osteonecrosis may benefit from a total hip arthroplasty (THA), patients with SCD have a higher proportion of complications and implant failure. Therefore, THA is not commonly performed in pediatric patients with SCD and osteonecrosis of the femoral head.[12-15]

In our current experience, children and adolescents with SCD presenting with hip pain typically undergo an anterior-posterior pelvic plain radiograph and a frog-leg lateral radiograph in addition to a contrast-enhanced MRI that helps in establishing the percentage of femoral head involved by necrosis process. Radiographic progression has been reported to be directly associated with the size and location of the necrotic lesion.[2,4,6,16] Although management of children with osteonecrosis secondary to SCD is controversial, with reports of relatively good functional outcome following nonsurgical and surgical treatment,[17] our preferred method of treatment is decompression by multiple epiphyseal drilling along with bone marrow autologous cell implantation.

Clinical Scenario

A 15-year-old Nigerian male with SCD and high hemolytic rate (HbSS) presented with right hip pain and a limp. His symptoms had been worsening for the past month. AP and frog-leg lateral radiographs reveal a localized sclerotic rim, suggesting osteonecrosis (**Figure 18.1.**). Coronal T1 postcontrast MRI revealed more than 50% of the femoral head was involved, and decompression by multiple epiphyseal drilling along with autologous bone marrow cell implantation was recommended (**Figure 18.2.**).

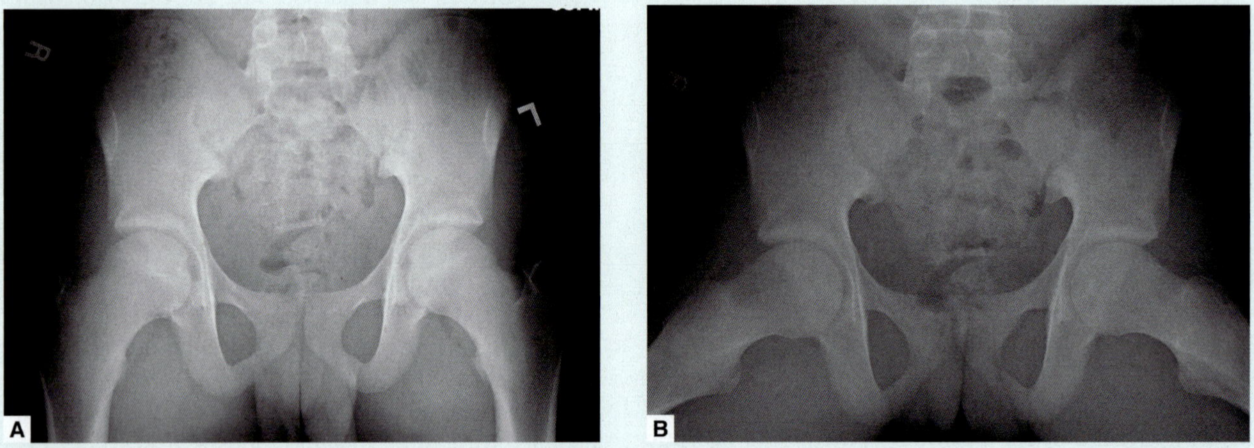

FIGURE 18.1. Anteroposterior (A) and frog-leg (B) radiographs of a 15-year-old male with sickle cell disease (HbSS) who presented with severe pain and limp for the past month. The radiographs are abnormal with sclerosis of the right femoral head without subchondral collapse (Steinberg stage II).

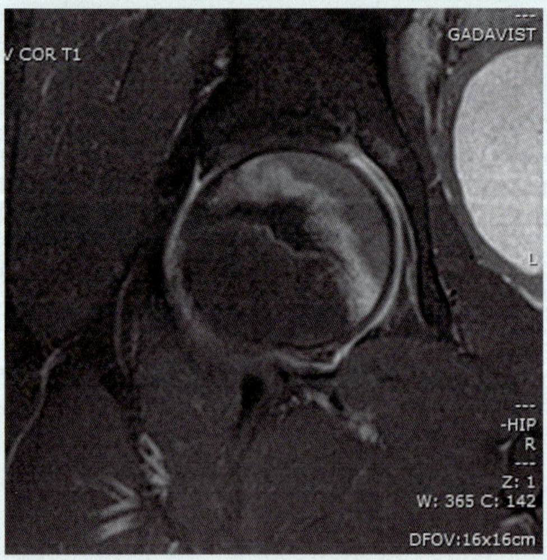

FIGURE 18.2. Coronal T1-post contrast-enhanced magnetic resonance imaging showing more than 30% (severe) involvement of the femoral head (Steinberg stage IIC).

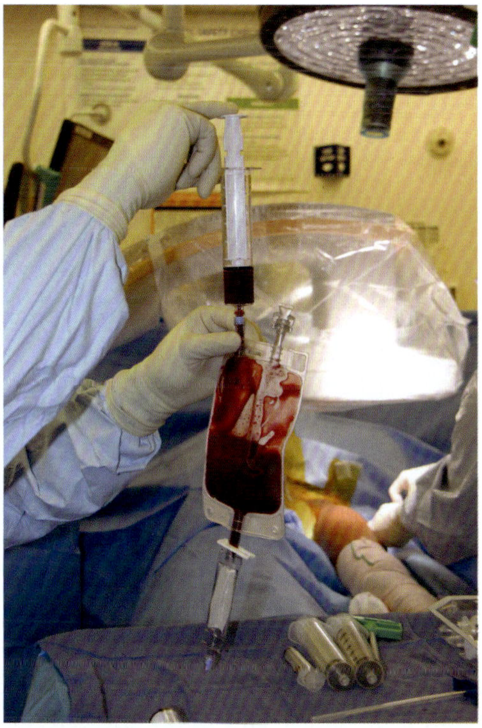

FIGURE 18.3. Intraoperative photograph showing the 60 mL of iliac bone aspirate transferred to a sterile bag for a total of 120 mL.

SURGICAL TECHNIQUE

The patient is positioned supine with a radiolucent bump under the ipsilateral shoulder to allow a slight shift of the ipsilateral trunk so that the lower extremity is in neutral rotation, with the patella facing forward and pointing toward the ceiling. The entire hemipelvis along with the ipsilateral lower extremity is prepared and draped free. A puncture wound is performed at the level of the iliac crest just above the anterior superior iliac spine. An eight-gauge needle is inserted deep into the ileum, carefully avoiding plunging through the inner or outer table of the ilium. About 120 mL of aspirated bone marrow cells is aspirated in a stepwise fashion. After about each 10 mL of aspiration, the needle should be rotated 90° with additional 10 mL of bone marrow aspirated. This will be followed by retraction of 1 cm in order to improve the number of bone marrow cells aspirated and reduce the volume of pure blood. Each syringe contains 60 mL of aspirated iliac marrow, and the content should be transferred to a prepared bag for a total of 120 mL (**Figure 18.3.**). Once the desired volume of 120 mL is achieved, iliac aspirated is transferred to a recipient for centrifugation (Harvest Technologies Corporation, Plymouth, MA) in the operating room (**Figure 18.4.**). While the bone marrow cells aspirated is processed, the multiple drilling of the epiphysis is performed.

Under C-arm fluoroscopy, a 2.8-mm guide wire for the 6.5-mm cannulated screw system is percutaneously inserted through the lateral cortex of the femur into the osteonecrotic area.

Another additional 2.8-mm guide wire is introduced, and then either a third wire is placed or the second wire reinserted using a different path to allow for multiple drilling of the epiphysis (**Figure 18.5.**). We then select the guide wire most centrally located in the necrotic area to be used as a guide for a perforating eight-gauge bone marrow biopsy needle. (Harvest Technologies Corporation, Plymouth, MA). The guide wire is removed and exchanged with the biopsy needle. This combination of guide wire and injection needle is chosen to get a tight fit around the bone because the injection is under pressure

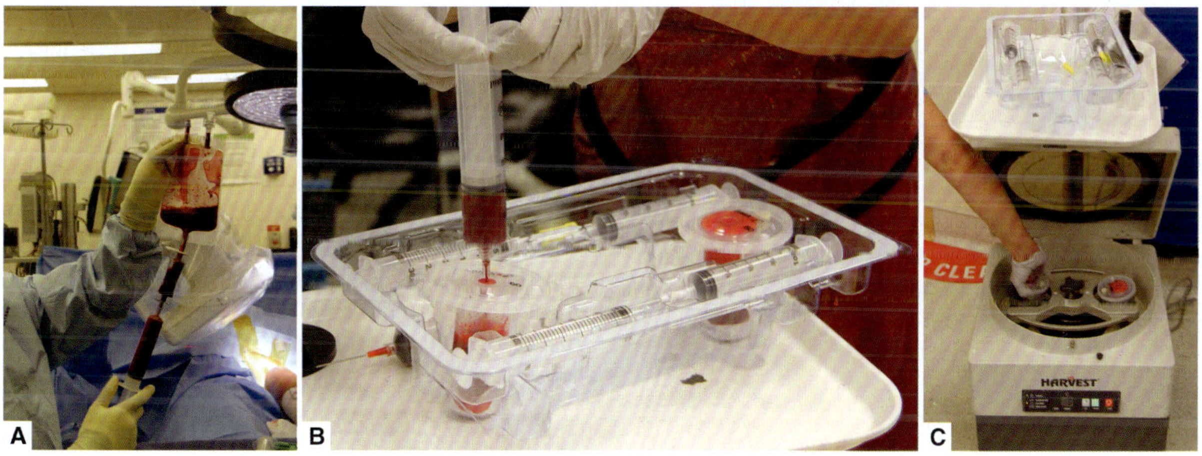

FIGURE 18.4. (A) Intraoperative photograph showing the aspirate being recollected from the sterile bag, and then (B) it is transferred into the recipient that will be placed into the (C) centrifugation system (Harvest Technologies Corporation, Plymouth, MA).

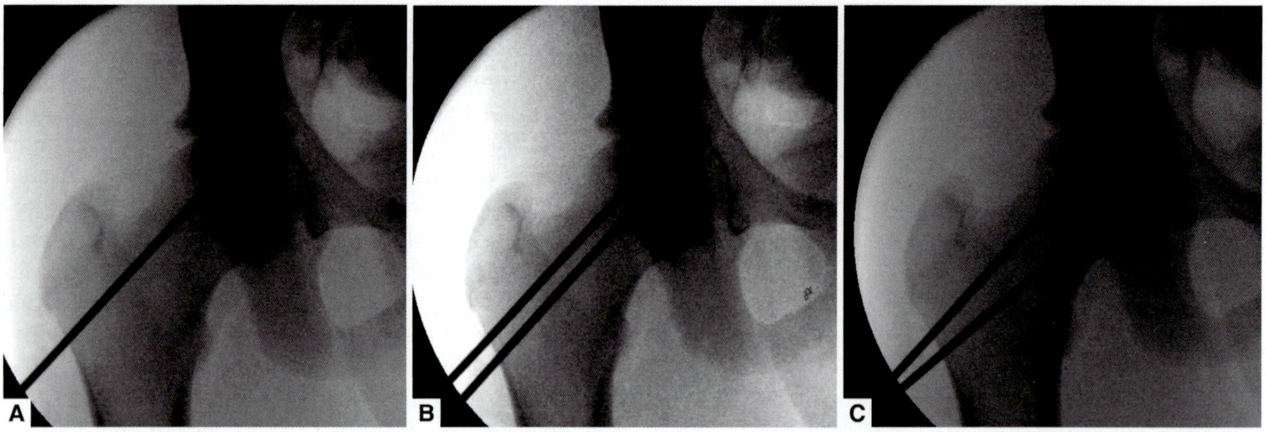

FIGURE 18.5. A, Intraoperative picture showing a guide wire for the cannulated system introduced percutaneously in the lateral aspect of the femur. B, Intraoperative fluoroscopy imaging showing the position of the initial guide wire. C, Intraoperative fluoroscopy imaging showing a different path for the guide wire is used to allow for multiple drilling of the epiphysis.

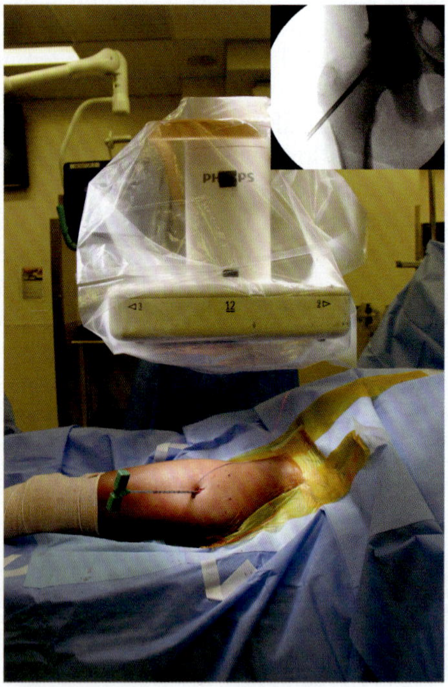

FIGURE 18.6. Intraoperative picture showing an eight-gauge bone marrow biopsy needle (Harvest Technologies Corporation, Plymouth, MA) inserted into the lateral aspect of the femur through the previously placed guide wire. In the top right-hand corner is the correspondent fluoroscopy image. The concentrated bone marrow cells are injected through the biopsy needle.

(**Figure 18.6.**). The concentrated marrow is injected into the femoral head slowly and under pressure to reduce leakage. The trocar and Steinman pins are then removed, and the small wounds are closed.

The protocol for treatment of patients with SCD includes admission to hematology service the day prior to surgery. The patient hemoglobin level is optimized for surgery, and the goal is to avoid a hemolytic crisis. With this goal in mind, during surgery the room temperature is kept slightly warmer than usual. Postoperatively, patients are admitted for 24 hours for hydration, pain management, and observation. We do not use any bracing or immobilization. Patients are instructed to follow a non-weight-bearing protocol for 6 weeks. Then, the patients progress to weight-bearing on the affected extremity with a physical therapy assisted rehabilitation program.

We have reported our preliminary results showing that multiple epiphyseal drilling with autologous bone marrow cell implantation brings about short-term clinical improvement and limits radiographic progression of osteonecrosis of the femoral head associated with SCD in children with minimal morbidity.[18] The patient described experienced improvement in his postoperative pain and limp over the first 2 years after his surgery (**Figure 18.7.**). Although he had some limitation of internal rotation with the hip flexed during his examination in clinic, he was mostly asymptomatic and had no specific complaints at his 2-year follow-up visit. Patients with SCD may have

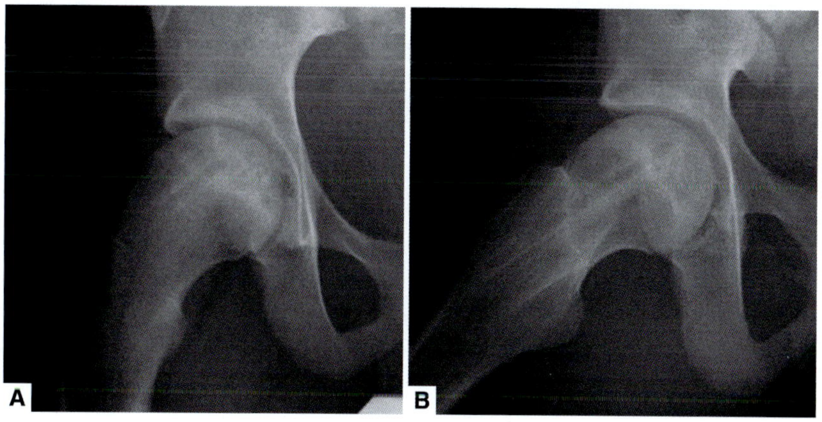

FIGURE 18.7. Postoperative image obtained 2 years after surgery showing that there has been no further progressive collapse of the femoral head.

residual deformity at skeletal maturity related to the osteonecrosis during adolescence or childhood, despite treatment with multiple epiphyseal drilling and implantation of autologous bone marrow concentrate. Therefore, routine follow-up and patient education is important. Residual deformities can be treated to improve the morphology of the femoral head-neck junction using arthroscopic or open approaches.

REFERENCES

1. Milner PF, Kraus AP, Sebes JI, et al. Sickle cell disease as a cause of osteonecrosis of the femoral head. *N Engl J Med.* 1991;325(21):1476-1481.
2. Kerboul M, Thomine J, Postel M, Merle d'Aubigne R. The conservative surgical treatment of idiopathic aseptic necrosis of the femoral head. *J Bone Joint Surg Br.* 1974;56(2):291-296.
3. Mose K. Methods of measuring in Legg-Calve-Perthes disease with special regard to the prognosis. *Clin Orthop Relat Res.* 1980(150):103-109.
4. Steinberg ME, Hayken GD, Steinberg DR. A quantitative system for staging avascular necrosis. *J Bone Joint Surg Br.* 1995;77(1):34-41.
5. Hernigou P, Galacteros F, Bachir D, Goutallier D. Deformities of the hip in adults who have sickle-cell disease and had avascular necrosis in childhood. A natural history of fifty-two patients. *J Bone Joint Surg Am.* 1991;73(1):81-92.
6. Hernigou P, Habibi A, Bachir D, Galacteros F. The natural history of asymptomatic osteonecrosis of the femoral head in adults with sickle cell disease. *J Bone Joint Surg Am.* 2006;88(12):2565-2572.
7. Gupta R, Adekile AD. MRI follow-up and natural history of avascular necrosis of the femoral head in Kuwaiti children with sickle cell disease. *J Pediatr Hematol Oncol.* 2004;26(6):351-353.
8. Neumayr LD, Aguilar C, Earles AN, et al. Physical therapy alone compared with core decompression and physical therapy for femoral head osteonecrosis in sickle cell disease. Results of a multicenter study at a mean of three years after treatment. *J Bone Joint Surg Am.* 2006;88(12):2573-2582.
9. Gangji V, Hauzeur JP, Matos C, De Maertelaer V, Toungouz M, Lambermont M. Treatment of osteonecrosis of the femoral head with implantation of autologous bone-marrow cells. A pilot study. *J Bone Joint Surg Am.* 2004;86(6):1153-1160.
10. Gangji V, De Maertelaer V, Hauzeur JP. Autologous bone marrow cell implantation in the treatment of non-traumatic osteonecrosis of the femoral head: five year follow-up of a prospective controlled study. *Bone.* 2011;49(5):1005-1009.
11. Hernigou P, Daltro G, Filippini P, Mukasa MM, Manicom O. Percutaneous implantation of autologous bone marrow osteoprogenitor cells as treatment of bone avascular necrosis related to sickle cell disease. *Open Orthop J.* 2008;2:62-65.
12. Acurio MT, Friedman RJ. Hip arthroplasty in patients with sickle-cell haemoglobinopathy. *J Bone Joint Surg Br.* 1992;74(3):367-371.
13. Bishop AR, Roberson JR, Eckman JR, Fleming LL. Total hip arthroplasty in patients who have sickle-cell hemoglobinopathy. *J Bone Joint Surg Am.* 1988;70(6):853-855.
14. Hanker GJ, Amstutz HC. Osteonecrosis of the hip in the sickle-cell diseases. Treatment and complications. *J Bone Joint Surg Am.* 1988;70(4):499-506.
15. Moran MC, Huo MH, Garvin KL, Pellicci PM, Salvati EA. Total hip arthroplasty in sickle cell hemoglobinopathy. *Clin Orthop Relat Res.* 1993(294):140-148.
16. Mont MA, Zywiel MG, Marker DR, McGrath MS, Delanois RE. The natural history of untreated asymptomatic osteonecrosis of the femoral head: a systematic literature review. *J Bone Joint Surg Am.* 2010;92(12):2165-2170.
17. Mallet C, Abitan A, Vidal C, et al. Management of osteonecrosis of the femoral head in children with sickle cell disease: results of conservative and operative treatments at skeletal maturity. *J Child Orthop.* 2018;12(1):47-54.
18. Novais EN, Sankar WN, Wells L, Carry PM, Kim YJ. Preliminary results of multiple epiphyseal drilling and autologous bone marrow implantation for osteonecrosis of the femoral head secondary to sickle cell disease in children. *J Pediatr Orthop.* 2015;35(8):810-815.

CHAPTER 19

Principles of Management of Hip Deformity in Cerebral Palsy

INTRODUCTION

Cerebral palsy (CP) is the most common cause of physical disability affecting children in developed countries.[1] CP describes a group of permanent disorders of the development of movement and posture, causing activity limitation, which are attributed to nonprogressive disturbances that occurred in the developing fetal or infant brain.[2,3] CP is defined by the presence of a static neurologic injury, with associated progressive musculoskeletal pathology.[4-6] Hip displacement in children with CP is the second most common deformity after spastic equinus of the ankle and may progress from initial silent lateral subluxation to painful dislocation when left untreated.[5,7,8]

The most useful development in the classification of CP in recent years has been the creation of the Gross Motor Function Classification System (GMFCS).[1] The GMFCS is a five-level ordinal grading system based on the assessment of self-initiated movement with emphasis on function with regard to sitting and walking. The risk of progression from hip displacement to dislocation is related to severity of neurologic involvement,[9,10] walking ability,[11,12] and is directly related to gross motor function as graded by the GMFCS[7] (**Figure 19.1**).

Historically, the incidence of CP has been reported to range from 1.5 to 2.5 per 1000 live births in several well-designed, population-based studies.[13] However, with recent improved resuscitation and care of the premature infant, a modest increase (3 per 1000 live births) has been reported in North America.[14] A series of authors have reported that the prevalence of hip displacement in CP is related to the degree of body involvement, ranging from very low risk in children with spastic hemiplegia (1%) to very high risk in children with spastic quadriplegia (75%).[8,11] Three large population-based studies have calculated that the overall prevalence of hip displacement is approximately 35% across a population of children with CP.[7,15,16]

PATHOPHYSIOLOGY

The majority of children with CP are born with anatomically "normal" hips without evidence of hip displacement or dislocation.[17] However, the natural history of spastic hip disease places children at risk for progressive lateral hip displacement.[18] In children with CP, this displacement is commonly referred to as "silent subluxation" as children

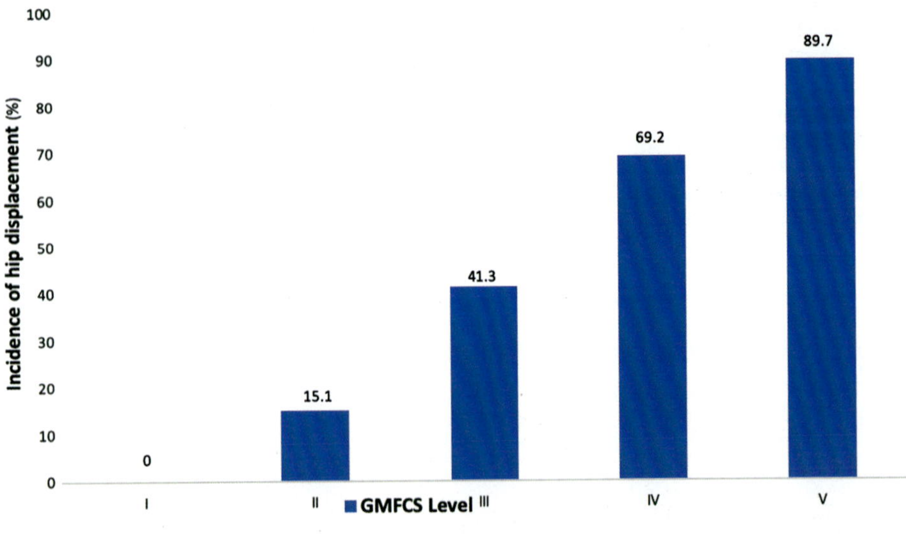

FIGURE 19.1. The relationship between hip displacement (Reimers index >30%) versus gross motor function classification system (GMFCS) level. Adapted from Soo et al.[7]

are often not symptomatic until the hip is dislocated and painful.

The altered brain function characteristic of CP includes loss of selective motor control, abnormal muscle tone, imbalance between agonists and antagonists, and impaired body balance mechanisms. The neurologic lesion associated with CP manifests as a nonprogressive or static encephalopathy; however, the associated musculoskeletal pathology is progressive, resulting in contractures of muscle tendon units, bony torsional deformity, and ultimately joint instability.[5,19] Asymmetric muscle spasticity and power has long been felt to be a major contributor to hip instability in children with CP. Sharrard et al[20] demonstrated progressive limitation of abduction, often associated with flexion deformity, was an indicator of early instability of the hip. In their study, they found that no hip with radiologic evidence of subluxation had abduction greater than 45°, suggesting limited abduction plays some role in the development of hip instability.

Two critical components to proximal femoral anatomy are anteversion of the femoral neck in the transverse plane and the femoral neck-shaft angle (NSA) in the coronal plane.[21,22] Robin et al[23] demonstrated that these two deformities were closely related to a child's GMFCS level. In their study, they propose that increased femoral anteversion and NSA may be caused by persistent fetal alignment because of delayed walking and limitations in gross motor function. The combination of elevated femoral neck anteversion and NSA contributes to the increased risk of hip displacement. A proper understanding of this cascade helps in formulating a treatment plan (**Figure 19.2**).

Soo et al[7] demonstrated a linear relationship between the rate of hip displacement and a child's GMFCS level. In their population-based study, GMFCS V children demonstrated an incidence of hip displacement of 90%, whereas there were no cases of hip displacement in 114 children with CP who were GMFCS level I. Hägglund et al[24] came to very similar conclusions with respect to his population-based study of children with CP in Sweden. Much can be learned from these population-based studies; knowledge and identification of groups of children with "hips at risk" for displacement are critical for planning surveillance programs and initiating early intervention.[7,25,26]

In establishing a hip surveillance protocol, reliance on clinical examination alone is not sufficient; regular radiographic examination is also important.[27] Early indicators for hip displacement include a patient's GMFCS level, age, gait classification, and migration percentage (MP).[28] Not surprisingly, isolated techniques to reduce spasticity or address adductor contracture alone have been ultimately disappointing in preventing hip displacement in higher level GMFCS children.[29-31] Hip surveillance identifies children with progressive hip displacement but does not dictate the timing or type of intervention.[32] Treatment must be tailored for the individual child taking into consideration all the factors mentioned in this section.

IMAGING AND CLASSIFICATION

Decisions for treatment regarding spastic hip displacement must be made in conjunction with a well-taken anteroposterior (AP) radiograph of the pelvis and hip joint in the supine position.[33,34] For hip surveillance to be successful, a standardized radiographic technique must be followed, ensuring the reliability between interval radiographs and between patients.[35] Recognition and positional correction of excessive femoral anteversion, hip flexion, and adduction contractures are necessary to generate accurate and reliable radiographs.[23,34] Unrecognized hip flexion contracture will create a lordotic pelvis (increased anterior pelvic tilt), which can be corrected by raising the legs on pillows to flatten the lumbar spine.[25] Positioning the legs parallel to each other will address the

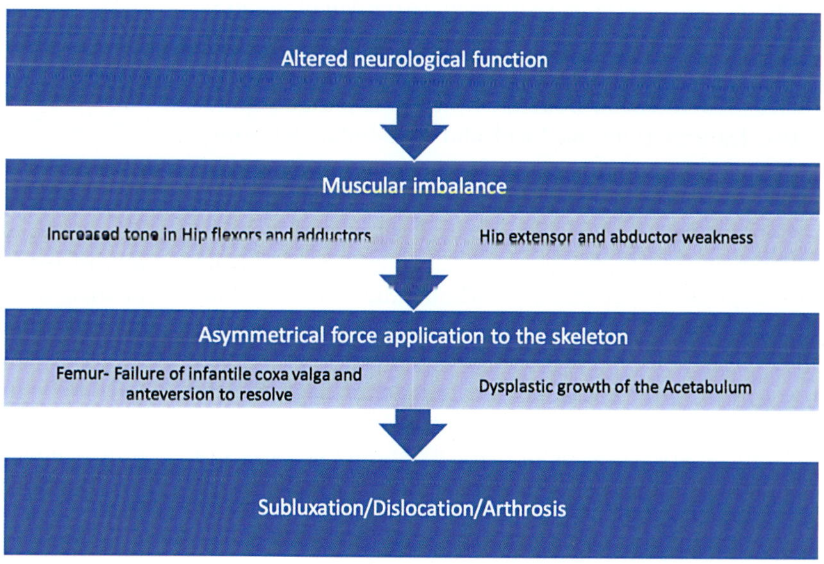

FIGURE 19.2. Pathophysiology associated with spastic hip subluxation.

adduction or abduction contractures, and pointing the patella upward will correct for excessive femoral anteversion.[26] A film-focus distance of 115 cm has been suggested to standardize film magnification between patients.[10]

The most accepted and reproducible measurement for spastic hip displacement is Reimers' MP,[36,37] which is a measure of the femoral head's containment within the acetabulum in the coronal plane.[38] This measurement is obtained identifying both Hilgenreiner and Perkin lines and then measuring, as a percentage, the amount of the ossified femoral head that has migrated laterally beyond Perkin line. In cases of severe displacement, there is often a "gothic arch" deformity of the lateral acetabular margin, and in these cases, the midpoint of the lateral acetabular margin is used instead of Perkin line.[37] The continuous measurement of the MP has proven to be valid, reliable, and useful in measuring hip displacement in children with CP.[27,36,39,40]

The definition of a hip "at risk" of instability is defined as having an MP greater than 30%.[36] Miller and Bagg[39] found that children (2 to 18 years) whose MP was greater than 60% progressed to dislocation (MP >90%) during childhood. Furthermore, those children (2 to 18 years) with an MP between 30% and 60% had equal rates of hip displacement (25%) and recommended close surveillance and surgical intervention to prevent hip dislocation. Settecerri and Karol[41] noted that a preoperative MP greater than 50% was associated with poor results and a higher revision rate. Oh et al[42] reported similar results using an MP greater than 50%, regardless of whether children were treated with femoral and pelvic osteotomy or femoral osteotomy in isolation. Terjesen[43] examined a population-based cohort of 334 children with CP in Norway and found that the mean yearly progression in MP increased markedly with decreasing functional level, from 0.2% for GMFCS I to 9.5% for GMFCS V.

The trajectory of hip development in children and adolescents with CP can be described using a variety of tools, including serial measurement of the MP of Reimers, head shaft angle, and hip morphology at skeletal maturity. In 2008, a new CP hip classification scheme was introduced that included both quantitative (MP) and qualitative features (femoral head and acetabular deformity, pelvic obliquity, and break in Shenton line) of femoroacetabular deformity.[44,45] The Melbourne CP Hip Classification System (MCPHCS) is a six-level ordinal grading scheme applied to children at skeletal maturity (closure of the triradiate cartilage).[45] Although designed for children at skeletal maturity, Gose et al[46] recently validated the MCPHCS for hip disease in children with CP between the ages of 2 and 7 with open triradiate cartilage. Recent studies have demonstrated the correlation between poor hip morphology at skeletal maturity and higher levels of pain and dysfunction.[47] In more advanced dysplasia, CT provides essential information about the extent and location of acetabular deficiency.[48]

HIP SURVEILLANCE

Hip surveillance refers to systematic periodic clinical and radiographic assessment of the hips of children with CP, to detect hip displacement when it is early and more effective management options are available.[33] Because of the increased risk of hip displacement in children with CP who do not walk, the first screening radiograph is usually advised at age 12 months and continued every 6 to 12 months until skeletal maturity.[34,49,50] Surveillance may need to be continued after skeletal maturity if the hips remain unstable, especially in the presence of symptomatic displacement, pelvic obliquity, and progressive scoliosis. Hip surveillance programs have demonstrated the ability to identify early indicators of progressive hip displacement and, with appropriate and timely surgical intervention, prevent hip dislocation and the need for salvage surgery.[33,34,49,50] Available surveillance guidelines on the Internet include the Australian Hip Surveillance Guidelines for Children with Cerebral Palsy (2014),[51] the Swedish CPUP Radiographic Follow-Up to Prevent Hip Dislocation,[52] the British Columbia Hip Surveillance Program,[53] and the American Academy of Cerebral Palsy and Developmental Medicine Hip Surveillance Care Pathway.[54]

In establishing a hip surveillance protocol, reliance on clinical examination alone is not sufficient; regular radiographic examination is also important.[27] Early indicators for hip displacement include a patient's GMFCS level, age, gait classification and migration percentage (MP).[28] Not surprisingly, isolated techniques to reduce spasticity or address adductor contracture alone have been ultimately disappointing in preventing hip displacement in higher level GMFCS children.[29-31] Hip surveillance identifies children with progressive hip displacement but does not dictate the timing or type of intervention.[32] Treatment must be tailored for the individual child taking into consideration all of the above-mentioned factors. Our Boston Children's Hip surveillance guidelines were developed in 2013 and is used across our enterprise to standardize the practice of radiographic hip surveillance for children with neuromuscular conditions (**Figure 19.3**).

TREATMENT OPTIONS

Treatment of the hip needs to be considered in the context of overall management of the child, in the context of their family, and in the presence of multiple medical comorbidities. Tone reduction has a primary place in all treatment strategies. Medical comorbidities that may need to be investigated and managed prior to any form of hip surgery include the movement disorder, respiratory illness, epilepsy, bone health, nutrition, and gastrointestinal function. In particular, optimization of the movement disorder using various combinations of oral medications, neurolytic blocks, and occasionally intrathecal baclofen

Until every child is well™

Hip Surveillance Screening Schedule

Boston Children's Hospital
Orthopedic Center
bostonchildrens.org/cp
617-355-6021

Using the **Gross Motor Function Classification System (GMFCS)**, a five-level ordinal classification system based on activities like walking and standing, Boston Children's Cerebral Palsy team are following a comprehensive screening schedule for hip surveillance, according to the severity of gross motor involvement.

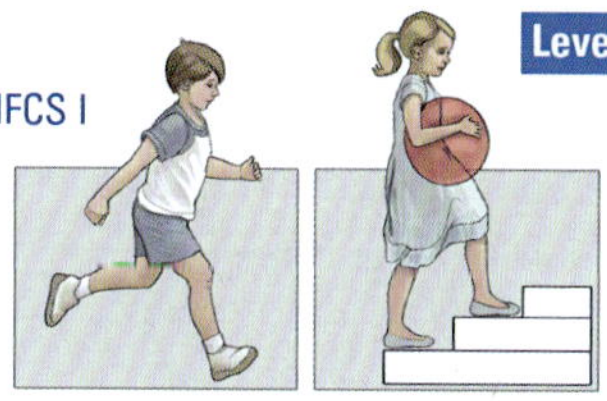
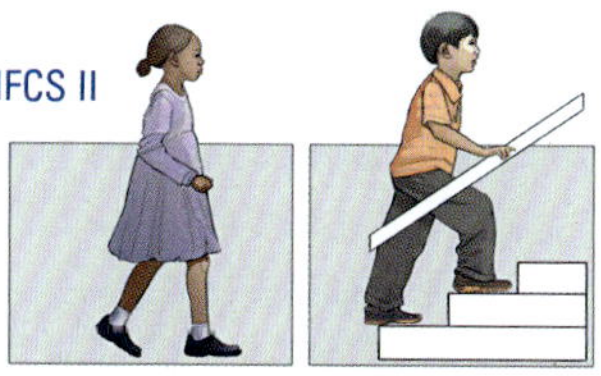
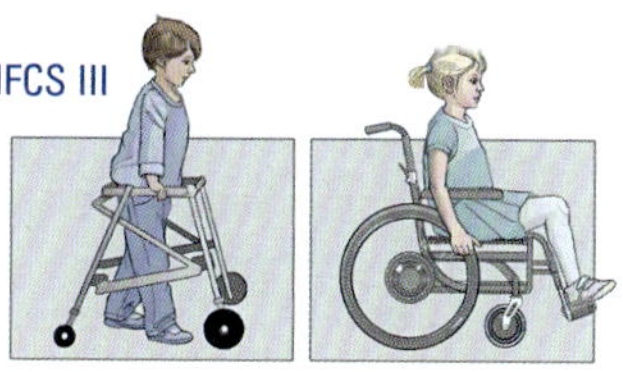
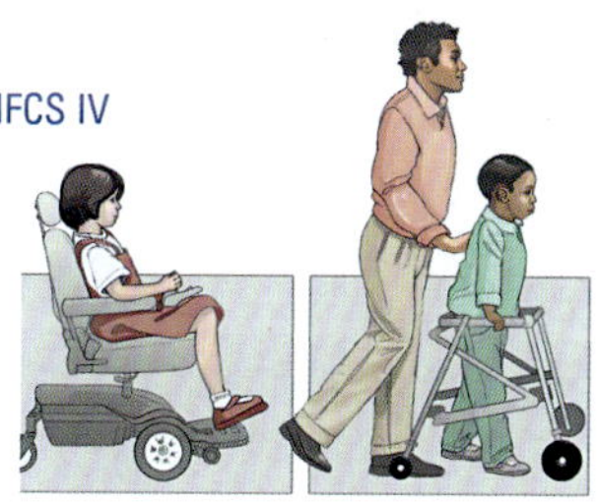
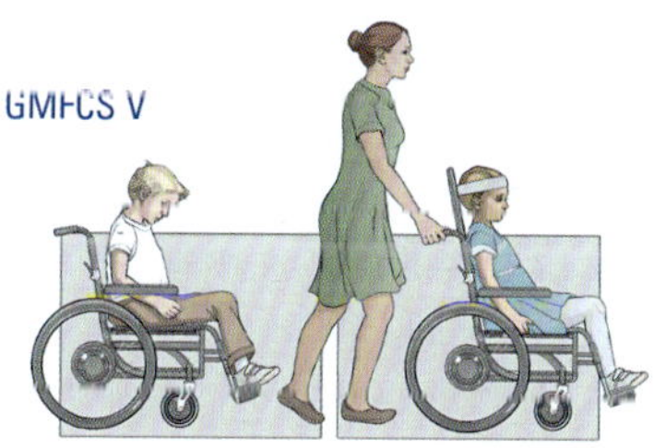

Level	Time period	Frequency of surveillance
GMFCS I	Younger than 2	All patients should have a clinical examination and assessment of GMFCS level
	3 years old	Repeat clinical examination and reassessment of GMFCS level and repeat AP pelvic x-ray
	6 years old	Repeat clinical examination, reassessment of GMFCS level, and repeat AP pelvic x-ray; may discharge from hip surveillance if asymptomatic without other significant signs of symptoms
GMFCS II	Younger than 2	All patients should have a clinical examination with AP pelvic x-ray at initial examination
	Annually	Repeat yearly clinical examination and AP pelvic x-ray if initial x-ray is normal, or clinical examination changes significantly
	6 years old	Repeat clinical examination, reassessment of GMFCS level, and repeat AP pelvic x-ray
	8 to 10 years old	If stable, review with clinical examination and AP pelvic x-ray; if unremarkable discharge, if abnormal continue yearly surveillance
GMFCS III	Younger than 2	All patients should have a clinical examination with AP pelvic x-ray at initial examination
	Every 6 months	If the MP is abnormal or unstable, repeat clinical examination and AP pelvis x-ray every 6 months until the MP stabilizes
	6 years old	Verify GMFCS level, and at each visit thereafter, if GMFCS level changes, modify surveillance accordingly
	Annually	Once MP stabilizes, reduce to annual clinical examination and AP pelvis x-ray; continue yearly surveillance until skeletal maturity
GMFCS IV	Younger than 2	All patients should have a clinical examination with AP pelvic x-ray at initial examination
	Every 6 months	If the MP is abnormal or unstable, repeat clinical examination and AP pelvis x-ray every 6 months until 6 years of age
	6 years old	Verify GMFCS level, and at each visit thereafter, if GMFCS level changes, modify surveillance accordingly
	Every 6 months	Until MP stabilizes, continue with repeat clinical examination and AP pelvis x-ray every 6 months until MP stabilizes
	Annually	Once MP stabilizes, reduce to annual clinical examination and AP pelvis x-ray and continue surveillance until skeletal maturity
GMFCS V	Younger than 2	All patients should have a clinical examination with AP pelvic x-ray at initial examination
	Every 6 months	If the MP is abnormal or unstable, repeat clinical examination and AP pelvis x-ray every 6 months until 6 years of age
	6 years old	Verify GMFCS level, and at each visit thereafter, if GMFCS level changes, modify surveillance accordingly
	Every 6 months	If MP remains unstable, continue with repeat clinical examination and AP pelvis x-ray every 6 months until MP stabilizes
	Annually	Once MP stabilizes, reduce to annual clinical examination and AP pelvis x-ray and continue surveillance until skeletal maturity
Hemiplegia (Winters and Gage)	Younger than 2	Surveillance as per the guidelines for GMFCS II
	6 years old	Repeat clinical examination, reassessment of the GMFCS level, repeat AP pelvis x-ray and continue yearly surveillance until skeletal maturity

FIGURE 19.3. Boston Children's Hospital Cerebral Palsy Hip surveillance guidelines. AP, anteroposterior; GMFCS, gross motor function classification system; MP, migration percentage.

Boston Children's Cerebral Palsy Hip Surveillance Screening Guide

Boston Children's Hospital
Orthopedic Center
bostonchildrens.org/cp
617-355-6021

The incidence of hip displacement is approximately 35 percent in children with cerebral palsy. This hip surveillance screening guide can help detect which patients may be at risk for spastic hip displacement or dislocation.

This hip surveillance guide provides direction on gathering medical history, conducting a physical examination and using the comprehensive screening schedule *(see reverse)*.

GATHER MEDICAL HISTORY AND CONDUCT PHYSICAL EXAMINATION

1. Does the child experience pain related to the hip? If yes, is there pain or discomfort with diaper changes, seating and positional changes or during other activities of daily living?
2. Does stiffness or pain around the child's hips limit the parent's ability to provide regular care for the child, such as perineal care, dressing, bathing and seating?
3. Has there been a recent deterioration in the child's lower extremity function, such as decreased sitting or standing tolerance?

If yes to the questions above, is there an orthopedic surgeon, physiatrist or pediatrician who is managing the child's hips?

CONDUCT A PHYSICAL EXAMINATION

Tardieu Scale

Measure hip abduction range of motion with hips at 0° and 90° flexion, according to the Modified Tardieu Scale (R1-dynamic and R2-static values)

The Tardieu Scale is a clinical measure of muscle spasticity for patients with neuromuscular conditions. This scale attempts to differentiate between muscle contracture (fixed muscle length) and muscle spasm (velocity-dependent muscle contraction).

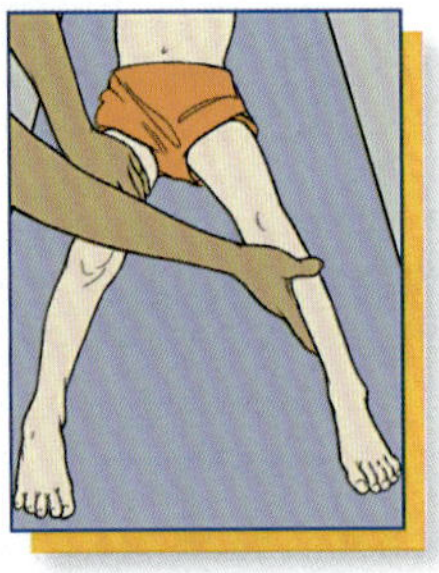

Thomas Test

Assess for presence of hip flexion contracture via Thomas Test

The patient lies flat (supine) on the examination table and brings one knee to the chest to flex the hip, while the other leg remains extended (straight).

The test is positive if the opposite (extended leg):

- hip flexes = tight iliopsoas
- hip abducts = tight tensor fascia lata
- knee extension = tight rectus femoris muscle

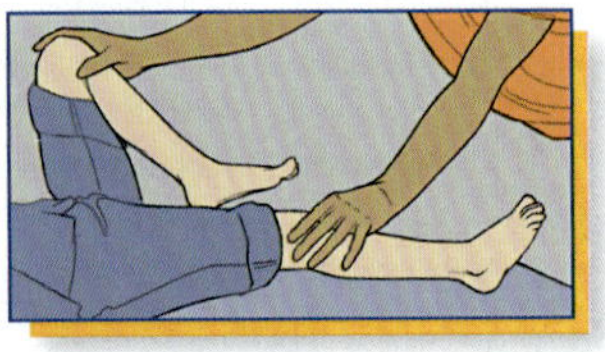

Galeazzi Test

Assess for leg length discrepancy via Galeazzi test

The patient lies flat on the examination table with knees flexed so that the feet are flat on the examination table; if the knees are not level then the test is positive, indicating potential hip instability or dislocation.

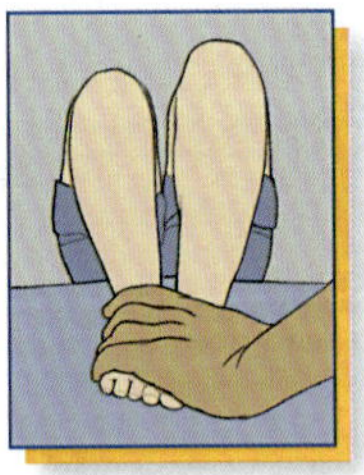

CRITERIA FOR REFERRING TO AN ORTHOPEDIC SURGEON

1. If the migration percentage is greater than 30 percent on x-ray.
2. If the hip abduction end range (R2) is less than 30 degrees.
3. If the Thomas Test or Hip Abduction Test shows deterioration or asymmetry.
4. If the patient/family answers yes to the three clinical questions described in medical history.

BOSTON CHILDREN'S HOSPITAL OFFERS ORTHOPEDIC CARE AT LOCATIONS IN BOSTON, WALTHAM, LEXINGTON AND PEABODY, MA.

FIGURE 19.3. *(continued)*

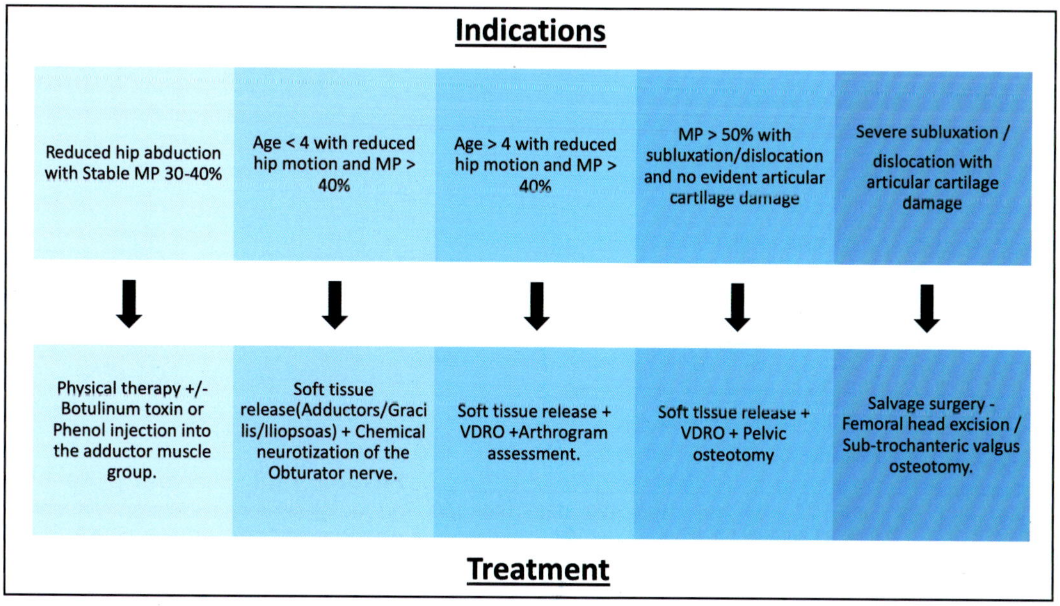

FIGURE 19.4. A general treatment guideline for the management of spastic hip subluxation. MP, migration percentage; VDRO, varus derotation osteotomy.

may result in less postoperative pain and fewer complications than in children in whom movement disorder management has not been optimized. Broad treatment guidelines are shown in **Figure 19.4**.

Preventative Surgery

Preventative hip surgery for the nonambulant child with CP applies to surgical procedures that involve lengthening of some of the hip adductors and may also involve lengthening of the hip flexors and occasionally phenolization to the anterior branch of the obturator nerve or anterior-branch obturator nerve neurectomy.[55-57] Accepted indications for preventative surgery include an MP greater than 40% or an increase in MP greater than 10% in under 1 year and hip abduction less than 30°.[12,26,39]

Studies with mainly short term follow up have reported that early preventative soft tissue surgery was successful in 80% of children, in achieving "good" or "fair" outcomes.[58] Yet the reported percentage of good results following adductor surgery in children with CP ranges from 32%[31] to 90%.[59] Long-term follow up has been reported by Presedo et al,[60] with 67% favorable results with isolated soft tissue release at 10.8 years of follow-up. This wide variation in success rate is believed to be the result of study heterogeneity regarding age of intervention, preoperative MP, surgical technique, definitions of surgical success, duration of follow-up, and population gross motor function.[31] As a result, after an extensive review of the literature surrounding the effect of adductor releases in children with CP, Stott et al[61] concluded that the current evidence base was poor and that it was difficult to draw definitive conclusions.

Recently, Shore et al[31] published the relationship between GMFCS and outcome of hip adductor surgery to prevent hip displacement in children with CP. The authors reported an overall success rate (absence of subsequent surgical procedures during the study period) of 32% over 7 years. However, in nonambulant children, the success rate decreased to 27% and 14%, respectively (GMFCS IV and GMFCS V) (**Figure 19.5**). This study illustrated the current paradox surrounding the management of hip displacement in nonambulant children with CP, in that children most affected and needing the surgery the most have the poorest results from isolated soft tissue lengthening.[31] As a result of this study, current strategies for nonambulatory children employ preventative soft tissue surgery as an intervention to "buy time" or allow the child to grow prior to performing a reconstruction procedure, and few pediatric surgeons would expect isolated soft tissue releases to be effective as an isolated surgery for the treatment of hip displacement in nonambulant children with CP.[31,62]

Boston Children's Hospital (BCH) Technique

The patient is positioned supine elevated on sheets, arms wrapped in blankets to allow anesthesia easy access to the arms (**Figure 19.6**). We utilize small vertical incisions about 3 cm in length, 1 cm lateral to the pubic tubercle. Sharp dissection through skin and subcutaneous tissue is performed (**Figure 19.7A, B**). Using electrocautery, we transversely open the adductor longus sheath from the pubic tubercle out laterally approximately 4 cm. With a combination of blunt and sharp dissection, the superior and inferior planes of the adductor longus are identified before a right angle clamp is passed from inferior to

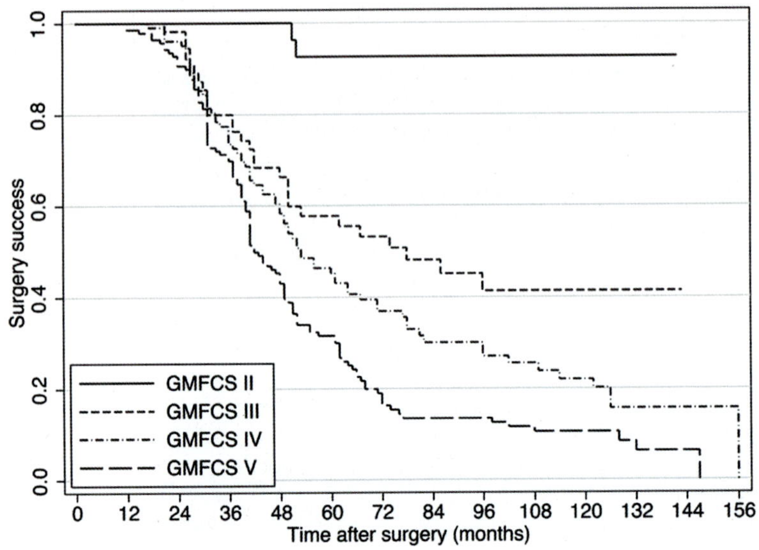

FIGURE 19.5. Survivorship over 8 years of adductor surgery in children with cerebral palsy (CP). Adapted from Shore et al.[31]

superior as close to the tendon as possible (**Figure 19.8**). We often attempt to identify the anterior branch of the obturator nerve first, which lies deep to adductor longus on the adductor brevis muscle at the interval between brevis and pectineus muscle (**Figure 19.9**). If phenol is to be applied to the anterior branch of the obturator nerve, we use 5% phenol and often just a few drops directly on the nerve. If lengthening of the iliopsoas at the less trochanter is indicated, the interval between adductor brevis and pectineus is exploited, keeping the nerve on the adductor brevis muscle belly. An obwegeser retractor is used to elevate the pectineus cranially to expose the iliopsoas tendon. We use a series of peanuts to expose the tendon and then use electrocautery to perform our tenotomy close to the insertion on the lesser trochanter (**Figure 19.10**).

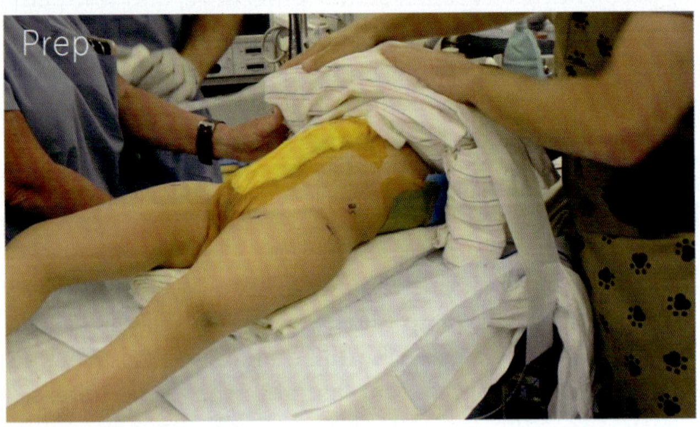

FIGURE 19.6. Typical positioning for neuromuscular hip reconstruction. Note the child is elevated on two pillows to allow for bilateral access to hip and pelvis. The arms are wrapped so that anesthesia is able to access the arms without disrupting the drapes.

Reconstructive Surgery

Surgical dosing is related to where the child is along the cascade of evolving hip pathology. Focal tone management does not alter hip subluxation once it has started, especially if the MP is more than 50%. Tone reduction may reduce the number of children experiencing hip dysplasia

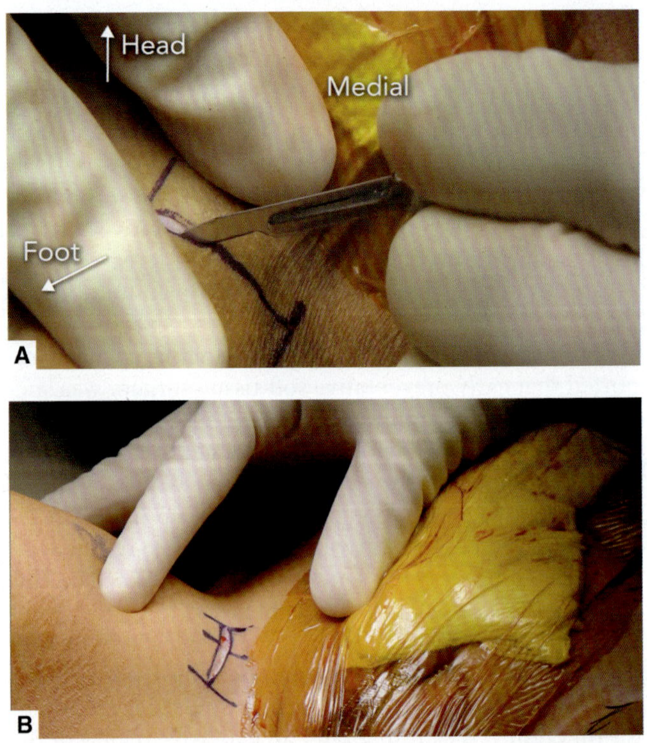

FIGURE 19.7. Illustration of the steps associated with an adductor and iliopsoas lengthening. A, A small 3 to 4 cm vertical incision is made 1 cm lateral to the pubic tubercle (B).

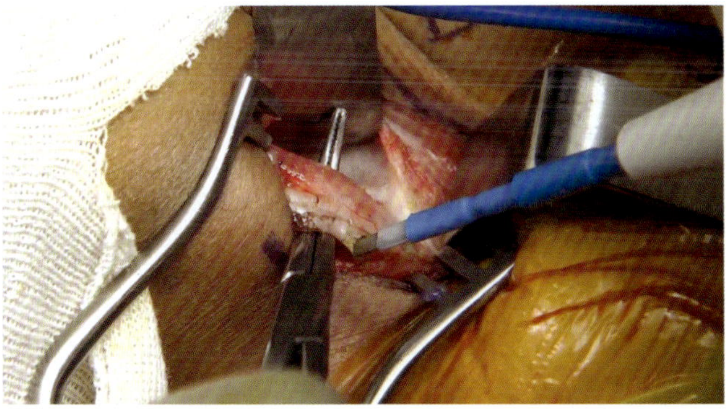

FIGURE 19.8. Illustration of the steps associated with an adductor and iliopsoas lengthening. The adductor longus is tenotomized close to the medial tendon border.

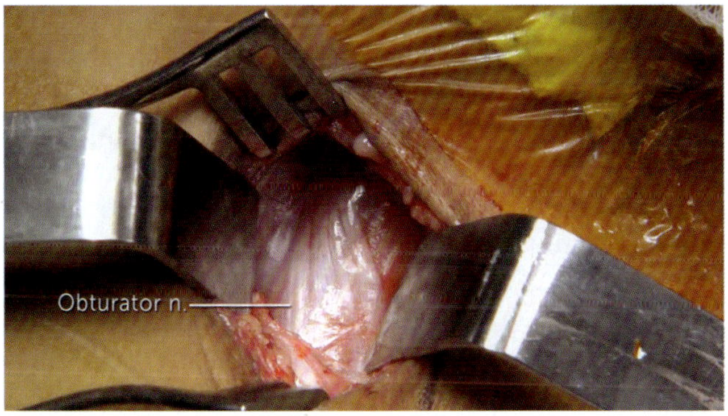

FIGURE 19.9. The branches of the obturator nerve can be visualized on the belly of the adductor brevis muscle. Note that at this level the nerve arborizes into 4-5 branches.

and will ease surgical recovery while reducing the likelihood of recurrent contracture and subluxation. Surgical hip reconstruction in nonambulatory children with CP is challenging for the child, the family, and the surgeon. The decision when to perform a proximal femoral varus derotation osteotomy (VDRO) alone or in concert with an open reduction and pelvic osteotomy has frequently been debated in the literature.[12,63] Reconstructive hip surgery is indicated when the MP is greater than 50% and there is evidence of hip subluxation or early dislocation without evidence of femoral head degenerative changes.[64] For correction of osseous hip deformity, VDRO is a proven, effective technique to improve hip joint reduction, redirect the femoral neck, and correct excessive anteversion commonly present in nonambulant GMFCS IV and V children with hip subluxation.[42,65-67] Several authors have suggested that combined proximal femoral and acetabular procedures for spastic hip displacement have been shown to yield positive results,[67-70] but it is not clear whether a pelvic osteotomy is needed in all nonambulatory CP patients.[12,64]

In addition to coxa valga and anteversion, nonambulant children with CP and spastic hip subluxation suffer

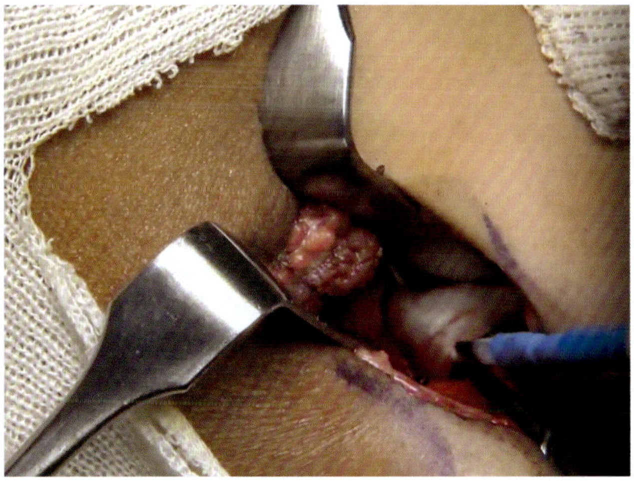

FIGURE 19.10. The iliopsoas tendon is lengthened through the adductor incision, exploiting the interval between the pectineus/adductor brevis muscle intervals. A series of peanuts are used to clear the soft tissue off the lesser trochanter to bluntly expose the iliospoas for tenotomy.

from posterolateral acetabular deficiency, which often requires a concomitant pelvic osteotomy.[70] The standard innominate osteotomies that have been used successfully in patients with developmental hip dysplasia are not recommended for those who have neuromuscular hip dysplasia.[71] Various corrective pelvis osteotomies have been advocated based on the degree of acetabular dysplasia and the state of the triradiate cartilage.[67,69,72,73] However, the recommendations for pelvic osteotomy in this patient population are less clear than for VDRO. Mazur et al[74] looked at the remodeling of the proximal femur and recommended adding a pelvic osteotomy to all nonambulatory patients over 8 years of age, because of the limited acetabular remodeling after isolated VDRO. Song and Carroll[75] recommended that patients with an MP greater than 70% undergo concomitant acetabular procedures, whereas Oh et al[42] recommended a pelvic osteotomy once the MP was greater than 80%. In general, most surgeons employ a sequential "a la carte" approach to the reconstruction for subluxated or dislocated hips in nonambulatory children with CP.[76] This approach involves performing firstly a soft tissue release to regain a full range of hip abduction and extension, a VDRO, and assessment of reduction aided with fluoroscopy and arthrogram if necessary. If inadequate reduction is appreciated, open reduction and/or pelvic osteotomy can be performed as indicated.[12]

In 1969 Dega[77] described his incomplete transiliac osteotomy, in which the cut penetrated the anterior and middle portions of the inner cortex of the ilium, leaving an intact hinge posteriorly consisting of the intact posteromedial iliac cortex and sciatic notch. The theoretical location of the hinge in the Dega osteotomy can involve, to varying degrees, the sciatic notch, the posterior portion of the inner pelvic cortex, the horizontal limb of the triradiate cartilage, and the symphysis pubis. This reshaping osteotomy has been proven to be effective in congenital[78-81] and neuromuscular hip dysplasia.[81-85] Mubarak et al[67] and McNerney et al[70] described their modification of the Dega as the "San Diego acetabuloplasty," where the semicircular osteotomy extends from the anterior inferior iliac spine to the sciatic notch. The osteotomy extends from the lateral cortex to, but not through, the medial wall of the pelvis.[67] This procedure in concert with soft tissue release and shortening VDRO has demonstrated excellent medium to long-term results regarding hip stability[70,86,87] and is a typical surgical prescription adopted by the coauthors for nonambulatory children with moderate to severe spastic hip subluxation and concomitant acetabular dysplasia.

A redirectional periacetabular osteotomy of the pelvis is another treatment option for children with severe acetabular deformity, where an acetabuloplasty is insufficient or counterproductive. Rebello et al[73] described the results of a modified Bernese triple pelvic osteotomy for children with neuromuscular conditions. More than half of their cohort had CP, yet few were GMFCS IV and V. In our experience, although the concept of a redirectional osteotomy is sound, we reserve this procedure for the ambulant GMFCS I-III children as the bone stock of the pelvis in GMFCS IV and V children is poor, making mobilization and fixation of the pelvic fragment very challenging in redirectional osteotomies.

In nonambulatory children who are skeletally mature with severe acetabular dysplasia and hip subluxation, limited reconstruction options are available. The Chiari pelvic osteotomy has been described as a salvage procedure performed after the triradiate cartilage has closed,[88] relying on reduction of the femoral head into the acetabulum and metaplasia of the superior capsule, with good results in children with CP.[89-91] In our hands, we define this procedure as a late reconstruction rather than a true salvage procedure for the neuromuscular child. Furthermore, Robb and Brunner[92] describe good results in performing a modified Dega osteotomy in nonambulatory patients with a closed triradiate cartilage, and this technique has been used by the authors particularly in GMFCS V children with poor bone stock who are not candidates for redirectional or Chiari osteotomy.

Despite the success of reconstructive surgery in the treatment of hip subluxation, the optimal treatment and timing of surgical intervention are controversial. Although VDRO is an accepted procedure for the treatment of spastic hip displacement in nonambulant children with CP, preforming early VDRO (in patients <6 years) has been criticized because of the transient nature of the correction achieved.[66,93-95] Brunner and Baumann[93] found that remodeling of the NSA after VDRO was related to the child's age, with the greatest femoral remodeling occurring during the initial 5 years after surgery. Shore et al[64] investigated the midterm results of VDRO in children with CP and found that younger age at initial surgery was a risk factor for revision hip surgery. Specifically, the mean age of the revision group was 2 years younger than the nonrevision group. On the acetabular side, there is evidence to suggest that early VDRO has the ability to remodel the growing acetabulum. Eilert and MacEwen[66] reported that acetabular dysplasia in children with CP may reverse when VDRO is performed before the age of 8 years. However, Shore et al,[95] during an 8-year study period, demonstrated that children under 6 years of age experienced the greatest degree of acetabular remodeling; yet, the greatest rebound coxa valga was seen in the same age group. Historically, there has been significant controversy surrounding unilateral hip reconstruction surgery in nonambulatory children with unilateral hip dysplasia. Some investigators advocate unilateral reconstruction only,[68,96-98] whereas others believe that bilateral reconstruction should always be carried out as unilateral reconstruction leads to progressive migration of the contralateral hip.[36,99,100] Several studies have demonstrated the phenomenon that in nonambulatory children with CP with primarily unilateral involvement, contralateral hip subluxation may occur after unilateral reconstructions.[65,68,101,102] Predictors for failure after unilateral hip reconstruction in nonambulant children include lack of contralateral soft tissue release, reversal of pelvic obliquity, and an initial MP greater than 25% and younger age (under 8 years).[101] A recent decision analysis by Park et al[103] demonstrated that a prophylactic VDRO on the contralateral stable hip for GMFCS IV and V children was beneficial from a medical perspective in children less than 10 years of age. As a result of the literature above, we would recommend bilateral femoral and/or pelvic reconstructions in the majority of nonambulatory children with CP. Consideration for unilateral surgery can be made in older children (>10 years), with minimal pelvic obliquity and hip subluxation.

BCH Technique

Our approach to hip reconstruction usually consists of performing a soft tissue release that involves lengthening of a combination of the adductor longus and gracilis most of the time as described earlier. Occasionally, the adductor brevis and/or the iliopsoas can be lengthened proximally if the adduction and flexion are very limited. This is followed by assessment of the proximal femur to determine the true NSA and anteversion. The VDRO is performed just proximal to the lesser trochanter, with the goal to achieve 10° to 15° of femoral anteversion and 110° of NSA. We use guidewires up the femoral neck and at the distal femur to assess our intraoperative version (**Figure 19.11A, B**). Depending on the functional level, a 1 to 1.5 cm wedge of bone is removed at the level of the lesser trochanter. Either a cannulated blade plate or locking plate is used to facilitate our reduction and we

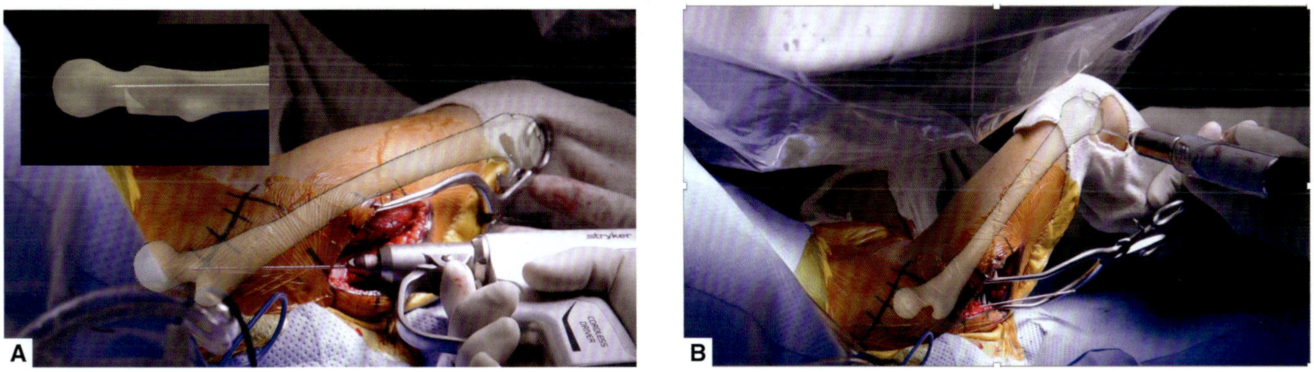

FIGURE 19.11. A and B: To perform our femoral osteotomy, guidewires are placed up the proximal femur and perpendicular to the distal femur to assess our intraoperative version.

typically use the 100° or 110° plate (**Figure 19.12A**, B). We then perform an arthrogram to assess the stability and coverage of the femoral head within the acetabulum. The most common acetabular augmentation that we perform in the CP patient is a modified Dega osteotomy (**Figures 19.13 and 19.14**). The osteotomy will exist at the level of the sciatic notch, and great care will be taken to ensure that the posterior aspect of the osteotomy is wedged open more than the anterior aspect of the pelvis (**Figure 19.15A**-D). Our goal is to improve posterior and lateral coverage. Typically, we do not use any fixation and a child is placed in a foam wedge and knee immobilizers at the end of the procedure (**Figure 19.16**).

Salvage Surgery

The goal of performing hip reconstructive surgery is to achieve and maintain a mobile, painless, and reduced hip. Salvage surgery is often required when reconstructive surgery fails or is precluded due to delayed presentation and/or advanced joint degeneration. Salvage options include proximal femoral resection (PFR)-interposition arthroplasty (Castle or Girdlestone procedure), valgus osteotomy (pelvic support osteotomy) with or without resection of the femoral head and neck (McHale procedure), hip joint arthrodesis, and total joint replacement or prosthetic interposition. A systematic review of salvage options for the CP hip suggests all of the above-mentioned surgeries

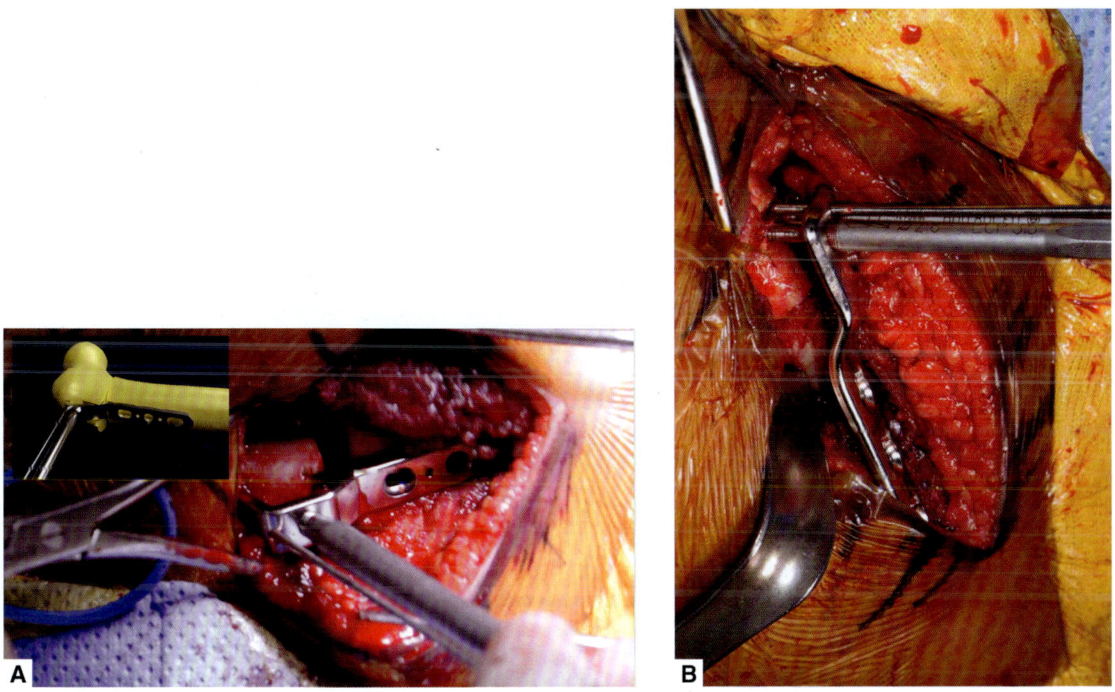

FIGURE 19.12. A and B: Either a locking hip plate or blade plate is used to fixate the osteotomy at either 100° or 110°.

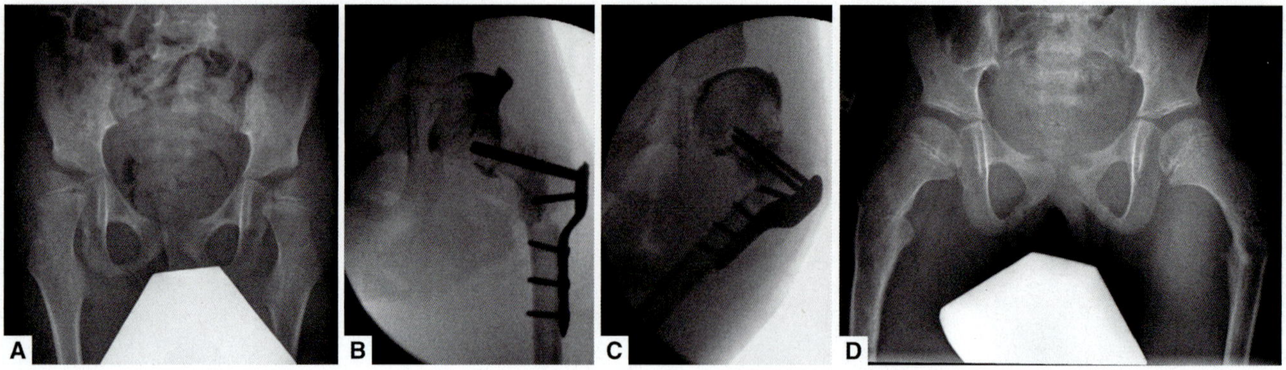

FIGURE 19.13. A 6-year-old child with spastic quadriparesis, Gross Motor Function Classification System (GMFCS) V. A, Bilateral hip deformity. B and C, Intraoperative arthrograms revealed no instability at the end of soft tissue release and varus derotation osteotomy (VDRO). D, Hips at 2-year follow-up.

provide good pain relief and increased range of motion except arthrodesis with comparable complication rate.[104] Hwang et al reported a significant improvement in most Caregiver Priorities and Child Health Index of Life with Disabilities (CPCHILD) and PedsQL subsection scores at a mean follow-up of 56 months with the least complications in the PFR group.[105]

We perform salvage surgery on patients who have hips that are subluxed/dislocated chronically and are not amenable to reconstruction, because of severe femoral head deformity. The preferred procedure historically was PFR (Castle procedure) but because of the problem of excessive heterotopic ossification (HO), we then moved to the McHale procedure since the last 10 years.

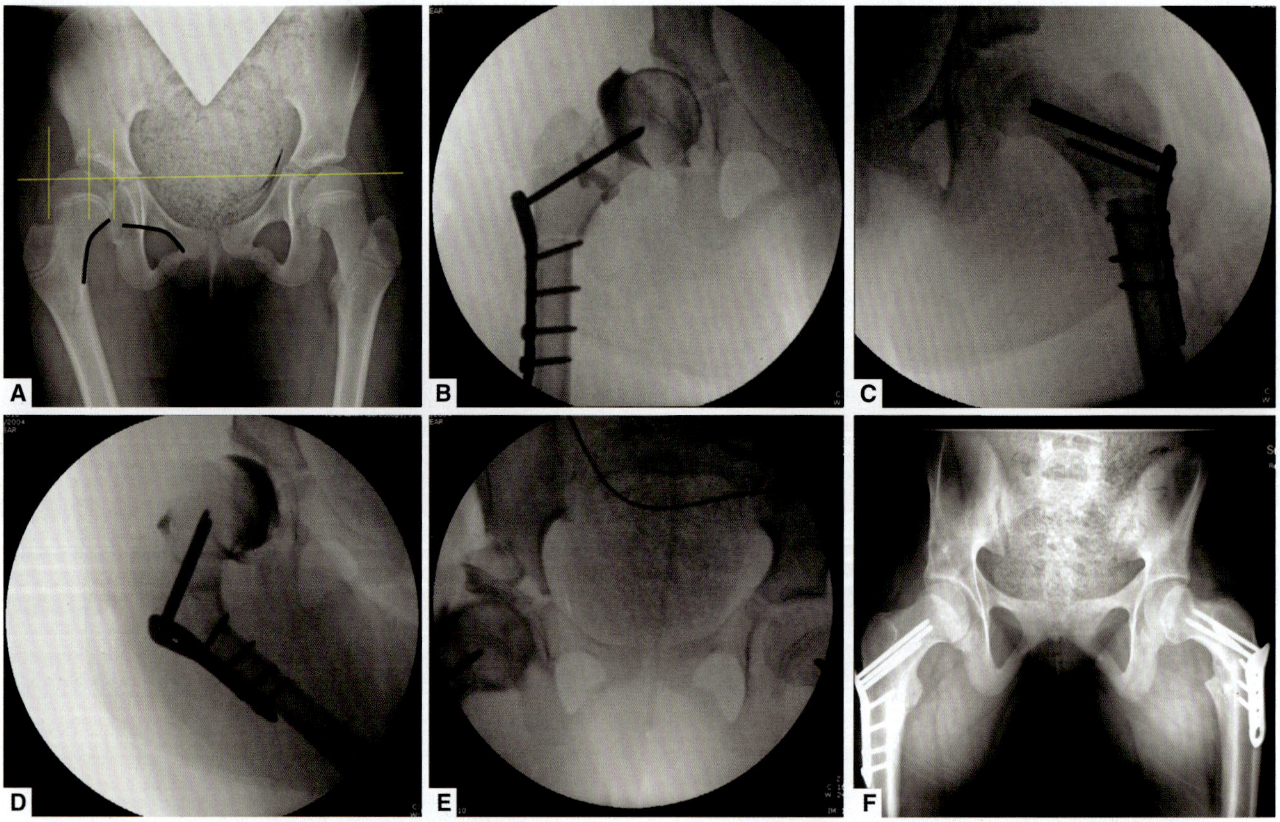

FIGURE 19.14. An 11-year-old child with spastic quadriparesis, Gross Motor Function Classification System (GMFCS) IV. A, Right hip subluxed. B and C, Intraoperative picture after soft tissue release and varus derotation osteotomy (VDRO). D, Intraoperative dynamic arthrogram demonstrating hip instability. E, Intraoperative picture after pelvic osteotomy. F, Hips at 2-year follow-up.

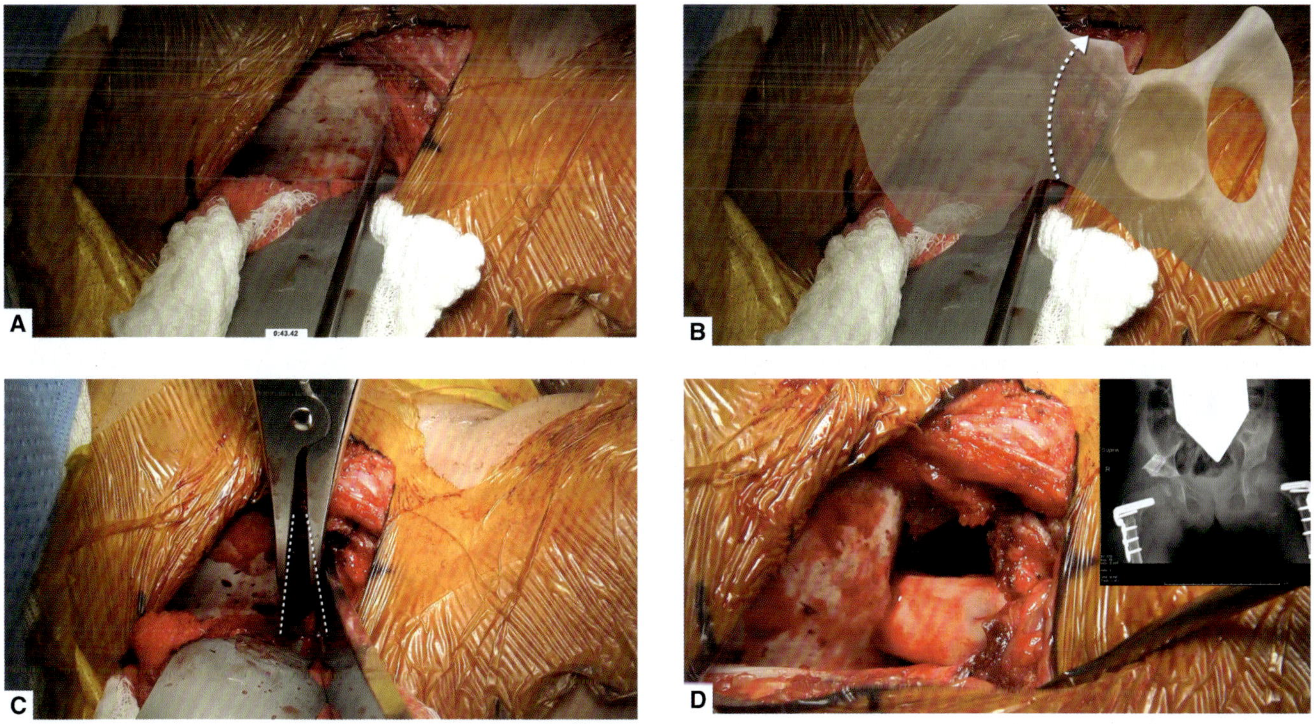

FIGURE 19.15. A–D, A modified Dega pelvic osteotomy is preferred for the management of spastic hip subluxation. A semicircular osteotomy is made from the sciatic notch to the level of the anterior inferior iliac spine (AIIS; A and B). Care is taken to create a wider wedge posterior than anterior with the laminar spreader (C). The final wedge is stable and does not require fixation (D).

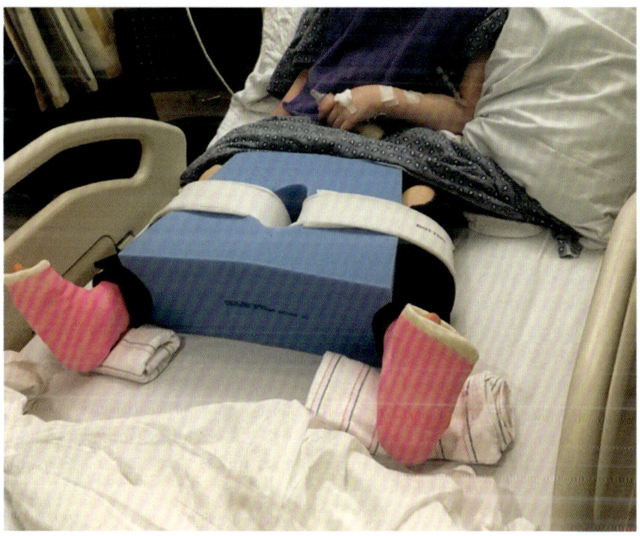

FIGURE 19.16. Children are typically immobilized in a foam wedge and knee immobilizers without the use of spica cast of A-frame casts.

OUTCOMES

The CPCHILD was developed in the early 2000s and constructed from recommendations from caregivers, health care providers, and review of other measures. This disease-specific measure of health status and well-being was developed specifically as an outcome measure of caregivers' perspectives on health status, comfort, well-being, and ease of care of children with severe developmental disabilities (GMFCS IV/V). The CPCHILD has been shown to be a reliable and valid measure of caregiver's perspectives on health status,[106] and crucially it has been shown to be responsive to hip reconstruction in children with CP.[107]

Recently, DiFazio et al[107] reported on the relationship between MP and health-related quality of life (HRQOL) as measured by the CPCHILD in GMFCS IV and V children undergoing hip reconstruction surgery. The authors identified a negative correlation between preoperative MP and CPCHILD scores and found that those children whose preoperative MP was higher than 50% had worse CPCHILD scores postoperatively.

REFERENCES

1. Palisano R, Rosenbaum P, Walter S, Russell D, Wood E, Galuppi B. Development and reliability of a system to classify gross motor function in children with cerebral palsy. *Dev Med Child Neurol.* 1997;39(4):214-223.
2. Stanley F, Blair E, Alberman E. *Cerebral Palsies: Epidemiology and Causal Pathways.* London, UK: Mac Keith; 2000.
3. Rosenbaum P, Paneth N, Leviton A, et al. A report: the definition and classification of cerebral palsy April 2006. *Dev Med Child Neurol Suppl.* 2007;109:8-14.
4. Graham HK, Selber P. Musculoskeletal aspects of cerebral palsy. *J Bone Joint Surg Br.* 2003;85:157-166.

5. Graham HK. Painful hip dislocation in cerebral palsy. *Lancet.* 2002;359(9310):907-908.
6. Graham HK. Mechanisms of deformity. In Scrutton D, Damiano D, Mayston M, eds. *Management of the Motor Disorders of Children with Cerebral Palsy.* London, UK: Mac Keith Press; 2004:105-129.
7. Soo B, Howard JJ, Boyd RN, et al. Hip displacement in cerebral palsy. *J Bone Joint Surg Am.* 2006;88(1):121-129. doi:10.2106/JBJS.E.00071.
8. Bagg MR, Farber J, Miller F. Long-term follow-up of hip subluxation in cerebral palsy patients. *J Pediatr Orthop.* 1993;13(1):32-36.
9. Howard CB, McKibbin B, Williams LA, Mackie I. Factors affecting the incidence of hip dislocation in cerebral palsy. *J Bone Joint Surg Br.* 1985;67(4):530-532.
10. Terjesen T. Development of the hip joints in unoperated children with cerebral palsy: a radiographic study of 76 patients. *Acta Orthop.* 2006;77(1):125-131. doi:10.1080/17453670610045803.
11. Lonstein JE, Beck K. Hip dislocation and subluxation in cerebral palsy. *J Pediatr Orthop.* 1986;6(5):521-526.
12. Flynn JM, Miller F. Management of hip disorders in patients with cerebral palsy. *J Am Acad Orthop Surg.* 2002;10(3):198-209.
13. Prevalence and characteristics of children with cerebral palsy in Europe. *Dev Med Child Neurol.* 2002;44(9):633-640.
14. Christensen D, Van Naarden Braun K, Doernberg NS, et al. Prevalence of cerebral palsy, co-occurring autism spectrum disorders, and motor functioning—Autism and Developmental Disabilities Monitoring Network, USA, 2008. *Dev Med Child Neurol.* 2014;56(1):59-65. doi:10.1111/dmcn.12268.
15. Hägglund G, Andersson S, Düppe H, Lauge-Pedersen H, Nordmark E, Westbom L. Prevention of dislocation of the hip in children with cerebral palsy. The first ten years of a population-based prevention programme. *J Bone Joint Surg Br.* 2005;87(1):95-101.
16. Connelly A, Flett P, Graham HK, Oates J. Hip surveillance in Tasmanian children with cerebral palsy. *J Paediatr Child Health.* 2009;45(7-8):437-443. doi:10.1111/j.1440-1754.2009.01534.x.
17. Cornell MS, Hatrick NC, Boyd R, Baird G, Spencer JD. The hip in children with cerebral palsy. Predicting the outcome of soft tissue surgery. *Clin Orthop Relat Res.* 1997;(340):165-171.
18. ILetts M, Shapiro L, Mulder K, Klassen O. The windblown hip syndrome in total body cerebral palsy. *J Pediatr Orthop.* 1984;4(1):55-62.
19. Bax M, Goldstein M, Rosenbaum P, et al. Proposed definition and classification of cerebral palsy, April 2005. *Dev Med Child Neurol.* 2005;47(8):571-576.
20. Sharrard WJ, Allen JM, Heaney SH. Surgical prophylaxis of subluxation and dislocation of the hip in cerebral palsy. *J Bone Joint Surg Br.* 1975;57(2):160-166.
21. Dunlap K, Shands AR Jr, Hollister LC Jr, Gaul JS Jr, Streit HA. A new method for determination of torsion of the femur. *J Bone Joint Surg Am.* 1953;35(2):289-311.
22. Laplaza FJ, Root L, Tassanawipas A, Glasser DB. Femoral torsion and neck-shaft angles in cerebral palsy. *J Pediatr Orthop.* 1993;13(2):192-199.
23. Robin J, Graham HK, Selber P, Dobson F, Smith K, Baker R. Proximal femoral geometry in cerebral palsy: a population-based cross-sectional study. *J Bone Joint Surg Br.* 2008;90(10):1372-1379. doi:10.1302/0301-620X.90B10.20733.
24. Hägglund G, Lauge-Pedersen H, Wagner P. Characteristics of children with hip displacement in cerebral palsy. *BMC Musculoskelet Disord.* 2007;8:101. doi:10.1186/1471-2474-8-101.
25. Scrutton D, Baird G. Surveillance measures of the hips of children with bilateral cerebral palsy. *Arch Dis Child.* 1997;76(4):381-384.
26. Dobson F, Boyd RN, Parrott J, Nattrass GR, Graham HK. Hip surveillance in children with cerebral palsy. Impact on the surgical management of spastic hip disease. *J Bone Joint Surg Br.* 2002;84(5):720-726.
27. Cooke PH, Cole WG, Carey RP. Dislocation of the hip in cerebral palsy. Natural history and predictability. *J Bone Joint Surg Br.* 1989;71(3):441-446.
28. Wynter M, Gibson N, Kentish M, Love S, Thomason P, Graham HK. The consensus statement on hip surveillance for children with cerebral palsy: Australian Standards of Care. *J Pediatr Rehabil Med.* 2011;4(3):183-195. doi:R35707H76U808563.
29. Graham HK, Boyd R, Carlin JB, et al. Does botulinum toxin A combined with bracing prevent hip displacement in children with cerebral palsy and "hips at risk"? A randomized, controlled trial. *J Bone Joint Surg.* 2008;90(1):23-33. doi:10.2106/JBJS.F.01416.
30. Krach LE, Kriel RL, Gilmartin RC, et al. Hip status in cerebral palsy after one year of continuous intrathecal baclofen infusion. *Pediatr Neurol.* 2004;30(3):163-168. doi:10.1016/j.pediatrneurol.2003.08.006.
31. Shore BJ, Yu X, Desai S, Selber P, Wolfe R, Graham HK. Adductor surgery to prevent hip displacement in children with cerebral palsy: the predictive role of the Gross Motor Function Classification System. *J Bone Joint Surg.* 2012;94(4):326-334.
32. Wynter M, Gibson N, Kentish M, Love S, Thomason P, Graham HK. The development of Australian Standards of Care for Hip Surveillance in Children with Cerebral Palsy: how did we reach consensus? *J Pediatr Rehabil Med.* 2011;4(3):171-182. doi:9326243N1K85548Q.
33. Hägglund G, Alriksson-Schmidt A, Lauge-Pedersen H, Rodby-Bousquet E, Wagner P, Westbom L. Prevention of dislocation of the hip in children with cerebral palsy: 20-year results of a population-based prevention programme. *Bone Joint J.* 2014;96(11):1546-1552. doi:10.1302/0301-620X.96B11.34385.
34. Wynter M, Gibson N, Willoughby KL, et al. Australian hip surveillance guidelines for children with cerebral palsy: 5-year review. *Dev Med Child Neurol.* 2015;57(9):808-820. doi:10.1111/dmcn.12754.
35. Shore B, Spence D, Graham HK. The role for hip surveillance in children with cerebral palsy. *Curr Rev Musculoskelet Med.* 2012;5(2):126-134. doi:10.1007/s12178-012-9120-4.
36. Reimers J. The stability of the hip in children. A radiological study of the results of muscle surgery in cerebral palsy. *Acta Orthop Scand Suppl.* 1980;184:1-100.
37. Parrott J, Boyd RN, Dobson F, et al. Hip displacement in spastic cerebral palsy: repeatability of radiologic measurement. *J Pediatr Orthop.* 2002;22(5):660-667.
38. Scrutton D, Baird G, Smeeton N. Hip dysplasia in bilateral cerebral palsy: incidence and natural history in children aged 18 months to 5 years. *Dev Med Child Neurol.* 2001;43(9):586-600.
39. Miller F, Bagg MR. Age and migration percentage as risk factors for progression in spastic hip disease. *Dev Med Child Neurol.* 1995;37(5):449-455.
40. Faraj S, Atherton WG, Stott NS. Inter- and intra-measurer error in the measurement of Reimers' hip migration percentage. *J Bone Joint Surg Br.* 2004;86(3):434-437.
41. Settecerri JJ, Karol LA. Effectiveness of femoral varus osteotomy in patients with cerebral palsy. *J Pediatr Orthop.* 2000;20(6):776-780.
42. Oh CW, Presedo A, Dabney KW, Miller F. Factors affecting femoral varus osteotomy in cerebral palsy: a long-term result over 10 years. *J Pediatr Orthop B.* 2007;16(1):23-30. doi:10.1097/01.bpb.0000228393.70302.ce.
43. Terjesen T. The natural history of hip development in cerebral palsy. *Dev Med Child Neurol.* 2012;54(10):951-957. doi:10.1111/j.1469-8749.2012.04385.x.
44. Murnaghan ML, Simpson P, Robin JG, Shore BJ, Selber P, Graham HK. The cerebral palsy hip classification is reliable: an inter-and intra-observer reliability study. *J Bone Joint Surg Br.* 2010;92(3):436-441. doi:10.1302/0301-620X.92B3.23105.
45. Robin J, Graham HK, Baker R, et al. A classification system for hip disease in cerebral palsy. *Dev Med Child Neurol.* 2009;51(3):183-192. doi:10.1111/j.1469-8749.2008.03129.x.
46. Gose S, Sakai T, Shibata T, Akiyama K, Yoshikawa H, Sugamoto K. Verification of the Robin and Graham classification system of hip disease in cerebral palsy using three-dimensional computed tomography. *Dev Med Child Neurol.* 2011;53(12):1107-1112. doi:10.1111/j.1469-8749.2011.04130.x.
47. Wawrzuta J, Willoughby KL, Molesworth C, et al. Hip health at skeletal maturity: a population-based study of young adults with cerebral palsy. *Dev Med Child Neurol.* 2016;58(12):1273-1280. doi:10.1111/dmcn.13171.
48. Chang CH, Kuo KN, Wang CJ, Chen YY, Cheng HY, Kao HK. Acetabular deficiency in spastic hip subluxation. *J Pediatr Orthop.* 2011;31(6):648-654. doi:10.1097/BPO.0b013e318228903d.

49. Wynter M, Gibson N, Kentish M, Love S, Thomason P, Graham HK. The development of Australian Standards of Care for Hip Surveillance in Children with Cerebral Palsy: How did we reach consensus? *J Pediatr Rehab Med.* 2011;4:1-12.
50. Kentish M, Wynter M, Snape N, Boyd R. Five-year outcome of state-wide hip surveillance of children and adolescents with cerebral palsy. *J Pediatr Rehabil Med.* 2011;4(3):205-217. doi:10.3233/PRM-2011-0176.
51. Wynter M, Gibson N, Kentish M, et al. The Australian hip surveillance guidelines for children with cerebral palsy. 2014. www.ausacpdm.org.au/professionals/hip-surveillance.
52. Hägglund G. Radiographic follow-up in CPUP to prevent hip dislocation. 2013. http://cpup.se/wp-content/uploads/2013/07/CPUPprevent_hip_dislocation20130210.pdf.
53. Duivestein J, Lanphear N, Matthews M, et al. Hip surveillance program for children with cerebral palsy. 2016. https://childhealthbc.ca/sites/default/files/clinical_booket_hip_surveillance_march_2018.pdf.
54. https://www.aacpdm.org/publications/care-pathways/hip-surveillance.
55. Kalen V, Bleck EE. Prevention of spastic paralytic dislocation of the hip. *Dev Med Child Neurol.* 1985;27(1):17-24.
56. Banks HH, Green WT. Adductor myotomy and obturator neurectomy for the correction of adduction contracture of the hip in cerebral palsy. *J Bone Joint Surg Am.* 1960;42:111-126.
57. Turker RJ, Lee R. Adductor tenotomies in children with quadriplegic cerebral palsy: longer term follow-up. *J Pediatr Orthop.* 2000;20(3):370-374.
58. Miller F, Cardoso Dias R, Dabney KW, Lipton GE, Triana M. Soft-tissue release for spastic hip subluxation in cerebral palsy. *J Pediatr Orthop.* 1997;17(5):571-584.
59. Onimus M, Allamel G, Manzone P, Laurain JM. Prevention of hip dislocation in cerebral palsy by early psoas and adductors tenotomies. *J Pediatr Orthop.* 1991;11(4):432-435.
60. Presedo A, Oh CW, Dabney KW. Soft-tissue releases to treat spastic hip subluxation in children with cerebral palsy. *J Bone Joint Surg.* 2005;87(4):832-841. doi:10.2106/JBJS.C.01099.
61. Stott NS, Piedrahita L, AACPDM. Effects of surgical adductor releases for hip subluxation in cerebral palsy: an AACPDM evidence report. *Dev Med Child Neurol.* 2004;46(9):628-645.
62. Graham HK, Rosenbaum P, Paneth N, et al. Cerebral palsy. *Nat Rev Dis Primers.* 2016;2:15082. doi: 10.1038/nrdp.2015.82.
63. Huh K, Rethlefsen SA, Wren TA, Kay RM. Surgical management of hip subluxation and dislocation in children with cerebral palsy: isolated VDRO or combined surgery? *J Pediatr Orthop.* 2011;31(8):858-863. doi:10.1097/BPO.0b013e31822e0261.
64. Shore BJ, Zurakowski D, Dufreny C, Powell D, Matheney TH, Snyder BD. Proximal femoral varus derotation osteotomy in children with cerebral palsy: the effect of age, gross motor function classification system level, and surgeon volume on surgical success. *J Bone Joint Surg Am.* 2015;97(24):2024-2031. doi:10.2106/JBJS.O.00505.
65. Noonan KJ, Walker TL, Kayes KJ, Feinberg J. Varus derotation osteotomy for the treatment of hip subluxation and dislocation in cerebral palsy: statistical analysis in 73 hips. *J Pediatr Orthop B.* 2001;10(4):279-286.
66. Eilert RE, MacEwen GD. Varus derotational osteotomy of the femur in cerebral palsy. *Clin Orthop Relat Res.* 1977;(125):168-172.
67. Mubarak SJ, Valencia FG, Wenger DR. One-stage correction of the spastic dislocated hip. Use of pericapsular acetabuloplasty to improve coverage. *J Bone Joint Surg Am.* 1992;74(9):1347-1357.
68. Gordon GS, Simkiss DE. A systematic review of the evidence for hip surveillance in children with cerebral palsy. *J Bone Joint Surg Br.* 2006;88(11):1492-1496. doi:10.1302/0301-620X.88B11.18114.
69. Miller F, Girardi H, Lipton G, Ponzio R, Klaumann M, Dabney KW. Reconstruction of the dysplastic spastic hip with peri-ilial pelvic and femoral osteotomy followed by immediate mobilization. *J Pediatr Orthop.* 1997;17(5):592-602.
70. McNerney NP, Mubarak SJ, Wenger DR. One-stage correction of the dysplastic hip in cerebral palsy with the San Diego acetabuloplasty: results and complications in 104 hips. *J Pediatr Orthop.* 2000;20(1):93-103.
71. Salter RB, Dubos JP. The first fifteen year's personal experience with innominate osteotomy in the treatment of congenital dislocation and subluxation of the hip. *Clin Orthop Relat Res.* 1974;(98):72-103.
72. Robb JE, Hägglund G. Hip surveillance and management of the displaced hip in cerebral palsy. *J Child Orthop.* 2013;7(5):407-413. doi:10.1007/s11832-013-0515-6.
73. Rebello G, Zilkens C, Dudda M, Matheney T, Kim Y-J. Triple pelvic osteotomy in complex hip dysplasia seen in neuromuscular and teratologic conditions. *J Pediatr Orthop.* 2009;29(6):527-534. doi:10.1097/BPO.0b013e3181b2b3be.
74. Mazur JM, Danko AM, Standard SC, Loveless EA, Cummings RJ. Remodeling of the proximal femur after varus osteotomy in children with cerebral palsy. *Dev Med Child Neurol.* 2004;46(6):412-415.
75. Song HR, Carroll NC. Femoral varus derotation osteotomy with or without acetabuloplasty for unstable hips in cerebral palsy. *J Pediatr Orthop.* 1998;18(1):62-68.
76. Hsu C-C, Sandford B. The Delphi technique: making sense of consensus. *Pract Assess Res Eval.* 2007;12(10).
77. Dega W. Selection of surgical methods in the treatment of congenital dislocation of the hip in children. *Chir Narzadow Ruchu Ortop Pol.* 1969;34(3):357-366.
78. Lalonde FD, Frick SL, Wenger DR. Surgical correction of residual hip dysplasia in two pediatric age-groups. *J Bone Joint Surg Am.* 2002;84(7):1148-1156.
79. Reichel H, Hein W. Dega acetabuloplasty combined with intertrochanteric osteotomies. *Clin Orthop Relat Res.* 1996;(323):234-242.
80. Thomas SR, Wedge JH, Salter RB. Outcome at forty-five years after open reduction and innominate osteotomy for late-presenting developmental dislocation of the hip. *J Bone Joint Surg Am.* 2007;89(11):2341-2350. doi:10.2106/JBJS.F.00857.
81. Karlen JW, Skaggs DL, Ramachandran M, Kay RM. The Dega osteotomy: a versatile osteotomy in the treatment of developmental and neuromuscular hip pathology. *J Pediatr Orthop.* 2009;29(7):676-682. doi:10.1097/BPO.0b013e3181b7691a.
82. Grudziak JS, Ward WT. Dega osteotomy for the treatment of congenital dysplasia of the hip. *J Bone Joint Surg Am.* 2001;83(6):845-854.
83. Barrie JL, Galasko CS. Surgery for unstable hips in cerebral palsy. *J Pediatr Orthop B.* 1996;5(4):225-231.
84. Chomiak J, Dungl P. Pelvic osteotomy in the neurogenic unstable hip. *Orthop Trauma Rehabil.* 2006;8(1):48-56.
85. Gordon JE, Capelli AM, Strecker WB, Delgado ED, Schoenecker PL. Pemberton pelvic osteotomy and varus rotational osteotomy in the treatment of acetabular dysplasia in patients who have static encephalopathy. *J Bone Joint Surg Am.* 1996;78(12):1863-1871.
86. Mallet C, Ilharreborde B, Presedo A, Khairouni A, Mazda K, Pennecot GF. One-stage hip reconstruction in children with cerebral palsy: long-term results at skeletal maturity. *J Child Orthop.* 2014;8(3):221-228. doi:10.1007/s11832-014-0589-9.
87. Braatz F, Staude D, Klotz MC, Wolf SI, Dreher T, Lakemeier S. Hip-joint congruity after Dega osteotomy in patients with cerebral palsy: long-term results. *Int Orthop.* 2016;40(8):1663-1668. doi:10.1007/s00264-015-3013-2.
88. Chiari K. Medial displacement osteotomy of the pelvis. *Clin Orthop Relat Res.* 1974;(98):55-71.
89. Debnath UK, Guha AR, Karlakki S, Varghese J, Evans GA. Combined femoral and Chiari osteotomies for reconstruction of the painful subluxation or dislocation of the hip in cerebral palsy. A long-term outcome study. *J Bone Joint Surg Br.* 2006;88(10):1373-1378. doi:10.1302/0301-620X.88B10.17742.
90. Osterkamp J, Caillouette JT, Hoffer MM. Chiari osteotomy in cerebral palsy. *J Pediatr Orthop.* 1988;8(3):274-277.
91. Zenios M, Hannan M, Zafar S, Henry A, Galasko CS, Khan T. Clinical and radiological outcome of combined femoral and Chiari osteotomies for subluxed or dislocated hips secondary to neuromuscular conditions: a minimum of 10-year follow-up. *Musculoskelet Surg.* 2012;96(2):101-106. doi:10.1007/s12306-012-0201-8.

92. Robb JE, Brunner R. A Dega-type osteotomy after closure of the triradiate cartilage in non-walking patients with severe cerebral palsy. *J Bone Joint Surg Br*. 2006;88(7):933-937. doi:10.1302/0301-620X.88B7.17506.
93. Brunner R, Baumann JU. Long-term effects of intertrochanteric varus-derotation osteotomy on femur and acetabulum in spastic cerebral palsy: an 11-to 18-year follow-up study. *J Pediatr Orthop*. 1997;17(5):585-591.
94. Persson-Bunke M, Hägglund G, Lauge-Pedersen H. Windswept hip deformity in children with cerebral palsy. *J Pediatr Orthop B*. 2006;15(5):335-338.
95. Shore BJ, Powell D, Miller PE, Matheney TH, Snyder BD. Acetabular and femoral remodeling after varus derotational osteotomy in cerebral palsy: the effect of age and gross motor function classification level. *J Pediatr Orthop B*. 2016;25(4):322-330. doi:10.1097/BPB.0000000000000322.
96. Noonan KJ, Walker TL, Kayes KJ, Feinberg J. Effect of surgery on the nontreated hip in severe cerebral palsy. *J Pediatr Orthop*. 2000;20(6):771-775.
97. Hoffer MM, Stein GA, Koffman M, Prietto M. Femoral varus-derotation osteotomy in spastic cerebral palsy. *J Bone Joint Surg Am*. 1985;67(8):1229-1235.
98. Carr C, Gage JR. The fate of the nonoperated hip in cerebral palsy. *J Pediatr Orthop*. 1987;7(3):262-267.
99. Samilson RL, Tsou P, Aamoth G, Green WM. Dislocation and subluxation of the hip in cerebral palsy. Pathogenesis, natural history and management. *J Bone Joint Surg Am*. 1972;54(4):863-873.
100. Silver RL, Rang M, Chan J, de la Garza J. Adductor release in nonambulant children with cerebral palsy. *J Pediatr Orthop*. 1985;5(6):672-677.
101. Shukla PY, Mann S, Braun SV, Gholve PA. Unilateral hip reconstruction in children with cerebral palsy: predictors for failure. *J Pediatr Orthop*. 2013;33(2):175-181. doi:10.1097/BPO.0b013e31827d0b73.
102. Canavese F, Emara K, Sembrano JN, Bialik V, Aiona MD, Sussman MD. Varus derotation osteotomy for the treatment of hip subluxation and dislocation in GMFCS level III to V patients with unilateral hip involvement. Follow-up at skeletal maturity. *J Pediatr Orthop*. 2010;30(4):357-364. doi:10.1097/BPO.0b013e3181d8fbc1.
103. Park MS, Chung CY, Kwon DG, Sung KH, Choi IH, Lee KM. Prophylactic femoral varization osteotomy for contralateral stable hips in non-ambulant individuals with cerebral palsy undergoing hip surgery: decision analysis. *Dev Med Child Neurol*. 2012;54(3):231-239. doi:10.1111/j.1469-8749.2011.04172.x.
104. Kolman SE, Ruzbarsky JJ, Spiegel DA, Baldwin KD. Salvage options in the cerebral palsy hip: a systematic review. *J Pediatr Orthop*. 2016;36(6):645-650. doi:10.1097/BPO.0000000000000501.
105. Hwang JH, Varte L, Kim HW, Lee DH, Park H. Salvage procedures for the painful chronically dislocated hip in cerebral palsy. *Bone Joint J*. 2016;98(1):137-143. doi:10.1302/0301-620X.98B1.35202.
106. Narayanan UG, Fehlings D, Weir S, Knights S, Kiran S, Campbell K. Initial development and validation of the Caregiver Priorities and Child Health Index of Life with Disabilities (CPCHILD). *Dev Med Child Neurol*. 2006;48(10):804-812. doi:10.1017/S0012162206001745.
107. DiFazio R, Shore B, Vessey JA, Miller PE, Snyder BD. Effect of hip reconstructive surgery on health-related quality of life of non-ambulatory children with cerebral palsy. *J Bone Joint Surg Am*. 2016;98(14):1190-1198. doi:10.2106/JBJS.15.01063.

CHAPTER 20

Traumatic Injuries to the Hip: Femoral Neck Fracture and Posterior Dislocation

BACKGROUND

Traumatic injuries involving the hip in children and adolescents, including femoral neck fracture, posterior hip dislocation, and acetabular wall fractures are relatively rare and usually associated with a high-energy mechanism. As these injuries are associated with severe complications such as osteonecrosis of the femoral head, understanding the principles that guide surgical treatment is crucial to achieve the best outcomes.

Femoral Neck Fractures

Pediatric femoral neck fracture is a rare injury typically associated with high-energy trauma, which accounts for less than 1% of all pediatric fractures.[1-3] The diagnosis is based on a history of trauma and examination, revealing a shortened and externally rotated lower extremity complemented by imaging. Radiographs should include an anteroposterior view of the pelvis and a cross-table lateral view of the femur. Frog-leg lateral imaging should be avoided because of further displacement and pain. Rarely, advanced imaging, including a computed tomography (CT) or magnetic resonance imaging (MRI), is used for a suspected occult fracture.

Femoral neck fractures in children and adolescents are classified on the basis of the anatomic location of the fracture according to the four-part system described by Delbet and popularized by Colonna[4] (**Figure 20.1**). The classification is important because of its correlation with the development of osteonecrosis of the capital femoral epiphysis. Type I is a fracture through the capital femoral epiphysis growth plate, which can be associated with dislocation of the hip joint. These fractures have a high rate of complications. Virtually, 100% of the type I fractures associated with a dislocation of the hip (type IB) complicate with osteonecrosis. Type II fractures are truly transcervical fractures, whereas type III fractures or basocervical fractures occur through the base of the femoral neck. It is essential to distinguish between the transcervical (type II) versus the basocervical (type III) because the risk of osteonecrosis of the femoral head is higher following a type II fracture. Type IV fractures are intertrochanteric fractures, which have a much lower risk of osteonecrosis. However, type IV fractures may complicate with malunion if not well reduced and appropriately fixed. Although widely used because of the association with the risk of osteonecrosis, the Delbet-Colonna classification system is incomplete because it does not take into consideration the degree of displacement of the fracture and the inclination of the fracture through the neck. Fracture displacement and the angle of fracture from the horizontal are important features for classifying femoral neck fracture in adults.[5,6] The severity of displacement and angulation of the fracture should be taken into consideration for pediatric fractures because of their association with osteonecrosis of the femoral head and malunion, respectively.[7]

Treatment of femoral neck fractures in children and adolescents is surgical. Although nondisplaced and incomplete fractures may be amenable to nonoperative treatment with cast immobilization in the very young child, our preference is for percutaneous fixation to avoid malunion. In toddlers, fixation may be achieved with smooth Kirschner wires, followed by spica cast immobilization.

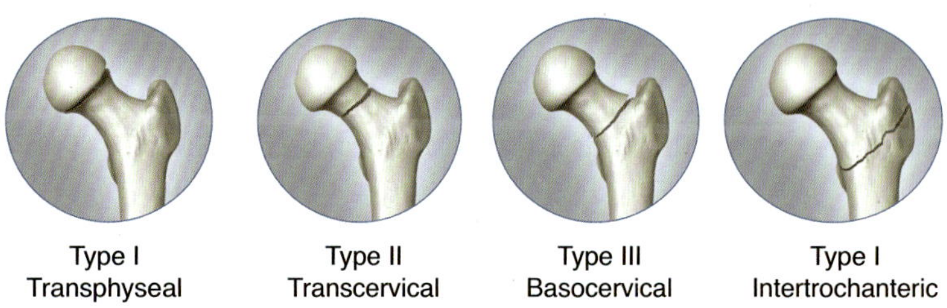

FIGURE 20.1. Delbet-Colonna classification of femoral neck fractures in children.

In older children, fixation of nondisplaced femoral neck fractures should be performed with cannulated screws or a pediatric hip sliding screw. In general, a fracture of the femoral neck should be fixed with mechanical stability of the fixation in mind. For this reason, it is often necessary to include fixation of the fracture that includes the capital femoral epiphysis growth plate to enhance stability of the fixation. Rarely, slipped capital femoral epiphysis has been described following fixation of a femoral neck fracture preserving the growth plate.[8] This catastrophic complication is to be avoided by including fixation of the capital femoral epiphysis into the construct of a femoral neck fracture fixation. After surgical treatment, children younger than 6 years of age may benefit from a spica cast immobilization. In older children, an abduction foam immobilizer should be sufficient. Patients are recommended to remain non–weight-bearing for a minimum of 6 to 8 weeks and then transition to weight-bearing with a walker or crutches. Femoral neck fractures should be followed for a minimum of 2 years because of the risk of late osteonecrosis.

Minimally displaced and angulated fractures may be treated by closed reduction using an operative traction table and percutaneous or internal fixation. Decompression of the intracapsular hematoma has been suggested as an adjunct to closed reduction. However, the role of decompression to decrease the risk of osteonecrosis remains controversial. Our preference for displaced femoral neck fractures is to perform an open reduction to achieve anatomic reduction of the fragments. Two types of surgical approaches can be used for the open treatment of femoral neck fractures. The anterior approach through the Smith-Petersen modified incision and dissection between the sartorius and tensor fascia lata allows adequate exposure of the anterior aspect of the femoral neck for reduction. Fixation of the fracture is then performed through a small lateral approach for the placement of cannulated screws or a sliding hip screw. We favor the use of an anterolateral approach described by Watson-Jones (**Figure 20.2**). Our technique for the treatment of femoral neck fractures using the Watson-Jones approach is similar to that described for the treatment of acute unstable slipped capital femoral epiphysis in Chapter 7. The rationale for using the Watson-Jones approach is that it allows full exposure of the superior, anterior, and medial aspects of the femoral neck and fixation through the same incision. Briefly, the patient is positioned in a sloppy lateral position with a bump under the ipsilateral scapula and the gluteal muscles. A curvilinear incision is made about 1 or 2 cm distal and lateral to the anterior superior iliac spine, aiming toward the greater trochanter and curved down to the lateral aspect of the thigh. The fascia lata is incised in line with the skin incision. The interval between the gluteus medius and the tensor fascia lata is dissected. It is easier to start the dissection distally and move proximally. Attention is required to avoid injury to nerve branches from the superior gluteal nerve which innervates the tensor fascia lata. Small vessels in this area can be ligated or cauterized as needed. We start the dissection by identifying the interval between the gluteus medius and the vastus lateralis distal in the trochanteric region and move proximally, retracting the gluteus medius proximally and laterally. As the dissection moves proximally, the gluteus minimus is identified and elevated from the posterosuperior aspect of the hip capsule. The iliocapsularis muscle is also elevated but in the anterior and medial direction. This allows full exposure of the hip capsule. A good reference for adequate exposure is visualization of the indirect head of the rectus femoris tendon. The joint capsule is then open longitudinally in line with the femoral neck up to the level of the acetabular labrum. The capsule is open medially and laterally just distal to the labrum for about a centimeter and a half for a final T-shaped capsulotomy. The fracture hematoma is evacuated, and the fracture fragments are cleaned using a curette. Reduction is gently achieved by manual traction to the lower extremity along with slight internal rotation by an assistant while the surgeon can guide the rotation using a ball spike instrument or a small bone hook. Rarely, reduction is achieved by insertion of a Schanz pin into the fragments to facilitate the manipulation. Once the fracture is anatomically reduced, provisional K-wires are introduced to hold the fixation in place while definitive fixation is planned. Definitive fixation can be achieved by sliding a hip screw with the addition of an antirotational screw or with cannulated partially threaded screws for compression with one fully threaded screw to avoid shortening of the neck. The choice of the implant is based on the fracture classification and obliquity. As a general rule, types I and II fractures are fixed with cannulated screws, whereas types III and IV fractures are fixed with a pediatric sliding hip screw with an antirotational screw. (**Figure 20.3**) We preferred the sliding hip screw rather than a fixed angle locking plate for fixation of femoral neck fractures, but in rare instances, where patients may have an associated metabolic condition with pathologic bone fragility, a locking device with fixed angle may be appropriate.

The most challenging aspect of treating a femoral neck fracture is the high proportion of complications, previously reported to be as high as 94%.[9] Reported complications include osteonecrosis of the femoral head, malunion, nonunion, premature physeal growth arrest, infection, leg length discrepancy, and implant failure. The most worrisome complication is osteonecrosis of the femoral head. Numerous factors have been implicated in the development of osteonecrosis, including age,[10,11] fracture type,[10,12,13] displacement,[9,12,14] surgical timing,[10,12,15,16] surgical fixation,[6,17] treatment type (open versus closed),[16,18] and quality of reduction.[11] Nevertheless, the best treatment strategy to reduce the occurrence of osteonecrosis remains controversial. Some reports suggest that open reduction and internal fixation (ORIF) reduces the risk,[7,18,19]

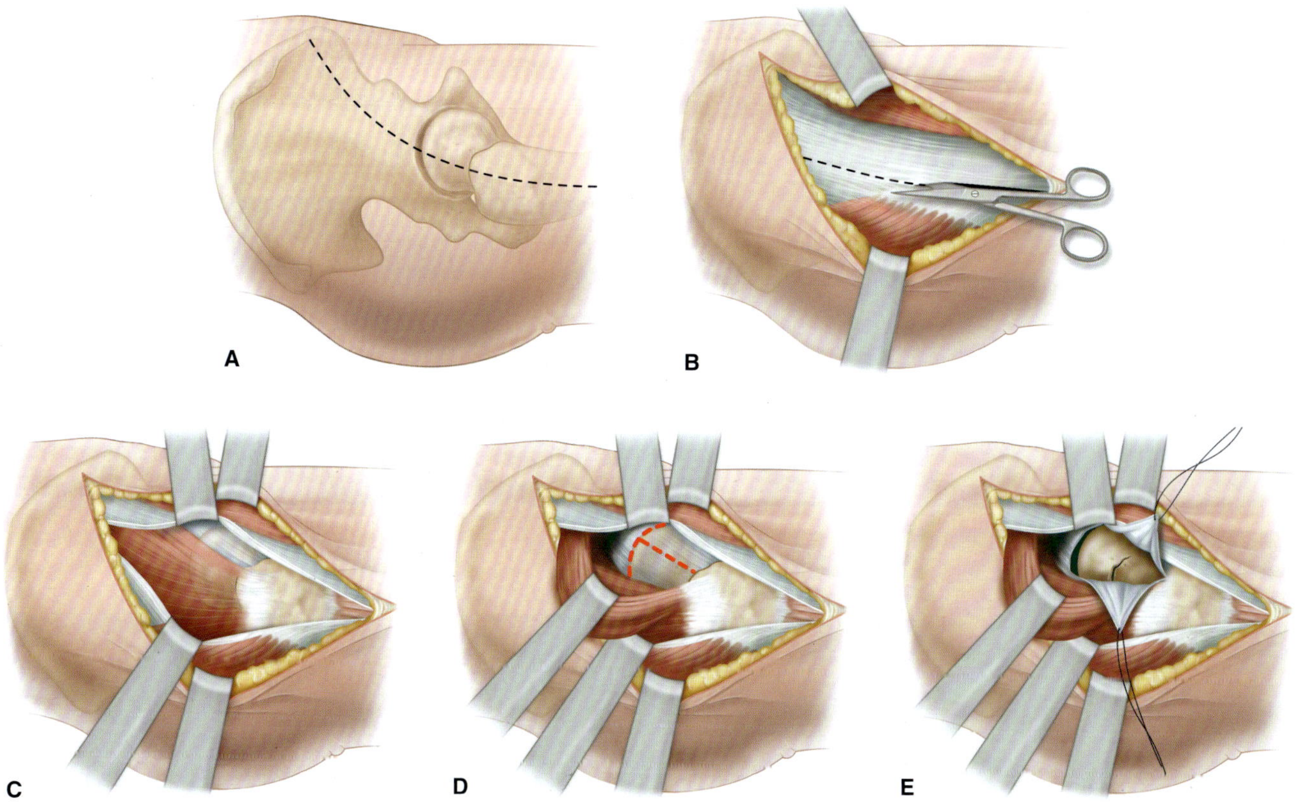

FIGURE 20.2. The Watson Jones approach. Adapted from Operative Techniques in Orthopedic Surgery. A, An incision is made for the Watson-Jones approach about 2.5 cm distal and lateral to the anterior superior iliac spine curved distally to the tip of the greater trochanter and along the anterior margin of the trochanter. B, The fascia lata should be split longitudinally in line with the incision. C, The interval between the tensor fascia lata and the gluteus medius is dissected. The dissection is technically easier if performed in the middle of the interval compared to distally. D, The anterior aspect of the hip capsule is exposed, and a capsulotomy is performed. Red lines mark the T-shaped capsulotomy. E, The anterior aspect of the femoral neck and fracture fragments are exposed. The fracture can be reduced under direct visualization and fixed appropriately. Sam Wiesel editor in chief – Tech Fig 1 – Volume 2 – Part 4 Pediatrics – Section 1 Trauma – Chapter 14 Pediatric Hip Fractures. Wiesel SW. *Operative Techniques in Orthopaedic Surgery*. 2nd ed. Philadelphia, PA: Lippincott Williams & Wilkins; 2015.

while others, report an increased incidence of ON associated with open treatment[16,20] However, in adult patients, the quality of reduction has been shown to be the most important factor for favorable fracture healing. Notably, the best outcomes have been reported when anatomic reduction and stable internal fixation are implemented.[6,21]

Posterior Traumatic Hip Dislocation

Traumatic dislocation of the hip joint is rare in children and adolescents.[22] Although during the first decade of life dislocations can happen following a low-energy mechanism, in adolescence high-energy trauma is often the mechanism of a hip dislocation. The most traditional mechanism for a traumatic posterior dislocation of the hip is a motor vehicle accident with a dashboard injury when a direct force is applied to the knee with corresponding axial force through a flexed and adducted hip. Recently, however, sports-related posterior dislocation of the hip following a relatively low- or moderate-energy trauma in association with femoral acetabular impingement (FAI) has been described.[23,24] Both cam-type morphology[25] and pincer morphology with acetabular retroversion[23] have been reported in adolescence with sports-related posterior dislocation of the hip. Anterior impingement secondary to a cam or pincer morphology limited the motion in flexion, adduction, and internal rotation. The impact from the femur into the anterior acetabulum may create a fulcrum that leads to the posterior instability.

Posterior dislocation of the hip joint in adults is typically associated with a posterior wall fracture of the acetabulum. Although controversy remains about the specific percentage of the posterior wall involvement, it is widely accepted that the larger posterior wall fragment may lead to instability of the joint. In adolescents and children, however, the posterior wall is often not completely

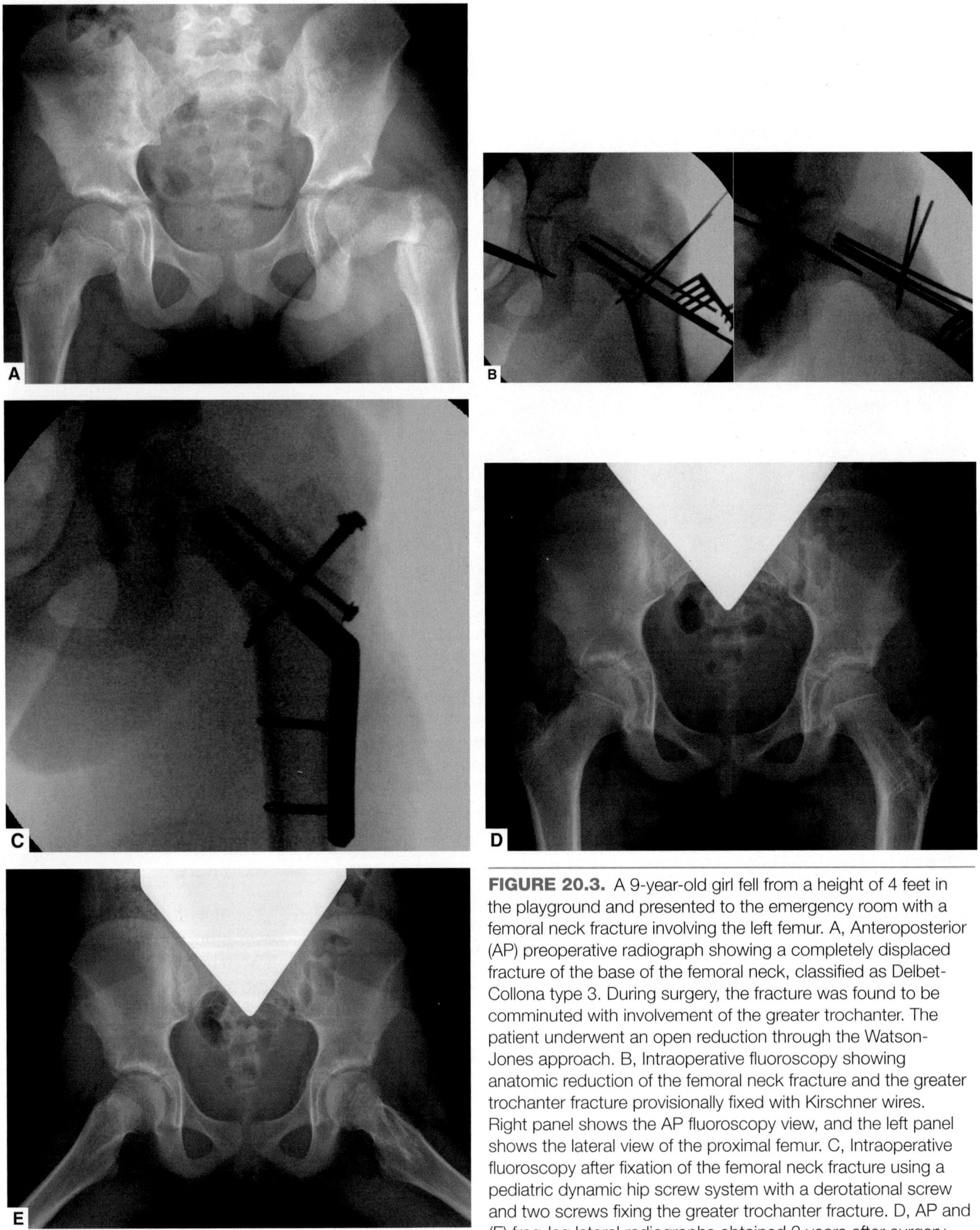

FIGURE 20.3. A 9-year-old girl fell from a height of 4 feet in the playground and presented to the emergency room with a femoral neck fracture involving the left femur. A, Anteroposterior (AP) preoperative radiograph showing a completely displaced fracture of the base of the femoral neck, classified as Delbet-Collona type 3. During surgery, the fracture was found to be comminuted with involvement of the greater trochanter. The patient underwent an open reduction through the Watson-Jones approach. B, Intraoperative fluoroscopy showing anatomic reduction of the femoral neck fracture and the greater trochanter fracture provisionally fixed with Kirschner wires. Right panel shows the AP fluoroscopy view, and the left panel shows the lateral view of the proximal femur. C, Intraoperative fluoroscopy after fixation of the femoral neck fracture using a pediatric dynamic hip screw system with a derotational screw and two screws fixing the greater trochanter fracture. D, AP and (E) frog-leg lateral radiographs obtained 3 years after surgery shows anatomic alignment of the proximal femur without signs of osteonecrosis.

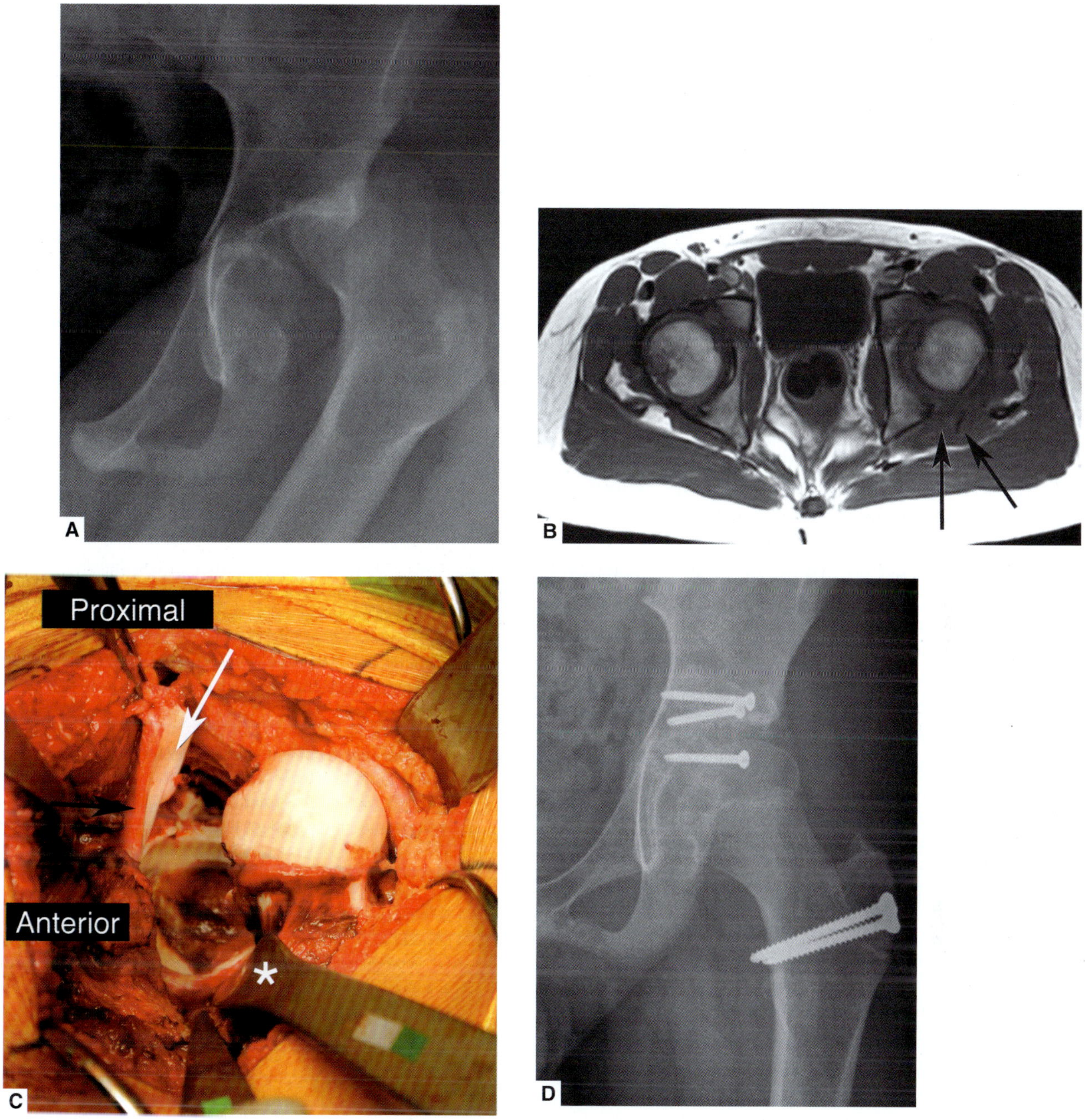

FIGURE 20.4. A 12-year-old boy fell while running during physical education class and was unable to bear weight on the left lower extremity and presented with severe pain in the left hip. A, Anteroposterior pelvic radiograph shows a posterior dislocation of the left hip. B, Magnetic resonance imaging (Axial T1-weighted) demonstrates a displaced, large fragment of the incomplete ossified posterior wall (arrow). C, Intraoperative pictures show a severe avulsion of the labrum (black arrow), including an intra-articular fracture of the posterior wall (white arrow) from superior to anterior. An asterisk marks the Hohmann retractor positioned inferior to the transverse acetabular ligament. We used suture anchors to reattach the labrum with interfragmentary screws for the posterior wall. D, Postoperative radiograph at 1.5 years after surgery shows anatomic reduction of the hip without avascular necrosis of the femoral head.

ossified[26] (**Figure 20.4**). The ossified posterior wall of the acetabulum creates an atypical pattern of injury observed in adolescents with a posterior dislocation of the hip. Although variations of the extent of soft tissue and bone pathology cannot be observed, there is typically an avulsion of the posterior acetabular labrum with rupture of the posterior capsule and complete tear of the thick periosteum combined with the fracture of the cartilaginous posterior wall.

Because of the extended involvement of soft tissues, diagnostic evaluation of adolescents with a posterior hip dislocation differs from skeletally immature patients. Initially, an anteroposterior supine pelvic radiograph along with the oblique views described by Judet (obturator and iliac views) should be obtained for accurate diagnosis. Traditionally, CT scan has been the most commonly performed imaging post reduction. However, we have found that MRI is a better imaging modality to evaluate the soft tissue pathology, including injury to the acetabular labrum and chondral damage.[27,28] Specifically, MRI is better in order to identify an inverted labrum that may be present after reduction and is not typically identified by x-rays or CT.[28] MRI is also better in order to evaluate the percentage of involvement of the posterior wall that may play a role in the stability of the hip.[27]

Treatment of a posterior traumatic hip dislocation depends on the energy involved with the trauma, the patient's age, and the associated injuries, including a fracture of the posterior wall and a potential fracture of the femoral head. As a general rule, the hip should be reduced as early as possible to avoid increased risk of avascular necrosis of the femoral head. The occurrence of avascular necrosis is associated with the interval between the injury and the reduction. Although it may be practical to obtain reduction in the emergency room under conscious sedation, our current preference is to reduce the hip under general anesthesia. Acute fracture through the growth plate may happen in combination with the traumatic hip dislocation. However, the maneuver to achieve a closed reduction of a posteriorly dislocated hip in an immature skeleton poses the risk of iatrogenic fracture through the growth plate, which carries a high risk of avascular necrosis.[29,30] Therefore, we strongly recommend general anesthesia with full muscular relaxation in the operating room when performing a closed reduction of the hip. Finally, excursionized imaging assessment is recommended to determine whether the growth plate may be involved before attempting a reduction.

In children younger than 10 years following a low-energy mechanism of dislocation, a closed reduction followed by spica cast immobilization is typically enough to maintain a stable hip if the MRI does not reveal a severely displaced cartilaginous posterior wall. For children older than 10 years, careful assessment of the postreduction CT or preferably MRI is recommended. If the hip is stable after reduction in the operating room and concentrically reduced without any asymmetry of the joint space or intra-articular chondral or osseous fragments, then nonsurgical treatment is warranted. However, the hip may be unstable because of a fracture of the cartilaginous posterior wall, or the labrum may be entrapped in the joint after reduction leading to a nonconcentric reduction.[27,28,31] In such cases, surgical treatment should be performed. Classically, treatment of posterior hip dislocation and posterior acetabular wall fractures has been performed through a posterior approach using the Kocher-Langenbeck technique. However, we prefer to perform the surgery through the surgical hip dislocation approach.[24,32] The surgical hip dislocation approach allows full exposure of the femoral head and neck for the treatment of associated fractures of the femoral head and complete exposure of the acetabular rim and posterior wall for surgical fixation. In young children, we often do not need to use plate fixation, and fixation of the posterior wall with intrafragmentary screws suffices. In older adolescents, a spring plate or a plate through the posterior column is usually recommended. Clinical and functional outcomes of this approach have been very good overall, with patients achieving good clinical and functional scores in the short term.[24,33]

REFERENCES

1. Bagatur AE, Zorer G. Complications associated with surgically treated hip fractures in children. *J Pediatr Orthop B.* 2002;11(3):219-228.
2. Canale ST, Bourland WL. Fracture of the neck and intertrochanteric region of the femur in children. *J Bone Joint Surg Am.* 1977;59(4):431-443.
3. Patterson JT, Tangtiphaiboontana J, Pandya NK. Management of pediatric femoral neck fracture. *J Am Acad Orthop Surg.* 2018;26(12):411-419.
4. Colonna PC. Fracture of the neck of the femur in children. *Am J Surg.* 1929;6(6):793-797.
5. Garden RS. Reduction and fixation of subcapital fractures of the femur. *Orthop Clin North Am.* 1974;5(4):683-712.
6. Ly TV, Swiontkowski MF. Treatment of femoral neck fractures in young adults. *J Bone Joint Surg Am.* 2008;90(10):2254-2266.
7. Stone JD, Hill MK, Pan Z, Novais EN. Open reduction of pediatric femoral neck fractures reduces osteonecrosis risk. *Orthopedics.* 2015;38(11):e983-e990.
8. Li H, Zhao L, Huang L, Kuo KN. Delayed slipped capital femoral epiphysis after treatment of femoral neck fracture in children. *Clin Orthop Relat Res.* 2015;473(8):2712-2717.
9. Forlin E, Guille JT, Kumar SJ, Rhee KJ. Complications associated with fracture of the neck of the femur in children. *J Pediatr Orthop.* 1992;12(4):503-509.
10. Moon ES, Mehlman CT. Risk factors for avascular necrosis after femoral neck fractures in children: 25 Cincinnati cases and meta-analysis of 360 cases. *J Orthop Trauma.* 2006;20(5):323-329.
11. Shrader MW, Jacofsky DJ, Stans AA, Shaughnessy WJ, Haidukewych GJ. Femoral neck fractures in pediatric patients: 30 years experience at a level 1 trauma center. *Clin Orthop Relat Res.* 2007;454:169-173.
12. Morsy HA. Complications of fracture of the neck of the femur in children. A long-term follow-up study. *Injury.* 2001;32(1):45-51.
13. Togrul E, Bayram H, Gulsen M, Kalaci A, Ozbarlas S. Fractures of the femoral neck in children: long-term follow-up in 62 hip fractures. *Injury.* 2005;36(1):123-130.
14. Canale ST. Fractures of the hip in children and adolescents. *Orthop Clin North Am.* 1990;21(2):341-352.
15. Flynn JM, Wong KL, Yeh GL, Meyer JS, Davidson RS. Displaced fractures of the hip in children. Management by early operation and immobilisation in a hip spica cast. *J Bone Joint Surg Br.* 2002;84(1):108-112.
16. Yeranosian M, Horneff JG, Baldwin K, Hosalkar HS. Factors affecting the outcome of fractures of the femoral neck in children and adolescents: a systematic review. *Bone Joint J.* 2013;95-B(1):135-142.
17. Ng GP, Cole WG. Effect of early hip decompression on the frequency of avascular necrosis in children with fractures of the neck of the femur. *Injury.* 1996;27(6):419-421.
18. Song KS. Displaced fracture of the femoral neck in children: open versus closed reduction. *J Bone Joint Surg Br.* 2010;92(8):1148-1151.
19. Song KS, Kim YS, Sohn SW, Ogden JA. Arthrotomy and open reduction of the displaced fracture of the femoral neck in children. *J Pediatr Orthop B.* 2001;10(3):205-210.
20. Dendane MA, Amrani A, El Alami ZF, El Medhi T, Gourinda H. Displaced femoral neck fractures in children: are complications predictable? *Orthop Trauma Surg Res.* 2010;96(2):161-165.

21. Florschutz AV, Langford JR, Haidukewych GJ, Koval KJ. Femoral neck fractures: current management. *J Orthop Trauma.* 2015;29(3):121-129.
22. Epstein HC, Wiss DA, Cozen L. Posterior fracture dislocation of the hip with fractures of the femoral head. *Clin Orthop Relat Res.* 1985(201):9-17.
23. Novais EN, Ferrer MG, Williams KA, Bixby SD. Acetabular retroversion and decreased posterior coverage are associated with sports-related posterior hip dislocation in adolescents. *Clin Orthop Relat Res.* 2019;477(5):1101-1108.
24. Novais EN, Heare TC, Hill MK, Mayer SW. Surgical hip dislocation for the treatment of intra-articular injuries and hip instability following traumatic posterior dislocation in children and adolescents. *J Pediatr Orthop.* 2016;36(7):673-679.
25. Mayer SW, Abdo JC, Hill MK, Kestel LA, Pan Z, Novais EN. Femoroacetabular impingement is associated with sports-related posterior hip instability in adolescents. a matched cohort study. *Am J Sports Med.* 2016;44(9):2299-2303.
26. Fabricant PD, Hirsch BP, Holmes I, et al. A radiographic study of the ossification of the posterior wall of the acetabulum: implications for the diagnosis of pediatric and adolescent hip disorders. *J Bone Joint Surg Am.* 2013;95(3):230-236.
27. Mayer SW, Stewart JR, Fadell MF, Kestel L, Novais EN. MRI as a reliable and accurate method for assessment of posterior hip dislocation in children and adolescents without the risk of radiation exposure. *Pediatr Radiol.* 2015;45(9):1355-1362.
28. Thanacharoenpanich S, Bixby S, Breen MA, Kim YJ. MRI is better than CT scan for detection of structural pathologies after traumatic posterior hip dislocations in children and adolescents. *J Pediatr Orthop.* 202040(2):86-92.
29. Herrera-Soto JA, Price CT, Reuss BL, Riley P, Kasser JR, Beaty JH. Proximal femoral epiphysiolysis during reduction of hip dislocation in adolescents. *J Pediatr Orthop.* 2006;26(3):371-374.
30. Kennon JC, Bohsali KI, Ogden JA, Ogden J 3rd, Ganey TM. Adolescent hip dislocation combined with proximal femoral physeal fractures and epiphysiolysis. *J Pediatr Orthop.* 2016;36(3):253-261.
31. Blanchard C, Kushare I, Boyles A, Mundy A, Beebe AC, Klingele KE. Traumatic, posterior pediatric hip dislocations with associated posterior labrum osteochondral avulsion: recognizing the acetabular "fleck" sign. *J Pediatr Orthop.* 2016;36(6):602-607.
32. Siebenrock KA, Keel MJB, Tannast M, Bastian JD. Surgical hip dislocation for exposure of the posterior column. *JBJS Essent Surg Tech.* 2019;9(1):e2.
33. Podeszwa DA, De La Rocha A, Larson AN, Sucato DJ. Surgical hip dislocation is safe and effective following acute traumatic hip instability in the adolescent. *J Pediatr Orthop.* 2015;35(5):435-442.

Index

Note: Locators followed by the letter '*f*' and '*t*' refers to figures and tables respectively.